Introduction to Clinical Pharmacology

Introduction to Clinical Pharmacology:

From Symptoms to Treatment

Edited by

Victor Uteshev,
Daniel Llano,
Edward Shadiack III

Cambridge
Scholars
Publishing

Introduction to Clinical Pharmacology: From Symptoms to Treatment

Edited by Victor Uteshev, Daniel Llano and Edward Shadiack III

This book first published 2023

Cambridge Scholars Publishing

Lady Stephenson Library, Newcastle upon Tyne, NE6 2PA, UK

British Library Cataloguing in Publication Data
A catalogue record for this book is available from the British Library

ISBN (10): 1-5275-2530-9
ISBN (13): 978-1-5275-2530-6

TABLE OF CONTENTS

Preface vii
Victor Uteshev

Chapter 1 1
The Concept and Brief History of Pharmacology
Katherine Hernandez

Chapter 2 6
General Principles of Pharmacology, Pharmacodynamics, Pharmacokinetics and Pharmacovigilance
Ben D. Richardson and Carl L. Faingold

Symptoms 1 – Immuno-Infectious Symptoms to Treatment

Chapter 3 20
Drugs for Infections
Diego Marin, Madhu Suryadevara and David P. Siderovski

Chapter 4 98
Allergic Rhinitis and Difficulty Breathing
Karen Woodfork

Chapter 5 110
Asthma and Chronic Obstructive Pulmonary Disease (COPD)
Karen Woodfork

Chapter 6 133
Cough and Excessive Mucus
Leah Hammer and Karen Woodfork

Chapter 7 150
Liver Disorders
Monte Troutman and Victor V. Uteshev

Chapter 8 167
Nausea and Vomiting
Monte Troutman and Victor V. Uteshev

Chapter 9.1 178
Joint Pain and Drugs for Gout
Knox Van Dyke and David P. Siderovski

Chapter 9.2 187
Joint Pain and Drugs for Arthritis
Robert Luedtke, Edward Shadiack and Victor V. Uteshev

Symptoms 2 – Cardio-Renal-Respiratory Symptoms to Treatment

Chapter 10 222
Cardiac Arrhythmias and Treatment
Rachel Pittman and Robert Allen

Chapter 11 242
Cardiovascular Chest Pain and Treatment
Robert Allen and Rachel Pittman

Chapter 12 252
Drugs for Hyperlipidemia
David P. Siderovski and Kendra Unger

Chapter 13.1 267
Hypertension
Anthony Shadiack and Keisa Mathis

Chapter 13.2 277
Hypotension
Anthony Shadiack

Symptoms 3 – Musculoskeletal Symptoms to Treatment

Chapter 14 288
Low Back Pain
Leah Hammer and Ryan Seals

Symptoms 4 – Neurological Symptoms to Treatment

Chapter 15 304
Excessive Thirst, Hunger, and Urination in Diabetes
Nancy S. Gregory

Chapter 16 324
Ataxia, Dizziness and Balance Problems
Daniel A. Llano

Chapter 17 345
Mental Health – Depression, Anxiety, and Suicidal Thoughts
Kathleen Bottum and Shelley Tischkau

Chapter 18 391
Seizures
Lauren Skalomenos, Charles Akos Szabo and Carl L. Faingold

Chapter 19 404
Drugs for Neurodegenerative Dementias
Meharvan Singh and Daniel Adolfo Llano

Symptoms 5 – Endo-Repro-Gastrointestinal Symptoms to Treatment

Chapter 20 416
Abdominal and Esophageal Pain
Monte Troutman and Victor V. Uteshev

Chapter 21 432
Constipation and Diarrhea
Monte Troutman and Victor V. Uteshev

Chapter 22 444
Abdominal Pain or Abnormal Uterine Bleeding and Drugs for Female Reproductive Disorders and Contraception
Shelley A. Tischkau and Kathleen M. Bottum

Miscellaneous – Benzodiazepines – Opioids

Chapter 23 476
Benzodiazepines
Leah W. Hammer

Chapter 24 486
Opioid Analgesics and Antagonists
Kendra E. Unger, MD and Leah W. Hammer, PhD

PREFACE

VICTOR UTESHEV

The teacher-centric didactic method of learning excessively focuses on memorizing data and has been viewed as inadequate for medical education. (Neufeld and Barrows 1974) As a result, the student-centric self-direct learning method termed Problem-Based Learning (PBL) has been introduced as a superior strategy (Barrows 1983) which facilitates the acquisition of pre-clinical knowledge and skills and allows medical, professional, and graduate students to learn how to approach and solve real-world problems. (Barrows and Tamblyn 1980) In 1965-1968, an innovative concept of *simulated patients* was developed for pre-clinical teaching of medical students by Dr. Howard S. Barlow and colleagues. (Barrows 1968) Those efforts gradually led to the PBL. Following the PBL guidance, in this textbook, each chapter is built around patient presentation advancing from symptoms through diagnosis to treatment as anticipated in clinical practice.

It is anticipated that this textbook will give medical, pharmacy, and graduate students a guided understanding of how practicing physicians think when facing symptoms and determining treatments by working through multiple steps including differential diagnoses, imaging, and lab results before achieving a final diagnosis. Tracking the pharmacology of a particular type of drug as pertaining to specific symptoms is a unique feature of this book. Each section discusses specific symptom-based mechanisms and drug treatments followed by relevant cases/questions. The main objective is to provide concise, focused information on pharmacological treatments and mechanisms of action as related to specific symptoms and patient presentation. The prime target audience includes medical students preparing for the United States Medical Licensing Examination (USMLE), the Comprehensive Osteopathic Medical Licensing Examination (COMLEX) in the United States, or similar exams in other countries, pharmacy students, pharmacology/physiology students, practicing physicians and pharmacists, and pre-medical students preparing for medical school. Certain important topics are not covered in this edition including oncology, dermatology, and substance abuse. These and other subjects will be addressed in future editions.

This textbook is an invited contribution of world experts in medical research and education. As this project is approaching its final stage, I am pleased to see that this tribune generously offered by Cambridge Scholars Publishing was enthusiastically used by the authors and I hope that their efforts will find an adequate positive response among medical, professional, and graduate students around the world.

Victor V. Uteshev, PhD
Vice President for Discovery Sciences
Epigen Biosciences Inc.
Fort Worth, Texas
November 25th, 2022

References

Barrows, H. S. 1968. Simulated patients in medical teaching. *CMAJ: Canadian Medical Association Journal* 98 (14):674-676.

Barrows, H. S. 1983. Problem-based, self-directed learning. *JAMA* 250 (22):3077-3080.

Barrows, H. S., and R. M. Tamblyn. 1980. *Problem Based Learning: An Approach to Medical Education.* New York: Springer.

Neufeld, V. R., and H. S. Barrows. 1974. The "McMaster Philosophy": an approach to medical education. *J Med Educ* 49 (11):1040-1050.

CHAPTER 1

THE CONCEPT AND BRIEF HISTORY OF PHARMACOLOGY

KATHERINE HERNANDEZ

University of North Texas Health Science Center, Fort Worth, Texas, USA

Pharmacology is the study of the composition, potential therapeutic effects and toxicity, therapeutic index, molecular mechanisms, cellular interaction, and overall impact of chemicals on the body. The two components that make up pharmacology are pharmacodynamics (what the drug does to the body) and pharmacokinetics (what the body does to the drug) of the chemical component (see Chapter 2). Pharmacology is essential for the drug development process. Pharmaceutical scientists create novel therapeutic compounds, whereas pharmacologists study the absorption, distribution, metabolism, excretion, and chemical effects on the body. The pharmacologist then can begin to understand the mechanism of the drug action by looking at the side effects, drug interactions, effects on pregnancy, age- and sex-dependent dosages, and the effects on different races, sexes, and ethnicities before any of the novel compounds make it to clinical trials (U.S. Department of Health and Human Services 2021).

The usage and search for therapeutic chemical components have been around for thousands of years worldwide. The precursors of this field trace back to the oldest known medicinal texts. These include the Sumerian clay slab from Nagpur, The Pen Ts'ao (a Chinese medicinal book written by Emperor Shen Nung) (Petrovska 2012), and The Ebers Papyrus, an Egyptian medical scroll that dates back to 1552 B.C., containing remedies to cure illnesses (Major 1930). These texts include recipes for drugs that use various herbs and plants available to their respective civilizations at the time of writing, demonstrating that humans have used various naturally occurring chemical compounds to cure and treat diseases for most, if not all, of recorded history.

Many people influenced the field of pharmacology and toxicology as we know it today. This dates back to Philippus Aureolus Theophrastus Bombastus von Hohenheim, a German-Swiss physician and alchemist, known as Paracelsus (1493-1541) (Michaleas et al. 2021). Born in Einsiedeln, Switzerland, he played a significant role in shaping our modern understanding of toxicology. Following the death of his mother, the family moved to Villach in Carinthia, where his father Wilhelm Bombast von Hohenheim, a physician and an alchemist (Borzelleca 2000), taught chemistry. While in Villach, Paracelsus worked in the mines. This gave Paracelsus knowledge of metallurgy, which likely influenced his later discoveries. In 1507, Paracelsus began traveling through Europe in search of world-renowned professors. During this time, Paracelsus attended various universities. Finally, in 1510, he received his baccalaureate in medicine from the University of Vienna, and in 1516 received his doctoral degree from the University of Ferrara. This is when he began using the name Paracelsus (Michaleas et al. 2021).

Paracelsus was disappointed with his academic endeavors as he believed, in his own words, "the universities do not teach all things" (Borzelleca 2000). He began to broaden his education by traveling through Europe, ultimately becoming an army surgeon (Hartmann 1896). During this search, he expanded his knowledge of alchemy and how to use what he termed "the latent forces of Nature." This experience led him to question the fundamental medical ideologies of the time (Cintas 2003). In 1524, Paracelsus returned to Villach, was appointed the town's physician, and became a lecturer at the University of Basel. His reputation for curing disease led to his lectures being well attended. In his classes, Paracelsus discussed the healing powers of nature. He also denounced several methods of treatment, which caused him to dispute with the local doctors, causing him to leave Basel in 1528 and travel once again. It was then when Paracelsus contributed significantly to the field of medicine. He went against the treatments of the time and described new treatment options. An example of this was when he used specified mercury compound doses to treat Syphilis, making him a pioneer in the application of minerals and metals for medicinal purposes. He emphasized that "a poison in the body would be cured by a similar poison," but the dosage is what makes it therapeutic. He expanded on this idea of dose responses in his work "Third Defense." Paracelsus greatly influenced toxicology with his ideology of learning and understanding that "the dose determines that a thing is not a poison" (Borzelleca 2000).

The study of pharmacology has progressed greatly from the times of Paracelsus to our current understanding of modern experimental pharmacology. Almost 300 years later, Rudolf Buchheim (1820-1879) set up the first pharmacology laboratory and later established an institute of pharmacology. Buchheim was a medical student when he began working as a research assistant to Ernst Heinrich Weber (1795-1878), a famous physiologist (Muscholl et al. 1995). His supervisor, Karl Gotthelf Lehmann (1812-1863), introduced him to the medicinal aspect of chemicals, leading him to his future studies. His scholastic endeavors allowed him to become a professor at the University of

Dorpat, where he lacked funding and decided to build a laboratory in the basement of his house. In 1860, he relocated to the newfound institute of pharmacology, where he mentored many students, some of whom became his successors (Scheindlin 2001). Buchheim established the basics of pharmacology by establishing that physiology and pathology are the roots of pharmacology. He correctly believed that a chemical's processes controlled an organism's functions and classified them by their mechanisms of action rather than their chemical class and origin (Muscholl et al. 1995).

Although Buchheim established the basic principles of pharmacology, his student Oswald Schmiedeberg (1838-1921) is recognized as the father of modern experimental pharmacology. Schmiedeberg was a devoted scientist who first introduced pharmacodynamics and pharmacokinetics, making pharmacology an autonomous scientific discipline (Pokrovskii et al. 2017). He received his Doctor of Medicine from Dorpat after submitting his thesis about chloroform measurements in the blood and succeeded Buchheim at Dorpat in 1869 (Scheindlin 2001).

In 1872, after receiving government funding and building an astonishing pharmacology institute, Schmiedeberg became a professor of pharmacology at the University of Strassburg. He taught there for 46 years, where he excelled in the field. It was during this time that he identified that muscarine evoked similar effects on the heart as the vagus nerve, used urea derivatives as a hypnotic, discovered nicotine's ability to block cardiac vagal ganglia, and found the toxic activity of heavy metals, among other findings (Muscholl et al. 1995). He also trained numerous successful pharmacologists. One of his apprentices was John Jacob Abel (1857-1938), the first chair of pharmacology at the University of Michigan, who later went to Johns Hopkins University, where he accomplished isolating epinephrine from extracts of adrenal glands and histamine isolation from the pituitary (Scheindlin 2001).

But The Best Treatment is Prevention

Chronic diseases such as heart disease, stroke, and diabetes are the leading causes of death and disabilities. In 2014, 60% of the adult population in America had one chronic condition, and 42% had multiple chronic diseases. These diseases affect the quality of life of the patient and their families. A person with a chronic illness has various limitations, which can lead to depression and losing their ability to cope with pain, resulting in worse disease outcomes. People with chronic diseases are also more likely to spend more on prescription drugs than those without. These diseases can also make it difficult for the patients to work, coinciding with lower incomes and, thus, impacting their finances (Levine et al. 2019).

Chronic diseases are the driving force of the rising costs of health care, which are expected to increase dramatically in the next few decades. It is estimated that 86% of healthcare-related expenses are due to the treatment of chronic diseases (Holman HR 2020). In 2016, treatment costs were more than $1 trillion, with Diabetes, Alzheimer's, and Osteoarthritis being the leaders of the increased costs. As the world population ages, these costs are projected to increase. Over 80 million Americans will have at least three chronic diseases by 2030 (Levine et al. 2019).

The prevention of disease requires drastic lifestyle changes and education across the general public, as the cause of disease is largely in part due to human behavior, including fitness and health considerations. The best course of action is to stop the onset of disease before it progresses, as there are lasting emotional and physical impacts from disease, which for some, can amount to death.

The degrees of clinical preventative strategies for disease consist of primary, secondary, and tertiary prevention. In primary prevention, healthcare providers intervene before the appearance of disease. In secondary prevention, health providers detect the disease in the early stages and begin treatment. Finally, in tertiary prevention, healthcare providers work with the patient to reduce or stop the progression of disease (Levine et al. 2019). These interventions can mitigate the detrimental implications of disease on the body. However, the lack of implementation of these preventive measures further contributes to disease progression. Nonetheless, chronic diseases can be prevented by healthier lifestyle routines such as exercising, healthy eating habits, refraining from excessive alcohol, and avoiding tobacco use.

Dietary changes help prevent and manage chronic diseases, such as Type 2 Diabetes, as well as cardiovascular diseases. This includes having a balanced diet with various vegetables, lean proteins, fruits, and whole grains. Additionally, limiting food high in sugars, sodium, and saturated fats will have a positive impact on health. In addition, eating balanced meals has been shown to improve insulin sensitivity. Whereas, having a diet with a high intake of processed meats (hot dogs, deli meats, etc.) has been shown to increase the risk of cardiovascular diseases, and high consumption of unprocessed red meats has an associated increased rate of colon cancer and cardiovascular mortality. A diet based on fish, poultry, and unprocessed red meat thus serves as a healthier alternative (Yu et al. 2018). This kind of preventative care is medically and financially beneficial, as heart disease costs the United States roughly $219 billion annually (Office of the Associate Director for Policy and Strategy 2021).

Observational trials show that exercise contributes to the primary and secondary prevention of cardiovascular disease. Health benefits can be seen with light to moderate intensity exercise on most days of the week for about 20 to 60 minutes, averaging at least 150 minutes per week (Warburton et al. 2008). Regular physical activity can decrease a patient's blood pressure and improve cholesterol. This can reduce the risk of developing Type 2 Diabetes. If a patient does muscle-strengthening activities such as weightlifting, they can increase strength, muscle, and bone density, decreasing the risk of Osteoporosis (Centers for Disease Control and Prevention 2022). Increased physical activity has a plethora of health benefits, even for a short time, as it can help prevent and manage existing chronic diseases.

Limiting tobacco and alcohol use can aid in lowering the risk of various comorbidities that can lead to chronic diseases. For example, excess drinking can lead to liver disease, stroke, high blood pressure, and heart disease. This can be reduced by decreasing alcohol intake. Smoking can also lead to serious health problems. By quitting smoking, individuals are reducing the risk of lung disease, Type 2 Diabetes, and the risk of heart disease (Centers for Disease Control and Prevention, 2022).

Using Drugs Only as The Last Resort

People generally require more medications as they age. These can include statins to lower cholesterol levels, alpha-blockers for high blood pressure, proton-pump inhibitors for acid reflux, and painkillers for pain management related to injury, among other medications. All medications carry risks, resulting in unwanted or unexpected side effects, which can range from headaches, dizziness, fatigue, rash, and nausea to more severe side effects such as liver failure, abnormal heart rhythms, and increased risk of bleeding. A few of these medications can be avoided through dietary lifestyle changes.

When taking prescribed drugs, a patient can also risk experiencing unwanted side effects due to drug interactions. The interactions can appear in the form of two drugs interacting together, such as aspirin and blood thinners. It can also occur with drugs and food, such as eating grapefruit, an inhibitor of cytochrome p450 CYP3A4, which can increase the toxicity of statins, such as atorvastatin; thus, consumption of grapefruit juice should be avoided while on CYP3A4-sensitive medications (Ramkumar et al. 2016). There are also drug and supplement interactions that can occur. For example, taking ginkgo (a dietary supplement) and blood thinners can cause an interaction resulting in adverse side effects (U.S. Department of Health and Human Services 2020). Interactions with drugs and medical conditions can also occur, such as taking aspirin while having stomach ulcers, furthering the risk of stomach bleeding. Therefore, patients must go over medications with their doctors and pharmacists to avoid problems with drug interactions.

Due to genetic polymorphism (different genetic makeup of individuals, which can cause them to metabolize drugs differently), prescription drugs can work differently for each individual, even if it is the same dose. For example, isoniazid is a drug used to treat tuberculosis that is metabolized by acetylation. However, the rate of acetylation varies from one individual to another due to genetic differences, which define the amount of unmetabolized isoniazid available for therapeutic effects (Ramachandran and Swaminathan 2012). Another example is clopidogrel, a blood-thinning prodrug metabolized to its active form by CYP2C19. Decreased response to clopidogrel has been noticed in Asian communities due to genetic polymorphisms that cause an inadequate metabolism of the drug (Brown et al., 2018).

Although drugs can help treat diseases, the outcomes are only sometimes beneficial or pleasant. Therefore, it is advantageous for the patient to use medications only as a last resort and instead attempt to prevent the diseases to avoid the need for medications and, thus, potential toxicity and side effects.

"All Drugs are Toxic, It's the Dose that Makes Them Therapeutic" (Paracelsus)

It was Paracelsus who first realized the importance of the dose in determining the drug's therapeutic effects and toxicity. Thus, even a poison can be therapeutically effective if given at an appropriately low dose. An important parameter called the therapeutic index, determines how appropriate and risky a drug is for clinical use. The therapeutic index is defined as a ratio of LD50 (lethal dose of a drug for 50% of the population) over ED50 (the minimum effective dose for 50% of the population). The dose window between the LD50 and the ED50 depends on the medication. The wider the window (i.e., the greater the ratio, LD50/ED50), the safer the drug (Tamargo et al. 2015). However, if the window is small, the drug has little difference between its therapeutic and toxic doses. Nevertheless, that does not eliminate certain drugs or drug classes from clinical use, as long as the patient takes certain precautions. For example, most general anesthetics have a low therapeutic index, yet clinical practices widely use them. Other drugs with a small therapeutic index are warfarin, phenytoin, and levothyroxine. Using medications with a low therapeutic index requires exceptional vigilance (see Chapter 2) and should be individualized for each patient. Note that the TD50 (toxic dose for 50%) instead of the LD50 can be used to define the therapeutic index (see Chapter 2).

In summary, pharmacology was created under the influence of various great physicians and scientists, including Paracelsus, who created the idea of using drugs for treatment and differentiating between the quantity that makes such treatments toxic or therapeutic, and Oswald Schmiedeberg, who introduced pharmacodynamics and pharmacokinetics. The combined ideas of these individuals, among others, led to the formation of this field. Although there are ways to prevent the necessity of drug treatment, such as eating a well-balanced diet and exercising, science has increased the benefits and progressively reduced the risk of using prescribed medication under observation from a medical provider, as this remains the best option to aid in the treatment of a patient. As Paracelsus said, "All drugs are toxic. It is the dose that makes them therapeutic," which defines the role of a pharmacologist to study drugs in order to understand how they can best be therapeutic to a patient (see Chapter 2).

References

1) U.S. Department of Health and Human Services. 2021. Why is pharmacology research important? Eunice Kennedy Shriver National Institute of Child Health and Human Development. U.S. Department of Health and Human Services. December 20, 2021.
https://www.nichd.nih.gov/health/topics/pharma/conditioninfo/important.
2) Petrovska BB. 2012. Historical review of medicinal plants' usage. Pharmacogn Rev. 2012 Jan;6(11):1-5. doi: 10.4103/0973-7847.95849. PMID: 22654398; PMCID: PMC3358962.
3) Major RH. 1930. “The Papyrus Ebers”. Ann Med Hist. 2(5):547-555. PMID: 33944361; PMCID: PMC7945839.
4) Hartmann F. 1896. “The life of Philippus Theophrastus Bombast of Hohenheim, known by the name of Paracelsus: and the substance of his teachings concerning cosmology, anthropology, pneumatology, magic and sorcery, medicine, alchemy and astrology, philosophy and theosophy”. London: Kegan Paul, Trench, Trübner, & Co. Ltd; revised and enlarged.
5) Michaleas SN, Laios K, Tsoucalas G, Androutsos G. 2021.“Theophrastus Bombastus Von Hohenheim (Paracelsus) (1493-1541): The eminent physician and pioneer of toxicology”. Toxicol Rep. 2021 Feb 23;8:411-414. doi: 10.1016/j.toxrep.2021.02.012. PMID: 33717994; PMCID: PMC7920879.
6) Cintas, P. 2003. “FRANCIS BACON: AN ALCHEMICAL ODYSSEY THROUGH THE NOVUM ORGANUM. BULLETIN FOR THE HISTORY OF CHEMISTRY”. 28(Number 2).
7) Borzelleca JF. 2000. Paracelsus: herald of modern toxicology. Toxicol Sci. 2000 Jan;53(1):2-4. doi: 10.1093/toxsci/53.1.2. PMID: 10653514.
8) Muscholl E. Second W.D.M. 1995. Paton Memorial Lecture. The evolution of experimental pharmacology as a biological science: the pioneering work of Buchheim and Schmiedeberg. Br J Pharmacol. 1995 Oct;116(4):2155-9. doi: 10.1111/j.1476-5381.1995.tb15047.x. PMID: 8564242; PMCID: PMC1908990.
9) Scheindlin, Stanley. 2001. A brief history of pharmacology. Modern Drug Discovery High-Throughput Screening. May 2001.
https://pubsapp.acs.org/subscribe/archive/mdd/v04/i05/html/05timeline.html.
10) Pokrovskii M, Avtina T, Zakharova E, Belousova Y. 2017. OSWALD SCHMIEDEBERG –THE “FATHER” OF EXPERIMENTAL PHARMACOLOGY. Research Results in Pharmacology. 2017 Dec; 3(4): 3-1. doi: 10.18413/2313-8971-2017-3-4-3-19
11) Levine S, Malone E, Lekiachvili A, Briss P. 2019. Health Care Industry Insights: Why the Use of Preventive Services Is Still Low. Prev Chronic Dis. 2019 Mar 14;16:E30. doi: 10.5888/pcd16.180625. PMID: 30873937; PMCID: PMC6429690.
12) Holman HR. 2020. The Relation of the Chronic Disease Epidemic to the Health Care Crisis. ACR Open Rheumatol. 2020 Mar;2(3):167-173. doi: 10.1002/acr2.11114. Epub 2020 Feb 19. PMID: 32073759; PMCID: PMC7077778.
13) Yu E, Malik VS, Hu FB. 2018. Cardiovascular Disease Prevention by Diet Modification: JACC Health Promotion Series. J Am Coll Cardiol. 2018 Aug 21;72(8):914-926. doi: 10.1016/j.jacc.2018.02.085. PMID: 30115231; PMCID: PMC6100800.
14) Office of the Associate Director for Policy and Strategy. 2021. Health topics - heart disease - polaris. Centers for Disease Control and Prevention. Centers for Disease Control and Prevention. August 17, 2021.
https://www.cdc.gov/policy/polaris/healthtopics/heartdisease/index.html.
15) Warburton DE, Nicol CW, Bredin SS. 2008. Prescribing exercise as preventive therapy. CMAJ. 2006 Mar 28;174(7):961-74. doi: 10.1503/cmaj.1040750. Erratum in: CMAJ. 2008 Mar 11;178(6):731-2. PMID: 16567757; PMCID: PMC1405860.
16) Centers for Disease Control and Prevention. 2022. Benefits of physical activity. Centers for Disease Control and Prevention. June 16, 2022.
https://www.cdc.gov/physicalactivity/basics/pa-health/index.htm.
17) Centers for Disease Control and Prevention. 2022. How you can prevent chronic diseases. Centers for Disease Control and Prevention. September 1, 2022.
https://www.cdc.gov/chronicdisease/about/prevent/index.htm.
18) Ramkumar S, Raghunath A, Raghunath S. 2016. Statin Therapy: Review of Safety and Potential Side Effects. Acta Cardiol Sin. 2016 Nov;32(6):631-639. doi: 10.6515/acs20160611a. PMID: 27899849; PMCID: PMC5126440.
19) U.S. Department of Health and Human Services. 2020. Ginkgo. National Center for Complementary and Integrative Health. U.S. Department of Health and Human Services.
https://www.nccih.nih.gov/health/ginkgo

20) Ramachandran G, Swaminathan S. Role of pharmacogenomics in the treatment of tuberculosis: a review. Pharmgenomics Pers Med. 2012;5:89-98. doi: 10.2147/PGPM.S15454. Epub 2012 Sep 13. PMID: 23226065; PMCID: PMC3513231.
21) Brown SA, Pereira N. 2018. Pharmacogenomic Impact of CYP2C19 Variation on Clopidogrel Therapy in Precision Cardiovascular Medicine. J Pers Med. 2018 Jan 30;8(1):8. doi: 10.3390/jpm8010008. PMID: 29385765; PMCID: PMC5872082.
22) Tamargo J, Le Heuzey JY, Mabo P. 2015. Narrow therapeutic index drugs: a clinical pharmacological consideration to flecainide. Eur J Clin Pharmacol. 2015 May;71(5):549-67. doi: 10.1007/s00228-015-1832-0. Epub 2015 Apr 15. PMID: 25870032; PMCID: PMC4412688.

CHAPTER 2

GENERAL PRINCIPLES OF PHARMACOLOGY, PHARMACODYNAMICS, PHARMACOKINETICS AND PHARMACOVIGILANCE

BEN D. RICHARDSON, PHD AND CARL L. FAINGOLD, PHD

Southern Illinois University School of Medicine, Springfield, IL 62702

General Background

Pharmacology is the study of agents that are capable of altering the body's physiological processes in a manner that may be therapeutic and/or toxic. The application of pharmacology ranges from drug discovery/design to clinical practice. The clinical application of pharmacology rests on three major components or pillars: the **ABCs of Pharmacology**. These three pillars are **A) Pharmacodynamics (PD)** – knowledge of what a drug does to affect the pathophysiology, **B) Pharmacokinetics (PK)** – knowledge of how the body processes a drug, and **C) Pharmacovigilance (PV)** – knowledge of the adverse and toxic effects of a drug. Understanding the ABCs of a given drug and the relevant characteristics of a specific patient, such as age or sex, are essential to reach an acceptable balance between the benefits and risks of a particular drug in that particular patient. Using the ABCs of Pharmacology, as detailed below, can help assure the rational use of drugs in the treatment of specific patient disorders while limiting untoward effects on the patient. Most drugs are given systemically to improve a pathology at a specific organ system, such as the heart, but a majority of drugs exert additional direct or indirect effects on other organ systems of the body beyond the systems being targeted. Therefore, as the father of pharmacology, Paracelsus, wrote over 500 years ago, it is critical to emphasize that even the most effective drugs are poisons if the dose is too high (see Chapter 1).

Pharmacology is a highly dynamic field due, in part, to the frequent introduction of new drugs with novel mechanisms of action, which has recently been occurring at the rate of over 50 novel agents a year. So, in addition to consulting with textbooks and online drug information sources, it is useful for each practitioner to develop their conceptual scaffold or **Tree of Pharmacology Knowledge** (Figure 1) to mentally map out the various classes of drugs targeting specific types of medical conditions and organ systems. Pharmacology knowledge can then be acquired into a mental database or conceptual scaffold that includes drug class, names, mechanism of action, pharmacodynamics (PD), and critical adverse events or toxicities (PV), allowing any new drug to be placed within this database to build onto their existing knowledge of familiar drugs. Thus, each novel drug becomes a new leaf on the specific branch of this tree that applies to the medical conditions in the mental database of the practitioner. The intentional and well-reasoned development of such a mental database/conceptual scaffold establishes an integrated understanding of pharmacology and facilitates the assimilation of new knowledge.

Often pharmacological knowledge is considered secondary to developing an understanding of pathophysiology, but this delay in developing a pharmacological knowledge base is a missed opportunity. Rather, once basic anatomical and physiological knowledge is in place, actively developing pharmacological reasoning and a knowledge base for treatment (and/or diagnosis) in parallel to understanding pathophysiology and disease can be mutually beneficial. For example, a clear understanding of why angiotensin receptor blockers are effective in heart failure facilitates an integrated view of smooth muscle contraction, intracellular signal transduction mechanism, neurohormonal control of blood pressure, the renin-angiotensin-aldosterone system, cardiac output, and hypertension, among others.

Integrating the Three Pillars in the ABCs of Pharmacology

Once the diagnosis is established and treatment goals are identified, the drug category needed to treat the patient's condition or the specific branch on the Tree of Pharmacology Knowledge is identified. For example, if a patient is diagnosed with an infectious disease and the causative organism is established by microbiological techniques, the specific chemotherapeutic branch on the Tree that specifies the agent useful to treat that infection will be selected. Then the three major pillars of pharmacology are addressed individually based on the options within that branch: What drugs are available that are therapeutically effective? What are their pharmacological properties at the dosages administered? What are the potential risks to the patient? Here, each question is the overarching question answered by an understanding of PD, PK, and PV. Within these pillars, important factors can be evaluated by working through a series of additional questions designed to address the most important issues within each pillar to eventually answer the important broader question: How do the potential benefits outweigh the risks of an implemented drug treatment to improve a patient's health and well-being? More details and an overview of practical considerations for the ABCs are listed below, but drug-specific information and safety should always be consulted when questions or uncertainty are present (Faingold and Dunaway, 2002; Dunaway and Faingold, 2002).

A. Pharmacodynamics (PD)

The first pillar of pharmacology is **pharmacodynamics (PD)**, referring to the actions of a drug on the body or a system. This is typically the first guiding principle of drug choice based on a leading **diagnosis** of the pathophysiological state.

Diagnosis

Incorporating *presentation, associated signs and symptoms, risk factors, lab tests, and exams*, is the key to choosing the correct drug to treat the accurately diagnosed pathophysiological condition to be addressed. Successful drug therapy is directly dependent on a thorough understanding of the pathophysiology underlying the presenting medical problem(s) that require(s) pharmacological intervention. Also, note that a comprehensive pharmacological knowledge base may be useful in developing a diagnosis by evaluating patient responses to specific drugs (e.g. administering a bronchodilator or bronchoconstrictor after obtaining baseline pulmonary function test values to identify obstructive lung diseases). Upon obtaining a diagnosis with the clearest possible understanding of the driving pathophysiology, goals for treatment should be developed. In many cases, these treatment goals may be able to provide a curative approach resulting in a complete correction of the pathophysiological state. In other cases, there may be no curative option, and a pharmacological approach that limits symptoms or delays mortality may be the sole option. Using the questions below, consider how drug action, specificity, and compensatory changes that may occur are used to refine the list of drug options.

1. *What drug classes are available that exert pharmacological effects needed to achieve treatment goals?*

Regardless of the condition, drugs within specific classes are identified based on their ability to affect change in certain systems to achieve identified goals, whether curative, preventive, or palliative. These drug-induced changes correspond to the biological sites where each drug acts, typically by binding to a site to produce some change in or interfere with an ongoing process, collectively referred to as the drug's mechanism of action.

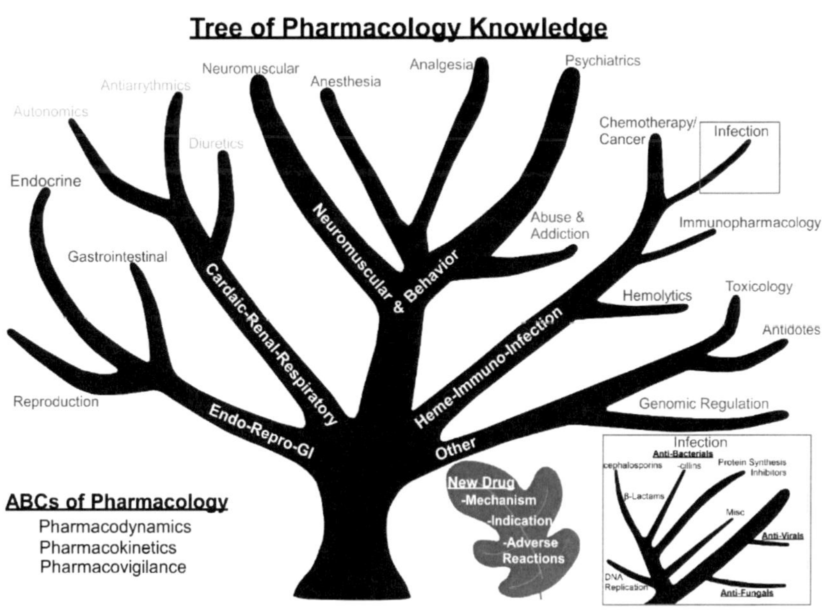

Figure 1. Tree of Pharmacology Knowledge

2. *What are the mechanisms of action of this drug?*

a. specificity/selectivity of the drug-receptor interaction

Guided by the need to induce specific changes in system function, the understanding of that system's physiology is essential to guide the choice of drug class based on the site and nature of that drug's interaction with the system(s) targeted for manipulation. In a case where a process may need to be enhanced, activating a receptor that drives such a process may be beneficial. Also, inhibiting a different opposing mechanism that slows that same process may be just as beneficial or even more so to achieve the desired effects. In addition to the direction of change, each class of drug should be evaluated based on its specificity or the drug's ability to affect only the intended signaling/system with little-to-no change in other signaling/systems. Drugs in clinical use today fall within an incredibly broad spectrum, ranging from monoclonal antibodies that selectively bind specific epitopes on specific receptor subtypes to small molecule neuropsychiatric medications that interact with several major signaling pathways within the nervous system. It is also important to distinguish within the latter, a drug that interacts with multiple effector classes (e.g. atypical antipsychotic clozapine) relative to drugs that interact with specific receptors/effectors that happen to be widely expressed (e.g. fentanyl and mu-opioid receptors or digoxin and Na+/K+-ATPase).

Across this spectrum of drugs that produce highly specific to non-specific effects, there is a general correlation with a drug's ability to affect change, where many drugs with poor selectivity are often the ones most effective at altering or restoring normal physiological status. However, increased off-target interactions of drugs with reduced binding specificity lead to more adverse or unintended effects. It is at this stage that the first risk-benefit analysis must be conducted to identify whether changes due to non-specific interactions of a drug are acceptable based on the potential to reach treatment goals. Doing so will further refine treatment options to those that will be best tolerated and/or produce only limited or acceptable adverse drug effects.

b. *dose-response relationship, effective dose versus toxic dose*

In most cases, higher drug doses/concentrations more readily produce the desired effects to achieve treatment goals. Unfortunately, the specificity of a drug is often reduced with increasing drug dose/concentrations. To quantify flexibility and safety across the dose range for a specific drug, a **therapeutic index (TI)** for each drug is determined as a ratio of the TD50/ED50. The ED50 (effective dose for 50%) is the concentration at which a drug produces a desired effect in 50% of the population whereas the TD50 (toxic dose for 50%) is the dose at which 50% of the population experiences toxic or adverse effects. Similarly, the dose range between where beneficial effects emerge but before toxic or adverse effects are observed is considered to be the **therapeutic window** of a drug for the population for which data are available. Using these population-based values of the therapeutic index and therapeutic window, which increases with lower doses needed to achieve effects or with higher doses needed to reach toxicity, a starting point and flexibility across a drug dose range can be considered to include/exclude a drug or choose a starting dose. Because these values are derived from populations that may have considerable variability, an individual may need to increase or decrease doses of a specific drug to simultaneously produce the greatest benefit with the fewest adverse effects that occur more frequently at higher doses.

c. *cell signaling*

Limitations or refinement of a potential list of drugs to produce a particular result may be significantly limited by drug specificity and therapeutic index. Therefore, it is valuable to consider a broader view of the pathophysiology and the multiple factors that can shape a physiological change. As indicated in section A.2.a., producing a particular effect may be achieved in several ways, including direct activation of a receptor or enzyme, inhibition of an opposing receptor or enzyme, and actions at distinct stages downstream or upstream of the site of disruption. One example of a system with multiple targetable cellular and molecular sites to achieve an intended result is blood pressure. Lowering blood pressure may be achieved by multiple approaches that include blocking the generation of angiotensin II, directly antagonizing the angiotensin receptor, preventing the degradation of cAMP, activating alpha 2 adrenergic receptors that reduce the release of norepinephrine, and stimulating nitric oxide production. With an integrated view of system physiology, cellular signaling mechanisms, and sites that may be targeted by specific drugs, treatment options may be expanded to rationally target a mechanism to produce an effect that may reduce adverse drug reactions (side effects) and needs to use higher doses/concentrations.

B. Pharmacokinetics

3. *What pharmacokinetic-related factors can alter the patient's responsiveness to a drug?*

Once any drug or agent is administered to the body, the body and organ systems will immediately begin to redistribute it into certain compartments and/or change its molecular structure or composition. These actions the body takes on the drug are unique to each compound and are referred to as the **pharmacokinetic (PK)** properties of a drug. Drug PK, or what the body does to the drug, is characterized by four major processes that include **absorption**, **distribution**, **metabolism**, and **elimination** (i.e. **ADME**). Each of these components may be shaped by either active or passive processes and may vary greatly between individuals based on their age, sex, mass, genetics, health status, and exposure to other experiences or substances. These individual variations within components that shape these processes may produce cumulative or synergistic effects on how much drug remains within the body or compensate for one another.

Generally, the cumulative effects of each of these processes are quantified by assessing the concentration of the drug in the plasma at regular intervals. Other reservoirs may be more appropriate in some cases (e.g. cerebrospinal fluid).

This evaluation of drug concentration over time after a single dose, repeated doses, or continuous delivery (pump or transdermal) is used to evaluate the time it takes for a specific amount of active drug to be removed from the body or that reservoir. This change in drug concentration follows one of two patterns: zero-order kinetics or first-order kinetics. In the case of **zero-order kinetics**, the processes involved in the body's ability to reduce the amount of the drug are saturated and only a finite *amount* of the drug is removed per unit of time (e.g., alcohol). In the case of **first-order kinetics**, the processes involved in changing the concentration of the drug are dependent on the concentration present, i.e. a fixed *proportion* or *percentage* of the drug is removed per unit of time rather than an amount. In other words, with first-order kinetics, the more drug present in the body means that a greater amount will be removed in a given time, whereas less drug in the body results in a lower amount of drug removed in a given time. Generally, drugs with zero-order elimination kinetics tend to bring a higher risk of overdose since the processes involved in drug removal are saturated, whereas drugs eliminated with first-order kinetics carry less overdose risk since the body removes more drug when more drug is present.

Regardless, variations from the "average" patient due to any of the above factors may require a change in drug dose and/or drug choice. Below are major physiological determinants of drug pharmacokinetic profiles to consider in drug and dosage choice. This list is not comprehensive, but rather a general guideline for thinking critically about each concept.

a. site and route of administration

Chemical limitations to the compound formulation and compound stability in certain states (aqueous, solid, etc.) that also facilitate the body's ability to absorb a drug (see below) together determine the possible formulations for all compounds, molecules, peptides, antibodies, etc. that may be administered to patients as drugs. These determinants and other aspects related to controlling the temporal component of drug delivery then limit whether a drug may be administered through intravenous, subcutaneous, transdermal, inhaled, intramuscular, and/or oral routes. This combination of a drug's state and its route of administration both impact the **bioavailability** of a drug, or the percentage of drug administered that is retained by the body. By definition, drugs that are delivered intravenously are considered to be 100% bioavailable since the serum is the common reference for the concentration of drugs in the body. Relative to intravenous administration, other routes of administration typically result in a lower bioavailability of a given drug.

b. drug absorption

Drug absorption refers to the mechanism, rate, and capacity for a drug to transition from its administered form to being present within biological tissues and fluid reservoirs or compartments. One major determinant of drug absorption is its ionization (or charged) state, which may differ based on its environment, especially pH, with the latter varying wildly based on the site of administration (e.g. gastric pH ~ 1.5, blood pH ~7.4). Using pH as an example, several factors may affect environmental pH and absorption, as is the case for gastric pH following oral administration or diabetes and subsequent metabolic acidosis in the case of blood pH. A second major determinant of drug absorption is the mechanism by which drugs move through biological barriers like membranes. Drugs may move passively (e.g. diffusion) or actively (e.g. transporter proteins) across barriers or compartments, the degree to which is a function of the interaction between the drug state and availability of requisite biological processes or environments.

c. drug distribution in the body

Once a drug is absorbed at its site of administration, some proportion of the drug may remain there and some may move to other compartments. These compartments include those where the drug remains free or in an aqueous state, bound to specific proteins, or some combination of the two. For example, some drug present in the blood may be free or unbound to any protein and a separate fraction may be bound to albumin. In this case, changes in blood pH may change the charge of the drug to make it more or less likely to remain free or be transported across membranes, while changes in albumin levels (e.g. glomerulonephritis) will alter the capacity of the drug to remain in the blood and bound rather than free. Other compartments where a drug may accumulate or redistribute include cerebrospinal fluid, intracellular space, interstitial/extracellular space, binding to specific proteins (e.g. serum albumin), fat in the case of lipophilic drugs, and bone, among others. This is largely governed by an interaction between a drug's chemical or thermodynamic properties and biological processes. Differences across individuals that affect such processes may produce individual variability in how a drug distributes within the body and in which compartments it accumulates. Therefore, an understanding of how underlying genetic (e.g. mutations in a transporter protein gene), environmental exposure (e.g. other prescription drugs), or pathophysiological conditions (e.g. hormone-secreting tumors/paraneoplastic syndromes) may be important to understanding how a drug appropriately or inappropriately distributes within the body of an individual to impact the amount of drug available to interact with the therapeutic site.

d. drug metabolism/biotransformation

For many drugs or exogenous compounds to be eliminated from the body, they must first be modified by a biological process in the body to reach routes of elimination (discussed below). This process of modifying drugs to facilitate their removal from the body is collectively referred to as drug **metabolism** or biotransformation and is typically the most significant determinant of how much active drug is available in the body and shapes zero- or first-order kinetic. In addition to inactivating or promoting the elimination of drugs, some may need to be modified by the body after administration to render them pharmacologically *active* or able to interact with and alter targeted biological processes. This group of drugs that require some biological transformation (biotransformation) to be active are administered as **prodrugs**. Whether for metabolism or biotransformation, the chemical or structural alteration of drugs occurs through a multitude of processes, but most often involves two phases. Phase 1 reactions involve the addition of a functional group through reduction, oxidation, or hydrolysis to inactivate/activate a drug, whereas Phase 2 reactions involve the conjugation of an additional molecule to promote water solubility for elimination. The enzymes responsible for Phase I and transferases for Phase 2 reactions are differentially expressed through the body and organ systems but are most abundant in the gastrointestinal system and liver. It is the primary role of enzymes found in the liver in metabolizing so many drugs that often cause a major proportion of drugs to be eliminated rather quickly after intravenous administration giving rise to what is called the 'first pass effect'. It is important to keep in mind that changes in the anatomy or physiology of the gastrointestinal, hepatic, or other systems that are important sites of metabolism/biotransformation of a particular drug may result in major changes in drug concentration for an individual given a particular dose. Because the rate and mechanism of drug metabolism are specific and the largest determinant of drug concentration and lifetime in the body, factors that affect these processes, whether genomic (e.g. pharmacogenomics) or pathophysiological (e.g. hepatitis, surgical removal), are important to consider in establishing drug choice and dose.

e. drug elimination from the body

While some drugs require metabolism by the body to reach a route that facilitates their removal or **elimination** from the body, many may be eliminated in the same form in which they are initially administered. Regardless of their form, nearly all drugs or their metabolites are removed from the body by being accumulated into waste compartments either in the urine by the kidneys or feces by the gastrointestinal and biliary tracts, with only a limited amount accumulating in other compartments for removal (e.g. sweat, breast milk, lungs etc.). As discussed previously, the movement into and accumulation of drugs or their metabolites in compartments may be passive or active, which will affect the capacity for drug elimination. For example, any changes (genomic or pathological) in glomerular filtration rate (e.g. as in hypertension or chronic kidney disease) or the environment and transporter activity in the proximal (drug secretion) or distal tubule (drug reabsorption) and collecting duct will alter how much drug is moved to and retained in the urine for eventual elimination. Similar mechanisms for diffusion and transport that accumulate drugs into the gastrointestinal lumen and/or packaging of drugs or metabolites with bile for recycling or excretion are also sensitive to disruption in these physiological processes (e.g. increased motility, cholecystectomy).

f. pharmacogenomic determinants of drug action

Pharmacogenomics refers to how individual variability in functionally-relevant genes that encode either drug targets or processes involved in establishing a drug's pharmacokinetic profile can determine the potency, efficacy, specificity, and temporal nature of the drug and body/system interaction. Whether single or multiple nucleotide insertions, deletions, substitutions, or translocations are present, any functionally-relevant change or mutation in a gene encoding for a particular protein may affect its function(s) in an individual. Mutated genes that encode sites at which drugs interact to produce some functional change may impact drug pharmacodynamics by increasing or decreasing the ability of the drug to bind or the degree to which downstream effectors are activated. Similarly, mutations in genes that encode transporters and enzymes responsible for drug absorption, distribution, metabolism, or excretion may increase or decrease the amount of drug present in the body or affect how long it takes the body to reduce the concentration of a drug. One of the most common sites where genomics affects pharmacokinetic properties is in mutations of genes encoding any one of the 12 major cytochrome P450 (CYP450) enzymes, which is a superfamily of proteins responsible for phase I metabolic reactions for many kinds of drugs or exogenous compounds. The presence of a dominant or homozygous loss of function mutations in CYP450 genes may easily go undetected for a lifetime until an individual experiences a toxic accumulation of a novel drug due to the reduced metabolism of that drug by a deficient CYP450 enzyme. The area of pharmacogenomics is complex and evolving, but awareness of potential genomic determinants of drug actions may be used to identify potential genetic causes of aberrant responses to a particular drug or screen preventively for mutations associated with such aberrant responses in the larger population, which is well outside the scope of this chapter.

g. race or ethnicity

Similar to pharmacogenomics but more wide-reaching, many unique functionally-relevant differences in genes encoding drug-relevant proteins are common within some groups having shared ethnic, racial, or regional backgrounds (e.g., the anticonvulsant, carbamazepine in certain Asian populations). Databases and references are available to guide drug choice or dose based on these commonly occurring variations in genes that encode drug targets or mechanisms for metabolism or elimination. However, be aware that some rationales for differentiating pharmacotherapeutic approaches based on racial or ethnic background persist in the literature despite a lack of appropriately powered and controlled studies, the implementation of which may lead to health disparities. Therefore, caution should be exercised when factoring in the rationale for drug choice and dose changes based on patient background.

h. target organ/effector cell sensitivity

Primarily considered a component of pharmacodynamics, changes in the sensitivity of a drug target or some component of the downstream effector (e.g. second messenger) of that target may vary between individuals or over time in a given individual due to genetics or experience. In addition to previously discussed pharmacogenomic implications (see B.3.f), genetic determination of a drug's affinity, potency, or efficacy at the target site may require increases or decreases in dosing to achieve the goal. An individual's history of exposure to prescribed or recreational drugs also affects drug targets and related signaling (see sections B.4 and C.7.b).

i. hypersensitivity (allergy) or idiosyncratic reactions of the patient

Some drug hypersensitivity or allergic reactions can be characterized as immunologic if they are mediated by immunoglobulins. They can be further classified into those that are rapid and mediated by immunoglobulins such as IgE (Type I) and those that are delayed and mediated by non-IgE (Type II-IV). In contrast, non-immunogenic/pseudo-hypersensitivity reactions are mediated by other known or unknown (idiopathic) mechanisms that are drug/class dependent, not by immunoglobulins. An individual's hypersensitivity or allergic reaction to a drug is often considered a clear contraindication for that drug and will require the identification of an alternative. Because drugs of a similar class often share a similar chemical structure, it may be ideal to choose a drug from an alternative class to achieve the treatment goal to avoid provoking a reaction by similar compounds (e.g. sulfa-containing drugs). In some instances, the hypersensitivity or allergic reaction is specific to one drug within a class and not the entire class, and using another drug within that class may still be safe. In other cases where a hypersensitivity reaction is not severe, uncertain, or delayed (Type II-IV) and the benefits of the drug are profound, it may be reasonable to implement the use of that drug with appropriate supervision, support, and/or a second drug to reduce the adverse effect. Sensitivity testing and a protocol to develop desensitization of the immune response to a drug may also be useful if the use of a specific drug or class of drugs is unavoidable.

j. weight of the patient

As individual body mass varies, so does the overall water volume, size of specific compartments and reservoirs, and a drug's general **volume of distribution**. Generally, an individual with lower total body mass will require less drug to achieve an effective concentration of that drug as it has a smaller volume over which to be distributed. Except for some extreme variations in individual total body mass, most adults may be administered a standard initial dose for a particular drug or started on a low dose, especially for drugs with limited acute adverse reaction profiles. Then, based on the progress toward a treatment goal and any observed adverse drug reactions, the dose may be increased or decreased from what is given initially. Likewise, those with greater body mass will likely require higher doses to achieve the necessary therapeutic concentrations. Of course, relative to a typical adult, children have lower body mass and body mass often decreases in the elderly. Separate from age-specific considerations (discussed below), the dose of many drugs may need to be reduced from a typical adult dose to account for body mass changes alone.

k. body composition of the patient (normal, lean, or obese)

Body composition referring to the relative percentage of an individual's mass made up of fat is primarily a determinant of drug distribution. Lipophilic drugs, unlike hydrophilic drugs, accumulate in adipose tissue and leave little in the plasma/blood/water volume. This effectively raises the volume of distribution and potentially sequesters away drug from non-adipose sites of action. As a result, lipophilic drugs will likely have an increased volume of distribution and reduced efficacy in obese individuals, while the opposite is true for leaner individuals. Although not a consideration for a majority of patients, those with body composition extremes of obese and very lean, their composition should be considered especially for lipophilic drugs (e.g. diazepam, propranolol, estrogen).

l. age of the patient

In addition to changes in body mass throughout the aging process, many other physiological parameters (e.g. muscle, fat composition) and physiological processes (e.g. kidney function/glomerular filtration rate) change throughout the lifetime. Pediatric and geriatric populations are not simply differently sized adults – there are significant changes that occur in the pharmacodynamic and pharmacokinetic properties of many drugs across the lifespan. As such, incorporating patient age as one variable to determine drug choice and dose is an essential consideration, especially early and late in life.

In addition to differences in body mass of children relative to adults mentioned previously, the underlying physiology of children is often still developing and produces quite different PK and PD profiles for certain drugs relative to adults. Mechanisms affecting drug absorption and distribution (muscle/fat ratio, transporter function, volume of distribution, protein binding), metabolism (e.g. CYP450, transferase expression), and elimination (e.g. glomerular filtration rate) have all been found to vary across childhood and adolescence in addition to being different from adults depending on the drug used (Batchelor and Marriott, 2015). Children are also uniquely susceptible to specific drug-induced adverse reactions or toxicities, including opioid-induced respiratory depression (e.g. codeine) or damage to tooth enamel by tetracyclines, making the use of these and other drugs in pediatric populations problematic despite a favorable safety profile in adults.

Geriatric populations pose a particular set of pharmacological challenges due to changes in pharmacokinetic and pharmacodynamic properties, but also due to the challenge of polypharmacy as dysfunction of systems accumulates with age. A few examples of pharmacokinetic considerations in older populations include the decrease in the muscle/fat ratio that impacts the volume of distribution for lipophilic drugs (e.g. fentanyl) and how drugs that require hepatic (e.g. metoprolol) or renal (e.g. gabapentin) mechanisms may be cleared from the body more slowly and accumulate. While it is arguably more difficult to predict the pharmacodynamic properties that change with age consistently, one common observation is the elevated sensitivity of older individuals to the anticholinergic adverse effects of many drugs, especially drugs that are commonly prescribed to treat aging-related conditions (e.g. antihistamines, antipsychotics, antidepressants, among others). Further complicating drug choice and dosing in geriatric populations is the need to achieve multiple goals like reducing blood pressure, improving depression, relieving pain, treating heart failure, and/or improving sleep. Achieving these goals often requires the administration of drugs unique to those goals, with some drugs exacerbating underlying issues, producing additive adverse reactions, or even provoking an entirely new problem. This issue of polypharmacy, occurring at greater rates with advancing age, is a longstanding problem. However, efforts to increase monitoring of an individual's complete medication list and identify drugs that are particularly problematic for older individuals (Beers Criteria, Merck Manual on Drug Therapy in Older Adults) are the first steps in reducing the unnecessary or inappropriate use of drugs or drug classes in elderly patients.

m. sex of the patient

Pharmacokinetic and pharmacodynamic properties of many drugs may vary based on sex since the underlying physiology of males and females is unique and those that are transitioning or have transitioned to one sex or the other may display drug-relevant aspects of each (Soldin and Mattison, 2009). Some important factors that affect drug absorption and distribution include body mass, body water, the fraction of extracellular/intracellular water, muscle/fat ratio, changes due to menopause or pregnancy, and the presence of soluble drug-binding proteins. Drug absorption, distribution, and metabolism are also unique based on sex-specific variations in transporter and enzyme activity (e.g. alcohol dehydrogenase).

n. preexisting or concurrent diseases

The impact of concurrent pathophysiology on drug effects and pharmacokinetic profiles has been mentioned above in other contexts and can be a major determinant of drug efficacy, adverse reactions, and potential for excessive accumulation of drugs in the body. Although this may seem obvious, it is often overlooked. For example, individuals with reduced kidney function should be cautiously administered certain antibiotics with regular assessment of plasma drug concentrations while others should avoid nephrotoxic antibiotics like aminoglycosides when possible. Individuals with diabetes should not be administered corticosteroids, thiazide diuretics, or beta-blockers due to their hyperglycemia-inducing properties. A list of drug-disease interactions is beyond the scope of this chapter, but the most important aspect of accounting for drug interactions with preexisting conditions is for the provider and potentially the pharmacist to have a comprehensive understanding of an individual's pathophysiological state and condition. The time taken to develop this understanding will help ensure drugs or drug classes are avoided that may be problematic in a given setting.

4. *What factors alter target cell responsiveness over time for this drug?*

Much of this chapter so far has discussed the implementation of a pharmacological regimen in a static context, i.e. the situation is not changing. However, the physiology of an individual almost always changes in response to drug administration. This arises from the efforts of the body to maintain a homeostatic balance and 'set point', which often produces unintended consequences that may be misinterpreted as an additional disease or disorder. So, when this imbalance is corrected by drug administration the body will work to restore the situation to a pre-drug state even if this state is pathophysiological. This reconfiguring of its systems and function in the setting of a new drug or drugs are often referred to as plasticity or adaptation. The mechanisms that can change to produce adaptation in response to the drug are extensive and encompass pharmacokinetic and/or pharmacodynamic changes based on the administered drug(s).

While many of the adaptive responses to a drug can be complex and affect multiple systems, one of the most common observations is **tolerance** – a reduced response to a drug over time. Drug tolerance may develop due to pharmacokinetic or pharmacodynamic changes. Pharmacokinetic changes that may produce drug tolerance can include increased expression of a transporter that enhances the movement of the drug to the gastrointestinal renal tubule lumen to promote excretion. Commonly, the expression of an enzyme essential for drug metabolism may increase with increasing exposure to a drug (e.g. alcohol dehydrogenase in chronic alcohol use). Both situations would facilitate more rapid degradation of this drug so that its effects on physiological systems are reduced. Tolerance to other drugs may rely on changes in the drug's pharmacodynamic properties, as there may be a reduction in the receptors and/or its downstream effectors that are being targeted, or there may be an increase in a separate system that compensates for the actions of the drug. One classic example of pharmacodynamic adaptations that occur to produce tolerance is **desensitization** in opioid receptor signaling. This involves a decrease in mu-opioid receptor expression and an increase in adenylyl cyclase/cAMP/protein kinase A (PKA) expression to compensate for the overactivation of mu-opioid receptors and inhibition of adenylyl cyclase. Similarly, the loop diuretic furosemide is often much more effective in the first few days of administration than it is weeks later due to an increase in expression of the NKCC2 transporter that is blocked by furosemide and increases in ion reabsorption at other sites within the renal tubule. Similar compensatory adaptations to produce tolerance do, or have the potential to occur, with almost every drug in use today, resulting in the need to escalate the dose and/or introduce additional drugs to achieve the treatment goal over time.

Drug-specific mechanisms that promote tolerance develop over time, because the continued presence may alter the function of the targeted system. As a result, the physiological state of the system/body is reliant upon the presence of the drug, also known as **dependence**. In addition to the need for a higher dose or other drugs to achieve the treatment goal, this 'new normal' in the presence of the drug also means that when the drug is withheld, the homeostatic balance of the system will be lost because the receptor desensitization and compensatory adaptations that developed over time will be unopposed in absence of the drug. **Withdrawal** refers to the physical or psychological symptoms due to the activation of dependence mechanisms and processes in the absence of a drug. This may vary from mildly uncomfortable to life-threatening, depending on the drug and duration of exposure. For example, a potentially life-threatening withdrawal condition can occur when the antihypertensive drug and alpha 2 adrenergic agonist, clonidine, is withheld. Continual activation of alpha 2 adrenergic receptors by clonidine causes desensitization through downregulation of the receptor, which is physiologically important to provide feedback inhibition of norepinephrine release. As a result, reduced receptor number without continual activation by an administered drug results in excessive norepinephrine release without the same degree of feedback inhibition, causing a hypertensive crisis. Unfortunately, drug tolerance, desensitization, dependence, and withdrawal are unavoidable consequences of pharmacotherapy in many instances, but with time and attention, it is possible to manage these risks to ensure patient safety and health.

C. Pharmacovigilance

In addition to the multitude of factors that comprise the pharmacodynamic and pharmacokinetic properties of a drug, it is essential to also account for the safety profile of a drug. Pharmacovigilance (PV) refers to the incorporation of a drug's toxic or adverse effects into the rationale for choosing a drug and its dose. As discussed previously, drug toxicity and adverse drug reactions stem from a drug's pharmacodynamic and/or pharmacokinetic properties, underscoring the interdependent nature of the three ABCs of Pharmacology. In some cases, adverse drug reactions arise due to non-specificity or off-target binding of a drug to produce a physiological response in a system outside of the one that is targeted for therapeutic benefit, as noted above. In other instances, the amount of drug in the body may accumulate to toxic levels due to decreases in the activity of an enzyme responsible for that drug's metabolism, either due to genetics, disease, or environmental factors. It is also important to note that pharmacovigilance is not a static factor or one that only needs to be considered only when initiating a new treatment regimen. Rather, it is dynamic, and an individual's therapeutic response to a drug must continually be weighed relative to the development of any adverse reactions. The need for continual pharmacovigilance is because the body's or system's status quo is continually changing over time. This may involve changes in underlying physiological processes, the emergence of new pathologies, the administration of a new drug to treat a new or different condition, or sensitized immune responses.

5. *What is the Risk/Benefit ratio of therapy (therapeutic index) of this drug?*

As discussed in detail in section A.2.b, the relationship between the dose at which adverse drug reactions or toxicities and the concentration of a drug at which beneficial changes occur is important to understand the potential risk/benefit of a given drug. The further apart these therapeutic and toxic dose ranges are, the wider the **therapeutic window** and the greater the **therapeutic index**. In contrast, when these concentrations are closer the therapeutic window and index both decrease. This means that it will be more difficult to find a concentration of a drug that is capable of achieving therapeutic goals without causing too many untoward effects. Ideally, the therapeutic window/index should be as large as possible to allow the most flexibility in choosing the maximally beneficial drug dose with minimal adverse drug reactions.

6. *What are the contraindications (absolute/relative) of this drug?*

In addition to common mild adverse reactions, which occur with the use of almost every drug in the general population, some drugs have been found to induce adverse reactions in specific settings. Sometimes these contraindicated situations are physiological (e.g. age), pathophysiological (e.g. renal failure), or due to interaction between two drugs (see below). Depending on how frequently a drug is used in a problematic setting, data collected during clinical trials or over years of use in clinical practice are what determine whether a contraindication exists and is listed in drug packaging and on professional databases (e.g. UpToDate, Medscape, Clinical Pharmacology, Drugs.com). Some of these contraindications are 'relative contraindications' that will produce mild adverse reactions if a drug is administered in the presence of that contraindication. Other contraindications are 'absolute' and administration of a drug in that setting could be life-threatening or fatal (e.g., ventricular fibrillation for digoxin). Regardless, a significant aspect of pharmacovigilance is the awareness and communication of drug contraindications, which again is a shared responsibility of a provider and pharmacist.

7. What adverse (side) effects are caused by this drug?

According to the Institute of Medicine (US) Committee on Quality of Health Care in America, adverse drug reactions (ADRs) are a major public health problem. Recent Centers for Disease Control and Prevention (CDC) data indicate that more than 700,000 Emergency Department visits (120,000 hospitalizations) for ADRs occur per year, with adults over 65 twice as likely to visit the Emergency Department for ADRs, often due to overdose. Roughly half of the medical error causes of death are drug-related, and ADRs are the 5th-8th leading cause of death in U.S. hospitals. ADRs may occur immediately (e.g. allergic reaction) or take months to years to develop (e.g. amiodarone-induced pulmonary fibrosis). They also may range from mild to life-threatening, and they stem from physiological, pathophysiological, or environment/experience-dependent changes in pharmacodynamic (see section B.3.h) or pharmacokinetic (B.3.a-e) processes. Some adverse effects are also difficult to predict due to the complex and dynamic physiological changes that occur over time in the presence of other drugs or exposures, as previously discussed (see Section B.4). Regardless, awareness and continual monitoring of adverse drug effects are essential to responsible drug prescribing and patient safety.

a. hypersensitivity and pseudo-hypersensitivity

Many types of adverse effects (side effects) have been mentioned above. One of the major concerns with the initial administration of a new drug or class of drugs to an individual is the possibility that an immune-mediated hyperreactivity reaction may occur that produces an immunoglobulin-mediated Type I-IV response. Often drugs with shared functional groups (e.g. sulfa-containing drugs) may induce similar reactions based on host immune detection of like antigens, despite falling in different pharmacotherapeutic classes (e.g. glipizide for Type II diabetes mellitus and the antibacterial sulfamethoxazole). Therefore, appropriate pharmacovigilance requires awareness of allergic reactions to drugs that may fall within different therapeutic classes but have shared chemical structures. In addition to awareness of hypersensitivity/allergic reactions, other drugs may cause pseudo-hypersensitivity in some individuals due to direct stimulation of a system (e.g. complement pathway) that mimics an immune-mediated reaction (Zhang et al., 2018). The groups of agents that trigger pseudo-hypersensitivity typically fall into a limited group of clinically relevant drugs, including opioids and non-steroidal anti-inflammatory drugs (NSAIDs). Note that, in some cases, it is the metabolite of a drug that triggers its hypersensitivity/hyperreactivity, which may result in a delayed reaction.

b. drug-drug interactions

One of the most common environment/experience-dependent causes of an adverse drug effect is due to interactions between two drugs. These drug-drug interactions do not necessarily refer to physical interactions of two substances, but rather the effects of one drug that impact the pharmacokinetics or pharmacodynamics of another drug. Regarding pharmacodynamics, drugs of one class may directly or indirectly affect the site of action or the effector mechanism for another drug. In individuals with asthma who use drugs that activate beta-adrenergic receptors (e.g. albuterol) to produce bronchodilation, administration of a non-selective beta-adrenergic receptor blocker (e.g. propranolol) to treat hypertension will antagonize this effect and exacerbate asthma. In addition to pharmacodynamically antagonistic drug-drug interactions, others may be pharmacodynamically additive. This can occur with the combined administration of a selective serotonin reuptake inhibitor like fluoxetine for depression and the anti-migraine drug sumatriptan because they both enhance the activity of serotonin (5-hydroxytryptamine) receptors and increase the risk of potentially life-threatening serotonin syndrome. Fortunately, a clear understanding of the drug mechanism of action makes it possible to predict and account for pharmacodynamic drug-drug interactions.

In contrast, drugs that interact to affect the pharmacokinetic properties of one another often do so by more complicated and less obvious mechanisms that may have to do with drug absorption, distribution, elimination, or metabolism. For example, commonly prescribed gastric proton pump inhibitors (e.g. omeprazole) work by decreasing gastric proton concentration, which negatively affects the absorption and eventual effectiveness of certain drugs that require an acidic environment (e.g. antifungal posaconazole). Reductions in drug elimination may cause elevations in drug concentrations that exceed therapeutic concentrations and reach toxic levels. For example, renal elimination of methotrexate, a cancer chemotherapeutic agent, is reduced when glomerular filtration rates decline in response to NSAIDs (e.g., aspirin), producing a drug-drug interaction that results in nausea, vomiting, and/or myelosuppression. While pharmacokinetic drug-drug interactions that occur through induced changes in absorption, distribution, or elimination may be simpler to predict, incorporating an understanding of interactions that alter drug metabolism is more challenging. This challenge stems from the fact that many of the metabolic processes or enzymes responsible for drug activation or inactivation are dynamic and not static. The activity of enzymes (CYP450s or transferases) responsible for drug transformation may be inhibited or induced, and their expression levels may be increased or reduced by several factors, especially other agents or drugs. As a result, concentrations of drugs that rely on a specific transferase or CYP450s to be metabolized for excretion may be elevated to toxic if those enzymes are inhibited or their expression is reduced. In contrast, elevation in the activity or expression of these enzymes may prevent that same drug from reaching therapeutic levels. Decades of data are now available that describe which drugs inhibit or induce specific enzymes/processes responsible for drug metabolism. Known CYP2C9 inhibitors like amiodarone or fluoxetine may cause prolonged elevation of CYP2C9 substrates like carvedilol or losartan. Likewise, CYP3A4 inducers like rifampin may lead to reduced levels of the antihypertensive drug, amlodipine, requiring higher amlodipine doses to achieve appropriate blood pressure control.

Whether due to pharmacodynamic or pharmacokinetic changes, drug-drug interactions become more common in older individuals and individuals with significant pathophysiologies, since both situations require administration of different drugs/classes to address accumulating pathologies. Therefore, the need to consider drug-drug interactions becomes more important as more drugs are administered. Accounting for and avoiding drug-drug interactions is complex, but the regular reference of drug-drug interactions in package inserts, available databases, and working closely with pharmacists are all approaches that should be leveraged to maximize patient benefits and safety.

c. overdose toxicity

As noted previously (see above and Chapter 1), Paracelsus, who is credited as the father of toxicology, made it clear that every drug is a poison if the dose is excessive. Even water can be toxic if taken in excessive doses, which can result in fatal cerebral edema, and water drinking games and excessive water intake related to athletic competitions have resulted in death even in relatively young and previously healthy individuals. The drugs associated with the highest rates of fatalities include opiates, which are a severe public health problem. In addition, other drugs of abuse, sedative-hypnotics, antipsychotics, CNS stimulants, alcohol, cardiovascular drugs, and even acetaminophen are all associated with a large degree of fatalities. For example, acetaminophen, also known as paracetamol, is a safe drug in therapeutic doses. However, it is found in a great number of over-the-counter products for pain and also in cold remedies, in which it is a major ingredient. These products have been taken together for decades, which has resulted in fatal overdose toxicity involving liver failure. A drug that has a toxic dose that is relatively close to its therapeutic dose is considered to have a low therapeutic index, as described above. The organ system that mediates the toxicity is often not the organ system that is the therapeutic target, as seen with acetaminophen which targets the nervous system for pain relief but targets the liver to produce toxicity.

8. What drug-related disease-like symptoms (including those due to drug abuse) can be mistaken for additional disease symptoms?

Many drug-induced changes in system processes or functions have the potential to mimic certain disease states or other problematic issues with acute or chronic use. For example, anticoagulants may appear to mimic spousal abuse. An adverse effect of these drugs is extensive bruising of the skin (ecchymosis). A patient with a history of marital discord taking an anticoagulant for a clotting problem who is consulting with a new healthcare professional could be erroneously thought to be suffering from spousal abuse. The key to mitigating this problem is the awareness of these possibilities based on understanding drug pharmacodynamic properties and potential adverse events, along with accumulation of data on an individual.

9. What alterations of clinical laboratory tests can be caused by this drug?

Just as many drugs can produce other pathologies, based on their mechanism of action it is possible to also predict how laboratory test values may be affected. Therefore, when a new drug has been added to the regimen and laboratory data suggest a deviation from previous or typical values, it is often best to first determine whether a drug may be the cause. For example, a patient who has a routine blood test that shows hypokalemia or low potassium might be taking a thiazide diuretic, since this is an adverse response to this class of drugs.

References

1. Batchelor HK, Marriott JF. Paediatric pharmacokinetics: key considerations. Br J Clin Pharmacol. 2015 Mar;79(3):395-404. doi: 10.1111/bcp.12267. PMID: 25855821; PMCID: PMC4345950.
2. Bullers K. Merck Manuals. J Med Libr Assoc. 2016 Oct;104(4):369–71. doi: 10.3163/1536-5050.104.4.028. PMCID: PMC5079511.
3. Dunaway G.A, Faingold C.L., Development and implementation of a multidisciplinary sophomore medical curriculum: integration of pharmacology with basic and clinical science. Pharmacologist 43:83-90, 2001.
4. Faingold CL, Dunaway GA. Teaching pharmacology within a multidisciplinary organ system-based medical curriculum. *N.S. Arch. Pharmacol.* 2002;366:18-25.
5. Institute of Medicine (US) Committee on Quality of Health Care in America. To Err is Human: Building a Safer Health System. Kohn LT, Corrigan JM, Donaldson MS, editors. Washington (DC): National Academies Press (US); 2000. PMID: 25077248.
6. Soldin OP, Mattison DR. Sex differences in pharmacokinetics and pharmacodynamics. Clin Pharmacokinet. 2009;48(3):143-57. doi: 10.2165/00003088-200948030-00001. PMID: 19385708; PMCID: PMC3644551.
7. Zhang B, Li Q, Shi C, Zhang X: Drug-Induced Pseudoallergy: A Review of the Causes and Mechanisms. Pharmacology 2018;101:104-110. doi: 10.1159/000479878

Acknowledgment

Earlier versions of the ABCs of Pharmacology were originally developed by William H. Cline Jr.

Quiz Questions

1. Pharmacovigilance issues do NOT include:

   A. Drug toxicity
   B. Drug adverse effects
   C. Drug-drug interactions
   D. Drug mechanism of action
   E. Drug-induced symptoms that resemble another disease

2. Which of the following is NOT true about adverse drug effects in the hospital?

   A. Lead to ED visits and hospitalizations
   B. Cause half of the medical error-induced death in the US
   C. Always occur within 1-2 hrs of drug administration
   D. Cause hospitalization most commonly in the older adult demographic

3. Which of the following will have the greatest effect on the pharmacokinetic profile of a drug?

   A. Downregulation of drug-activated effector mechanism
   B. Reduced drug binding affinity due to mutation in the drug binding site
   C. Inhibition of a phase I type enzyme activity responsible for prodrug transformation
   D. Increases in target enzyme expression with prolonged administration of a drug

4. Which of the following changes in pharmacokinetic properties may lead to drug toxicity?

   A. Decreased absorption to due elevated gastric pH
   B. Increased volume of distribution due to elevated adipose tissue levels
   C. Increased rate of drug metabolism due to induction of CYP2C9
   D. Decrease in renal elimination due to dysfunctional organic anion transporter 3

5. Which of the following necessitates a re-evaluation of drug choice or dosage when they occur after initiation of a new pharmacotherapeutic regimen?

   A. Thrombocytopenia
   B. Pulmonary fibrosis
   C. Cough
   D. Orthostatic Hypotension
   E. Anaphylaxis
   F. All the above

Quiz Answers

1. D. Pharmacovigilance refers to the knowledge of what contributes to the adverse effects of a drug. Option D refers to a drug's mechanism of action, which is typically considered a pharmacodynamic concept as it deals with what the drug does to the body, but not necessarily what leads to an adverse event or negative reaction to a drug.

2. C. All options are true for adverse drug effects or events in the US, except C. Adverse drug events may occur in the short term and/or over long periods of time due to accumulating effects of a drug over weeks, months, or years.

3. C. Options A and B refer to changes that would primarily impact a drug's pharmacodynamic properties, while option D refers to pharmacodynamic changes that occur with drug exposure – none of which will necessarily affect absorption, distribution, metabolism, or elimination (pharmacokinetics) of a drug.

4. D. For drug toxicity to develop, it is implied that the drug concentration in the body must increase. Therefore, anything that leads to an increase in drug concentration in the body may cause toxicity. Options A-C would all decrease the amount of free drug in the body and therefore reduce the potential for toxicity to develop. Decreasing the elimination of a drug will likely lead to unexpected accumulation of the drug in the body and lead to potential toxicity.

5. F. The occurrence of any new physiological change after beginning a new drug should always be evaluated further as potentially being caused by the new drug, whether serious (anaphylaxis) or mild (cough). Even in the case of mild adverse events/effects, this may signify an individual's natural high sensitivity to or reduced ability to eliminate a drug. The emergence of these adverse events indicates a need to consider other drugs or changes in dose to ensure patient safety.

SYMPTOMS 1 –

IMMUNO-INFECTIOUS SYMPTOMS TO TREATMENT

CHAPTER 3

DRUGS FOR INFECTIONS

DIEGO MARIN, DO[1], MADHU SURYADEVARA, MD[2] AND DAVID P. SIDEROVSKI, PHD[3]

[1] HCA Florida Westside Hospital, Fort Lauderdale, FL
[2] The Family Health Center at Newark Beth Israel Medical Center, Newark, NJ
[3] University of North Texas Health Science Center, Fort Worth, TX

Symptoms: Immuno-Infectious
Musculoskeletal
Neurological

ANTIBACTERIAL DRUG LIST

Penicillins:
β-lactam ring-containing bacterial cell wall synthesis inhibitors
penicillin G
given intramuscular or intravenously; PBP transpeptidase inhibitor
penicillin V
given orally; PBP transpeptidase inhibitor
ampicillin
an aminopenicillin with an extended spectrum; given with **sulbactam**
amoxicillin
an aminopenicillin with an extended spectrum; given with **clavulanate**
piperacillin
"anti-pseudomonal" penicillin; often given with **tazobactam**
nafcillin, oxacillin, dicloxacillin
"anti-staphylococcal" penicillins; PBP transpeptidase inhibitors

Cephalosporins:
β-lactam ring-containing cell wall synthesis inhibitors
cefazolin, cephalexin, cephalothin
1st generation cephalosporins; PBP transpeptidase inhibitors
cefuroxime, cefoxitin, cefotetan
2nd generation cephalosporins; PBP transpeptidase inhibitors
ceftriaxone, cefotaxime, ceftazidime
3rd generation cephalosporins; PBP transpeptidase inhibitors
cefepime
4th generation cephalosporin; PBP transpeptidase inhibitor
ceftaroline fosamil
5th generation cephalosporin; PBP transpeptidase inhibitor

Carbapenems:
β-lactam ring-containing cell wall synthesis inhibitors
imipenem
given with **cilastatin** (anti-dehydropeptidase adjuvant)
doripenem, ertapenem, meropenem
broad-spectrum inhibitors of bacterial PBP transpeptidases

Monobactams:
β-lactam ring-containing cell wall synthesis inhibitors
aztreonam
monocyclic; narrow spectrum PBP transpeptidase inhibitor

Non-β-lactam drugs:
Inhibitors of cell wall synthesis / membrane integrity
vancomycin
glycopeptide; binds and blocks peptidoglycan precursors
bacitracin
cyclic peptide; inhibits peptidoglycan precursor delivery
polymyxin B
cyclic peptide; alters bacterial membrane permeability

Folate antagonists:
Inhibitors of bacterial purine production / DNA synthesis
sulfamethoxazole (SMX),
sulfadiazine, mafenide
sulfonamides ("**sulfa**" drugs) that inhibit dihydropteroate synthase
trimethoprim (TMP)
dihydrofolate reductase inhibitor; usually given as **TMP-SMX** combination
pyrimethamine
dihydrofolate reductase inhibitor; usually given in combination with a **sulfa**

Tetracyclines:
Inhibitors of bacterial protein synthesis
tetracycline
30S ribosomal subunit inhibitor
doxycycline
30S ribosomal subunit inhibitor
minocycline
30S ribosomal subunit inhibitor
tigecycline
30S ribosomal subunit inhibitor; broader spectrum
sarecycline
30S ribosomal subunit inhibitor; narrower spectrum

Aminoglycosides:
Inhibitors of bacterial protein synthesis
streptomycin
30S ribosomal subunit inhibitor
gentamicin
30S ribosomal subunit inhibitor
tobramycin
30S ribosomal subunit inhibitor
amikacin
30S ribosomal subunit inhibitor; successor to kanamycin
neomycin
30S ribosomal subunit inhibitor; topical agent only
paromomycin
30S ribosome inhibitor; antiparasitic and anthelmintic uses
chloramphenicol:
inhibitor of bacterial protein synthesis via 50S subunit

Macrolides and Ketolides:
Inhibitors of bacterial protein synthesis
erythromycin
50S ribosomal subunit inhibitor
azithromycin
50S ribosomal subunit inhibitor
clarithromycin
50S ribosomal subunit inhibitor
telithromycin
50S ribosomal subunit inhibitor; ketolide
clindamycin (a lincosamide):
inhibitor of bacterial protein synthesis via 50S subunit
mupirocin (a mixture of pseudomonic acids):
inhibitor of bacterial isoleucine-tRNA ligase; used topically
fidaxomicin (a macrocyclic):
inhibitor of bacterial RNA polymerase; used for *C. diff* only

Fluoroquinolones:
Inhibitors of bacterial DNA gyrase and topoisomerase IV
ciprofloxacin
levofloxacin
a "respiratory fluoroquinolone"
moxifloxacin
a "respiratory fluoroquinolone"
gemifloxacin
a "respiratory fluoroquinolone"
nitrofurantoin (a nitrofuran):
reduced to highly reactive intermediates damaging to bacterial DNA;
concentrated in the urine to bactericidal levels

Nitroimidazoles:
DNA-damaging drugs (anaerobic bacteria / protozoa)
metronidazole
forms reactive nitroso radical within reducing environment
tinidazole
forms reactive nitroso radical within reducing environment

ANTIMYCOBACTERIAL DRUG LIST

First-line drugs for tuberculosis

- **isoniazid (INH)**
- **Rifamycins: rifampicin** (a.k.a. **Rifampin), rifapentine**
- **ethambutol**
- **pyrazinamide**

Second-line drugs for MDR-/XDR-tuberculosis

- Fluoroquinolones: **levofloxacin, moxifloxacin**
- Add-on agents: **bedaquiline; delamanid;** ***p*-aminosalicylic acid**
- Injectables: **amikacin, streptomycin; capreomycin; carbapenems + clavulanate**
- **pretomanid + bedaquiline & linezolid**

First-line drugs for Hansen's disease ("leprosy")

- **dapsone**
- **rifampicin**
- **clofazimine**

ANTIFUNGAL DRUG LIST
terbinafine:
inhibitor of ergosterol biosynthesis
azoles:
inhibitors of ergosterol biosynthesis
ketoconazole
imidazole, fungal CYP450 inhibitor; generally a topical application
miconazole
imidazole, fungal CYP450 inhibitor; generally a topical application
clotrimazole
imidazole, fungal CYP450 inhibitor; generally a topical application
fluconazole
triazole, fungal CYP450 inhibitor; narrower spectrum (~*Candida*)
itraconazole
triazole, fungal CYP450 inhibitor; broader spectrum (+*Aspergillus*)
voriconazole
triazole, fungal CYP450 inhibitor; broader spectrum (+*Aspergillus*)
posaconazole
triazole, fungal CYP450 inhibitor; broader spectrum (+*Aspergillus*)
isavuconazole
triazole, fungal CYP450 inhibitor; broader spectrum (+*Aspergillus*)

Polyenes:
Ergosterol binders / fungal cell membrane destabilizers
amphotericin B (AmB)
first-line option for many serious systemic fungal infections
nystatin
reserved for topic use in oral, esophageal, & vaginal infections

Flucytosine:
inhibitor of fungal DNA & RNA synthesis

Echinocandins:
Inhibitors of β-glucan synthesis / fungal cell wall destabilizers
caspofungin
inhibitor of fungal 1,3-β-glucan synthase
micafungin
inhibitor of fungal 1,3-β-glucan synthase
anidulafungin
inhibitor of fungal 1,3-β-glucan synthase
atovaquone:
alone for PCP fungal pneumonia (with proguanil for malaria)
griseofulvin:
inhibitor of fungal microtubule dynamics

ANTIHELMINTHIC DRUG LIST

Benzimidazoles:
Inhibitors of helminthic microtubule dynamics
albendazole
binds worm β-tubulin to inhibit microtubule polymerization
mebendazole
binds worm β-tubulin to inhibit microtubule polymerization
triclabendazole
binds worm β-tubulin to inhibit microtubule polymerization
thiabendazole/tiabendazole
may inhibit the helminth-specific enzyme fumarate reductase
pyrantel pamoate
helminth-selective depolarizing neuromuscular blocking agent
ivermectin
helminth-selective glutamate-gated chloride channel agonist
praziquantel
helminth-selective calcium permeability enhancer
niclosamide
tapeworm-selective glucose uptake inhibitor
diethylcarbamazine
filarial-selective inhibitor of arachidonic acid metabolism
paromomycin
see Antibacterial aminoglycoside-class drugs

ANTIPARASITIC AND ANTIPROTOZOAN DRUG LIST

metronidazole
see Antibacterial (anaerobes) nitroimidazole-class drugs
paromomycin
see Antibacterial aminoglycoside-class drugs
permethrin
topical; neuronal inhibitor for lice and scabies mites
pentamidine
poorly understood mechanism of action: dependent on the target organism

melarsoprol
highly toxic, arsenic-containing prodrug; inactivates pyruvate kinase
suramin
poorly understood mechanism of action; inhibits energy metabolism
nifurtimox
a nitrofuran with a similar mechanism of action to the nitroimidazoles
eflornithine
irreversible inhibitor of trypanosomal ornithine decarboxylase
benznidazole
has a similar mechanism of action to the nitroimidazoles
diloxanide furoate
prodrug of diloxanide, toxic to *E. histolytica* trophozoites
iodoquinol
iodine-containing chelator of ferrous ions essential for metabolism
miltefosine
toxic lipid interactions (has a phosphorylated fatty-acid structure)

ANTIMALARIAL DRUG LIST

Prophylaxis (and Treatment)

chloroquine
formation of heme-chloroquine toxin in susceptible *Plasmodium spp.*
mefloquine
malarial protozoan 80S ribosome inhibitor
primaquine
also kills liver-stage *P. vivax* and *P. ovale*; unknown mechanism of action
tafenoquine
also kills liver-stage *P. vivax* and *P. ovale*; unknown mechanism of action
doxycycline
see Antibacterial tetracycline-class drugs
atovaquone-proguanil
malarial cytochrome bc_1 complex inhibitor with folate antagonist pro-drug

Treatment

artemisinin,
artesunate, artemether
active metabolite dihydroartemisinin produces vacuolar toxic free radicals
lumefantrine
used in combination with artemether as "co-artemether"

ANTIVIRAL DRUG LIST

HIV antivirals

fostemsavir
viral attachment / fusion inhibitor (prodrug of temsavir)
ibalizumab
viral attachment / fusion inhibitor (antibody against CD4)
maraviroc
viral attachment / fusion inhibitor (CCR5 receptor antagonist)
enfuvirtide
viral attachment / fusion inhibitor (polypeptide against viral gp41)
azidothymidine (AZT)
nucleoside (nucleotide) reverse transcriptase inhibitor (NRTI)
abacavir
nucleoside (nucleotide) reverse transcriptase inhibitor (NRTI)
emtricitabine
nucleoside (nucleotide) reverse transcriptase inhibitor (NRTI)
lamivudine
nucleoside (nucleotide) reverse transcriptase inhibitor (NRTI)

tenofovir DF
nucleoside (nucleotide) reverse transcriptase inhibitor (NRTI)
doravirine
non-nucleoside reverse transcriptase inhibitor (NNRTI)
efavirenz
non-nucleoside reverse transcriptase inhibitor (NNRTI)
etravirine
non-nucleoside reverse transcriptase inhibitor (NNRTI)
nevirapine
non-nucleoside reverse transcriptase inhibitor (NNRTI)
rilpivirine
non-nucleoside reverse transcriptase inhibitor (NNRTI)
bictegravir
inhibitor of the viral DNA integrase protein
cabotegravir
inhibitor of the viral DNA integrase protein
dolutegravir
inhibitor of the viral DNA integrase protein
elvitegravir
inhibitor of the viral DNA integrase protein
raltegravir
inhibitor of the viral DNA integrase protein
atazanavir
inhibitor of viral protease
darunavir
inhibitor of viral protease
fosamprenavir
inhibitor of viral protease
ritonavir
inhibitor of viral protease
saquinavir
inhibitor of viral protease
tipranavir
inhibitor of viral protease

Influenza A/B antivirals

oseltamivir
inhibitor of viral neuraminidase
peramivir
inhibitor of viral neuraminidase
zanamivir
inhibitor of viral neuraminidase

baloxavir marboxil
inhibitor of cap-dependent endonuclease activity

COVID-19 antivirals

remdesivir
inhibitor of SARS-CoV-2 RNA polymerase
nirmatrelvir (+ ritonavir)
inhibitor of SARS-CoV-2 protease
molnupiravir
promotes deleterious mutagenesis by SARS-CoV-2 RNA polymerase

Broad spectrum antiviral

ribavirin
guanosine analogue; may inhibit RNA synthesis & mRNA capping

Herpes family virus (HSV, VZV, CMV) antivirals

acyclovir
triphosphate form inhibits viral DNA polymerase
valacyclovir
triphosphate form inhibits viral DNA polymerase
ganciclovir
triphosphate form inhibits viral DNA polymerase
vidarabine
triphosphate form inhibits viral DNA polymerase

Hepatitis virus (HBV, HCV) antivirals

interferon α2b
immune system modulator; activator of host antiviral enzymes
peginterferon α2a
immune system modulator; activator of host antiviral enzymes

daclatasvir
inhibitor of HCV NS5A protein involved in viral replication and assembly
elbasvir
inhibitor of HCV NS5A protein involved in viral replication and assembly
ledipasvir
inhibitor of HCV NS5A protein involved in viral replication and assembly
ombitasvir
inhibitor of HCV NS5A protein involved in viral replication and assembly
velpatasvir
inhibitor of HCV NS5A protein involved in viral replication and assembly

sofosbuvir
inhibitor of HCV NS5B RNA polymerase
dasabuvir
inhibitor of HCV NS5B RNA polymerase

grazoprevir
inhibitor of HCV NS3/4A protease
paritaprevir
inhibitor of HCV NS3/4A protease
simeprevir
inhibitor of HCV NS3/4A protease

Infectious Disease – Bacteria – General Background

Bacteria are all around us, literally. Unless you work under laboratory conditions, the vast majority of surfaces you interact with, including your own skin, are covered in a wide array of bacteria. Although it may seem that there are quite a number of bacterial organisms that cause disease in humans, they represent a small minority of all bacterial species. The term "virulence" refers to the ability of a particular organism to infect and cause disease in another organism. Virulent bacteria are technically quite rare in comparison to all existing bacteria, but they are known to cause disease when they infect us.

One of the fundamental ways in which bacterial infections can be categorized is something called a Gram stain. This particular laboratory stain is used by the pathology department and has not only clinical but also pharmacologic implications depending on its results. Although a multitude of laboratory stains exist, the Gram stain is easily the most well-recognized and most performed of all stains in medicine. Gram staining is performed on various bodily fluid samples (such as blood, sputum, and urine), and positivity is due to the uptake of the stain by the bacterial cell wall. Bacteria that take up the stain show up as purple (termed "Gram positive") on microscopic examination. Bacteria that do not take up the strain will appear pink or red (termed "Gram negative") due to the counterstain safranin. Gram "positive" organisms lack an outer membrane and have a thick bacterial wall of peptidoglycans that retain the crystal violet stain. In contrast, Gram "negative" organisms have a thinner peptidoglycan layer of their bacterial cell wall that does not retain the stain. Bacterial microorganisms can then be further categorized based on their morphological appearance on microscopic examination. Various descriptive shapes are routinely seen, including circular/spherical (coccus), rods (bacilli), amongst other patterns. Employing the two categorizations in conjunction (e.g. Gram positive cocci or Gram negative rods) usually provides a presumptive diagnosis, and antibiotic choices can be tailored to match the suspected bacterial organism. (Burnham and Storch 2020)

Diagnosis

Leukocytosis, or an increase of white blood cells above normal levels, can be suggestive of infection but can also occur in other circumstances. Fevers can also suggest an infectious etiology but are not 100% specific to any particular infection. Like most diagnoses in medicine, obtaining a thorough history, performing a thorough physical exam, and sometimes sending samples for laboratory testing are fundamental steps in making the diagnosis of a bacterial infection. Definitive diagnosis of a bacterial infection routinely involves obtaining a body fluid sample that can then be stained, examined under the microscope, and cultured for identification. While bacterial cultures are considered the "gold standard" for diagnosis, there are many issues with this approach. There is a significant time delay with most cultures, often multiple days. Newer technologies, including genome-based polymerase chain reaction (PCR) testing, can help identify the causative organism much faster, sometimes in just a few hours. The availability of this technology is not uniform, and there is always the possibility of false positives or false negatives. If a sample can be obtained, microscopic examination and Gram staining can be performed, providing a presumptive diagnosis quickly, also in just a few minutes. Although this is ideal, there are many clinical implications to obtaining certain types of samples, such as performing blood draws, catheterizations, bronchoscopies, endoscopies, or lumbar punctures. These all require certain skill levels and sometimes medical specialists to perform. In clinical practice, utilizing a combination of anatomical, demographic, and historical data can help guide antibiotic drug choices when medical attention is sought. (McAdam and Onderdonk 2018)

Central Nervous System (CNS) Infections

Presentation

Bacterial infections of the central nervous system (CNS) are often quite severe. Anatomical areas of interest are the meninges (the brain's outer layer), the brain tissue itself, the fluid-filled areas of the brain called the ventricles, and the space around the spinal cord. Specific infectious diagnoses would be meningitis (infection of the meninges), encephalitis (infection of the brain tissue), meningoencephalitis (from meninges spreading to brain tissue), a brain abscess (a pocket of pus around the brain tissue), ventriculitis (infection of the ventricles), or an epidural abscess (a pocket of pus on the outside layer of the spinal cord). The classic triad of headache, fever, and neck stiffness is often mentioned when discussing meningitis, and these three symptoms would highly suggest this type of infection. In the real world, however, all three are rarely present. Patients may also present with other neurological signs such as altered mentation, confusion, seizures, focal neurologic deficits, or even coma. Significant morbidity and mortality are associated with these infections, given the delicate nature of the CNS. Mortality can range from 6-10% in developed countries and as high as 54-58% in underdeveloped ones. The incidence of infection also varies widely by region and country, from as little as 0.7 to 0.9 cases per 100,000 people to as much as 10 to 40 cases per 100,000 people. (Hasbun 2022)

Risk factors

Immunosuppression of any kind is a universal risk factor for all types of infection across all organ systems. Infections near the CNS, such as in the ears, nose, throat, or bloodstream, can also provide a route of entry into the CNS. While the brain does have a layer of protection in place called the blood-brain barrier, any disruption in this barrier can significantly increase the risk of CNS infections. This risk can be seen in both traumatic causes, such as cranial injuries, or after neurosurgical surgery when elements of the CNS may be exposed (either cranial or spinal). Certain organisms can also infect from person to person through infectious oral secretions or droplets, such as *Neisseria meningitidis*, which makes highly populated areas such as army barracks and college dorms prime locations for outbreaks of meningitis. Other risk factors may be more specific to certain types of infections, such as intravenous drug abuse as a risk factor for brain abscess. Diabetes, renal disease, alcoholism, and malignancy can all also be risk factors for CNS infections. Asplenia, a lack of a functional spleen, can predispose to infections from encapsulated organisms such as *Neisseria meningitidis*.

Pathophysiology

Bacteria can arrive at the CNS in a variety of ways. Direct exposure or penetrative trauma can expose all areas to bacteria. Bacteria may also move along adjacent regions, such as the nasal mucosa or the auditory canals. Bacteria may also embolize from other sources, such as in the case of infectious endocarditis, where chunks of bacteria may fly to other body areas via the bloodstream. Once there the nutrient-rich CNS provides the resources for bacteria to begin to replicate. Depending on the particular type of bacteria and area infected, damage can occur from toxin production and/or local compression. Pressure can build in the cranium resulting in headaches as increased protein in the cerebral spinal fluid (CSF) and white blood cells block CSF absorption by the arachnoid villi. (Rosenberg 2022) As an immune response is initiated, fevers can ensue.

Examination

Physical examination can vary depending on the site of infection. As discussed above, the triad of fever, neck stiffness, and headache should prompt evaluation for possible meningitis. Of note, one study found the three were only seen in 44% of cases. (van de Beek et al. 2004) Two physical exam signs, Brudziński's and Kernig's signs, are classically taught as findings seen in meningitis. Brudziński's sign (or "neck sign") is when there is a reflexive knee and hip flexion to passive flexion of the patient's neck (due to discomfort from meningeal stretch), while Kernig's sign is when there is an inability or patient discomfort with extending the leg when the hip is flexed (involving the same meningeal stretch mechanism). In children, Brudziński's sign has a 66% sensitivity and Kernig's sign has a 53% sensitivity. (Curtis et al. 2010) In adults, sensitivity can be much lower, and one study found only a 5% sensitivity for these tests. (Thomas et al. 2002) Symptoms of altered mentation and headaches alone should add a CNS infection to the list of differential diagnoses. Focal neurologic symptoms are rare in meningitis and encephalitis. Still, they can be seen in patients with cerebral abscesses depending on their anatomical location due to pressure in specific areas of the brain tissue. Seizures are also potentially suggestive, particularly in patients without a prior history. Back pain and sensory deficits, as well as involuntary loss of urine or feces, may be caused by pressure from abscesses along the spinal cord. These epidural abscesses are considered medical emergencies that can lead to permanent paralysis and disability. (Walker et al. 2020)

Laboratory findings

Leukocytosis is an increase in the concentration of white blood cells on a blood sample and is commonly seen in many different types of infections, not just bacterial ones. A lack or presence of leukocytosis does not entirely exclude or include the presence of an infection though. Depending on multiple factors, some patients may in fact have leukopenia, which is a low white blood cell count. In general, a predominance of neutrophils (a particular type of white blood cell) may suggest a bacterial diagnosis but does not guarantee that there is one. (Leukocytosis and Leukopenia 2020) Laboratory analysis of CSF, which requires a lumbar puncture, is much more specific in diagnosing a CNS infection. Cultures from a CSF sample are considered the gold standard for diagnosing CNS infections but may not always grow an organism. (Hasbun 2022)

Imaging

A computed tomography (CT) scan of the head may show a predisposition to CNS infection from nearby areas, such as the sinuses. Magnetic resonance imaging (MRI) is much more sensitive and specific for CNS infection, and the anatomical regions affected can even provide clues into particular disease entities. Early CT or MRI of the head and brain can be completely normal in the case of meningitis. In the case of CNS abscesses, these can be clearly visualized by a CT scan or MRI. (Hasbun 2022)

Associated symptoms/conditions

Infectious endocarditis can be associated with CNS abscesses. Diabetes mellitus is also associated with various infections, including cranial and spinal abscesses. Smoking has also been associated with meningococcal disease. Anatomical skull and cranial deformities may also cause insufficient protection from the blood-brain barrier and can be associated with recurrent infections. (Hasbun 2022) Otitis media (commonly known as an inner ear infection), mastoiditis (infection of the mastoid air spaces), and sinusitis (sinus infection) can all be associated with CNS infections, particularly abscesses. (Walker et al. 2020)

Diagnosis

Lumbar puncture remains a critical part of diagnosing meningitis and other CNS infections. Characteristic findings in bacterial infection include an elevated leukocyte count, neutrophil predominance, high protein, and low glucose. Imaging can aid in the diagnosis of meningitis and can quickly diagnose a cerebral or spinal abscess. Imaging can sometimes be completely normal, as previously discussed. As with most diagnoses, a combination of history, physical exam, and lab/imaging findings can lead to a final diagnosis. Rapid meningitis panels are available and can quickly provide a causative bacterial agent. (Hasbun 2022)

Treatment

A sampling of CSF should be performed before initiating antibiotics, but initiation of empiric antibiotics should not be delayed, as CNS infections often carry a significant risk of morbidity and mortality. Bactericidal agents should be utilized, given the severity of these infections. Third-generation cephalosporins such as ceftriaxone are often used due to their broad coverage, but overt risk factors for Gram-positive bacteria such as methicillin-sensitive *Staph. aureus* (MSSA) and methicillin-resistant *Staph. aureus* (MRSA) should prompt the use of agents such as vancomycin. Cranial or spinal instrumentation and intravenous drug abuse can increase the suspicion of these bacteria. Fourth-generation cephalosporins, such as cefepime, and carbapenems, such as meropenem, may be indicated, particularly if there is a concern for *Pseudomonas aeruginosa*. (Hasbun 2022) Once a causative organism is identified, antibiotics can be tailored.

Management

Antibiotics are the mainstay of treatment for most bacterial CNS infections, although neurosurgical drainage may be required in cases of cerebral and spinal abscesses. Neurosurgical consultation should be obtained immediately in patients with CNS abscesses. Some patients may require admission to the intensive care unit given the high likelihood of complications such as paralysis from spinal cord compression or the development of seizures. Most patients receive antibiotics for as long as six to eight weeks, depending on the organism. (Walker et al. 2020)

Upper and Lower Respiratory Infections

Presentation

Upper and lower respiratory tract infections are incredibly common and contribute significantly to outpatient and inpatient medical visits. These infections often present with a variety of symptoms depending on the areas affected. Upper respiratory infections (URIs) may present with a sore throat, increased mucus production, nasal congestion, sinus pressure, sneezing, headaches, ear fullness, or pain, amongst other symptoms. Fever may be seen in bacterial airway infections of all types. Otitis media is quite common in children, as their eustachian tubes are not only small and narrow, causing impaired drainage, but also relatively horizontal compared to the downsloping angle seen as we progress through the teenage years and into adulthood. Small children, in particular, may tug at their ears or be irritable. Sinusitis, an infection of a sinus, can present with sinus pressure and pain, purulent drainage, or even decreased sense of smell. The patient may interpret sinus pressure as merely a headache. Pharyngitis, or a throat infection, is almost always caused by viruses. Still, the bacteria *Streptococcus pyogenes* is responsible for the disease process commonly known as "Strep throat" and can be the causative organism in about 10% of pharyngitis cases. *Corynebacterium diphtheriae,* as a cause of pharyngitis, is now rarely seen thanks to vaccination. (Ryan 2022) Laryngitis, or inflammation of the vocal cords, may present with hoarseness or even inability to speak. Epiglottitis, or inflammation of the epiglottis, carries a significant risk of airway loss and requires prompt medical attention. Symptoms of epiglottitis may include pain or difficulty with swallowing. Tonsillitis, or inflammation of the tonsils, is quite common in children. Abscesses may also form behind the pharynx, termed retropharyngeal abscesses, or other areas of the airway. As we progress down the respiratory tract into the trachea and bronchi, tracheitis and bronchitis can also be seen but are rarely caused by bacteria. Pneumonia, or an infection of the lung parenchyma, may present with symptoms of cough, sputum production, and chest pain. It is not uncommon for infections that start in the upper airways to descend and cause disease in the lower airways. (Levinson et al. 2022) Tuberculosis can mimic acute bacterial pneumonia but usually has a more insidious, prolonged course with associated respiratory symptoms, and patients appear more chronically ill. (Musher 2020)

Risk factors

Whether acquired or congenital, immunosuppression can increase the risk of upper and lower airway bacterial infections. Close contact with someone with a bacterial infection may cause spread via airway secretions. Smoking may cause impaired ciliary function and thus impaired clearance of the airways, increasing the risk for all types of airway infections. Alcohol abuse may also be a risk, evoking similar impairments. Congenital/genetic mutations that affect mucus clearance, such as in patients with cystic fibrosis and other causes of bronchiectasis, may also increase the risk of bacterial airway infections. Oftentimes a bacterial upper and lower respiratory tract infection may first be preceded by a viral infection which then makes it easier for the bacteria to grow in what is termed a bacterial superinfection. Pneumonia may also manifest as a result of a prolonged need for mechanical ventilation or due to the hematogenous spread of bacteria, such as in cases of septic emboli in infective endocarditis. Incarceration and homelessness are risk factors for tuberculosis. (Musher 2020)

Pathophysiology

Any impairment in the normal mucociliary clearance of the airways can lead to bacterial overgrowth and subsequent clinical disease. Narrowed or obstructed openings of the Eustachian tubes can prevent normal drainage and allow for bacterial overgrowth, resulting in otitis media. This can cause discomfort from the increased pressure in the channel. The maxillary sinuses located in the bones of the cheeks are a common site of infection given their large size and multiple entry points for bacteria. The maxillary sinuses are located in a region of the face that is prone to trauma, which can increase the risk of sinusitis. In sinusitis, normal drainage of these sinuses into the nasal passages becomes impaired due to excessive mucus production, resulting in the closure of the space and an increase in pressure that causes characteristic sinus pain.

Pharyngitis and tonsillitis can result from the person-to-person spread of organisms through contact with oral secretions. Bacterial growth in these areas can cause local inflammation and discomfort. Retropharyngeal and other abscesses are rare and usually the result of traumatic infiltration of the area. Pneumonia can result in impaired ciliary clearance and has multiple etiologies. Common bacterial organisms responsible for upper and lower airway infections include *Streptococcus pneumoniae*, *Moraxella catarrhalis*, and *Haemophilus influenzae*. Direct inhalation of these organisms from respiratory droplets is possible, but this mechanism is more commonly seen in infections caused by *Mycobacterium tuberculosis* and *Bacillus anthracis*, which cause tuberculosis and anthrax, respectively. (Musher, 2020)

Examination

A physical examination can help significantly narrow down the differential diagnosis in patients with suspected upper or lower respiratory infections. However, it may not be specific to bacterial etiologies versus others. Pain upon palpation over a particular area, such as a specific sinus, may provide a clue to the diagnosis of sinusitis. Swollen or tender lymph nodes in a specific distribution can indicate the location of the infection, and identifying purulent secretions can also help narrow down the affected anatomical area, such as in tonsillitis. For example, with pharyngitis, the submandibular lymph nodes under the jaw may be swollen. It is important to note that swollen lymph nodes are not always present in pharyngitis and may not be necessary for making a diagnosis. Other symptoms, such as redness or swelling of the pharynx, can also indicate pharyngitis. Auscultation over the chest may reveal coarse rhonchi in the case of pneumonia. Examination with an otoscope can reveal erythematous and bulging tympanic membranes in the case of otitis media. In the context of a thorough history, a focused physical exam can help determine the correct diagnosis. (Levinson et al. 2022)

Laboratory

There are no specific laboratory findings for upper airway bacterial infections, but leukocytosis with a neutrophil predominance in the proper clinical setting can suggest this. There are no characteristic laboratory findings that will confirm many of these diagnoses, such as otitis media and pharyngitis. These diagnoses are primarily made based on clinical examination. A rapid Strep test can be used to identify *Streptococcus pyogenes* infection in the appropriate clinical context. Throat cultures can be done to aid in the diagnosis but antibiotic treatment should not be delayed while waiting for results, which may take multiple days. (Levinson et al. 2022) Gram staining of sputum and other secretions can help with identification but it is not routinely performed unless in an inpatient setting. Enzyme-linked immunosorbent assays (ELISA) for *Streptococcus pneumoniae* and *Legionella pneumophila* and PCR testing for *Chlamydia pneumoniae*, *Mycobacterium tuberculosis*, and *Mycoplasma pneumoniae* are available but are also not routinely used in the outpatient setting or even available. (Musher 2020)

Imaging

Imaging is not often obtained in cases of upper respiratory tract infections. In some rare instances, such as suspicion of a retropharyngeal abscess, a CT scan of the neck will aid in the diagnosis of an upper respiratory infection. A CT scan of the head may also reveal findings of sinusitis, such as fluid within a particular sinus. Plain radiographs of the chest are, by definition, needed to make the diagnosis of pneumonia where an infiltrate of the lung fields would be seen. A CT of the chest would very clearly delineate parenchymal involvement and consolidation in pneumonia. However, imaging is rarely obtained in most cases of upper and lower respiratory infections, as these are often complaints seen in the outpatient setting and managed medically without the need for imaging. More severe cases may need inpatient management at a hospital, and imaging is quickly and easily obtained there. Cavitary lung lesions, particularly in the upper lobes, may suggest infection with *Mycobacterium tuberculosis* or *Mycobacterium avium* complex (MAC). (Musher 2020)

Associated symptoms/conditions

Viral infections of the upper and lower respiratory tracts can be associated with bacterial superinfections. Immunocompromised states, such as those seen in patients with Common Variable Immunodeficiency or other congenital immunocompromising conditions like Wiskott-Aldrich, a rare X-linked disorder, can also increase the risk of bacterial infections. Wiskott-Aldrich results in issues with humoral immunity and can present clinically with recurrent otitis media, sinusitis, and pneumonia episodes. X-linked agammaglobulinemia patients may also first present with recurrent or chronic respiratory tract infections. (Tosi 2019)

Diagnosis

Making the diagnosis of an upper or lower respiratory tract infection will often combine findings from a thorough history, physical exam, and other results such as imaging and labs to make the final diagnosis. In the case of sore throat, the Centor Criteria can be used to aid in the diagnosis of strep throat from *Streptococcus pyogenes* infection. These criteria include tonsillar exudates, tender anterior cervical adenopathy, fever, and absence of cough. If all criteria are met, a rapid strep test should be performed and may confirm the diagnosis. (Levinson et al. 2022) The diagnosis of pneumonia requires a pulmonary infiltrate on chest imaging, and some of the above-mentioned ELISA and PCR tests can now quickly help make a diagnosis. An elevated procalcitonin level increases the chances of there being a bacterial infection, but a normal or low level does not exclude one. Although there is PCR testing for *Mycobacterium tuberculosis*, diagnosis is usually still made using a combination of history, tuberculin testing, interferon-gamma assays testing, sputum staining, and imaging findings. (Musher 2020)

Treatment

Antibiotic management is usually started broad to cover common organisms, as with most bacterial infections. While results from cultures would be ideal, the upper and lower respiratory tract is full of normal flora which will grow on culture mediums but may not necessarily be causing disease. Upper respiratory tract infections such as otitis media can often be managed with penicillins such as amoxicillin or cephalosporins like cephalexin in penicillin-allergic patients.

If there is a concern for resistance in the community, sometimes amoxicillin-clavulanic acid may be used first and provides wide coverage for usual organisms. For more concerning infections involving the sinuses or lower respiratory tract, antibiotics such as doxycycline or fluoroquinolones such as moxifloxacin or levofloxacin (colloquially termed the "respiratory fluoroquinolones") may be used. Beta lactams such as ceftriaxone and macrolides such as azithromycin could also provide adequate coverage for common organisms and are used quite often in clinical practice. (Musher 2020) Treatment of tuberculosis and MAC infections typically requires extended treatment regimens that are heavily monitored due to public safety concerns with input from pulmonologists and infectious disease consultants.

Management

The management of upper and lower respiratory illnesses is largely supportive. In addition to what is discussed above, symptomatic management is often achieved with non-steroidal anti-inflammatory medications (NSAIDs) and/or acetaminophen. Inhaled bronchodilators may help play a role in certain patients with pneumonia, such as those with obstructive lung diseases. Certain infections, such as tonsillar and retropharyngeal abscesses, may require surgical intervention from an otolaryngologist in order to control the infection. Recurrent otitis media infections or tonsillitis may also require an otolaryngologist referral for consideration of tonsillectomy or myringotomy tubes. (Hannallah et al. 2019) A certain degree of suspicion for inborn disorders in immunity should always be present, particularly in cases where a child has recurrent illnesses. (Tosi 2019)

Bacteremia and Infective Endocarditis (IE)

Presentation

Bacterial bloodstream infections and endocarditis are severe clinical infections that carry significant morbidity and mortality risks to patients. Acutely, patients may appear toxic and have high fevers and even rigors and chills. These patients are often septic, meaning they have a systemic response to infection. This is more common in acute infective endocarditis (IE), while subacute endocarditis may present more indolently and chronically over time. Patients with acute bacteremia may not have any specific visual findings at first. Intravascular infections that progress to IE, where particular areas of the heart like valve leaflets become a nidus for bacterial growth, may have symptoms of bacterial "septic" emboli. These embolic events may result in petechiae throughout the body, nail bed hemorrhages, Osler nodes (painful, raised, and tender purple or pink nodules seen on the fingers and toes), or Janeway lesions (hemorrhagic and painless lesions on the palms of the hands and the soles of the feet). Septic emboli can affect almost any part of the body and can lead to a wide array of complications depending on their location. Neurologic manifestations such as strokes and cerebral abscesses may occur, as well as left upper quadrant pain from splenic infarction or renal failure due to embolic occlusions. Patients may also have a new murmur present on chest auscultation. (Southwick 2020)

Risk factors

Any pre-existing damage to the endocardial surface can become a nidus for bacterial infection. Untreated group A streptococcus infections are now rare but are known to significantly increase the risk of rheumatic heart disease with subsequent increased risk for IE due to endocardial damage. Congenital heart defects such as valvular or septal malformations and prosthetic valves increase the risk of endocardial infection. Intravenous drug abuse increases the risk of bloodstream and cardiac bacterial infections, as non-sterile solutions are injected directly into the bloodstream. Foreign bodies in the vasculature, particularly medical catheters such as central lines and dialysis catheters, also provide a potential nidus for bacterial growth and biofilm formation that can cause systemic bloodstream infection and endocarditis. (Southwick 2020) As with other bacterial infections, immunocompromised states remain important risk factors.

Pathophysiology

While using sterile equipment and proper hygiene significantly decreases the risk of medical catheters becoming infected, the risk always exists with any type of foreign body usage. Injection of non-sterile fluids, such as during IV drug abuse, provides direct bacterial access to the bloodstream. In the case of IE, endocardial damage promotes the accumulation of platelets and fibrin, promoting the formation of nonbacterial thrombotic endocarditis (NBTE). Although this in and of itself is sterile, it provides a scaffolding for bacterial growth. Bacterial growth can also stimulate further platelet aggregation and create "platelet vegetations," which house a significant amount of bacteria and provide protection from the normal immune defense. Certain bacteria are more likely to adhere to these previously affected areas that are predisposed to colonization, such as Staphylococcus and Streptococcus. (Holland et al. 2020)

Examination

Physical examination can vary broadly in bloodstream infections. Early on, bacteremic patients may have little to no findings. High fevers, rigors, and chills should raise the suspicion of bloodstream infection, particularly in patients with recent catheter insertions or removals. Patients with a new heart murmur may also have vegetations on the valve associated with that heart sound. Skin findings of Osler nodes and Janeway lesions should also prompt investigation for IE. Septic emboli can lead to altered mental status, focal neurologic deficits, loss of pulses due to occlusion, abdominal pain, shortness of breath, or various other findings. A fundoscopic examination may reveal flame hemorrhages, retinal hemorrhages, petechial hemorrhages in the conjunctiva, or Roth's spots (a red spot with a pale center). (Southwick 2020)

Laboratory

White blood cell (WBC) counts may or may not be elevated in bacteremia and endocarditis. Subacute endocarditis is more likely to have a normal WBC count, while acute IE is more likely to have an elevated count. Anemia is a common finding but is also not very specific. Elevated erythrocyte sedimentation rate (ESR) and C-reactive peptide (CRP) can also be seen but are not specific to bacteremia or endocarditis. The most critical laboratory test in both entities will be blood cultures. In clinical practice, two to three cultures are usually obtained and provide a 90 to 99% sensitivity. Blood cultures should be obtained before antibiotics are administered, when sensitivity is the highest. Blood cultures will not only provide the causative bacteria but also allow for testing for antibiotic sensitivity, which will aid in tailoring antibiotic treatment. (Holland et al. 2020)

Imaging

While CT or MRI imaging does not usually have a significant role in cases of bacteremia and endocarditis, echocardiography should be performed in all suspected cases of endocarditis. Transthoracic echocardiograms (TTE) have a relatively lower sensitivity (44-63%) for detecting endocardial vegetations when compared to transesophageal echocardiograms (TEE) (94-100%). In clinical practice, a TTE is usually performed first as it is much less invasive than a TEE which requires anesthesia for conscious sedation. A positive TTE may be all that is needed, but a negative TTE does not rule out endocarditis, and thus a TEE may be needed. TEE is also much more sensitive at finding extravalvular manifestations, such as an extravalvular abscess (87% vs 28% sensitivity). (Southwick 2020) Not only do these echocardiograms help establish a diagnosis, but if surgical intervention is needed, they can provide crucial anatomical information that may need to be considered. (Holland et al. 2020)

Associated symptoms/conditions

Indwelling catheters are associated with an increased risk of bacteremia and/or endocarditis. Catheters used for total parenteral nutrition (TPN), dialysis, and even central venous catheters (CVC) or peripherally inserted central catheters (PICC) in chronically ill patients or those requiring extended IV antibiotic regimens are all associated with bacteremia and endocarditis. (Holland et al. 2020) Prosthetic heart valves are also associated with endocarditis. As mentioned before, although rare in developed countries, rheumatic heart disease is associated with endocarditis. Other implantable cardiac devices such as pacemakers and defibrillators also are associated with endocarditis as wires cause endocardial disruption and serve as a nidus for bacterial growth. (Southwick 2020)

Diagnosis

While diagnosing bacteremia requires the growth of bacteria from a blood sample, the diagnosis of IE has strict criteria. The modified Duke criteria are the most studied and widely used diagnostic criteria for IE. Definitive IE can be diagnosed either by pathologic criteria or clinical criteria. Definite IE by pathologic criteria requires that an organism be identified from the culture or histologic examination of either vegetation, septic emboli, or an intracardiac abscess specimen. Definite IE by clinical criteria requires that either two major criteria, one major criterion, and three minor criteria, or five minor criteria be met. There is a category of possible IE when there are one major and one minor criteria, or only three minor criteria.

The two major criteria categories are blood culture and endocardial echocardiogram findings. Blood culture criteria can be met by either:

- Two separate cultures showing typical bacteria (*Viridans streptococci*, *Streptococcus bovis*, *Staphylococcus aureus*, or one of the HACEK group of bacteria [genus Haemophilus, Aggregatibacter, Cardiobacterium, Eikenella, or Kingella]).
- Persistently positive blood cultures with the same organism.
- One single blood culture with *Coxiella burnetii.*

Endocardial involvement criteria on echocardiogram include:

- Oscillating intracardiac mass on a valve or supporting structure without an alternative anatomical explanation.
- Endocardial abscess.
- New partial dehiscence of a prosthetic valve.
- New valvular regurgitation.

Minor criteria include predisposition to IE (such as heart conditions or IV drug abuse), fever, vascular phenomena such as septic emboli and Janeway lesions, immunologic phenomena such as Osler nodes and glomerulonephritis, or microbiological evidence such as blood cultures that do not meet major criteria or serologic evidence of organisms known to cause IE. (Holland et al. 2020)

Treatment
Antibiotics are the mainstay of therapy for bacteremia and IE. The intravenous route is preferred over oral, and bactericidal agents should be used as bacteriostatic agents may be ineffective. Once blood cultures are drawn, empiric treatment should be initiated and tailored depending on risk factors. Combinations of vancomycin and ampicillin with gentamicin are one option. At the same time, concern for Gram-negative organisms in critically ill patients may instead prompt the use of vancomycin and a fourth-generation cephalosporin like cefepime or broad-spectrum penicillin with a beta-lactamase inhibitor such as piperacillin-tazobactam. Once an organism is identified and antibiotic sensitivity results are obtained, empiric antibiotic regimens can be narrowed. MSSA or coagulase-negative Staphylococcus can be managed with nafcillin, while MRSA will require vancomycin or daptomycin. Certain synergistic antibiotic combinations, such as penicillin (*e.g.*, ampicillin) with an aminoglycoside (*e.g.*, gentamicin, streptomycin), can produce rapid bactericidal effects against most Viridans streptococci and enterococci. While treatment duration for transient bacteremia without IE can be as short as two weeks, IE warrants an extended period of treatment of at least 4 to 6 weeks. (Holland et al. 2020)

Management
Apart from antibiotic management, other considerations arise in managing bacteremia and IE. Catheters should only be replaced as absolutely necessary, and those that may be infected should be removed. Cultures can be obtained from the tip of catheters when there is suspicion of infection. Cardiothoracic consultation is often indicated as surgical interventions such as valve replacement may be necessary. The onset of acute heart failure or cardiogenic shock, prosthetic valve dehiscence, rupture or perforation, persistent vegetations despite antibiotic management, or paravalvular abscess can prompt emergent surgical intervention. Electrocardiogram changes can suggest a paravalvular abscess, which can be a surgical emergency. The size of vegetations is sometimes used as surgical indications (often above 1cm in diameter), but overall indications are controversial and so multidisciplinary discussion between the medical team, cardiology, and cardiothoracic surgery is encouraged. (Holland et al. 2020)

Intra-Abdominal Infections

Presentation
There are multiple potential sites of infection within the abdominal cavity. Bacterial infections of the urinary tract include cystitis (infection of the urinary bladder), pyelonephritis (infection of the kidneys), or the generalized term of urinary tract infections: UTIs. Patients often present with painful or burning urination, but some may be asymptomatic. (Ryan 2022) While most infectious causes of food poisoning (gastroenteritis) and diarrhea are viral in nature, bacterial etiologies are also common. For example, *Clostridium difficile* infection (often termed *C. diff*) remains a significant cause of bacterial diarrhea, specifically colitis in outpatient and inpatient settings. Shigella, Salmonella, Yersinia, and Campylobacter species can present with bloody diarrhea. *Escherichia coli* can also cause diarrhea illness and is the causative organism in traveler's diarrhea, except in Southeast Asia where Campylobacter is more prevalent. (Gurram 2023) Peritonitis and intra-abdominal abscesses may present with severe abdominal pain and can be surgical emergencies as they could signal colonic perforation. These can be complications of appendicitis or diverticulitis, which can also present as vague abdominal pain. (Kisat and Haider 2020) *Helicobacter pylori*, a bacterial cause of gastritis, may only present with epigastric abdominal pain or symptoms of reflux. (Mahvi and Mahvi 2022) Fever can also be seen in all these infections. Sexually transmitted infections (STIs) with organisms such as chlamydia or gonorrhea can present with burning urination and urethral discharge. Syphilis, another STI, can present with painless skin ulcers termed chancres. (Frank 2022) One of the most common causes of bacterial infections presenting as abdominal pain, specifically in the right upper quadrant, is cholecystitis. Other bacterial infections like liver abscesses and cholangitis are rare but potentially life-threatening. Patients often present quite ill, septic/toxic-appearing, and potentially in shock. (Sifri and Madoff 2020)

Risk factors
Immunocompromised patients are at risk for all types of bacterial infections. Anatomical alterations, whether congenital or iatrogenic after surgery or foreign objects such as catheters, can predispose patients to infections such as UTIs. (Ryan 2022) Antibiotics can alter gut microdiversity and increase the risk for pathogenic bacteria to predominate and cause diseases, such as *C. diff* colitis. Diabetes also significantly increases the risk of many bacterial infections, including intra-abdominal ones. Obstruction of the normal flow of fluids by stones, such as in the urinary tract or biliary system, increases the risk of infection. Ascites, which can occur in patients with liver failure, increases the risk for peritoneal infections as it functions as a growth medium for bacteria. (Barshak and Kasper 2022)

Pathophysiology
Various mechanisms exist for intraabdominal infections. Flagella, or tail-like projections, are used by some bacteria to navigate their environment, allowing them to spread and cause infection. For UTIs, most disease is caused by Gram-negative rods, with the vast majority of these being *Escherichia coli*, which have flagella. Proteus, Klebsiella, and Enterococcus species are amongst other causes. (Ryan 2022) In the case of gastritis, *Helicobacter pylori* also has flagella, allowing it to navigate the mucosal surface of the stomach. (Mahvi and Mahvi 2022) STIs are, by definition, transmitted from person to person via sexual contact and clinical disease occurs from the effects of bacterial growth

within genitalia. The gastrointestinal (GI) system is also full of an entire ecosystem of bacteria ("*microbiome*") that often does not cause disease. Similar to the skin, the GI system is constantly exposed to the outside world via the food we eat. While the constituent bacterial species are harmless when contained within the lumen of the intestines and colon, the GI microbiome can cause significant illness if particular bacterial species within it extend to any areas outside of that. Most of these bacteria are anaerobes, requiring lower oxygen concentrations in the environment to replicate. The GI tract is therefore a prime environment for anaerobic growth. If a perforation of the GI tract allows for exposure of its contents into the peritoneal cavity, peritonitis and/or abscesses can occur. In these situations, infections are often polymicrobial. Most often *Escherichia coli*, Bacteroides species (predominantly *Bacteroides fragilis*), Peptostreptococcus, Prevotella, and Fusobacterium species are isolated when a culture can be obtained. (Cohen-Poradosu and Kasper 2020) In the case of acute cholecystitis, infection is not specifically thought to be a trigger. Still, cultures from bile are often positive, although polymicrobial as well. When there is an interruption of the normal flow of bile, such as in the case of cholelithiasis (commonly known as gallstones), there is an increased risk of cholangitis. This infection of the common bile duct usually occurs as a consequence of choledocholithiasis and patients become severely ill. (Sifri and Madoff 2020) In the case of pancreatitis, progression to necrotizing pancreatitis is also a life-threatening complication as this dead tissue can become infected and lead to multiorgan failure and death. (Besinger and Stehman 2020)

Examination

A physical examination can help to significantly narrow down the differential diagnosis in the patient with an intraabdominal infection. After a thorough history, a focused exam can help determine the next step in the patient's management. In UTIs, suprapubic fullness and tenderness can point towards cystitis, and costovertebral tenderness can suggest pyelonephritis. (Ryan 2022) Epigastric tenderness remains one of the vaguest physical exam findings in clinical medicine, but in the proper clinical context can point toward cholecystitis, gastritis, or pancreatitis. (Besinger and Stehman 2020) Bacterial diarrhea may just have diffuse abdominal tenderness. More concerning findings, like a rock-hard, stiff abdomen (termed an "acute abdomen"), can signal peritonitis, a medical emergency that is acutely life-threatening. (Barshak and Kasper 2022) Sexually transmitted infections may reveal urethral discharge in gonorrhea and chlamydial infections. The characteristic "painless chancres" or ulcers with clear margins on genitalia and associated swollen inguinal lymph nodes are highly characteristic of syphilis. (Frank 2022) Tenderness over the right lower quadrant can be associated with appendicitis, while left lower quadrant pain is more often seen in diverticulitis. (Barshak and Kasper 2022) Point tenderness of the prostate during a rectal exam can suggest prostatitis. (Gupta and Trautner 2022)

Laboratory

Laboratory findings for a lot of intraabdominal infections are rarely specific. Leukocytosis, similar to other bacterial infections, can be suggestive. Cultures are ideal in the proper clinical scenario but are sometimes not feasible without surgery as the number of bacteria may actually be quite low. Cultures are also often polymicrobial. For these reasons, antibiotic management is usually empiric in nature. Elevated alkaline phosphatase can be highly suggestive of biliary tree disease, but can also be seen in things like a liver abscess. (Barshak and Kasper 2022) Urine dipstick testing or urinalysis can aid in the diagnosis of urinary tract infection in the right clinical context, particularly if nitrite and leukocyte esterase are positive. Nitrites (a product of some but not all UTI-causing organisms) suggest an active bacterial breakdown of nitrate, and leukocyte esterase indicates the presence of white blood cells in the urine. (Gupta and Trautner 2022) In the case of *C. diff* as a cause of diarrhea, toxin-specific ELISA and PCR assays are available to help identify it in a fecal sample. (Gurram 2023)

Imaging

Ultrasound (US) can play an important role in diagnosing multiple infections and is commonly utilized in suspected cholecystitis. Findings of pericholecystic fluid (fluid around the gallbladder) and/or gallbladder wall thickening are suggestive of cholecystitis. Other infections visible using US include intraabdominal abscesses, liver abscesses, and emphysematous pyelonephritis, amongst others. In the case of biliary tree disease, radionuclide cholescintigraphy also termed a hepatobiliary iminodiacetic acid (HIDA) scan, can demonstrate a lack of normal biliary drainage which can suggest obstruction from choledocholithiasis. (Sifri and Madoff 2020) CT of the abdomen and pelvis is incredibly useful in diagnosing intra-abdominal infections as many etiologies can be visualized this way. Cholecystitis, colitis, diverticulitis, pyelonephritis, and many other infections that occur in the abdomen can be quickly identified on a CT scan. CT scans can also clearly identify abscesses in the liver or abdomen. (Barshak and Kasper 2022) MRI of the abdomen is rarely performed in clinical practice, particularly for infections, given that CT scans are cheaper, faster, and can aid in diagnosing most infections. A particular type of MRI termed magnetic resonance cholangiopancreatography (MRCP) is sometimes used in the diagnosis of certain liver and gallbladder diseases but is not specifically used to diagnose infections. (Besinger and Stehman 2020)

Associated symptoms/conditions

Immunocompromised states continue to be associated with all types of infections, including intraabdominal ones. Blockage of normal flow of bodily substances, such as in choledocholithiasis, bowel obstructions, ureteral stones, urinary retention, and even fecal impaction, can all be associated with abdomen infections. Diverticulosis is associated with diverticulitis, as the small outpouchings of the colon can become infected.

Diagnosis

Diagnosing an intraabdominal infection usually requires a combination of history, physical exam, and laboratory/imaging findings. For most infections, a positive fluid culture is the definitive way to make a diagnosis. Positive urine cultures in the proper clinical setting establish the diagnosis of a UTI. (Gupta and Trautner 2022) Pyelonephritis can be diagnosed with findings of UTI with signs and symptoms of upper urinary tract involvement. Imaging can be used to confirm the diagnosis but is not required. The diagnosis of bacterial diarrhea is usually clinical. Although cultures can be helpful, they are usually polymicrobial. Cultures may not even be positive if the diarrhea is caused by a toxin produced by a bacteria, such as in Staphylococcus-related bacterial diarrhea, *Bacillus cereus* diarrhea, and in enterohemorrhagic *E. coli* which produces a Shiga-like cytotoxin. Colitis from *C. diff* can be diagnosed with the help of toxin and/or PCR assays. Cholecystitis, colitis, appendicitis, pancreatitis, and diverticulitis are all diagnoses made clinically and can be supported by laboratory findings such as leukocytosis and imaging findings. Peritonitis, such as spontaneous bacterial peritonitis, can be diagnosed with positive cultures or ascites sampling showing a high number of polymorphonuclear cells. Peritonitis from colonic perforation with bacteria located in the peritoneal space is also a clinical diagnosis that can be supported by imaging and confirmed by positive cultures from the peritoneal space. Liver and intraabdominal abscesses are usually diagnosed with imaging, which clearly defines the abscess location and size, and cultures will yield the causative organism for final diagnosis. (Barshak and Kasper 2022) For STIs, Gram staining of genital discharge is often helpful for diagnosis. Nucleic acid/PCR amplification tests for gonorrhea and chlamydia can provide results faster than cultures and may be more sensitive. (Marrazzo and Holmes 2022) Diagnosing syphilis is somewhat more complex. Ideally, samples from chancres can be tested using PCR, antibody panels, or dark field microscopy. Positive antibodies in the blood may take weeks to develop. Serologic testing includes treponemal (*e.g.*, fluorescent treponemal antibody absorption [FTA-ABS]) and nontreponemal (*e.g.*, Venereal Disease Research Laboratory [VDRL] or rapid plasma reagin [RPR]) testing. Treponemal tests are more specific but may stay positive even if there is no active disease, while nontreponemal tests can have false positives and cross-react with other antibodies. Current recommendations are for "reverse sequence" testing in which a treponemal test is performed first and, if positive, is followed by a nontreponemal test. If both are positive, a third treponemal test different from the one first used should be tested to help confirm the diagnosis. (Frank 2022)

Treatment

Antibiotic treatment for intraabdominal infections usually begins empirically. A careful history will reveal any risk factors for resistant organisms, such as a history of previous hospitalization or recent antibiotic use. In the case of UTIs, uncomplicated cystitis can be managed in the outpatient setting with trimethoprim-sulfamethoxazole (TMP-SMX), ciprofloxacin, or nitrofurantoin. Cephalosporins are also appropriate and better options in pyelonephritis, as tissue penetration becomes more critical than bladder concentration. Treatment can be escalated to carbapenems such as meropenem in cases of resistant organisms. Duration of treatment will depend on multiple factors, from a few days for uncomplicated cystitis to 2 weeks in pyelonephritis. (Gupta and Trautner 2022) Gastritis from *H. pylori* requires extended treatment with what is known as triple therapy (proton pump inhibitor, clarithromycin, and amoxicillin or metronidazole) or quadruple therapy (proton pump inhibitor, bismuth, tetracycline, and metronidazole) depending on allergies, history of previous macrolide exposure, or known community resistance to clarithromycin. (Mahvi and Mahvi 2022) For other intra-abdominal infections, second- and third-generation cephalosporins, carbapenems, and beta-lactams with a beta-lactamase inhibitor are all appropriate choices as they cover the most common organisms mentioned earlier. Antibiotic regimens for cholecystitis, colitis, appendicitis, diverticulitis, and even peritonitis are quite similar because of the shared bacterial etiologies. Ideally, cultures will return within a few days and help narrow antibiotic choices but obtaining these cultures is only sometimes feasible. (Besinger and Stehman 2020) While many causes of diarrhea do not warrant antibiotics, identification via PCR of Shigella or Campylobacter usually warrants antibiotic use, as does a positive stool toxin assay for *C. diff*. Choices of treatment for *C. diff* include metronidazole, oral vancomycin, and fidaxomicin, depending on the severity of the illness. Enterohemorrhagic *E. coli* should not be treated with antibiotics as it increases the chance of developing one of its complications: hemolytic uremic syndrome. For STIs, the macrolide azithromycin is effective against *Chlamydia trachomatis* infection and is commonly used, while a third-generation cephalosporin like ceftriaxone is effective against *Neisseria gonorrhoeae* infections. (Marrazzo and Holmes 2022) For syphilis, penicillin G is preferred for all stages. It is so preferred, in fact, that syphilitic individuals with a penicillin allergy should undergo desensitization so they can receive penicillin G. (Frank 2022)

Management

Antibiotics are critically important in the management of intra-abdominal infection management, but they are sometimes not enough. In the case of intra-abdominal abscesses, source control is still recommended. Surgical consultation will help coordinate treatment efforts with surgical planning. In certain cases where surgery is not feasible, or the patient is considered too ill for surgery, interventional radiology may be able to insert a catheter percutaneously to drain the collection such as in abdominal abscesses or cholecystitis. (Barshak and Kasper 2022)

UTIs that are complicated due to kidney stones, particularly large stones that cannot be expelled, may also require urologic consultation and intervention. Stones can provide a surface for bacterial colonization and the creation of a biofilm that prevents infections from being cleared with treatment. This can lead to the development of resistant organisms as patients receive multiple antibiotic regimens without full clearance of the infection. Urology consultation should also be obtained for cystitis in men, as there may be anatomical or other variations that predispose to infection. (Gupta and Trautner 2022)

Bone and Joint Infections

Presentation

Bone and joint bacterial infections are often severe and carry a significant risk of morbidity and mortality. Bone infections are termed osteomyelitis and can destroy the bone leading to pain, instability, bacteremia, and sepsis. Patients may present with localized pain, tenderness, and possibly fever. The tissue overlying the affected bone may also be red, swollen, and tender. Sometimes symptoms may develop more slowly, and findings may be more challenging to elicit explicitly. Depending on the bones involved and the damage caused by the infection, there may be neurologic symptoms such as shooting pains in a dermatomal pattern. This can be seen in cases of osteomyelitis affecting the spine. (Matteson and Osmon 2020) Septic arthritis presents similarly with localized swelling and pain with movement of the joint and is often associated with fever. Depending on the organism, patients may have a protracted history of joint pain and sometimes even drainage of pus through the overlying skin. (Zimmerli 2022)

Risk factors

Immunocompromised state and diabetes remain significant factors for bone and joint infection. While there is a theoretical risk of infection from the instrumentation of joints such as in arthrocentesis or arthroscopy, sterile techniques used during these procedures make these cases quite rare. Hematogenous spread remains the most common cause, responsible for about 75% of cases. Thus, patients with indwelling catheters are at risk. Other risk factors include penetrating trauma, alcoholism, IV drug use, and arthritis. Recent STI with *Neisseria gonorrhoeae* can predispose to gonococcal septic arthritis. (Matteson and Osmon 2020) The presence of prosthetics, like in patients with knee replacements, complicates the clinical picture as this allows a place for bacteria to seed and makes eradication difficult. Local spread from skin ulcers, such as sacral osteomyelitis from sacral decubitus ulcers, is seen in bed-bound patients. Similarly, patients with diabetes, arterial disease, or neuropathies may have altered sensation and not be aware of foot injuries like fissures or ulcers, leading to the spread of infection from the overlying skin to the bones of the feet. (Zimmerli 2022)

Pathophysiology

Once bacteria arrive at the bone or joint via one of the aforementioned mechanisms, they replicate and cause disease. *Staphylococcus aureus,* in particular, can bind to the bone via fibronectin and collagen receptors and is the most common cause of bacterial osteomyelitis. Streptococcus and Gram-negative bacilli like *Escherichia coli* and Pseudomonas are other common etiological organisms. Coagulase-negative Staphylococcus is also sometimes seen, particularly in IV drug users and in patients with prolonged bacteremia from infected pacemakers. (Zimmerli 2022)

Examination

Tenderness over the affected bone can be seen depending on the location of osteomyelitis. Fever is common, and patients may appear quite ill in acute osteomyelitis or septic arthritis. Pain with the movement of a particular joint may be seen in septic arthritis and joints can appear swollen, erythematous, boggy to palpation, and warm. Immunocompromised and elderly patients may have milder and more subtle findings as they do not mount the same level of immune response to the infection. Some patients may present with full-on septic shock and appear moribund. (Zimmerli 2022)

Laboratory

Leukocytosis is likely to present with neutrophilia in cases of septic arthritis and osteomyelitis, but it is not very specific. (McGillicuddy et al. 2007) ESR and CRP are usually elevated, and each has a high sensitivity for osteomyelitis of about 91-97%, although specificity is low at around 70-78%. Their high sensitivity means that they can help rule out these infections. In cases of suspected septic arthritis, arthrocentesis (joint aspiration) should be performed for synovial fluid analysis. This fluid can be examined using Gram stain to obtain a preliminary bacterial identification and also sent for cultures. PCR testing exists for some organisms but is not always used. Measuring the WBC concentration in the synovial fluid can help rule out other differentials such as gout or pseudogout. In one study, patients with an elevated WBC above 50,000 per microliter had a diagnosis of septic arthritis 47% of the time, while those above 100,000 WBC per microliter had it 77% of the time. Like fever and other symptoms, immunocompromised patients may not have this high a level of WBC in synovial fluid despite having septic arthritis, so the results should be taken in the context of the patient and their history. (Matteson and Osmon 2020) In the case of osteomyelitis, a surgical biopsy can be sent for histopathological examination and culture. (Zimmerli 2022)

Imaging

Imaging is an essential tool in the diagnosis of bone and joint infections. Radiographs can be an excellent initial step in evaluating both, particularly if there is a history of trauma to the area and concern for possible retained foreign bodies. However, in acute osteomyelitis, plain radiographs have low sensitivity. CT scan of affected bone or joint will provide much more information about associated tissues but can also be falsely negative due to low sensitivity. MRI is the most sensitive for diagnosing osteomyelitis and remains the gold standard. MRI can also give important information in cases of septic arthritis but is not often needed for this diagnosis. A positron emission tomography (PET) scan can also be beneficial in diagnosing osteomyelitis but is only used if MRI is contraindicated. However, in patients with prosthetic joints or other orthopedic devices, CT and MRI may be falsely negative because of the imaging artifacts these devices can cause. Gallium scanning can be used in these scenarios. (Matteson and Osmon 2020)

Associated symptoms/conditions

Prosthetic joints such as knee replacements and other orthopedic devices (spinal fixation screws and rods) are associated with recurrent infections and sometimes resistant infections. These devices can become a nidus for bacterial growth, particularly *Staphylococcus aureus*, which can develop a biofilm that layers around the device and allows for protection against the immune system. Chronic vertebral osteomyelitis can be associated with such hardware. (Zimmerli 2022) Infections with rarer organisms, such as Gram-negative infections, can be associated with bladder or bowel disease. Rheumatoid arthritis and osteoarthritis have also been associated with septic arthritis. (Matteson and Osmon 2020)

Diagnosis

The diagnosis of septic arthritis and osteomyelitis is a combination of clinical, laboratory, and imaging findings. A high degree of suspicion should be present for these conditions in patients with pain on movement of a particular joint or pain over bone associated with redness, swelling, and fever. As mentioned, MRI is the gold standard for diagnosing osteomyelitis, but if a prosthetic is involved, a gallium scan should be used. (Zimmerli 2022) For the diagnosis of septic arthritis, arthrocentesis is indicated for analysis of the synovial fluid culture for speciation. Blood cultures should be obtained in all patients with suspected septic arthritis as they may be positive in up to 50% of cases, which makes sense considering the most common mechanism is hematogenous seeding of bacteria. (Matteson and Osmon 2020) In osteomyelitis and prosthetic joint infections, the diagnosis can be definitively made with a pathological examination of a tissue sample. (Zimmerli 2022)

Treatment

Antibiotics should be started empirically as soon as there is a strong suspicion of joint or bone infection, particularly as these patients may present quite septic. Targeting the most common organisms, coverage should include antibiotics against both Gram-positive and -negative organisms. Vancomycin can be used for Gram-positive coverage, particularly for suspected MRSA or MSSA, until cultures return. For Gram-negative coverage, antibiotics with Pseudomonas activity should be used and include choices such as cefepime, meropenem, and piperacillin-tazobactam. In the case of septic arthritis, a Gram stain of synovial fluid should aid in narrowing antibiotics depending on staining but is only positive in 50% of patients. Regimens vary from two to six weeks. (Matteson and Osmon 2020) For osteomyelitis, similar antibiotic regimens that cover the usual organisms can be used, and antibiotic duration is four to six weeks. (Zimmerli 2022)

Management

Blood cultures should be drawn for both bone and joint infections to help identify if the hematogenous spread was the original etiology. Aside from antibiotics, orthopedic consultation should be obtained and can assist in obtaining synovial fluid in the case of septic arthritis or bone biopsy if indicated for suspicion of osteomyelitis. This is even more important if any orthopedic hardware may be involved to determine if removal is necessary. General surgery consultation may also be required in cases where osteomyelitis is due to skin ulceration, such as sacral osteomyelitis from sacral decubitus ulcers. (Matteson and Osmon 2020) In other exceptional circumstances, such as osteomyelitis of the sternum associated with previous surgery/sternal wires, cardiothoracic surgery may need to be involved. Neurosurgery consultation should be obtained in the case of vertebral osteomyelitis. People with diabetes and poorly controlled sugar should have regimens adjusted to ensure euglycemia, as hyperglycemia can make both of these infections resistant to management. Podiatry consultation may be required in cases of foot osteomyelitis, which is also seen in poorly controlled diabetics. (Zimmerli 2022)

Skin and Soft Tissue Infections

Presentation

There are a variety of different infections that can affect the skin, its various layers, and the soft tissues underneath it. Superficial infections such as folliculitis, furuncles, erysipelas, and impetigo are usually very visible and symptomatic. Furuncles (or "boils") are skin abscesses caused by a bacterial infection involving a hair follicle and its surrounding tissue. Carbuncles are clusters of furuncles connected subcutaneously and are smaller and more superficial than subcutaneous abscesses but can cause more profound scarring than isolated furuncles. Deeper infections like cellulitis, subcutaneous abscesses, and necrotizing fasciitis may not be so clearly evident but can be quite symptomatic. Skin findings such as redness, purulence, pain, warmth, and swelling are shared amongst a variety of these clinical entities. Fever can sometimes be seen with some of the more severe, deeper infections, such as necrotizing fasciitis. (Stevens and Bryant 2022) Patients may present quite ill, often with sepsis or septic shock, and complain of excruciating pain despite the area not appearing abnormal visually. This scenario is a medical and surgical emergency requiring inpatient management. (Lew and Southwick 2020)

Risk factors

Any penetrating trauma or scratches/abrasions can introduce bacteria into the skin's deeper layers, which normally protects the body from outside infections. Multiple diseases, such as heart disease, diabetes, obesity, peripheral vascular disease, and liver disease, can all affect normal skin healing and the ability to heal and fight off infection normally. Prolonged immobilization can lead to decubitus ulcers at pressure points like the sacrum and hips, which can then become infected. Even surgical procedures can lead to these infections as they also disrupt the normal protective qualities of skin from the deeper structures underneath. (Ramakrishnan 2022) Immunosuppressed states and certain genetic diseases continue to be ubiquitous risk factors.

Pathophysiology

Bacterial overgrowth amongst different areas will result in various clinical entities affecting the skin and soft tissue. From the superficial into the deep, abnormal clearance of sebum from hair follicles can lead to bacterial overgrowth and folliculitis. Furuncles and carbuncles may complicate folliculitis. Superficial skin infections such as impetigo occur in exposed areas through abrasions or previous insect bites that then spread in pustules that crust over, a characteristic of impetigo. As infections go deeper, they can affect the dermis and subcutaneous tissue and form pus pockets, manifesting as abscesses. Erysipelas affects the deeper layers of the dermis and can spread quickly via lymphatics, usually causing a characteristic demarcation. (Lew and Southwick 2020) Cellulitis results from infection of the deeper subcutaneous tissues. (Ryan 2022) Necrotizing fasciitis and myonecrosis are severe, deep-tissue infections of the connective layers (fascia) and muscle, and can spread rapidly along tissue planes. These infections can affect vasculature leading to thrombosis of vessels and subsequent necrosis. (Stevens and Bryant 2022)

Examination

After a thorough history, a detailed exam can reveal a lot about most of these infections. Visible findings of redness, warmth, swelling, and purulence can quickly help guide diagnosis. Careful attention should be paid to the integrity of the skin, as even minor cuts and scrapes may have made way for bacterial entry. Folliculitis is usually clearly visible. Impetigo and erysipelas have very characteristic appearances: yellow crusting pustules and sharply demarcated red swollen skin, respectively. Cellulitis may also have redness and swelling but is not sharply demarcated and is warm to the touch. Palpation is integral to the exam, as carbuncles, furuncles, and abscesses can be palpated. (Lew and Southwick 2020) A feeling of crepitus may signal gas under the skin, a concerning finding for clostridial infection. Pain out of proportion to exam, or areas with hemorrhage, tense edema, and bullae, may be signs of necrotizing infection. (Ramakrishnan 2022) Patients with certain tick-borne illnesses, such as Rocky Mountain Spotted Fever (RMSF), may or may not initially have a rash. A careful exam should be performed, although the tick is often never found. (Wittler 2022)

Laboratory

Most skin infections do not require laboratory workup. Depending on the severity, patients may have leukocytosis with a left shift (shifted to more immature precursors) and elevated CRP or other inflammatory markers. These are often only seen in deeper, more severe infections and are not expected in milder superficial cases of infection like folliculitis and impetigo. Blood cultures should be obtained in critically ill patients who arrive with suspected sepsis or septic shock, which can be associated with deeper infections. Superficial skin cultures are often not recommended, but if there is purulence, such as in an abscess, it can be swabbed and sent to be cultured. Deep cultures can be obtained during surgery for necrotizing fasciitis, and Gram staining should be done to get a presumptive etiological organism. However, some of these infections can be polymicrobial and are termed Type 1 (in contrast, Type 2 infections have a single organism as the cause). Creatine phosphokinase (CPK) may be elevated in necrotizing fasciitis and myonecrosis, as it is released from muscle tissue after its destruction. (Lew and Southwick 2020) For patients with suspected RMSF, there are PCR tests available. (Wittler 2022)

Imaging

Imaging is usually not necessary for most of the less severe, superficial skin and soft tissue infections. Ultrasound, CT, and MRI may have roles in determining the severity of infection for deeper infections like necrotizing fasciitis but should not delay surgical intervention if indicated. (Ramakrishnan 2022) Ultrasound, in particular, may be useful in children and can also be used for deep abscesses.

Associated symptoms/conditions

Primary immunodeficiencies, particularly leukocyte adhesion defects, chronic granulomatous disease, and hyper-IgE syndrome can all present with recurrent skin infections such as abscesses, with *Staphylococcus aureus* as the most common cause. (Michaels et al. 2020) Diabetes is also often associated with all skin and deeper tissue infections, likely given diabetes-related barrier and immune dysfunctions, poor vascular flow, and the possibility of elevated glucose levels serving as a substrate for bacterial growth.

Diagnosis

Most skin and soft tissue infections are clinical diagnoses, made after a careful history and physical exam. Diagnosis of a particular organism is often only reached in some of the cases in which a culture is usually obtained, such as cases with purulence like an abscess or deep infections that require surgical intervention like necrotizing fasciitis where direct cultures can be obtained. (Ramakrishnan 2022) In Rickettsial diseases, a fourfold increase in IgG titers from acute to the convalescent stage can confirm this diagnosis, but this would be obtained 2-4 weeks after the onset of illness, so this diagnosis is also most often made clinically. Tissue biopsies with immunostains are 100% specific and 70% sensitive for RMSF. (Wittler 2022)

Treatment

The two most common causative organisms for skin and soft tissue infections are *Staphylococcus aureus* and beta-hemolytic Streptococcus. Thus antibiotic regimens usually target these two organisms. Mild superficial infections like folliculitis usually respond to warm compresses and topical mupirocin. Impetigo similarly may be treated with topical mupirocin when mild. Cefazolin or cephalexin, first-generation cephalosporins, or amoxicillin-clavulanate, and penicillin with a beta-lactamase inhibitor, are options that effectively cover MSSA and group A streptococcus (GAS). If MRSA is suspected, options may include TMP-SMX or clindamycin when an oral antibiotic is preferred, such as in the outpatient setting for managing diseases like abscesses and mild cellulitis. For more severe infections requiring hospitalization, vancomycin can effectively cover MRSA while cultures are pending, and penicillins with beta-lactamase inhibitors such as ampicillin-sulbactam or piperacillin-tazobactam can aid in extending coverage for Gram-negative organisms. Depending on risk factors and allergies, carbapenems like ertapenem may be used. Clindamycin, in particular, is often used with other antibiotics to treat necrotizing fasciitis, given its ability to suppress toxin production and increase phagocytosis of *Streptococcus pyogenes*. (Lew and Southwick 2020) Doxycycline is the first-line medication for treating tick-borne Rickettsial diseases like RMSF. Although chloramphenicol is another option, its side effects limit its use in clinical practice. (Wittler 2022)

Prevention of recurrent superficial infections often involves attention to personal hygiene and may require topical interventions like the scheduled use of mupirocin or chlorhexidine gluconate baths. (Lew and Southwick) In the case of necrotizing fasciitis, general surgery consultation should be obtained as soon as there is clinical suspicion, as debridement of tissue is imperative. Patients are often quite ill or may rapidly become so and require hospital management for careful monitoring and IV antibiotics. Critical care consultation is usually obtained early in the clinical course, if not immediately after surgery. Depending on how much tissue needs to be removed, closure may require extensive flaps and plastic surgery consultation may also be needed. (Ramakrishnan 2022)

General Treatment Strategies for Bacterial Infections

There are two types of antibacterial drugs: **bacteriostatic** (i.e., inhibiting growth but not overtly killing the organism) and **bactericidal** (*i.e.*, killing the susceptible organism). Generally, drugs that inhibit bacterial protein synthesis are bacteriostatic (except the bactericidal aminoglycosides). The following categories and specific antibacterial agents are generally bacteriostatic: macrolides, tetracyclines, chloramphenicol, clindamycin, linezolid, and trimethoprim/sulfamethoxazole. Bacteriostatic agents slow the bacterial growth rate to allow the immune system to respond and remove the illness-causing bacterial burden; given this dependency on an intact immune response, bacteriostatic agents are generally avoided as monotherapy for immuno-compromised patients (*e.g.*, avoid for an AIDS patient with poorly controlled HIV infection and [therefore] frank bacterial infection comorbidity). For this reason, *bactericidal* agents are required for infections in the immuno-compromised, and for patients with endocarditis, meningitis, or infections secondary to chemotherapy-induced neutropenia. Antibacterial drugs active against bacterial cell wall integrity are generally bactericidal (*e.g.*, the penicillins and the cephalosporins). Furthermore, synergistic bactericidal activity can be achieved by combination therapy; for example, penicillin in combination with an aminoglycoside (*e.g.*, gentamicin) will generate more-than-additive bacterial killing effects given the penicillin's actions in increasing the permeability of the aminoglycoside.

A second consideration when selecting antibacterial agents is their individual spectra. "Spectrum" or range of activity is generally categorized as narrow or broad. A **narrow-spectrum** antibacterial drug (Melander et al. 2018) will only inhibit growth or kill a specific type or types of disease-causing bacteria (*e.g.*, the tetracycline class-member sarecycline used solely for the treatment of acne vulgaris (Zhanel et al. 2019)). **Broad-spectrum** agents are useful in treating many different types of bacterial infections: for example, the tetracycline class-member doxycycline is used to treat bacterial pneumonia, chlamydia or syphilis infections, Lyme disease, cholera, and typhus. Broad-spectrum agents (and/or combination antibiotic therapy) are also required treatments for "super-infections": multiple types of bacteria collectively causing illness in a single patient.

The **drug sensitivity or resistance** borne by the targeted bacterial infection is a third factor when selecting antibacterial agents for treatment. Whether shown empirically by lab testing of patient-derived samples or suspected by national or local prevalence, the existence of infection by bacteria with an acquired ability to grow in the presence of a particular antibacterial drug will naturally eliminate choice among the drug classes. Indiscriminate usage of broad-spectrum antibacterial medicines in treating community-acquired bacterial infections (and even viral infections!), without attempts to culture or otherwise identify the causative agent of the illness, is thought to have contributed over time to the emergence of more drug-resistant bacterial strains. For this reason, narrow-spectrum agents are favorable because their application is less likely to select for resistance in non-targeted bacterial species and/or for multidrug resistance phenotypes. Broad-spectrum antibiotics are most appropriately used when the causative bacteria is empirically identified, when resistance to narrow-spectrum antibiotic(s) is empirically identified, or when a delay in treatment for such lab tests would result in the potential for the patient to elevate quickly into serious illness (*e.g.*, with the presentation of meningitis, in which a patient can become so ill that death could occur within hours if broad-spectrum antibiotics are not initiated immediately).

Pharmacological Treatments for Bacterial Infections

Penicillins

The penicillins share a central β-lactam ring structure (Figure 3.1). Their targets are bacterial transpeptidases that normally work to stitch together muropeptides (pentameric peptidoglycan precursors) into the lengthy macromolecules comprising the unique peptidoglycan cell wall that bacteria possess (but our own cells lack). These bacterial transpeptidases are called "penicillin-binding proteins (PBPs)". Penicillins bind and inhibit the PBP transpeptidases, thereby preventing further cross-linking of the peptidoglycan cell wall. Resultant cell wall structural weakening and the activation of local autolytic enzymes lead to lysis and bacterial death (hence, **penicillins are bactericidal**). Penicillins are generally safe drugs when considering possible adverse effects, with only allergy and hypersensitivity to consider. Patients with prior history of a hypersensitive or allergic reaction to penicillin may also show such responsiveness to other β-lactam ring-containing antibacterial agents (*e.g.,* the cephalosporins of the next section).

Figure 3.1 Structures of penicillins.

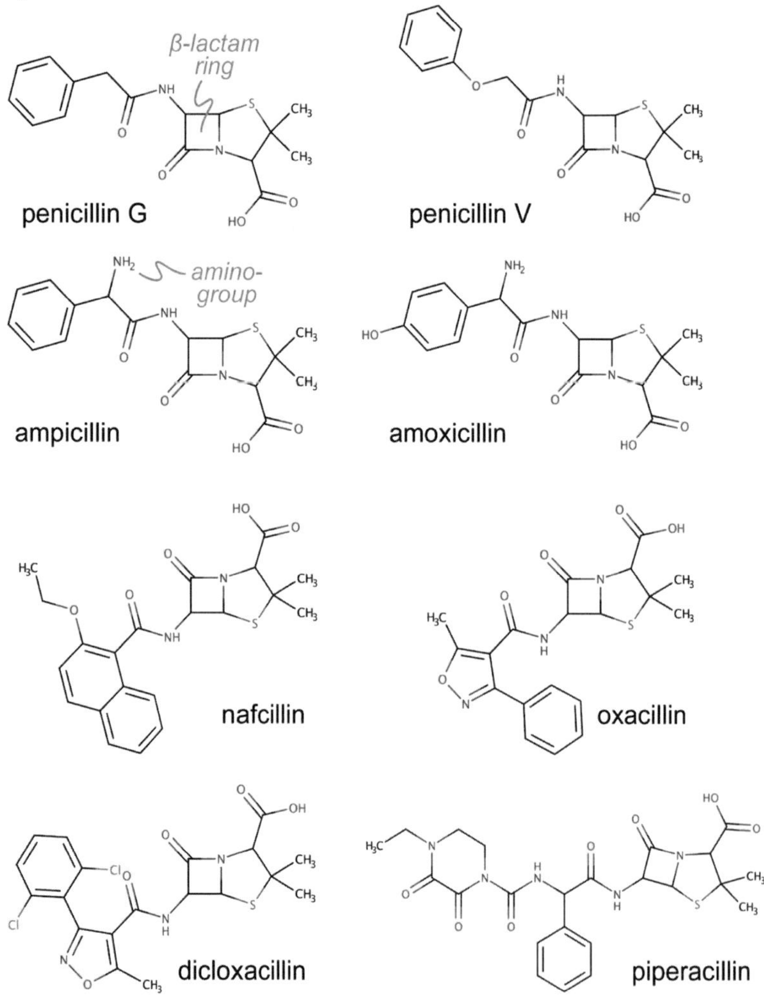

Penicillin G (a.k.a. benzylpenicillin) is destroyed by stomach acid and, therefore, must be given intravenously or via intramuscular injection (not orally). As a "first generation" penicillin produced naturally from penicillium fungus fermentation, it is inherently susceptible to inactivating hydrolysis by bacterially produced β-lactamase enzymes. Penicillin G has its most significant activity against Gram-positive bacteria, Gram-negative cocci, and non-β-lactamase-producing anaerobes (*i.e.*, bacteria that can live without free oxygen). The initiation of penicillin G therapy in patients with syphilis or other Gram-negative spirochetal infections (*e.g.*, Lyme disease) often can elicit an acute, self-limited, systemic febrile reaction, beginning one to two hours after therapy initiation and disappearing within 12 to 24 hours: namely, the **Jarisch-Herxheimer reaction**. It is characterized by fever, chills, myalgias, headache, exacerbation of cutaneous lesions, tachycardia, hyperventilation, vasodilation with flushing, and mild hypotension. Pathogenesis of the Jarisch-Herxheimer reaction is thought to arise from the release of heat-stable pyrogens from the dying spirochetes.

Penicillin V (a.k.a. phenoxymethylpenicillin) is more acid-stable than benzylpenicillin and therefore is given orally. Like benzylpenicillin, penicillin V can be inactivated by β-lactamase activity and thus is not useful against β-lactamase-producing "resistant" bacteria, which include many *Staphylococci* strains (Barber and Rozwadowska-Dowzenko 1948). Penicillin V still has modern utility against mild-to-moderate *Streptococcus pyogenes* infections of the skin, tonsils, or pharynx, as well as for odontogenic infections and prophylaxis against the development of rheumatic fever or pneumococcal spleen disorders.

The "extended-spectrum" aminopenicillins **ampicillin** and **amoxicillin** (Figure 3.1) retain the antibacterial spectrum of their parent benzylpenicillin but also have improved activity against Gram-negative rods. They are effective against most Gram-positive bacterial infections and Gram-negative infections such as *Escherichia coli* and *Haemophilus influenzae* (the latter being "Pfeiffer's bacillus," which was misnamed in Latin given that it actually does not cause influenza). As the aminopenicillins are also susceptible to β-lactamase inactivation, each is given with an adjuvant to inhibit β-lactamase activity: ampicillin is given with **sulbactam**, and amoxicillin is given with clavulanic acid (a.k.a. **clavulanate**).

This same adjunctive strategy is often employed with the "anti-pseudomonal" penicillin **piperacillin** (a member of the ureidopenicillin class). Combined with the β-lactamase inhibitor **tazobactam**, piperacillin has bactericidal activity against many Gram-positive and Gram-negative bacteria including *Pseudomonas aeruginosa* (the latter of particular medical importance given its multi-drug resistance and its association with serious illnesses such as ventilator-associated and cystic fibrosis-associated pneumonia). Piperacillin and other anti-pseudomonal penicillins are sometimes combined with an aminoglycoside or fluoroquinolone (see following sections), especially in infections outside of the urinary tract. (Tamma et al. 2012)

The "anti-staphylococcal" penicillins (including methicillin, **nafcillin, oxacillin,** and **dicloxacillin**) are all inherently resistant to inactivation caused by staphylococcal β-lactamases. They are therefore active against many Gram-positive *Staphylococci* and *Streptococci* species. They are drugs of choice for methicillin-*susceptible Staphylococcus aureus* (MSSA), but they are not useful against enterococci, anaerobes, Gram-negative cocci or rods, or methicillin-*resistant Staphylococcus aureus* (MRSA). (Chalmers and Wylam 2020) Bacteria can generate resistance (Hakenbeck and Coyette 1998; Chambers 1999), even against the anti-staphylococcal penicillins impervious to staphylococcal β-lactamases, by directly mutating the targeted PBP transpeptidases (*e.g.*, ref. (Ropp et al. 2002) for *Neisseria gonorrhoeae*). These resistance mechanisms can be shuttled from bacterium to bacterium via gene transfer; therefore, there are several heuristics to be applied in prescribing antibacterial drugs to control the further development and proliferation of bacterial resistance:

- Use an adequate dose and duration to *eliminate* the infecting organism
- Select antibacterial agent(s) for the infection according to *proven susceptibility* to those agent(s)
- Use *narrow-spectrum* antibiotics when possible
- Use antibacterial agents *in combination* across classes to prevent the emergence of resistant mutants
- Use antibacterial agents *prophylactically* when proven valuable, and *only for a short time* to avoid selection of resistance

Cephalosporins, Penems, and Monobactams (other β-lactam ring-based antibacterial drugs)
The **cephalosporins** share with the penicillins a central β-lactam ring structure (Figure 3.2). Like the penicillins, the cephalosporins bind and inhibit bacterial PBP transpeptidases, thereby weakening cell wall structural integrity to cause lysis and bacterial death (hence, **cephalosporins are bactericidal**). First-generation cephalosporins (*e.g.*, **cefazolin, cephalexin, cephalothin**; Figure 3.2) are predominantly active against Gram-positive bacteria, including *Staphylococcus* and *Streptococcus* strains (Cephalosporins 2012), and are therefore mainly used for skin and soft tissue infections and preventing hospital-acquired surgical infections. First-generation cephalosporins also have modest activity against some Gram-negative organisms (*e.g.*, *E. coli, Proteus mirabilis, Klebsiella pneumoniae*) and are thus still considered, for example, in cases of either uncomplicated or complicated urinary tract infections (UTIs) caused by Gram-negative bacteria (Diaz-Brochero et al. 2022). The successive generations of cephalosporins (Figure 3.2) possess increasing activity against Gram-negative organisms but often with reduced activity against Gram-

positive bacteria. Cephalosporins do not have activity against the "LAME" organisms: namely, *Listeria*, "atypicals" (like *Chlamydia trachomatis* and *Mycoplasma* species), methicillin-resistant *Staph. aureus* (MRSA), and enterococci; an exception to this LAME mnemonic is the clear effectiveness that fifth-generation cephalosporins exhibit against MRSA. (Duplessis and Crum-Cianflone 2011)

First- and second-generation cephalosporins are less susceptible than the penicillins, but not impervious, to inactivating hydrolysis by bacterially produced β-lactamase enzymes. In contrast, the third, fourth, and fifth-generation cephalosporins (Figure 3.2) are impervious to β-lactamase activity but can still be overcome by bacterial resistance: specifically, by direct mutations or expression level changes in their PBP transpeptidase targets. (Zapun et al. 2008) An additional noteworthy distinction between the first- and third-generation cephalosporins relates to their relative utility in treating bacterial meningitis: while the first-generation cephalosporins are ineffective owing to failure to cross the blood-brain barrier (BBB), the third-generation cephalosporins **ceftriaxone** and **cefotaxime** are effective against bacterial meningitis because they cross the BBB and are detected in high concentrations in the cerebral spinal fluid after administration. (Goldwater 2005)

Figure 3.2 Structures of five generations of cephalosporins.

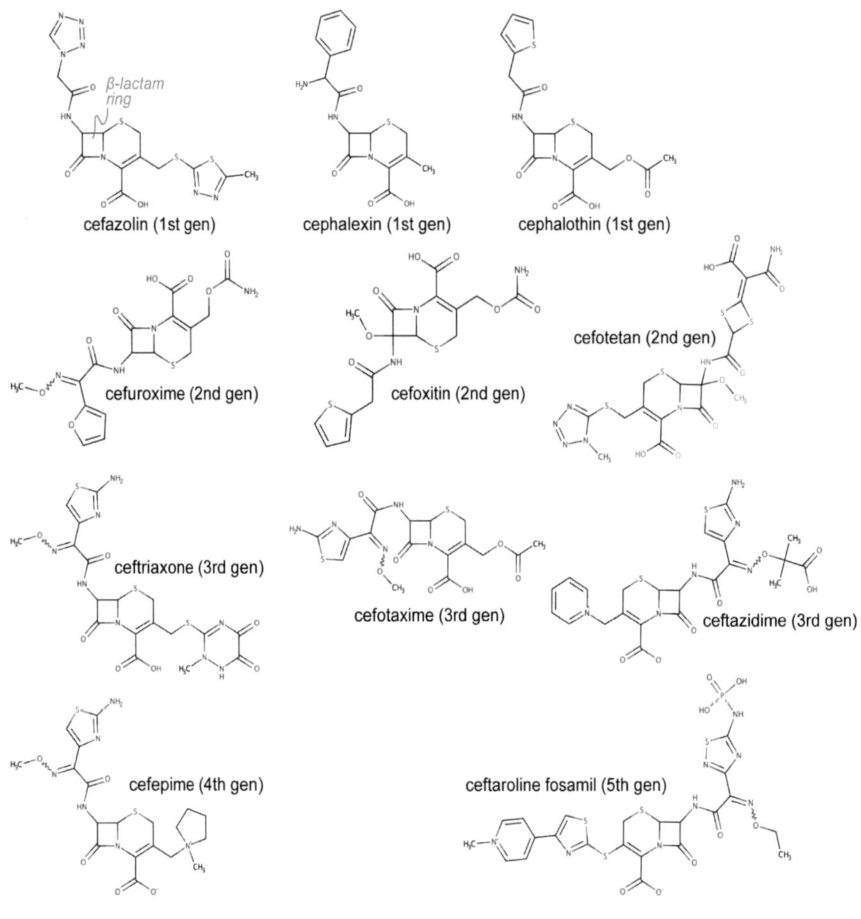

Patients with prior history of an allergic or hypersensitive reaction to penicillin may also show such adverse responses to cephalosporins, given their shared β-lactam ring-containing structures. However, original estimates of up to 10% cross-reactivity were formulated after considering reactions to early-generation cephalosporins; (Dash 1975) more recent epidemiological work has decreased this cross-reactivity rate estimate for second- and later generations. (Pichichero 2006)

Like penicillins and cephalosporins, the carbapenems **imipenem**, **doripenem**, **ertapenem**, and **meropenem** all share the central β-lactam ring structure (Figure 3.3) and share the same mechanism of action of inhibiting bacterial PBP transpeptidases. The carbapenems have shown broad coverage against Gram-negative organisms, including anaerobes (*e.g., Bacteroides fragilis* (Takesue et al. 2018)) and drug-resistant strains (*e.g., Pseudomonas aeruginosa*), but particular resistance to the carbapenem class is emerging; (Tenover et al. 2022) for example, carbapenems are often considered "drugs of last resort" against the *Enterobacteriaceae*, yet carbapenemase-producing *Escherichia coli*, *Enterobacter aerogenes*, *Enterobacter cloacae* complex, *Klebsiella pneumoniae*, and *Klebsiella oxytoca* are presenting an ever-increasing challenge in hospital-acquired infections. (*e.g.*, ref. (Landman et al. 2012))

Figure 3.3 Structures of carbapenems, the monobactam aztreonam, and the cyclic peptides vancomycin and bacitracin.

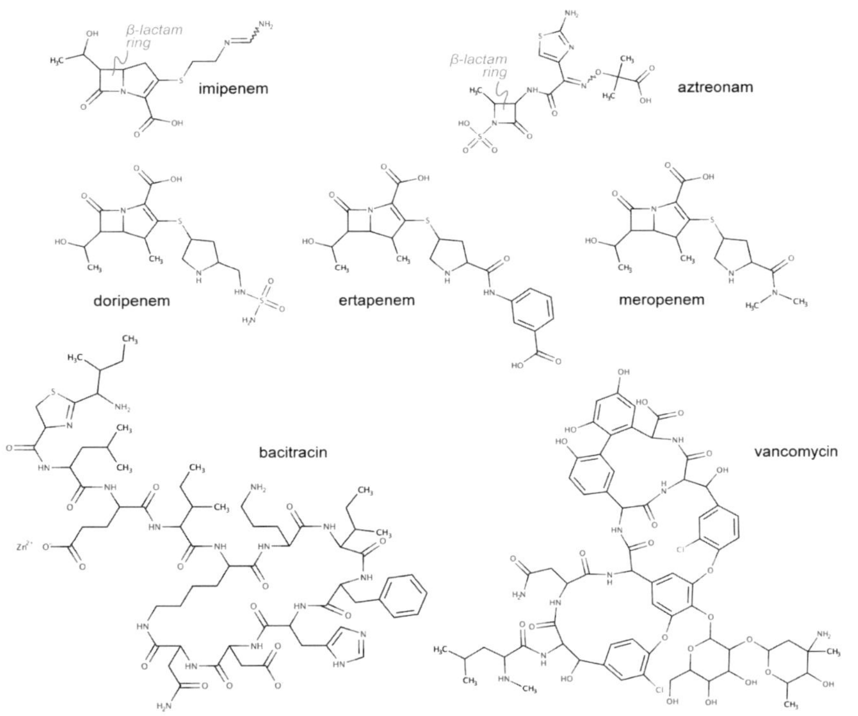

Imipenem, in both its intravenous and intramuscular formulations, is co-formulated with a dehydropeptidase inhibitor (cilastatin) to prevent its hydrolysis into a nephrotoxic intermediate by dehydropeptidase activity within the kidney. To combat emerging bacterial resistance, a β-lactamase inhibitor (relebactam) has now been approved for addition to the imipenem/cilastatin combination. (Papp-Wallace et al. 2020)

The sole commercially available monobactam is **aztreonam** (Figure 3.2), which is (as its "*mono-*" class-name suggests) a monocyclic, β-lactam ring-containing antibacterial drug. While sharing a core structural element and mechanism of action with the penicillins, cephalosporins, and carbapenems, the monobactam aztreonam is distinctly narrow-spectrum in its utility and thus generally restricted to clinical use against aerobic Gram-negative rods like *Pseudomonas aeruginosa* (although, again, mutation-based resistance to aztreonam is emerging. (Jorth et al. 2017)) Patients allergic to penicillins can tolerate aztreonam. (*e.g.*, ref. (Romano et al. 2016))

Vancomycin and Bacitracin (non-β-lactam bacterial cell wall synthesis inhibitors)

Pentameric peptidoglycan precursors (muropeptides), which bacterial PBP transpeptidases stitch together to form the peptidoglycan cell wall, end in a D-alanine-D-alanine dipeptide. This D-alanyl-D-alanine motif directly binds to the PBP transpeptidase. This critical binding event is inhibited by the covalent (irreversible) attachment of a β-lactam antibacterial drug to this PBP transpeptidase binding site. In contrast to this mechanism of action shared by the penicillins, the cephalosporins, the carbapenems, and the monobactams, the glycopeptide **vancomycin** (Figure 3.3) binds directly to the D-alanyl-D-alanine motif of the peptidoglycan precursors, preventing their incorporation into the long peptidoglycan strands of the bacterial cell wall. This ability to inhibit cell wall synthesis is only bactericidal to Gram-positive bacteria; given differences in how Gram-negative bacteria produce their cell walls and accessibility issues given the outer membrane of Gram-negative bacteria, vancomycin is not active against Gram-negative pathogens except for some nongonococcal *Neisseria* species. Therefore, clinical use of vancomycin is generally reserved for severe Gram-positive infections, including MRSA, drug-resistant *Streptococcus pneumoniae* (even in the severely ill), and the anaerobe *Clostridium difficile* (the latter usually treated with either oral vancomycin or metronidazole). However, bacterial resistance to vancomycin can develop: the pentameric peptidoglycan precursors can be formed with D-lactate instead of D-alanine at their termini, thereby abrogating vancomycin binding yet still permitting cell wall incorporation. For example, vancomycin-resistant *Staphylococcus aureus* (VRSA) strains (Cong et al. 2020) have been clinically isolated since 2002; infections with methicillin- and vancomycin-resistant strains usually evoke treatment with linezolid, tigecycline, or daptomycin (although resistance to the latter lipopeptide antibiotic is also now emergent (Jahan et al. 2022)) (Table 3.1).

Vancomycin is given orally for severe *C. difficile* colitis or intravenously for complicated skin or bloodstream infections, bone and joint infections, endocarditis, and MRSA-driven meningitis. (Liu et al. 2011) The latter route of administration, dependent on dose and rate of infusion, can elicit an acute anaphylactoid adverse effect (now called "*Vancomycin Flushing Syndrome*"): a pruritic, erythematous rash of the face, neck, and upper torso of the patient within 5 to 10 minutes of receiving intravenous vancomycin. (Martel et al. 2022)

Table 3.1. **Staging of possible pharmacotherapy upon diagnosis of *Staphylococcus aureus* infection**

Methicillin-sensitive?	*Methicillin-resistant (MRSA)?*	*Both Methicillin (MRSA)-and Vancomycin (VRSA)-resistant strains?*
An anti-staphylococcal penicillin: *e.g.*, **nafcillin, oxacillin,** or **dicloxacillin**	*MRSA is usually also resistant to cephalosporins, imipenem & meropenem, fluoroquinolones, and clindamycin* **vancomycin**	**linezolid**
cefazolin or **cephalexin**	**ceftaroline fosamil**	**daptomycin**
clindamycin	**tigecycline**	**tigecycline**
A fluoroquinolone		

Bacitracin is another complex, cyclical polypeptide antibiotic (Figure 3.3) that, like vancomycin, disrupts peptidoglycan cell wall synthesis in Gram-positive bacteria. Bacitracin interferes with the dephosphorylation of lipids that normally carry peptidoglycan monomers through the bacterial plasma membrane for insertion into the bacterial cell wall (Stone and Strominger 1971; Schneider and Sahl 2010). As it causes kidney damage if taken internally, bacitracin is primarily used as a topical ointment for localized skin and eye infections. Bacitracin-containing antibacterial ointments often contain other antibiotic agents, such as **neomycin** (see next section) and/or **polymyxin B**, a cyclic peptide with cationic detergent properties able to alter bacterial membrane permeability to a bactericidal result. Alone, polymyxin B is also employed by injection or inhalation to treat Gram-negative infections causing meningitis, pneumonia, sepsis, or UTIs; however, typical side effects of these non-topical routes of administration include fever, rash, pruritus, and renal and neurological problems.

Folate antagonists (inhibitors of purine production)

Bacteria are dependent on a folate biosynthetic pathway (Figure 3.4) that merges dihydropteridine with para-aminobenzoic acid (PABA) to produce the tetrahydrofolate (THF) ultimately required to form the purine building blocks of their DNA. In contrast, humans can also source folate directly from dietary items. Exploiting this metabolic difference between bacteria and humans, drugs that antagonize this folate biosynthetic pathway at one of two distinct steps are used as antibacterial agents, often in combination to achieve bactericidal action. The sulfonamides or "sulfa drugs" **sulfamethoxazole** (SMX), **sulfadiazine** (sometimes as the silver salt), and **mafenide** inhibit the first key enzyme of this pathway – dihydropteroate synthase. Alone, the sulfonamides are bacteriostatic and have utility in treating UTIs, conjunctivitis, and infected burns. Bactericidal activity is only achieved when the sulfa drug is combined with a second drug that inhibits the second key pathway enzyme of dihydrofolate reductase. For this reason, the dihydrofolate reductase inhibitor **trimethoprim** (TMP) is commonly used in combination with sulfamethoxazole as "**TMP-SMX**" or "co-trimoxazole." A related pyrimidine compound, **pyrimethamine** (Figure 3.4), is paired with a sulfa drug to treat toxoplasmosis, or with **dapsone** as a second-line combination treatment against *P. jiroveci* fungal pneumonia in people with HIV/AIDS.

Figure 3.4 Structures of the sulfa drugs sulfamethoxazole, sulfadiazine, and mafenide, and of the dihydrofolate reductase inhibitors trimethoprim and pyrimethamine, as well as an illustration of the bacterial folate biosynthetic pathway and where these antibacterial agents act.

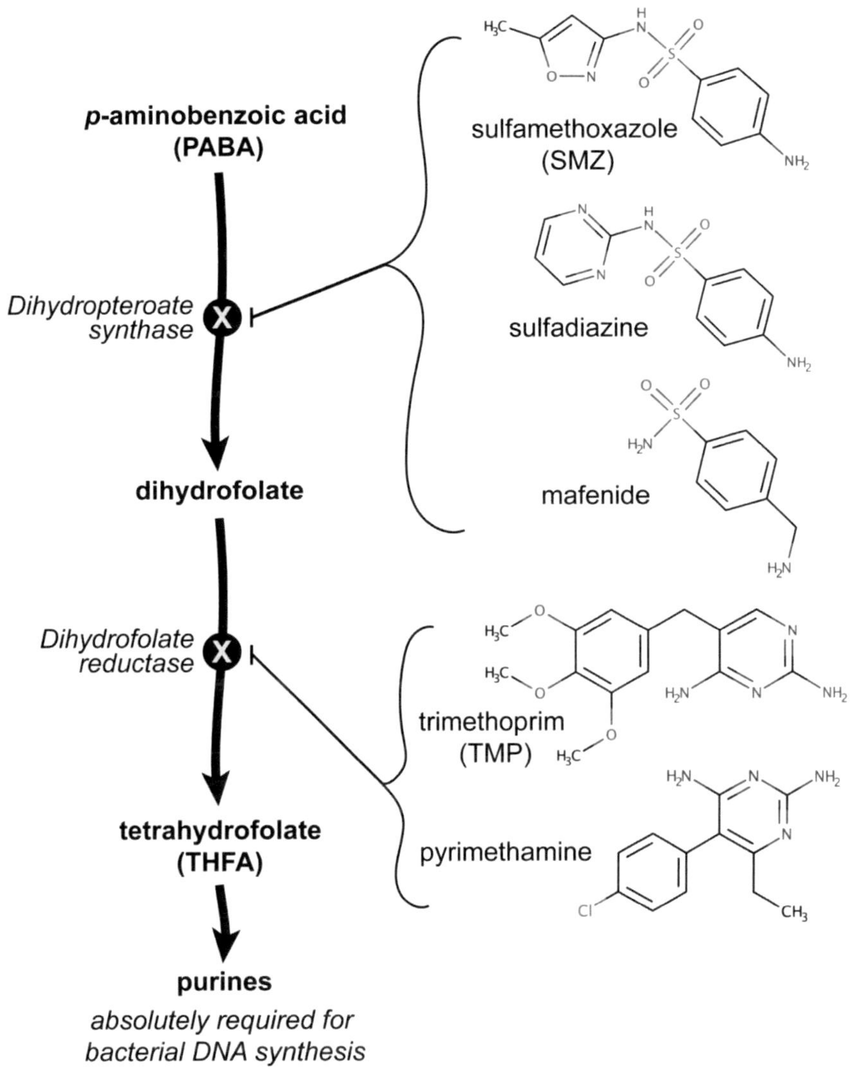

Bacteria can mount resistance against both arms of this folate antagonism strategy. To thwart the bacteriostatic action of sulfa drugs, bacteria can produce more of the pathway substrate PABA, destroy the sulfa drug by acetylation, or use alternative biosynthetic pathways to provide the required building blocks for DNA synthesis. To circumvent inhibition by trimethoprim or pyrimethamine, bacteria can overproduce the target enzyme dihydrofolate reductase (Hawser et al. 2006) or mutate the enzyme to reduce antibacterial agent binding affinity/activity. For example, the Gram-negative bacterium *Moraxella catarrhalis*, initially considered non-pathogenic but now known to infect the upper respiratory tract, middle ear, eye, joints, and the CNS, was found decades ago to be resistant to trimethoprim. (Winstanley and Spencer 1986)

The combination of a sulfa drug (usually SMX) with trimethoprim is commonly used for pediatric otitis media, acute infective exacerbations of chronic bronchitis, pulmonary or systemic nocardiosis, and uncomplicated UTIs (including urethritis, cystitis, pyelonephritis, and prostatitis) as caused by Gram-negative bacteria such as *Proteus mirabilis*, *Klebsiella pneumoniae*, and *E. coli* (Jancel and Dudas 2002; Hanlon et al. 2019). As folate antagonists, these combinations lead to a common adverse effect of folate deficiency; concomitant provision of folic acid can prevent this adverse effect while preserving antibacterial efficacy (as bacteria cannot use dietary folate). More serious adverse effects are numerous, with some identified early on after the advent of this folate antagonism strategy (*e.g.*, ref. (Sulfonamides and Vitamin K Deficiency 1945)). Trimethoprim-driven folate deficiency can lead to megaloblastic anemia, leukopenia, or granulocytopenia. Red blood cell depletion (anemia) can arise from the sulfa drug's effects in depressing hematopoiesis in the bone marrow (Sulfonamides and Vitamin K Deficiency 1945); a more severe and acute hemolytic anemia occurs if the patient has a genetic deficiency in glucose-6-phosphate dehydrogenase (G6PDH) activity (*e.g.*, estimated to be as high as 10% in African-Americans and 70% in Kurdish Jews; ref. (Beutler 1994)). Rarely, certain high-risk patients may respond to sulfa drug use with agranulocytosis (loss of leukocytes and other myeloid cells).

Sulfa drugs are also known to elicit **Stevens-Johnson syndrome**: a sudden onset of erosion of mucous membranes (e.g., oral mucosa, lips, conjunctivae) with widespread skin blistering; (*e.g.*, ref. (Taqi et al. 2012)) this severe allergic reaction can be accompanied by fever, polyarthritis, renal and multiple other organ failure(s). Sulfa drugs precipitating within urine can also cause crystalluria leading to renal failure. Sulfa drugs also have notable drug-drug interactions: (1) They act synergistically with sulfonylurea, which can lead to increased insulin release and reduced blood glucose levels, and (2) they can engender bleeding risks by displacing orally administered anticoagulant drugs from plasma albumin binding sites and by inhibiting warfarin's metabolism via cytochrome P450 isoform CYP2C9. Finally, sulfa drugs are contraindicated in pregnancy and for very young children, given the risk of driving bilirubin to accumulate in the CNS grey matter, thereby causing neuronal defects (*i.e.*, hyperbilirubinemia leading to **neonatal kernicterus**).

Tetracyclines (inhibitors of bacterial 30S ribosomal subunit)
Bacteria translate their messenger RNAs into polypeptides by the actions of a ribosome composed of 50S and 30S subunits; in contrast, mammalian cells have different (larger) ribosomes consisting of a 60S and 40S subunit pairing. As a bacteriostatic drug class, the **tetracyclines** (Figure 3.5) share a mechanism of action of binding to and thereby inhibiting the bacterial 30S ribosomal subunit, leading to selective inhibition of bacterial protein synthesis. Bacteria have demonstrated several means by which they can develop resistance to tetracyclines' bacteriostatic action (Grossman 2016), including enzymatic inactivation of the drugs via monooxygenase-mediated modification, out-competing their 30S binding by producing "ribosome-protecting" proteins, mutating the 16S ribosomal RNA that forms a vital component of the 30S target for the drugs, and/or impairing drug entry and even increasing active pumping out of the drugs via "Tet" transport pump protein expression.

Tetracyclines exert more overt toxicity than penicillins and cephalosporins, so their usage is generally more restricted. Tetracyclines, however, are the drugs of choice for tick- and flea-borne fevers and infections such as *Rickettsia* ("Rocky Mountain Spotted Fever"), *Yersinia pestis* ("The Black Plague"), and *Borrelia* ("Lyme Disease"). Other common clinical uses are in treating community-acquired pneumonia and mycoplasma pneumonia, infections with Gram-negative *Chlamydia*, *Vibrio cholera*, or *Helicobacter pylori* (*i.e.*, the infectious etiology of peptic ulceration), and uncomplicated cystitis and prostatitis (the latter being treated with **doxycycline** or **minocycline**, with alternatives being TMP-SMX or a fluoroquinolone [see next section]). **Doxycycline** has historically been a drug of second choice for prophylaxis against "Traveler's Diarrhea" (with drugs of first choice being fluoroquinolones); however, recent weighing of risks and benefits of this long-standing prophylaxis strategy (combined with the new development of vaccination strategies (Das et al. 2018)) has led for some to call for restricting this prophylactic usage of tetracyclines solely for select, high-risk travelers (*e.g.*, the immunosuppressed and/or those with comorbidities) and short-term, critical trips. (Diptyanusa et al. 2018) **Minocycline** is often added to TMP-SMX for those with nocardiosis unresponsive to the latter. Minocycline has historically been used to treat acne vulgaris. However, the newer **sarecycline** (Figure 3.5) has been specifically designed and tested as a narrow-spectrum tetracycline for acne treatment. (Zhanel et al. 2019) In contrast, **tigecycline** is broad spectrum and effective against otherwise tetracycline-resistant bacterial strains; for this reason, tigecycline is used for MRSA and vancomycin-resistant *Staphylococcus aureus* (VRSA) strains (Cong et al. 2020), as well as for multiple strains of *Streptococci* and vancomycin-susceptible *Enterococcus faecalis*. However, tigecycline use, especially against hospital-acquired pneumonia, increases mortality risk compared to other appropriate antibacterial treatments. (Dixit et al. 2014)

Figure 3.5 Structures of tetracyclines.

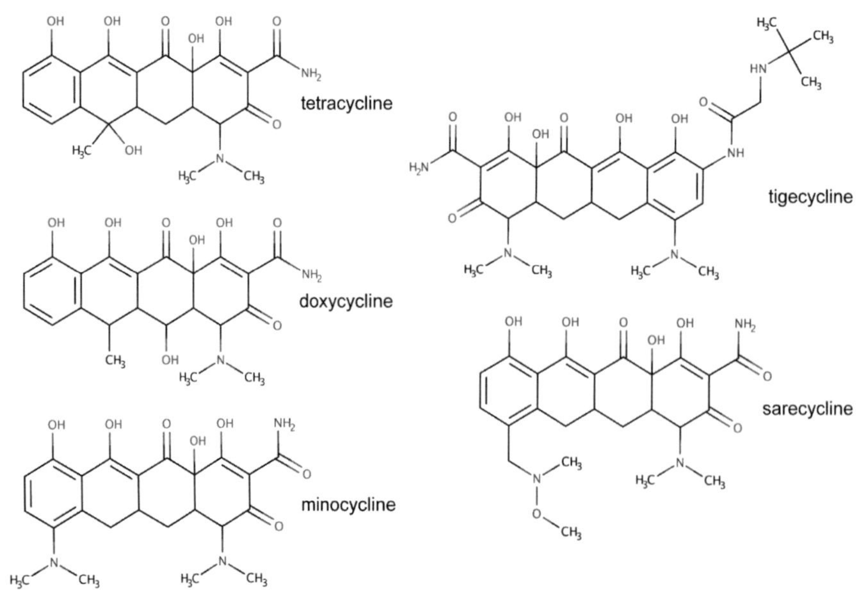

Tetracyclines are contraindicated for those who are pregnant (as these drugs cross the placenta). They are also avoided with children less than eight years of age owing to bone growth retardation and tooth developmental problems that can develop. Permanent discoloration of the teeth is a tell-tale sign of tetracycline use in early life. (Grossman et al. 1971) High-dose intravenous tetracycline was associated with acute fatty liver and severe hepatic dysfunction (Hooper and Jacoby 2016); this toxicity is rarely seen currently as tetracycline is no longer available in the parenteral form, and intravenous tetracycline use has been superseded by better tolerated and more effective broad-spectrum antibacterial agents. Tetracycline (but not the more lipid-soluble doxycycline or minocycline) can worsen renal dysfunction. Of particular note is **tetracycline-induced phototoxicity**: in combination with sunlight or other environmental light, the use of tetracycline can lead to itching, sunburn, and systemic fever (Hooper and Jacoby 2016). Given the broad spectrum nature of the tetracyclines, except for sarecycline (see above), the patient risks the development of **superinfection** ("suprainfection"), leading to secondary infection *in situ* and/or pathological changes in the overall makeup of the intestinal flora with potential pathologic overgrowth of *Proteus*, *Pseudomonas*, or *C. difficile* (*e.g.*, ref. (Yahav et al. 2011) for tigecycline).

Aminoglycosides (inhibitors of bacterial 30S ribosomal subunit functions)

Unlike the tetracyclines (*bacteriostatic* 30S subunit inhibitors), the **aminoglycosides** (Figure 3.6) are *bactericidal* in their action, a functional difference thought to result from multiple debilitating effects on bacterial 30S ribosomal subunit functions such as translational initiation, translocation, peptide chain (mis)coding, and termination. (*e.g.*, ref. (Aguirre Rivera et al. 2021)) Bacteria have evolved multiple strategies to overcome the aminoglycosides, including the trading of plasmid-encoded enzymes that adenylate, phosphorylate, or acetylate (and thereby inactivate) the aminoglycoside, the impairment of aminoglycoside accumulation via decreased permeability and/or increased efflux, and the chemical alteration of the 16S ribosomal RNA that represents a central target for aminoglycoside engagement within the 30S subunit. (Doi et al. 2016)

Figure 3.6 Structures of aminoglycosides.

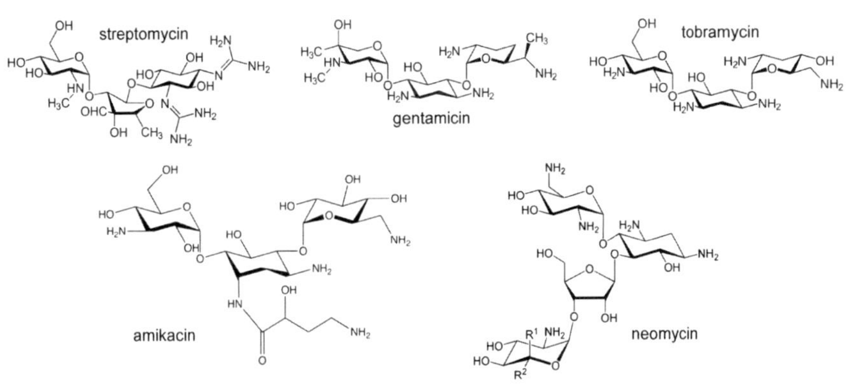

The aminoglycosides, administered by venous or intramuscular injection, are very effective in general against aerobic Gram-negative bacteria, especially when the patient is in sepsis and/or the bacteria involved are drug-resistant. **Gentamicin, tobramycin,** and **amikacin** are used on aerobic Gram-negative infections such as *Pseudomonas aeruginosa*, and **streptomycin** (the original aminoglycoside) is effective against plague, tularemia (Siderovski 2006), and drug-resistant tuberculosis. Streptomycin and gentamicin are also helpful against some Gram-positive bacteria, including *Enterococcus* species. However, neomycin is very toxic compared to the other aminoglycosides and is therefore reserved for topical uses only. The others are effectively used in combination with β-lactam antibacterial agents (see above), producing synergism (Kristich et al. 2014) and allowing for the reduction in dose (and therefore toxicity) of the aminoglycoside. When combined with a β-lactam antibiotic, the bactericidal action also has an extended spectrum (*e.g.*, effective use of penicillin and an aminoglycoside for Enterococcal endocarditis; ref. (Kristich et al. 2014)). Combining an aminoglycoside with antipseudomonal penicillin (*e.g.*, piperacillin) is an effective strategy for the Gram-negative *Pseudomonas aeruginosa*; the similar pairing of an aminoglycoside with ampicillin or a cephalosporin has often been seen for treating uncomplicated UTIs caused by *E. coli* or *Klebsiella pneumoniae* (although UTI treatment has become multifactorial in the face of advancing resistance development). (Bader et al. 2020)

Ototoxicity is a central, serious, and enduring toxicity associated with aminoglycoside usage. (Staecker 2021) If used in pregnancy, fetal exposure can lead to hearing loss in the newborn. The ototoxicity is not limited to causing auditory damage derived from hearing system neurotoxicity, but the vestibular system can also be damaged, leading to vertigo, balance loss, and ataxia. Aminoglycosides also exert neurotoxicity in other systems, are nephrotoxic, and can even cause neuromuscular blockade leading to respiratory paralysis at very high doses.

Chloramphenicol (inhibitor of bacterial 50S ribosomal subunit)
The single antibacterial agent **chloramphenicol** is broad spectrum but rather toxic and therefore restricted in its use to life-threatening infections. For example, chloramphenicol is a drug of last resort for penicillin-resistant bacterial meningitis cases: It is bacteriostatic against *Staphylococcus aureus* and family *Enterobacteriaceae* bacilli and bactericidal against *Haemophilus influenzae*, *Streptococcus pneumoniae*, and *Neisseria meningitidis* (Rahal and Simberkoff 1979). Chloramphenicol is also employed against *Rickettsia* and *Salmonella typhi* ("Typhoid Fever"), and (as a topical treatment) for eye infections. Bacteria develop chloramphenicol resistance primarily by trading amongst themselves a plasmid (circular DNA) encoding a chloramphenicol acetyltransferase protein, which acetylates (and thereby inactivates) chloramphenicol. (Schwarz et al. 2004)

The toxic nature of chloramphenicol is well-established and cannot be understated (Powell and Nahata 1982). It is rarely used outside the hospital setting and is contraindicated in pregnancy. Chloramphenicol can induce bone marrow hematopoiesis disturbances leading to anemia, reticulocytopenia, or, in rare yet fatal cases, aplastic anemia or pancytopenia. **"Gray Baby Syndrome"** (a.k.a. Gray or Grey syndrome) can affect children up to two years of age taking chloramphenicol and is of the highest risk for premature infants given hepatic insufficiency leading to impaired drug and metabolite clearance. This syndrome is characterized by circulatory collapse, presenting as a sudden blood pressure drop; given the lack of oxygenation, the skin and nails of the infant turn gray. If untreated, this circulatory collapse leads to poor feeding behavior, vomiting, vasomotor collapse, irregular respiration, and (ultimately) death.

Macrolides and the ketolide telithromycin (inhibitors of bacterial 50S ribosomal subunit)
The macrolides (**erythromycin, azithromycin, clarithromycin**; Figure 3.7) and the erythromycin-related ketolide **telithromycin** all target the bacterial 50S ribosomal subunit to inhibit protein synthesis; as they only inhibit bacterial protein synthesis, they are considered bacteriostatic, but at high enough doses, these antibacterial agents can achieve bactericidal action (Vazquez-Laslop and Mankin 2018). Bacteria can mount an effective resistance against these agents, such as modifying the ribosomal binding site, reducing membrane permeability and increasing active efflux to reduce active concentrations within the bacterium, and producing esterases to hydrolyze the drug.

Erythromycin and azithromycin have been the drugs of choice for community-acquired pneumonia (CAP), with a spectrum similar to that of penicillin G that includes *Streptococcus pneumoniae* and atypical causes of pneumonia (*e.g.*, *Mycoplasma* and *Legionella* species). Both macrolides are also effective against *Campylobacter jejuni* in cases of gastrointestinal (GI) upset or reactive arthritis. Azithromycin is a drug of second choice for sexually transmitted infections (STIs) of *Chlamydia trachomatis* and *Neisseria gonorrhea*. Clarithromycin is often part of combination pharmacotherapy (Zagari et al. 2021; Miftahussurur et al. 2017) for *Helicobacter pylori* (the infectious etiology of peptic ulceration): for example, "triple therapy" with amoxicillin and a proton-pump inhibitor (the latter to reduce stomach acidification) (Ierardi et al. 2019). The first clinically available ketolide in this grouping – telithromycin – is a drug of choice for macrolide-resistant bacterial strains, as these bacteria remain susceptible to the ketolide's structural modifications on the parental erythromycin chemotype (Figure 3.7). Adverse effects of these agents include GI intolerance due to direct stimulation of gut motility (although this is reduced with clarithromycin *versus* the prototypical erythromycin), and potential drug-drug interactions owing to erythromycin metabolites being able to inhibit cytochrome P450 enzymes.

Figure 3.7 Structures of macrolides and the ketolide telithromycin.

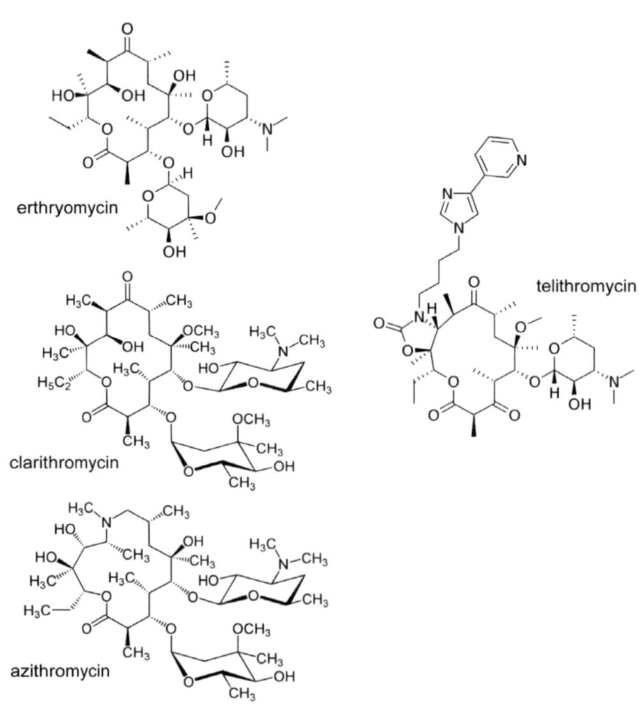

The lincosamide clindamycin (inhibitor of bacterial 50S ribosomal subunit)
Like the macrolides, **clindamycin** (the most prominent member of the lincosamide class) binds and inhibits the function of the bacterial 50S ribosomal subunit. Bacterial resistance to clindamycin arises similarly to macrolide resistance: modification of the 50S ribosomal binding site or enzymatic inactivation of the drug. Clinical uses for clindamycin include skin and soft tissue infections by *Streptococci* and *Staphylococci*, and infections involving anaerobes such as *Bacteroides fragilis*. Adverse side effects of clindamycin include diarrhea, nausea, skin rash, and impaired liver function (with or without the tell-tale sign of jaundice); more infrequently, clindamycin usage can lead to neutropenia.

Fluoroquinolones ("topoisomerase poisons"; inhibitors of DNA and RNA synthesis)
The fluoroquinolones block bacterial DNA synthesis by inhibiting their DNA gyrase and topoisomerase IV enzymes. These enzymes generate negative supercoils by untwisting DNA, relaxing the double-stranded helical DNA into an uncoiled state required for DNA replication and RNA transcription of encoded genes. The fluoroquinolones, as "topoisomerase poisons," trap these enzymes in a transient step of their catalytic cycle, leading to an accumulation of DNA replication forks and double-stranded breaks. The inhibitory action of the fluoroquinolone thereby prevents bacterial DNA and RNA synthesis, leading to broad-spectrum bactericidal activity against both Gram-positive and Gram-negative bacteria. Resistance to fluoroquinolones can arise via mutation to the enzymatic target(s) of fluoroquinolone (DNA gyrase, topo IV) or acquisition of increased expression of efflux pumps mediating fluoroquinolone export. (Hooper and Jacoby 2016)

While generally well tolerated, the fluoroquinolones can induce nausea, diarrhea, headache, dizziness, and/or confusion; if taken along with the asthma drug theophylline, the latter drug may increase in concentration owing to cytochrome P450 inhibition (Sarkar et al. 1990), leading to the potential for exceeding the induction threshold for seizures. Given the demonstrated risk of cartilage damage, fluoroquinolones are generally shunned for three demographic groups: those under 18 years of age (Playe 2007) and those who are pregnant (given fears of engendering an arthropathy or cartilaginous lesioning), as well as those over 60 years-of-age (given risk of cartilage erosion, tendinitis, and even tendon rupture).

As fluoroquinolones are generally well-tolerated and have broad-spectrum bactericidal action against both Gram-positive and Gram-negative bacteria, these antibiotics are used to treat a range of urinary tract, respiratory, gastrointestinal, and sexually transmitted infections, but usually as a second-line of defense. (Oliphant and Green 2002) Such usage includes cystitis, pyelonephritis, or prostatitis caused by multidrug-resistant UTI bacteria, penicillin-resistant syphilis or gonorrhea, and drug-resistant respiratory tract infections; indeed, given the latter, the fluoroquinolones **levofloxacin**, **moxifloxacin**, and **gemifloxacin** are nicknamed "respiratory fluoroquinolones". While useful for methicillin-*susceptible Staphylococcus aureus* infections (MSSA) (Beganovic et al. 2019), fluoroquinolones are not generally used with MRSA infections, as the acquisition of fluoroquinolone resistance is prevalent amongst MRSA strains. (Gade and Qazi 2013) Stockpiling and widespread distribution of **ciprofloxacin** were of particular concern (Josefson 2001) in the United States during the *Bacillus anthracis* (anthrax) domestic terrorism scare of 2001.

Metronidazole and Tinidazole (DNA-damaging nitroimidazoles)
In the reducing environment within anaerobic bacteria or protozoans, the nitroimidazole group found within **metronidazole** and **tinidazole** is converted into a reactive nitroso radical that can damage DNA and thereby inhibit the pathogen's ongoing DNA synthesis and proliferation. (Edwards 1980) Metronidazole and tinidazole are drugs of choice for managing infections caused by anaerobes (*e.g.*, *Bacteroides fragilis, Clostridium difficile*) and are also valuable for treating parasitic protozoal illnesses like Amebiasis, Giardiasis, Toxoplasmosis, and Trichomoniasis. Minor adverse effects of these agents include GI disturbances and a metallic or bitter taste in the mouth; significant CNS symptoms like dizziness, headache, and sensory/peripheral neuropathies are far more severe. In addition, these agents interfere with the metabolism of alcohol. Taken together, alcohol and metronidazole lead to disulfiram-like reactivity, including increased blood pressure, flushing, severe nausea, and vomiting. (*e.g.*, ref. (Alonzo et al. 2019))

Pharmacological Treatment of Mycobacterial Infections

Mycobacterial infections are highly persistent and thus considered separately, as unique drugs and drug combinations are employed, although some components often come from the antibacterial drug classes described earlier. The "Myco-" prefix means "*fungus*" in Greek, but these are indeed bacteria, not fungi; their observed, mold-like growth patterns on culture surfaces are reminiscent of fungal growth. Mycobacteria are classified as "Gram-positive" and, like other Gram-positive bacteria, lack an outer cell membrane; however, mycobacteria actually do not retain the crystal violet Gram stain *per se* and instead are stained red in "acid-fast" lab tests owing to retention of carbol fuchsin in their thick cell-wall peptidoglycan layers. (True *antifungal* drugs are considered in the subsequent section.)

Treating Mycobacterium tuberculosis infections
Mycobacterium tuberculosis complex (MTBC) consists of a closely related group of *Mycobacterium* species that cause tuberculosis (TB) in humans and other animals, including *M. tuberculosis*, *M. africanum*, *M. bovis*, and *M. bovis*

BCG. Latent tuberculosis is formally identified by a positive tuberculin skin test (PPD) or an interferon-gamma release assay (IGRA) (Kestler and Tyler 2022). Active tuberculosis is identified via chest radiograph evidence of lung infection, followed by laboratory confirmation of MTBC presence ("acid-fast red bacilli") in sputum smears. Both the latent and active stages are to be actively managed by combination pharmacotherapy with strict attention to patient adherence.

Latent TB Infection:
Standard treatments include months-long prescriptions of isoniazid and/or a rifamycin (*e.g*., rifapentine or rifampicin). **Isoniazid** (a.k.a. isonicotinic acid hydrate or "INH") has a unique bactericidal action against mycobacteria: inhibiting their synthesis of long fatty acids ("mycolic acids") that are uniquely required for building the mycobacterial cell wall. Mycobacterial species can resist the effects of isoniazid treatment by mutating or deleting their *katG* gene that encodes a catalase-peroxidase required to activate isoniazid and/or by overexpressing or mutating their *inhA* gene that encodes the enoyl reductase enzymatic target of activated isoniazid. Adverse effects of isoniazid treatment include elevated liver enzymes (AST, ALT) that can progress to frank hepatitis, peripheral neuropathy, and (more rarely) optic neuritis.

The rifamycins (*e.g*., **rifapentine**, **rifampicin**/rifampin) bind specifically to a beta-subunit of bacterial DNA-dependent RNA polymerase, blocking RNA synthesis by this enzyme. (Feklistov et al. 2008) Resistance to rifamycin action can develop within mycobacterial species, as mutation to their *rpoB* gene can reduce binding and blockade of RNA synthesis. (Shea et al. 2021) Rifamycin can cause bodily fluids, such as urine, sweat, and tears, to become orange-red in color, an innocuous side effect that nonetheless can be frightening if not forewarned. Health-adverse side effects of rifamycin usage include possible cholestatic jaundice and hepatitis, and the strong induction of cytochrome P450 enzymes, thereby increasing the degradation and elimination of several drugs/drug classes (*e.g*., warfarin, glucocorticoids, opioid analgesics, oral anti-diabetic drugs, and estrogen [the latter decreasing the effectiveness of oral contraceptives]).

Dosing these two drugs for latent TB can take on several different variations: *e.g*., nine months of daily isoniazid, or four months of daily rifampicin, or three months of weekly isoniazid plus rifapentine. The latter type of strategy (*i.e*., shorter duration with weekly, rather than daily, dosing) provides for better patient compliance, as the entire months-long duration of any one of these prescription strategies is vitally important for the patient to complete to eliminate the slow-growing MTBC infection.

Active TB Infection:
Even before lab tests are completed and analyzed, the presenting patient must begin a first-line, four-drug daily regimen of isoniazid, rifampicin, ethambutol, and pyrazinamide to counter the potential development of multi-drug resistant TB ("MDR-TB"). When lab tests are complete, unnecessary pyrazinamide treatment can be excluded from this regimen in confirmed cases of *M. bovis* or *M. bovis BCG* infection, since these two related mycobacterial strains are pyrazinamide resistant. In addition, ethambutol can be excluded if susceptibility testing confirms that the patient's isolate is sensitive to the first-line drugs of isoniazid and rifampicin.

Structurally related to nicotinamide (a.k.a. vitamin B3), **pyrazinamide** is a pro-drug that must be converted to pyrazinoic acid by a mycobacterial pyrazinamidase (encoded by the *pncA* gene). Pyrazinoic acid was initially thought to disrupt mycobacterial cell membrane metabolism and transport functions and, more recently, has been identified as targeting mycobacterial aspartate decarboxylase for destruction (Gopal et al. 2020); resistance to these actions can arise from loss-of-function mutation to the *pncA* gene or impairments to pyrazinamide uptake. Adverse reactions to pyrazinamide treatment include fever, nausea/vomiting, and joint pain. Resultant hyperuricemia may provoke acute gouty arthritis, and 1-5% of pyrazinamide users experience hepatotoxicity.

Ethambutol, similarly to how isoniazid acts, has a unique bacteriostatic action against mycobacteria: inhibiting their synthesis of specific arabinogalactans that are uniquely required for building the mycobacterial cell wall. Resistance can therefore develop by mutation to the mycobacterial *embB* gene within the *embCAB* operon that encodes the targeted arabinosyl transferase enzyme. Optic neuritis can develop when taking ethambutol, leading to a dramatic impairment in visual acuity and color vision.

Infection with Multi-Drug Resistant (MDR) TB:
Drug-resistant TB can occur when the regimens used to treat active or latent TB infections are misused or mismanaged, including lack of completion of an entire course of treatment, original prescription of the wrong treatment (*e.g*., wrong dosing, wrong length of time), or drug availability or quality issues. The formal definition of Multi-Drug Resistant (MDR) tuberculosis is demonstrated resistance to at least isoniazid and rifampicin (the two first-line drugs discussed above) and yet susceptibility to second-line anti-tuberculosis drugs. Formal diagnosis or suspicion of MDR TB (the latter based on geographical and epidemiological considerations) requires escalation of treatment duration, a more extensive combination of drugs (increasing adverse effect burden and potential for drug-drug interactions), and the evocation of specialized, second-line TB drugs that have more serious adverse effect potentials. An initial intensive treatment phase of five or more months involves at least five orally available anti-TB drugs (Table

3.2) plus at least one injectable agent (*i.e.*, amikacin, streptomycin, capreomycin, or carbapenem with clavulanate). A second, continuation phase of up to 21 additional months involves at least four drugs from among those listed in Table 3.2. Among this list, **cycloserine** is an older, simpler compound reminiscent of the structure of D-alanine and thus found to inhibit mycobacterial peptidoglycan synthesis. (Prosser and de Carvalho 2013) Two of the newer drugs available for this combination regimen are **bedaquiline**, a diarylquinolone that blocks mycobacterial ATP production, and **delamanid**, a nitroimidazole able to block the synthesis of mycolic acids. (Blair and Scott 2015)

Table 3.2. American Thoracic Society / CDC / European Respiratory Society / Infectious Disease Society of America recommendations(Nahid et al. 2019) for or against the use of individual agents in combination regimens to address drug-resistant tuberculosis

Drug (drug-class)	*Recommendation for MDR TB?*
Bedaquiline (diarylquinolone)	Strongly in favor
Moxifloxacin (fluoroquinolone)	Strongly in favor
Levofloxacin (fluoroquinolone)	Strongly in favor
Linezolid	Conditional
Clofazimine	Conditional
Cycloserine	Conditional
Ethambutol	Conditional
Pyrazinamide	Conditional
Delamanid (nitroimidazole)	Conditional
Amikacin (injectable; aminoglycoside)	Conditional
Streptomycin (injectable; aminoglycoside)	Conditional
Carbapenems + clavulanate (injectable)	Conditional
Kanamycin (injectable; aminoglycoside)	Against
Capreomycin (injectable; aminoglycoside)	Against
p-Aminosalicylic acid	Against
Ethionamide or **Prothioamide (thioamides)**	Against
Amoxicillin + clavulanate	Strongly against
Azithromycin or **Clarithromycin (macrolides)**	Strongly against

Infection with Extensively Drug-Resistant (XDR) TB:
Active, extensively drug-resistant (XDR) tuberculosis is rare, comprising ~5% of MDR TB cases. The formal definition of XDR TB is demonstrated resistance to isoniazid, rifampicin, any fluoroquinolone, and at least one of the second-line injectable drugs (Table 3.2). The American Food and Drug Administration (FDA) and European Medicines Agency (EMA) have both recently approved a new nitroimidazole drug, called **pretomanid** to reflect its origins from the Pretoria, South Africa non-profit group TB Alliance, to be used in combination with bedaquiline and linezolid for the treatment of extensively drug-resistant, treatment-intolerant, or non-responsive MDR tuberculosis. (Lenaerts et al. 2005)

Treating Hansen's Disease (Leprosy)
Hansen's disease (formerly called leprosy) is caused by long-term infection with *Mycobacterium leprae* or *Mycobacterium lepromatosis*. There are two types of infection observed: **Tuberculoid infection**, also called paucibacillary (*"few bacilli"*) leprosy, in which the patient's T-cells vigorously produce interferon-gamma enabling macrophages to kill intracellular microbes; and, **Lepromatous infection** or multibacillary ("many bacilli") leprosy in which the patient's immune response is dominated by IL-4 production to the detriment of interferon-gamma production. (Paludan 1998) Tuberculoid infection is treated with a combination of dapsone and rifampicin, whereas lepromatous infection adds clofazimine to the regimen. The sulfone **dapsone** is similar to the sulfonamides (described earlier; see Figure 3.4) in that it works as a folate antagonist, inhibiting the mycobacterial synthesis of dihydrofolic acid by competing with PABA for binding to dihydropteroate synthase. Red blood cell hemolysis (especially if the patient is G6PDH-deficient) is an adverse effect of dapsone shared with the sulfonamides; other adverse side effects of

dapsone usage include liver inflammation, skin rashes, and methemoglobinemia – the oxidation of hemoglobin from the ferrous (Fe^{2+}) to the ferric state (Fe^{3+}; the latter does not combine with oxygen). The drug **clofazimine** has been ascribed at least three different mechanisms of action: (i) binding guanine bases within mycobacterial DNA, (Morrison and Marley 1976) (ii) activating bacterial phospholipase A2 to release toxic lysophospholipids, (Arbiser and Moschella 1995) and (iii) inhibiting acid sphingomyelinase. (Kornhuber et al. 2011) Adverse effects of clofazimine usage include the development of skin discoloration (ranging from red-brown to nearly black) and (occasionally) GI intolerance.

Infectious Disease – Fungal/Parasitic – General Background

Fungal and parasitic infections are not as common as bacterial and viral infections but constitute a significant portion of infectious disease care. Depending on how they grow, fungi are classified as either yeast, mold, or dimorphic. Fungal infections are often only limited in nature, given the body's natural defenses and deeper infections affecting solid organs or other areas are rare in immunocompetent patients. (Lionakis and Edwards Jr 2022) Parasitic, protozoan, and helminthic infections are also quite rare, particularly in first-world countries where strict protocols are in place about water and food hygiene, inspection, and treatments. Many of the most common infections are in tropical and subtropical regions. (Mathison and Pritt 2022) The recent development of immunomodulating drugs and the use of steroids has increased the overall incidence of fungal and parasitic infections as they affect normal immune response mechanisms. Similarly, these infections are more prevalent in patients with HIV and acquired immunodeficiency syndrome (AIDS), as these also affect the immune system. (Anderson et al. 2022)

Diagnosis

Specific diagnostic pathways exist for fungi depending on what the presumptive diagnosis is. Cultures, unfortunately, may take weeks to grow and are not always sensitive enough to be useful in clinical practice. The best way to diagnose a fungal infection would be from a microscopic examination of a tissue showing invasion of a fungus into it, but this is not always achievable. Certain stains help identify fungi in microscopic samples, with the most common being periodic acid-Schiff (PAS) and Gömöri methenamine silver (GMS). There are now also antigen and serologic tests available for various fungi such as Blastomycosis, Coccidiomycosis, and Histoplasmosis. (Lionakis and Edwards Jr 2022)

Central Nervous System Infections

Presentation

Like bacterial and viral infections of the CNS, fungal and parasitic infections will have a variety of presentations that can include symptoms such as fever, headache, altered mentation, and possibly focal neurologic deficits. While bacterial meningitis usually has a more acute presentation, fungal meningitis from organisms like Cryptococcus, Aspergillus, Coccidioides, Blastomycosis, and Histoplasmosis are usually more subacute or insidious in nature. While immunocompromised states significantly increase the chances of these organisms, Cryptococcus and Coccidioides species are known to cause disease in patients with intact immune systems. Patients with focal neurologic signs raise concern more for cerebral abscess, and headache is a common symptom. Parasitic infections are uncommon, but *Toxoplasma gondii* is an important cause in immunocompromised patients such as those with HIV/AIDS. Toxoplasmosis can cause more subtle symptoms at first, such as changes in personality. Other etiologies, such as *Naegleria fowleri* (which causes primary amebic meningoencephalitis (Bosch et al. 2022)) and *Entamoeba histolytica* (which causes cerebral amebiasis (Bosch and Siderovski 2013)), can create symptoms similar to other causes of meningitis or meningoencephalitis and should be suspected in patients with recent exposures to untreated fresh water. Cerebral malaria causes encephalopathy and can lead to coma. Neurocysticercosis caused by *Taenia solium*, the pork tapeworm, can present with focal lesions of the CNS with focal neurologic findings; neurocysticercosis is a frequent cause of seizures, epilepsy, and other neurological morbidities in much of the world. (Bustos et al. 2021) Echinococcus species of parasites are also a rare cause of CNS lesions with focal findings. (Anderson et al. 2022) Neuroschistosomiasis, an infection of the CNS by a blood fluke of the genus Schistosoma, is common in tropical regions and can cause substantial neurological disability. (Ferrari and Moreira 2011)

Risk factors

Immunocompromised states remain a common topic, but even more so for fungal and parasitic infections. Exposure to certain animals (such as livestock), freshwater, recent intestinal amebiasis, and travel to or living in endemic areas are all risk factors for these infections. Certain organisms, like Candida species and Pneumocystis, rarely cause CNS disease unless there is disseminated disease. Although rare, given improvements in sterilization techniques, exposure of the CNS to the environment during surgical procedures or history of previous instrumentation of any part of the CNS are risk factors for these infections. Diabetes mellitus remains a significant risk factor for these infections as well, regardless of immune status. (Anderson et al. 2022)

Pathophysiology

Fungi and parasites arrive in the CNS in a variety of ways. Disseminated spread is one way to traffic to the CNS, in which a total body infection can spread via blood. Local extension, such as from the sinuses, is also seen. Fungal organisms like Blastomyces, Histoplasma, and Coccidioides are often inhaled and can spread from the lungs to the rest of the body. (Anderson et al. 2022) Fungi can cause overt disease in a variety of ways: fungal replication, leading to tissue invasion and disrupted tissue/organ function; elicitation of an immunopathological response (via cell-mediated or humoral responses); metabolic competition (*i.e.*, consuming local nutrient and energy stores to the exclusion of intended cellular recipients); and, production of toxic metabolites (*e.g.*, some Candida species produce carcinogenic acetaldehyde).

Parasitic infections can sometimes also be caused by inhalation, such as infection from *Naegleria fowleri* via accidentally "inhaling" contaminated water up the nose. Interestingly, the invasion from Naegleria is not from the lungs but via the olfactory nerve. More commonly, parasitic infections begin from ingesting the organism via the fecal-oral route from contaminated water or food, such as in the cases of *Entamoeba histolytica* and *Taenia solium* infections. (Koshy 2021)

Examination

The exam in patients with fungal or parasitic infections of the CNS does not differ from that of bacterial or viral infections. Patients may have altered mental status/confusion, headache, photophobia, and possibly fever. Focal neurologic findings should prompt concern for abscess, as meningitis/encephalitis cases cause more global effects. There are very few exam findings that may suggest fungal or parasitic etiology. In the case of *Taenia solium*, direct visualization may be possible on a fundoscopic exam. Other organ systems such as the lungs or GI tract being affected may signal disseminated disease from these sources. (Anderson et al. 2022)

Laboratory

Leukocytosis may or may not be present in fungal and parasitic infections. Still, there is often local and peripheral eosinophilia, as this subset of WBCs is involved in the defense from these organisms. Their presence is neither perfectly sensitive nor specific but could be a diagnostic clue in the right setting. Suspicion of an infection affecting the CNS will likely result in a lumbar puncture and various tests that can be performed on the resultant CSF specimen. Glucose is often decreased, protein is increased, and mononuclear pleocytosis often occurs. This is not specific either, but it can also begin to suggest the diagnosis. (Anderson et al. 2022) India ink smears can be performed and may diagnose cryptococcus. (Lionakis and Edwards Jr 2022) CSF cultures can be performed but may take weeks and be falsely negative. Various PCR, antigen, antibody, and enzyme immunoassays (EIA) tests are now available for infections like Cryptococcus, Coccidioides, and Histoplasma. Galactomannan and beta-D-glucan tests on the CSF are helpful to determine that there are fungal wall components but also are not specific to one type. Eosinophilic pleocytosis, where there is more than 10% CSF eosinophilia, can be from parasites *Taenia solium* and *Angiostrongylus cantonensis* (a cause of the entity eosinophilic meningitis). However, this finding is not unique to parasites, as it can also be found in infections from fungi like coccidioides, or even tuberculosis or sarcoidosis. (Anderson et al. 2022) If *Naegleria fowleri* infection is suspected, such as illness after swimming in a lake, a wet mount of CSF can be performed and may show the mobile trophozoites. (Koshy 2021)

Imaging

MRI and CT imaging of the CNS can provide valuable information on fungal and parasitic infections. Both imaging modalities can clearly identify focal lesions and can provide important diagnostic clues. Multiple different findings can be very specific, such as the cystic lesions with scolex (head of the tapeworm) of neurocysticercosis or the ring-enhancing lesions in the gray matter seen in toxoplasmosis. (Koshy 2021) Because these findings are related to the soft tissue, MRI with and without contrast is the preferred imaging modality, given a higher sensitivity and specificity. Fungal abscesses can also be visualized, although they may not differ in appearance from bacterial abscesses. (Anderson et al. 2022) Imaging can also be helpful when a biopsy needs to be performed. (Perfect 2021)

Associated symptoms/conditions

HIV and AIDS remain the most commonly associated conditions with fungal and parasitic infections of the CNS. Other immunocompromising conditions, such as solid organ transplants and neutropenia from chemotherapy, can be associated with fungal and parasitic infections. Infection of other organs, such as intestinal infection with *Entamoeba histolytica*, is associated with cerebral amebiasis. (Anderson et al. 2022)

Diagnosis

As is often the case, an official diagnosis is usually reached using a combination of history, physical exam, appropriate imaging, and laboratory testing. The presentation can give many diagnostic clues that help focus testing for a suspected diagnosis. Exposure to fresh water may prompt a wet mount or PCR testing of CSF for *Naegleria fowleri*, ingestion of undercooked pork may prompt fundoscopic examination, CSF antibody and MRI testing for possible neurocysticercosis, and travel to endemic areas can prompt MRI and serology/PCR testing for cerebral malaria from *Plasmodium falciparum* or cerebral amebiasis from *Entamoeba histolytica*. Many facilities now have a rapid meningitis panel including Cryptococcal antigen testing. Rarely, meningeal biopsies can be performed and histopathological examination is used for diagnosis. (Anderson et al. 2022)

Treatment

Infections of the CNS carry significant morbidity and mortality, and fungal and parasitic etiologies are no different. Various medication regimens exist depending on the organism responsible, and courses are usually longer than for bacterial infections. **Amphotericin B** is not used often in clinical practice due to side effects (mainly renal toxicity), except in these types of infections, given their severity. Some infections require a period of "induction," where aggressive treatment with amphotericin B is used and later transitioned to another antifungal with fewer side effects. It is used to manage cryptococcus, histoplasmosis, sporotrichosis, blastomycosis, and candidiasis. Azole antifungals are also commonly used across these regimens, such as **fluconazole**, **itraconazole** and **voriconazole**. (Anderson et al. 2022) **Fluconazole** remains one of the most commonly used antifungals in CNS infections and plays in role in treating cryptococcosis, coccidioidomycosis, blastomycosis, and candidiasis. The recent development of resistant Candida species requires the use of broader azoles like **voriconazole**, which is also commonly used. (Perfect 2021) Unlike bacterial meningitis, corticosteroids are not routinely used except in cases of immune reconstitution inflammatory syndrome (IRIS) in HIV patients and are most often seen with cryptococcal meningitis. (Anderson et al. 2022) Parasitic CNS infections have a wide array of treatments depending on the etiology. Given their rarity, contacting the Centers for Disease Control (CDC) is recommended. Treatment of Toxoplasmosis encephalitis with the folate antagonists **pyrimethamine** and **sulfadiazine** is recommended for immunocompromised patients. Cerebral malaria is managed as severe malaria with **artesunate**. Various regimens have been used for amebic meningoencephalitis, but there is no definite treatment given how few patients are diagnosed before death. Neurocysticercosis can be managed with the anthelmintic benzimidazole **albendazole** and corticosteroids when there are only one or two parenchymal viable cysts seen on imaging, but treatment requires the addition of **praziquantel** when there are more. Neuroschistosomiasis is similarly treated with **praziquantel** and corticosteroids. (Koshy 2021)

Management

Apart from medical antifungal or antiparasitic therapy, some infections require surgical intervention. Careful attention should be paid to signs of increased intracranial pressure in fungal CNS infections. If this is suspected, patients may require a ventriculostomy by a neurosurgeon to relieve the pressure and prevent herniation. Cerebral abscesses may also require neurosurgical intervention for drainage. Salvage therapy for refractory coccidioidomycosis requires intrathecal **amphotericin B** in combination with azole therapy. Cerebral amebiasis is usually treated with a combination of surgical drainage, **metronidazole**, and **paromomycin**. Neurocysticercosis affecting the eye should be managed with surgical removal of the cyst and sometimes when cysts are present in the spine or certain areas of the ventricles. (Koshy 2021)

Upper and Lower Respiratory Infections

Presentation

Fungal infections of the upper and lower respiratory tract do not often occur, particularly in immunocompetent patients. Therefore, patients may have a history of immunocompromising diseases like HIV/AIDS or be post-transplant. Candida species, particularly *Candida albicans*, are ubiquitous and normally present in our skin and GI tract. Thrush, a painless condition of white tongue patches, is caused by Candida and can be seen often in clinical practice. (Jameson et al. 2020) More severe infections with Candida are rare and related to disseminated disease. These include empyema, and airway and mediastinal infections. (Saullo and Alexander 2022) Other fungal infections of the airway may have indolent and long-standing symptoms, ranging from nasal congestion, epistaxis, shortness of breath, cough, fever, or hemoptysis. Given that most patients with these infections are immunocompromised, patients may present quite ill and require inpatient management or even intensive care unit care. Some infections may become disseminated and cause various symptoms relating to the airways and other body parts. Coccidioidomycosis, the organism responsible for Valley Fever, can present with subtle flu-like symptoms like fatigue and headache. As discussed, Blastomyces and Histoplasma are also often inhaled like Coccidioides and affect the lungs first. While the risk of progression to pneumonia and disseminated disease is present in certain patients, the disease is most often self-limited. Overall, symptoms can be very non-specific, and careful attention should be paid to particular geographic locations where patients may have been exposed. (Nosanchuk and Thompson 2022) *Pneumocystis jirovecii* is another commonly encountered fungus in clinical practice that causes pneumonia and is the most common AIDS-defining infection in the United States. (Crothers et al. 2022) Of note, *Pneumocystis jirovecii* pneumonia is sometimes referred to as "PCP" given that it was previously known as *Pneumocystis carinii*. (Jameson et al. 2020) Aspergillus, Mucor, and Rhizopus are opportunistic infections that can cause devastating diseases in patients with predisposing conditions. Mucor and Rhizopus are organisms attributed to mucormycosis, which can infect the airway from the nasal passages all the way down to the lung parenchyma. Aspergillus, Mucor, and Rhizopus species can lead to life-threatening hemoptysis as they are angioinvasive, which can cause thrombosis and necrosis of tissue. (Saullo and Alexander 2022) Parasitic airway infections are rare, but Ascariasis, Dirofiliriasis, Strongyloidiasis, tropical pulmonary eosinophilia from *Wucharia bancrofti*, Schistosomiasis, Amebiasis, and Trypanosomiasis are some of the entities that can present with a variety of nonspecific pulmonary symptoms like dyspnea, pleuritic chest pain, and fever. Many of these entities affect the lung only in disseminated cases. (Kim and Weiss 2022)

Risk factors
Immunosuppression is the most important of all factors for airway-related fungal and parasitic infections. HIV/AIDS and transplant patients make up a significant percentage of all patients with these infections, particularly those that are severe. Whether oral, parenteral or even inhaled, steroid therapy can also be a risk. (Nosanchuk and Thompson 2022) Diabetes, neutropenia, and malignancy also increase the risk of infections like mucormycosis. (Jameson et al. 2020)

Pathophysiology
As mentioned in CNS infections, most fungi enter the body via inhalation from the environment. Various factors, such as the virulence of the fungus, how many spores/yeast/mold cells are inhaled, host immune factors, and comorbidities, can impact whether the clinical disease progresses and to what severity. Some fungi are ubiquitous, such as Candida, Aspergillus, and Mucor species, are therefore termed opportunistic because they only cause clinical disease when there is an issue with normal host defense. (Saullo and Alexander 2022) Other fungi are termed endemic, meaning they are only present in certain geographic areas, so patients must have been in an area containing that organism to inhale them. Histoplasmosis, Blastomycosis, Coccidioidomycosis, and Paracoccidioidomycosis are all endemic fungi. These are also the fungi that can cause disease even in immunocompetent patients. Histoplasma is inhaled, phagocytosed, and migrates to the lymph nodes in the chest, where it can then spread via the blood. Similarly, Coccidioides is inhaled and forms the unique structure termed a spherule, which ruptures and can also spread via the lymphatics. Blastomyces are inhaled as conidia and transform into a "yeast form" at body temperature, which is more resistant than the conidia to immune response and can then spread out from the lungs via the blood or lymphatics. (Nosanchuk and Thompson 2022) *Pneumocystis jirovecii* is found worldwide and inhaled from the environment. Like the previously mentioned organisms, it reaches the alveolar spaces and proliferates there, causing an immune response that subsequently causes damage and impaired oxygen exchange. Pneumocystis pneumonia is seen almost exclusively in HIV/AIDS patients with a CD4+ T-cell count of fewer than 200 cells/mm^3, although most cases develop when CD4 counts are less than 100. (Jameson et al. 2020) Parasitic infections of the airway are rare and pulmonary infection is usually the result of hematogenous or local spread. Echinococcus, Toxoplasmosis, hookworms, and amebiasis are examples of parasites that can cause lung infection in disseminated disease. Helminths like Ascariasis, hookworms, Trichinosis, and Strongyloides cause disease as their larvae migrate from the lungs to the GI tract. They can cause an asthma-like syndrome with increased eosinophils and serum IgE levels. Filariae cause tropical pulmonary eosinophilia, but the pathophysiology is poorly understood. (Kim and Weiss 2022)

Examination
Fungal and parasitic infections of the nasal passages, pharynx, sinuses, and conducting airways are rare and may present with local symptoms. Thrush will show classic white plaques on the tongue. Mucormycosis can cause eye or facial pain, numbness, and swelling. Areas affected may show a black, necrotic eschar due to tissue thrombosis. Aspergillus can also cause invasive sinusitis with facial discomfort and discharge. Pulmonary infections by fungi will have nonspecific exam findings ranging from rhonchi, rales, wheezing, hypoxia, hemoptysis, and even sepsis. Patients with disseminated disease may have a wide range of findings, such as cutaneous or CNS changes. (Jameson et al. 2020)

Laboratory
Routine laboratory testing may show leukocytosis or leukopenia depending on multiple factors. Patients with neutropenia are susceptible to fungal and parasitic infections, so this finding may already be present. Increased lactate dehydrogenase is seen in Pneumocystis patients due to pulmonary damage but is neither specific nor sensitive. (Jameson et al. 2020) Beta-D-glucan, a fungal wall component, can be measured in the blood and is seen in invasive Candida, Aspergillus, and Pneumocystis. Cryptococcus and Mucormycosis are notable exceptions. False positives are known to happen with dialysis membranes, intravenous immunoglobulin infusions, and other blood products, making the test less useful in transplant populations who may require these interventions. Serum galactomannan is another component of fungal cell walls and is seen in Aspergillus but has cross-reactivity with other fungi such as Fusarium and Histoplasma. (Saullo and Alexander 2022) Bronchoalveolar lavage (BAL) performed during bronchoscopy by a pulmonologist or intensivist has significant utility in diagnosing invasive pulmonary aspergillosis, with a sensitivity of 87% and specificity of 89% on meta-analysis. (Zou et al. 2012) Histopathological evaluation of biopsy tissue using stains like hematoxylin and eosin (H&E), periodic acid-Schiff, and GMS can also aid in identifying the organism. Cultures are also crucial for the speciation of various fungi species, particularly Candida. Various other modalities, like PCR and antigen testing, are available for fungi like Histoplasma and Coccidioides and can also be run on BAL samples for suspected pulmonary disease. (Jameson et al. 2020) Parasitic infections may manifest with peripheral eosinophilia and may also cause increased sputum eosinophils. Sputum can also be stained and smeared for direct visual analysis by microscopy. Serologic testing is available for Strongyloides. (Kim and Weiss 2022)

Imaging
Fungal infections can have a variety of imaging findings on radiographs and CT scans. Mucormycosis and Aspergillosis affecting the upper respiratory structures such as the nose and pharynx can cause findings of bony and anatomical distortion and destruction, inflammatory changes, and extension of disease into the sinuses. (Jameson et al. 2020) Chest imaging may reveal nodules, mass-like consolidations, cavitations, and other nonspecific interstitial findings. A halo or reversed halo sign, where a ground glass opacity is surrounded by a ring of consolidation, is also

seen in Aspergillosis and Mucormycosis. Mediastinal and/or hilar lymphadenopathy can be seen in Histoplasmosis, Coccidioidomycosis, and Cryptococcosis. (Nosanchuk and Thompson 2022) Parasites can also have many of these findings, although given their increased size and movement, "tracks" of their movement across the lungs can be seen. Pleural effusions can occur and may also have an eosinophilic predominance. Hydatid cysts have a very particular appearance of daughter cysts within a larger cyst. Imaging can also reveal fistulas, a mechanism of the spread of Entamoeba from the liver to the pleural space. (Kim and Weiss 2022)

Associated symptoms/conditions

Like other fungal and parasitic infections, any immunocompromising condition can be associated with clinical disease. Interestingly, because so many of the aforementioned fungi are inhaled, soil disturbances such as sandstorms and construction can aerolize cells and cause outbreaks. (Nosanchuk and Thompson 2022) Toxoplasmosis sheds oocysts in cat feces and is thereby highly infectious to cat owners. Poor sanitization of food and raw, contaminated meats are associated with multiple parasites. (Kim and Weiss 2022)

Diagnosis

As with most medical diagnoses, fungal and parasitic infections are made from a combination of clinical findings and history. Thrush is probably the most straightforward diagnosis, given its characteristic white plaque appearance on the tongue. Diagnosis of other fungal upper or lower respiratory infections is best made with either culture or isolation of the fungus in infected tissue. Diagnosis is delayed in many cases due to nonspecific presentations and exam findings. Direct observation via microscope can provide a rapid diagnosis in some cases, and antigen testing also offers quick results. Blastomyces, Histoplasma, Cryptococcus, Coccidioides, and Paracoccidioides have antigen assays available that can be used on serum or sputum samples and aid in diagnosis. (Nosanchuk and Thompson 2022) As discussed in laboratory findings, beta-D-glucan and galactomannan can also be helpful, especially if present in BAL samples in the case of invasive pulmonary aspergillosis. Candida pneumonia can be difficult to diagnose given that Candida normally colonizes the airway, so positive cultures have a low positive predictive value for an actual infection. Findings of beta-D-glucan in the serum can suggest actual, invasive Candida species infection versus a colonizer. Clinical worsening without other explanation may also favor this diagnosis. Aspergillus can cause a range of pulmonary entities, including aspergilloma, nodules, invasive aspergillosis, chronic cavitary pulmonary aspergillosis, and chronic fibrosing pulmonary aspergillosis, and diagnosis is usually multidisciplinary. (Saullo and Alexander 2022) Parasitic infections of the airways are typically diagnosed with an examination of sputum or tissue under the microscope using a variety of stains, where they can be identified and speciated. PCR testing is available for Pneumocystis, Leishmania, and Entamoeba. (Kim and Weiss 2022)

Treatment

Antifungal management of upper and lower respiratory fungal infections varies with organism and severity. Thrush is usually managed with **nystatin** swish and spit regimens. (Jameson et al. 2020) Mild to moderate Histoplasmosis and Blastomycosis can be managed with **itraconazole**, with liposomal **amphotericin B** reserved for severe or disseminated disease. Acute pneumonia from coccidioides with mild to moderate illness does not warrant treatment in immunocompetent patients. **Fluconazole** or **itraconazole** is used in severe diseases, and **amphotericin B** is reserved for disseminated cases. Given the rarity of paracoccidioides, no single regimen has been recommended, but **itraconazole** and **ketoconazole** have been commonly used. (Nosanchuk and Thompson 2022) Treatment for Cryptococcus varies depending on other areas affected and immune status, with immunocompromised patients receiving induction therapy with liposomal **amphotericin B** followed by prolonged treatment with **fluconazole**. Given the variety of species of Candida and possible azole-resistance, echinocandins like **micafungin** or **caspofungin** are used initially until speciation and sensitivity results return and show whether treatment can be de-escalated to **fluconazole**. Medical treatment of aspergillus and its various presentations can vary, but **voriconazole** is often preferred. **Isavuconazole** is also first-line for the treatment of invasive aspergillosis. Mucormycosis can be life-threatening and has a high chance of mortality, so liposomal **amphotericin B** is the agent of choice. (Saullo and Alexander 2022) Pneumocystis can be managed with **trimethoprim-sulfamethoxazole (TMP-SMX)** for 14 days in non-HIV patients with mild disease and 21 days for all others. Patients with moderate to severe disease, which includes patients with an atmospheric-alveolar gradient higher than 35 or arterial oxygen tension of less than 70 on room air, should receive adjunctive glucocorticoids as it has been shown to improve survival rates. (Jameson et al. 2020) The anthelmintic benzimidazoles **albendazole** and **mebendazole** (Table 3.3) are used to treat a variety of roundworms/nematodes such as ascariasis, hookworm, and trichinosis infections. Ameba infections have no definitive, effective treatment, and their management can vary. **Ivermectin** is used for Strongyloides infections and is recommended in all patients, given the risk of autoinfection. Tropical pulmonary eosinophilia is managed with the antifilarial drug **diethylcarbamazine**. (Kim and Weiss 2022)

Management

Many fungal and parasitic infections require treatment outside of antifungal or antiparasitic agents. Given its proximity to the mediastinum, Histoplasmosis may cause mediastinal granulomas that require surgical removal. Histoplasmosis may also cause fibrosing mediastinitis, which sometimes requires intravascular stenting. Cavitary lesions, as a consequence of fungal infections, may also require surgical removal. (Nosanchuk and Thompson 2022)

Management of aspergillosis sometimes also warrants cardiothoracic consultation, such as in symptomatic aspergillomas (*e.g.*, hemoptysis). Interventional radiology consultation may also be needed in other cases of hemoptysis from fungal infections to embolize the responsible bronchial artery. Mucormycosis often requires surgical consultation for debulking the disease. (Saullo and Alexander 2022) Certain parasites also require surgical removal, such as *Dirofilaria immitis* (dog heartworm) and *Echinococcus granulosus* (Hydatid cyst). (Kim and Weiss 2022)

Table 3.3. Clinical utility, mechanisms of action, and adverse effects of several antihelminthic drugs

Drug:	**albendazole**	**mebendazole**	**pyrantel pamoate**	**ivermectin**	**praziquantel**	**niclosamide**
Clinical use	Nematodes Tapeworms	Nematodes Tapeworms	Nematodes	Nematodes	Flatworms Tapeworms	Tapeworms
Mechanism of action	Binds worm β-tubulin to inhibit microtubule polymerization (*higher dose?*) Uncouples oxidative phosphorylation	Binds worm β-tubulin to inhibit microtubule polymerization	Direct acetylcholine release & inhibits cholinesterases ↓ Depolarizing neuromuscular block causes worm paralysis (*Poor intestinal absorption of drug limits actions to worms, not host*)	Activates glutamate-gated Cl^- channels ↓ Tonic paralysis of worm musculature	Increases muscular activity, followed by spastic paralysis, possibly by increasing Ca^{++} permeability ↓ Affected worms detach from host tissues	Inhibits glucose uptake, oxidative phosphorylation, and anaerobic metabolism of tapeworm
Adverse effects	Mild (GI upset; dizziness, headache) **Contraindicated** in 1st trimester of pregnancy	Rare (GI upset) **Contraindicated** in pregnancy *(teratogenic)*	Mild (GI upset; dizziness, headache)	Mild for most; 1-3% get fever, hypotension, bronchospasm	Mild (GI upset; dizziness, headache)	Mild (GI upset)

Fungemia and Infective Endocarditis

Presentation

Fungal infections of the heart are rare but have grown in incidence, likely from increased access to healthcare, identification, and diagnosis, as well as the use of indwelling catheters and devices that could become a nidus for infection. These infections are often very severe, life-threatening, and require inpatient medical care. Patients may present very similarly to bacterial cases, with fevers, rigors, chills, and sepsis. (Holland et al. 2020) Fungal infective endocarditis (IE) patients may present with symptomatic embolic phenomena like stroke more commonly than bacterial IE. Fungal IE has a poor prognosis and outcomes. Fungemia may present insidiously with new fevers and malaise in patients receiving total parenteral nutrition or requiring long-term central venous access. (Southwick 2020)

Malaria remains one of the most common parasitic infections worldwide and the most common one that affects the bloodstream. Malaria patients have clearly defining features of "malarial attacks" or paroxysms where they will first get shaking chills, high fevers, sometimes above 40°C, and generalized diaphoresis that completely resolves. These attacks can last from six to ten hours and are related to the rupture of erythrocytes during the replication of the parasite; the timing of attack recurrence is dependent on the malarial parasite: "tertian" parasites *P. falciparum, P. vivax,* and *P. ovale* are classically considered to have attacks occurring every second day, whereas the "quartan" parasite *P. malariae* is considered to cause attacks every third day. Babesiosis also infects erythrocytes, but fevers and malaise have no specific pattern. Trypanosomiasis, or Chagas disease, can be mild or even asymptomatic and usually presents with fever, chills, malaise, and swelling around the eyes where "kissing bugs" may have bitten. These bugs defecate while feeding, and patients inadvertently scratch the parasite-infected feces into the bite. Chronic manifestations of Chagas disease include abnormal heart rhythm, dilated heart, mega-esophagus, and/or mega-colon. Although not the primary site of infection, many other parasites can disseminate through the blood, such as *Ascaris lumbricoides* (Ascariasis) and *Entamoeba histolytica* (Amebiasis), and cause disease distally from where they first enter the body. (Mathison and Pritt 2022)

Risk factors

Immunosuppression is present in many patients with fungemia and fungal IE. Other than host factors predisposing to infection, fungi must have a way to enter the bloodstream and cause disease. IV drug use is a significant risk factor associated with fungemia and fungal IE. Medical use of catheters, particularly central venous catheters, can be associated with fungemia. Candida is the predominant organism, given its ubiquitous presence on the skin. These catheters are also sometimes used for total parenteral nutrition/hyperalimentation, in itself, is a risk for fungal infection. Prosthetic valves are also at risk for infection. (Southwick 2020) Hospitalization, in general, can be a risk for fungal infections, as can antibiotic use and surgical procedures. (Hilmarsdottir et al. 2023) Travel to endemic areas is a risk factor for parasitic infections.

Pathophysiology

Once access to the bloodstream is obtained, fungi can still be easily killed by host defenses in most immunocompetent hosts. Colonization by Candida of areas like the lungs and genitourinary tract still does not equate to disease but provides a source for continuous inoculum. Candida can form a glycocalyx that helps it adhere to catheters and prosthetic valves, progressing to fungemia. (Southwick 2020) Other fungi also can have an original source of infection, like the lungs, and spread via the bloodstream in disseminated disease (*e.g.*, Histoplasma). (Saullo and Alexander 2022) Malaria species have life cycles that include mosquitoes as their definitive host and humans as an intermediate. Anopheles mosquitoes carry the infection and infect sporozoites directly into the bloodstream, which then travel to the liver and invade hepatic cells. They proliferate there and eventually cause rupture of hepatic schizonts that release merozoites back into the bloodstream. These merozoites infect erythrocytes and can grow trophozoites. These trophozoites then can either become erythrocytic schizonts which produce more merozoites and ruptured erythrocytes, which trigger the well-recognized malarial attacks, or form macrogametocytes (female) and microgametocytes (male) which are meant to be picked up by mosquitoes and begin a different cycle. Babesia species are transmitted by ticks such as Ixodes scapularis, known colloquially as deer ticks. Parasites multiply in erythrocytes by binary fission, producing trophozoites and gametes. American Trypanosomiasis (Chagas disease) starts by infecting cells near the bug bite and dividing into amastigotes. These fill the cell and become trypomastigotes released into the bloodstream when they cause cellular rupture. They continue the amastigote-trypomastigote cycle once in the bloodstream. When *Entamoeba histolytica* causes bloodstream infection, it originates from the intestinal wall, invading and spreading to other sites. (Mathison and Pritt 2022)

Examination

A physical examination can provide some clues in fungemic and fungal IE patients. Given the aforementioned risk factors, many of these patients may be chronically ill with multiple risk factors. If catheters are present, there may be erythema, tenderness, or swelling around the skin where it enters. A new murmur should always raise suspicion for IE of some kind. Skin and nail findings similar to bacterial IE can be seen. Fundoscopic exams may also have similar findings of Roth spots and flame-shaped hemorrhages. Patients may overall be toxic appearing and septic. (Southwick 2020) If the infection is disseminated, multiple findings are possible from the original infectious site. Malaria patients may have hepatomegaly on exam and appear pale due to anemia. Babesiosis patients may also appear anemic. (Mathison and Pritt 2022)

Laboratory

Like CNS and other fungal infections, WBC counts can vary. Many other findings, like anemia, are nonspecific. Blood cultures should be obtained for suspected fungemia and fungal IE but can be falsely negative. Recommendations remain that two to three sets of blood cultures from different sites should be obtained to increase sensitivity. Any fungi that grow on these cultures can then be sampled and stained to identify the species under a microscope. Matrix-assisted laser desorption ionization-time of flight mass spectrometry (MALDI-TOF MS) technology can provide identification of cultured organisms in minutes and is used for the speciation of Candida and other fungi. Serologic and molecular testing like PCR is also available, including PCR testing for seven major Candida species and Aspergillus. Galactomannan and beta-D-glucan testing can also guide diagnosis. (Hilmarsdottir et al. 2023) Suspected malaria, babesiosis, trypanosomiasis, leishmaniasis, and filariasis should prompt microscopic evaluation of thin and thick blood smears on a microscope for visual diagnosis. Certain malaria species, like *Plasmodium vivax* and *Plasmodium ovale*, will show Schüffner stippling: small uniform pink granules within infected erythrocytes. Babesiosis is known for the Maltese cross on the microscopic exam, a tetra formation of merozoites. (Mathison and Pritt 2022)

Imaging

Imaging of possibly originating sources, like the lungs, may be indicated for suspected disseminated fungal infections for fungemia. For fungal IE, transthoracic echocardiography is performed to identify possible vegetations or new valvular regurgitation. Transesophageal echocardiography is much more sensitive but requires anesthesia involvement and a certain degree of clinical stability. Embolic phenomena like strokes may also warrant CT or MRI of the brain. (Southwick 2020) Parasitic bloodstream infections usually do not warrant imaging.

Associated symptoms/conditions
Critical illness and prolonged hospitalization, medical comorbidities, immunocompromised states, neutropenia, transplant status, prior azole or echinocandin use, and advanced age are associated with fungal bloodstream infections and IE. (Hilmarsdottir et al. 2023)

Diagnosis
Clinical diagnosis of fungemia and fungal IE is often difficult. A high degree of suspicion is needed; sometimes, diagnosis can be delayed. Diagnosis of fungemia is made with the identification of fungal species on blood cultures or smears as discussed above in the Laboratory section. However, sometimes the diagnosis must be presumptive while cultures are pending to quickly begin empiric treatment depending on the patient's clinical status. An echocardiogram with vegetations would make the diagnosis of fungal IE highly suspicious in the setting of blood cultures growing fungi. The final diagnosis would be made from pathological examination of samples obtained from surgery, but some patients are too unstable to undergo cardiothoracic interventions. (Holland et al. 2020) Parasitic bloodstream infections similarly require a high degree of suspicion, usually from a thorough history with diagnostic clues such as travel to endemic areas or recent bug bites. Many patients do not recall or notice bites, however. Clinical suspicion should prompt clinicians to obtain blood smears which can be used to identify the parasite and guide treatment. (Mathison and Pritt 2022)

Treatment
In uncomplicated cases, Candida fungemia can be treated with echinocandins like **caspofungin** and **micafungin**. Patients with persistent fungemia or severe disease may need liposomal **amphotericin B** therapy. (Southwick 2020) If the brain, eye, or genitourinary tract is involved, **fluconazole** is preferred due to penetration into those areas. (Hilmarsdottir et al. 2023) **Fluconazole** can also be used as step-down therapy if the particular species is found to be susceptible. Disseminated Aspergillosis is managed with **voriconazole**. In patients with critical illness and not yet speciated fungal infection, **amphotericin B** is the treatment of choice and can be de-escalated later when sensitivities are obtained. (Ostrosky-Zeichner and Al-Obaidi 2019) **Artemisinin**-based combination therapy is recommended for malarial treatment unless the species is **chloroquine** sensitive. *Plasmodium vivax* or *P. ovale* infection also warrants adding **primaquine** or **tafenoquine** to ensure eradication of hepatic hypnozoites; however, patients at risk of having glucose-6-phosphate dehydrogenase (G6PD) deficiency should be tested before their use. Babesiosis does not warrant treatment in asymptomatic or immunocompetent patients. Patients with immunocompromising conditions at risk for severe disease are treated with **atovaquone** with **azithromycin** or **clindamycin** with **quinine**. Treatment of other rarer parasites may require consultation with the CDC and infectious disease specialists. (Mathison and Pritt 2022)

Management
Apart from antifungals and supportive management, fungemic patients need to have catheters like central lines or temporary dialysis catheters removed. There is a 10-15% risk of Candida endophthalmitis associated with candidemia, so ophthalmology needs to be consulted in all cases. (Southwick 2020) Fungal IE remains challenging to treat, and the prognosis is poor. Antifungals have poor penetration into vegetations, which tends to be large when compared to bacterial IE. Cardiothoracic surgery consultation plays an essential role in these patients as valve removal or replacement is indicated depending on the location of the vegetation. (Holland et al. 2020) Both fungal and parasitic bloodstream infections may require surgical consultation and intervention if there is an identifiable source elsewhere in the body. Consultation with local health authorities can provide important information about parasitic infections that are being seen locally. (Mathison and Pritt 2022)

Intra-Abdominal Infections

Presentation
Various fungal and parasitic organisms we have discussed in other sections can also infect structures of the abdomen, including the GI tract, solid organs, and the GU tract. These can be both the original site of entry or be involved in disseminated infections. Candida is the most common fungus in abdominal infections and can affect almost any organ system. It is the most common cause of fungal peritonitis, which presents with abdominal pain and tenderness. Fungal peritonitis can be further complicated by abscess formation. Candidal esophageal infection may present with pain upon swallowing or difficulty swallowing. Candida is also common in genital infections that can present with itching, burning upon urination, discomfort during intercourse, and whitish discharge. Candida can also rarely cause infections involving the liver and spleen with associated pain, fever, and likely sepsis. Aspergillus, Paracoccidioides, Mucormycosis, and Histoplasma can affect the GI tract and present with various symptoms like abdominal pain from ulcerations, diarrhea, bloody stools, and peritonitis. Paracoccidioidomycosis can cause enlargement of the liver and abdominal lymph nodes and may present with jaundice from the blocked flow of bile. Disseminated blastomycosis, histoplasmosis, and paracoccidioidomycosis can manifest as prostate, testicular, or other genital pain. (Hilmarsdottir et al. 2023) Multiple parasites are associated with GI tract infection. *Entamoeba histolytica* (Amebic dysentery), *Dientamoeba fragilis*, Giardia species, Cryptosporidium, *Strongyloides stercoralis* (Strongyloidiasis), hookworms, and a variety of other rarer parasites can all present with symptoms of nausea, bloody or non-bloody diarrhea, abdominal

pain, cramping, fever, and weight loss. Schistosoma infection of the urinary tract can first present with hematuria. (Mathison and Pritt 2022)

Risk factors

Immunosuppression remains a key risk factor in fungal infections throughout the body. Anything that exposes the peritoneum to the environment, be it peritoneal dialysis catheters or drains, surgery, or wounds, can increase the risk of a fungal infection. Fungi are part of the normal flora of the intestines, so any perforation that leads to leakage from the GI tract into the peritoneum can cause a fungal infection. Necrotizing pancreatitis is another risk factor. Hyperglycemia from diabetes also provides glucose for fungal growth and precipitates disease. (Hilmarsdottir et al. 2023) Traveling to endemic areas is the most significant risk factor for most parasitic infections of the abdomen, as well as ingesting contaminated meats or water. Outbreaks of Giardia, for example, have been seen in campers, travelers, and daycares. Ingestion of raw fish has also increased the incidence of fish nematode infections. (Mathison and Pritt 2022)

Pathophysiology

Since most fungal disease in humans is opportunistic, a fungal disease affecting the abdomen (and the multiple organs located there) is rare and most often seen in disseminated disease in immunocompromised patients. The lack of normal defenses from fungal organisms causes the overgrowth of fungal flora, leading to disease. Mucosal damage in patients undergoing specific chemotherapy regimens can facilitate the translocation of Candida and other fungi into the portal circulation. (Hilmarsdottir et al. 2023) Parasites, on the other hand, must be ingested to reach the mucosa of the GI tract, where many have mechanisms to attach to the intestinal walls and replicate. Giardia species multiply in the small bowel and adhere to the mucosa using a suction disk. Tapeworms and roundworms invade and then migrate through the intestinal walls, and adults can grow in the lumen. *Entamoeba histolytica* (Amebiasis) also invades the intestinal wall and causes dysentery. (Mathison and Pritt 2022)

Examination

Patients with limited infections of the GI tract may have mild symptoms like tenderness of the abdomen. Those with diarrheal presentations are expected to have increased bowel sounds, while those with peritonitis may have decreased bowel sounds. Fever is sometimes seen but may not be present, given the likelihood of immunosuppression. Infections of the peritoneal space will have more acute presentations with severe tenderness and guarding. Patients with disseminated infections may have a variety of physical exam findings outside of the abdominal area. Parasitic infections like Echinococcus that affect the liver may have findings of liver failure like ascites or splenomegaly. (Shuclick and Ibrahim-Zada 2020)

Laboratory

Like other fungal infections, intra-abdominal fungal infections can have a variety of insensitive laboratory findings like leukocytosis, leukopenia, neutropenia, or even anemia. Alkaline phosphatase can also be elevated. Various PCR, antibody, antigen, and other molecular tests are available to rapidly test suspected infections, particularly for disseminated cases. Many of these tests, including galactomannan and beta-D-glucan detection, can be run on various bodily fluids. Cultures can also be helpful but may be falsely negative. (Hilmarsdottir et al. 2023) Identification of parasites in fluid samples can be performed under a microscope. Diarrheal samples can be sent for ova and parasite examination and should ideally be as fresh as possible to ensure infective organisms can be identified. Eosinophilia can sometimes be seen in the serum. Cultures can be done for some parasites, but few laboratories perform them. (Mathison and Pritt 2022)

Imaging

Imaging of the abdomen can identify abdominal free air or areas of perforation. Plain radiographs are helpful in these cases and can show free air. Still, CT of the abdomen can provide more detailed information about the part of the GI tract affected and help identify if there are abscesses. If diarrhea is a symptom, a CT scan may show findings of colon inflammation. There is often little utility for imaging in fungal genitourinary tract infections unless there are complications like pyelonephritis or perinephric abscess formation. (Hilmarsdottir et al. 2023) Imaging is also not often used in diagnosing parasitic abdominal infections but, in some cases, may incidentally identify infections. Echinococcus infection may remain silent and be found on CT or US of the abdomen revealing hepatic lesions and cysts. (Shuclick and Ibrahim-Zada 2020) Amebic liver abscesses are the most common extraintestinal manifestation seen in *Entamoeba histolytica* and can be seen on CT or U/S. (Mathison and Pritt 2022)

Associated symptoms/conditions

Hematologic malignancy and neutropenia are associated with disseminated and abdominal fungal infections. (Saullo and Alexander 2022) Peritoneal dialysis is also associated with fungal peritonitis. (Hilmarsdottir et al. 2023)

Diagnosis

A combination of a thorough history, physical exam, diagnostic testing, and sometimes imaging is used to obtain a final diagnosis of a fungal intra-abdominal infection. Clinical suspicion is usually high as most patients have a history of immunocompromising conditions. Cultures make the definitive diagnosis but are sometimes not easily obtained or can be delayed. Surgical intervention provides an opportunity to obtain samples for culture in the case of peritonitis or intraabdominal abscess from fungi. Disseminated infections are diagnosed using the constellation of symptoms with serologic markers. In the case of fungal infections from perforations, diagnosis may be presumptive when patients do not improve with antibiotics, and many infections are polymicrobial. Fungal esophagitis can be seen and diagnosed on endoscopy. (Hilmarsdottir et al. 2023) Diagnosis of a parasitic infection also depends on a combination of the aforementioned and clinical suspicion for parasites. Ova and parasite examinations, like wet mounts, can be used to visualize parasites using a microscope and identify their various stages (*e.g.*, oocysts) in samples.

Treatment

Disseminated candida infections are treated with an echinocandin, usually **caspofungin**. Candida peritonitis (not from disseminated disease) is also treated the same way. Given the severity of disseminated infections from organisms like Aspergillus, Histoplasma, or Blastomyces and the delay in diagnosis, **amphotericin B** can be used empirically, given its comprehensive coverage. Once an etiologic diagnosis is made, therapy can be de-escalated. **Isavuconazole** and **posaconazole** represent newer azole antifungals that are sometimes utilized in refractory infections. (Ostrosky-Zeichner and Al-Obaidi 2019) Parasitic depends on the site and organisms causing infection. Many diarrheal illnesses caused by parasites like nematodes, hookworms, pinworms, and nematodes can be managed with **albendazole**, **mebendazole**, and sometimes **ivermectin** (Table 3.3). Strongyloides is the exception, for which the recommended treatment is **ivermectin**. Cestodes, colloquially known as tapeworms, such as Taeniasis, are treated with **praziquantel**. While other trematodes can also be managed with praziquantel, *Fasciola hepatica* (Fascioliasis) infection is controlled with the anthelmintic benzimidazole **triclabendazole**. (Mathison and Pritt 2022)

Management

Overall management of abdominal fungal infections is multifaceted, particularly in disseminated cases and those arising from colonic perforations. Surgical intervention is often required for source control in fungal peritonitis. Disseminated cases may also require surgical interventions for source control. Patients too ill for surgery should be evaluated by interventional radiology as percutaneous drainage can also be used in the same way. Patients with fungal esophagitis or colitis may require an endoscopy by a gastroenterologist to properly diagnose and repeat endoscopies to monitor for complications. (Hilmarsdottir et al. 2023) While many parasitic infections can be managed with antifungals alone, some require surgical removal. Anisakiasis is both diagnosed and treated with either surgical or endoscopic removal. (Mathison and Pritt 2022) Surgical consultation should be obtained for Echinococcus infections as there are many indications for surgical removal, like infected cysts or those communicating with the biliary tree, which can lower the risk of recurrent infections. (Shuclick and Ibrahim-Zada 2020)

Skin, Soft Tissue, and Bone Infections

Presentation

Fungal infections of the bone, skin, and soft tissues have a variety of clinical presentations. Bone and joint infections are rare but can be caused by either traumatic inoculation or hematogenous spread in disseminated disease. Patients may experience joint pain, swelling, redness and warmth, bone pain, or other localized findings. Candida, particularly *Candida albicans*, are the most common fungi responsible for fungal bone and joint infections. Almost all of the fungi we have discussed previously can infect the bones and joints. Hematogenously spread infections can involve the spine causing back pain or even radicular symptoms. Skin, hair, and nail fungal infections are the most common type of all fungal infections. Skin infections have many patterns, sometimes characteristic of their causative organism. Affected skin may appear a different color from the rest, sometimes darker or lighter, flaky, or scaly, and patients complain of itching. Colloquially, "ringworm" refers to the round or oval shape of the rash, but these are *fungal* infections, not parasites. These infections can affect any part of the skin, including the scalp. Onychomycosis, a fungal infection of the nails, will present with discoloration and thickening of the nails and separation from the nail plate. Complaints of painless nodules that appear to be making their way up from the hands to the arms in someone exposed to roses or other thorny bushes are characteristic of Sporothrix infections. (Hilmarsdottir et al. 2023) Parasitic infections of the bone and joints are often due to disseminated infection, like in visceral Leishmaniasis, Echinococcus, Trypanosomiasis, and amebiasis. Strongyloides and Schistosoma may directly penetrate the skin. However, the most commonly encountered skin parasites are scabies and hookworm infections causing cutaneous larva migrans. Patients will present with intense itching and complaints of red skin that may have linear lines where the parasites have burrowed. (Rajagopalan 2016)

Risk factors

Fungal infections of the skin and nails can affect just about anyone, unlike other organ systems. Persistently humid skin folds like in patients with hyperhidrosis or those living in hot and humid climates, occlusive shoes, poor grooming, smoking, diabetes mellitus, peripheral vascular disease, and of course, any immunocompromised states are risk factors for skin and nail infections by fungi. Certain professions like miners, soldiers, and athletes may have their feet in a hot and humid environment for extended periods and are at risk for onychomycosis. Bone, joint and soft tissue infections are most often due to disseminated disease, in which case most patients with disseminated disease have some kind of immunocompromised state. Direct inoculation, such as in the case of Sporothrix and the classic "rose bush gardener," are one-way fungi that may affect deeper spaces in immunocompetent patients. Similarly, intravenous drug abuse is associated with bone, joint, and soft tissue fungal infections. (Mathison and Pritt 2022) Risk factors for parasitic skin infections are mainly those individuals with direct contact with the environment where parasites are located. Traveling to endemic areas with warm and moist soils or sand or even exposure to sandboxes can be risk factors. Farmers, gardeners, and pest exterminators are all at risk for parasitic infections of the skin. (Rajagopalan 2016) Homelessness and poor hygiene are also associated with parasitic infections like scabies and lice. (Mathison and Pritt 2022)

Pathophysiology

Fungal skin and nail infections by dermatophytes occur in the right skin environment that is often hot, humid, and dark. Skin folds are a common site, particularly in between toes. The multiple species of dermatophytes metabolize the keratin present in the skin and nails. These dermatophytes can spread from person to person via flaked skin or hair, indirectly from objects like combs or hats, or shared areas like locker rooms and showers. They infect the outermost layer of skin called the stratum corneum, which contains this keratin, and replicate, causing local inflammation and irritation responsible for symptoms of itching. Candida and Malassezia species are usually present in human skin and also cause disease under the right conditions, particularly if there is any issue with the integrity of the normal skin barrier, like in burns, macerations, or abrasions. Candida can cause a wide array of infections, including intertrigo, folliculitis, angular cheilitis, and genital infections. Malassezia species cause pityriasis (tinea) versicolor, seborrheic dermatitis and folliculitis. Deeper infections of the subcutaneous tissues can occur from direct inoculation, like in Sporothrix, via thorns or from cuts that come into contact with contaminated soil. Mycetoma, a term used to describe a chronic granulomatous infection of the subcutaneous tissues, is caused by hyaline or melanized molds that usually enter the space via traumatic inoculation. Blastomyces, Coccidioides, Paracoccidioides, Cryptococcus, Aspergillus, and Sporothrix species can cause bone and joint infections through hematogenous seeding, usually from a primary lung infection. Other rarer organisms can only cause disease in cases where neutropenia or immunosuppression is present. (Hilmarsdottir et al. 2023) Scabies mites are obligate parasites that live in the epidermis, burrowing into superficial skin while laying eggs. Infected individuals usually have symptoms due to a delayed-type hypersensitivity reaction after a month from exposure to the mites, eggs, or mite feces. The various hookworms that can cause cutaneous larva migrans normally begin their life cycle in soil and penetrate the stratum corneum causing localized inflammation and symptoms. (Rajagopalan 2016) Lice species transferred from person to person through hats, combs, or other shared items suck blood from the attached area and cause itching and inflammation when they bite. Bed bugs and kissing bugs also cause weals and other skin reactions from their bites and saliva, to which patients may have varying sensitivity. (Mathison and Pritt 2022)

Examination

Skin affected by fungal infections is often scaly, slightly raised, and will have an erythematous border where the active infection is spreading outwards. This oval or round pattern is why terms like ringworm or the descriptive "tinea" term are used, which means worm or moth in Latin. This term was coined before it was known that fungi were the causative organism. Nails affected by fungal infections are discolored, thickened, and often will separate from the nail plate. Disseminated fungal infections causing osteomyelitis may present with tenderness over the affected bone and joint infections with pain with active and passive movements. When the spine is involved, there may be areas with muscle weakness or numbness. (Mathison and Pritt 2022) Fungal subcutaneous infections can form fistulas and drain pus, which may have characteristic fungal granules. (Hilmarsdottir et al. 2023) Parasitic skin infections will also have findings of irritated skin, erythema, intense pruritus, weals, vesicles, papules, or other local findings. Linear lesions, or burrows, are a pathognomonic sign of scabies and are intraepidermal tunnels created by the moving mite. Serpiginous lesions, which are slightly raised tunnels, are also seen in cutaneous larva migrans. (Rajagopalan 2016) Parasitic infections of the bone and joints are rare and will have local symptoms within a disseminated course, like in Echinococcus.

Laboratory

Fungal infections of the skin and nails are diagnosed clinically, and laboratory testing is usually warranted. Skin scrapings, nails, abscess pus, and other samples can be cultured if indicated and can also be stained for microscopic viewing. Culture from infected bones, joints, or synovial fluid is indicated and, along with microscopy, can often be diagnostic. Pityriasis versicolor patients can have skin scrapings stained with methylene blue to reveal a characteristic "spaghetti and meatballs" pattern, which are the hyphae and yeast forms. Fungal abscesses or other subcutaneous infections with draining pus can be cultured, but biopsy or surgical specimen cultures are preferred due to potentially contaminating flora. Bone biopsies can be visualized under a microscope and reveal invasive fungal infections. (Hilmarsdottir et al. 2023) Skin parasites may cause peripheral eosinophilia and increased IgE levels. Biopsy of affected tissue may show larvae, burrows, and eosinophils. (Rajagopalan 2016)

Imaging

Fungal and parasitic skin infections do not warrant imaging unless there is a concern for deep abscesses, where ultrasound may be beneficial. Blastomycosis can cause extrapulmonary disease, including bony involvement with focal osteolytic lesions without periosteal reactivity. (Nosanchuk and Thompson 2022) Other disseminated fungal or parasitic infections can have various imaging findings discussed in other sections.

Associated symptoms/conditions
Disseminated fungal infections are associated with bone and joint infections. Immunosuppression remains a common comorbidity for fungal skin infections. Homelessness, poverty, and poor personal hygiene are associated with parasitic skin infections like scabies and lice.

Diagnosis
Diagnosis of fungal skin and nail infections combines a thorough history and physical exam. As discussed above, typical skin findings of a scaly, oval, or round lesion with erythematous borders make clinical diagnosis straightforward. Pityriasis versicolor and Candida skin infections similarly will have characteristic appearances. Onychomycosis is not the only cause of nail dystrophy, so ideally, samples from affected nails can be sent for a wet mount with microscopy. As discussed above, skin scrapings can be used in suspected pityriasis versicolor, but a Wood's lamp can also demonstrate red or yellowish fluorescence of lesions. Subcutaneous infections and abscesses should undergo microscopy of both samples and culture. Bone and joint infections similarly involve the evaluation of imaging findings and histopathology and are often in the context of a more complex diagnosis of disseminated disease. (Hilmarsdottir et al. 2023) Parasitic skin infections are usually diagnosed clinically based on the appearance of the eruption. Definitive diagnosis entails skin biopsy samples showing causative organisms on light microscopy. (Rajagopalan 2016) Diagnosing head lice is straightforward as lice or nits can be visualized on hair or skin. (Smith 2022)

Treatment
Bone and joint fungal infections are often part of disseminated infection, and patients are treated based on the causative fungus. Given the severity of disseminated infections, most patients should receive **amphotericin B** until the fungus is identified and treatment tailored to the organism and its sensitivities to antifungals. Treatment regimens are often prolonged for weeks. Fungal skin infections, including the variety of tinea affecting different areas, are managed with topical antifungals such as **terbinafine** or an azole (**ketoconazole**, **miconazole**, or **clotrimazole**). Tinea capitis is an exception and requires systemic therapy to fully clear. Extensive skin infections may also warrant systemic antifungal treatment, but this is rare. It was initially thought that onychomycosis required oral antifungals to fully clear due to poor penetration of these drugs into the nail tissue. Topical application is still a valid approach, as is (in some cases) no antifungal treatment at all. (Falotico and Lipner 2022; Leung et al. 2020; Queller and Bhatia 2015) Pityriasis versicolor from Malassezia species can be managed with **terbinafine** and other topical azoles or orally, depending on severity. Topical **nystatin** preparations are used for Candida skin infections as well as drying agents to prevent worsening. Subcutaneous and other deeper infections often require a combination of oral azole treatment and surgery. (Hilmarsdottir et al. 2023) **Permethrin** cream is the treatment of choice for scabies and requires application two or more times about a week apart. Cutaneous larva migrans from the various hookworms are often self-limited in nature, but symptoms may prompt treatment with agents like the anthelmintic benzimidazoles **thiabendazole** or **albendazole**. (Rajagopalan 2016) Lice can be treated with 5% permethrin cream applied to affected areas. (Smith 2022)

Management
Depending on the affected areas, an orthopedic surgeon or neurosurgeon should evaluate fungal bone and joint infections involving any prosthetics like artificial knees or spinal instrumentation. Surgery may be needed for debridement, drainage, or to remove the prosthetics, which can remain a nidus for infection. Deep tissue infections may also require surgery and, in severe cases, amputation. (Hilmarsdottir et al. 2023) Parasitic infections like lice require thorough cleaning or discarding clothing or other potential sources of re-infection. Bed bugs are challenging to eradicate as they are not only present in bedding, but other areas, including cracks and even under carpeting and hardwood floors, and an exterminator is usually required. (Smith 2022)

Pharmacological Treatments for Fungal Infections

The incidence of invasive fungal infections seems to be ever-increasing, (Fisher et al. 2022) especially in immunocompromised patients (*e.g.*, those receiving cancer chemotherapy, or immunosuppressive drugs for autoimmune diseases or organ transplantation; those with uncontrolled or breakthrough HIV infection leading to acquired immunodeficiency syndrome [AIDS]). Fortunately, fungi have a unique lipid constituent in ergosterol (whereas humans have cholesterol instead), thereby posing ergosterol-centered attributes and pathways as Achilles' heels to be exploited pharmacologically. Other antifungal strategies have also been developed into clinically valuable agents.

Terbinafine (inhibitor of ergosterol biosynthesis)
Terbinafine inhibits ergosterol synthesis by inhibiting the fungal enzyme squalene epoxidase, which converts squalene into lanosterol (the immediate precursor of ergosterol). It is used orally or topically to treat dermatophyte infections, including tinea versicolor, fungal nail infections, and "ringworm" rashes like jock itch and athlete's foot.

Azoles (inhibitors of ergosterol biosynthesis)
An 'azole' is a compound bearing a five-membered heterocyclic ring containing at least one nitrogen and one or more additional non-carbon atoms (*e.g.*, nitrogen, sulfur, or oxygen; Figure 3.8A&B). As a drug class, the antifungal azoles are broadly active against various fungal pathogens and act by inhibiting the fungal cytochrome P-450 enzyme ("lanosterol 14-alpha-demethylase") responsible for ergosterol synthesis (Zhang et al. 2019). The resultant depletion of ergosterol levels damages the fungal cell membrane and causes lysis. The first azole to find clinical utility as an antifungal agent was the imidazole **ketoconazole**; however, the hepatotoxicity induced by its orally available, systemically disseminated form led to its subsequent restriction only for topical applications ("superficial mycoses") and for oral use only with endemic mycoses where alternatives are not available nor feasible (Gupta and Lyons 2015). Additional common adverse effects of oral ketoconazole are nausea, vomiting, and anorexia, as well as hepatotoxicity, adrenal suppression, and inhibition of testosterone synthesis. Like ketoconazole, the more recently developed imidazoles **miconazole** and **clotrimazole** are also generally restricted to topical use, or as a lozenge or other buccal-localized formulations for prophylaxis against, or treatment of, oropharyngeal candidiasis.

Figure 3.8 Structures of imidazole (A) and triazole (B) antifungal agents, and an example polyene antifungal agent (C).

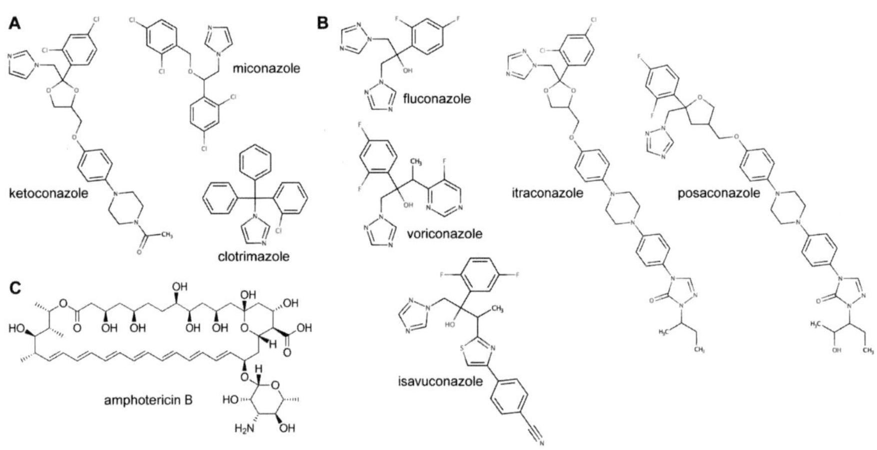

The second azole antifungal sub-class, the triazoles, is composed of **fluconazole**, **itraconazole**, **voriconazole**, **posaconazole**, and **isavuconazole** (Figure 3.8B). Given the triazoles' improved safety and more predictable absorption upon oral administration, this sub-class is preferred over the imidazoles when systemic treatment is required. Of the triazoles, fluconazole has a narrower spectrum of usage that includes most *Candida* species (except *C. krusei* and *C. glabrata*) and some dimorphic fungi and dermatophytes; fluconazole is used primarily for susceptible *Candida* species causing superficial or systemic infection and is often used for AIDS patients with cryptococcal meningitis (*e.g.*, ref. (Nayak et al. 2011)) after an initial course of intravenous treatment with **amphotericin B (AmB**; see below and Figure 3.8C). Resistance to fluconazole within *Candida* species can arise from mutation to the target 14-demethylase. (Fisher et al. 2022) The other triazole antifungal agents (Figure 3.8B) are broader in their antifungal spectrum than fluconazole and, in particular, have utility in aspergillosis where fluconazole does not. (Chang et al. 2017) **Itraconazole** is helpful in treating blastomycosis, chromoblastomycosis, coccidioidomycosis, histoplasmosis, sporotrichosis, and some cases of aspergillosis. IV formulation of itraconazole obviates its poor oral absorption, which traditionally required concomitant consumption of acidic drinks like orange juice or cola (Willems et al. 2001). In both IV and oral formulations, **voriconazole** has superior activity against invasive *Aspergillus* and fluconazole-resistant *Candida* species (Shirasawa and Nagino 2005), yet can lead to transient vision changes in ~30% of users and (more infrequently) rash, hepatotoxicity, or other adverse effects.

Amphotericin B and Nystatin (ergosterol binders)
The structurally related polyene antimycotics **amphotericin B (AmB**; Figure 3.8C) and **nystatin** each act by binding to ergosterol in the fungal cell membrane, thereby leading to leakage, lysis, and death. **AmB** is a first-line option for many serious systemic fungal infections, including systemic *Candida* infections, severe fungal pneumonia or systemic blastomycosis, histoplasmosis, or coccidioidomycosis, invasive aspergillosis, invasive sporotrichosis, mucormycosis, and cryptococcal meningitis (when it is often used in combination with **flucytosine**; see below). Side effects are numerous and can be severe. A common, serious febrile response can occur soon after an AmB infusion, characterized by fever, chills, headache, hypotension, nausea, vomiting, anorexia, dyspnea/tachypnea, and drowsiness. IV AmB is also associated with the risk of multiple organ damage, including nephrotoxicity, hepatotoxicity, electrolyte

imbalance, anemia, and cardiac arrhythmia. Newer lipid-based AmB formulations have reduced this risk, and AmB in the hospital setting is often given with aspirin or paracetamol/acetaminophen to reduce any febrile response. In contrast to the first-line utility of AmB for serious and systemic fungal infections, **nystatin** is generally too toxic for IV administration and thus reserved for topical use on skin and mucosal membranes in the treatment of oral, esophageal, and vaginal infections.

Echinocandins (inhibitors of fungal β-glucan synthesis)
The echinocandins **caspofungin**, **micafungin**, and **anidulafungin** are noncompetitive inhibitors of the fungal enzyme 1,3-β-glucan synthase, thereby reducing the levels of β-glucan critically required for fungal cell wall synthesis, leading to cell lysis. Given their limited oral bioavailability, these echinocandins are administered via intravenous infusion; they are effective against all *Candida* species (with only limited evidence of resistance development in *Candida* spp.) and are also used in patients who have failed conventional antifungal therapy for invasive aspergillosis.

Flucytosine (inhibitor of fungal DNA & RNA synthesis)
Flucytosine is a fluorinated pyrimidine analog and is therefore converted in the fungus both to 5-fluorodeoxyuridine monophosphate that inhibits fungal DNA synthesis and to 5-fluorouridine triphosphate that disrupts fungal RNA synthesis. Given the rapid development of fungal resistance, it is rarely used alone: most fungal pathogens are resistant to flucytosine, but *Cryptococcus* and *Candida* species are susceptible. Flucytosine is often given in combination with AmB, with the thought that the membrane-destabilizing effect of AmB facilitates the entry of flucytosine for the latter drug's intracellular metabolism and resultant DNA/RNA synthesis inhibitory effects (*c.f.*, ref. (Cuenca-Estrella 2004)). Adverse effects from flucytosine can include bone marrow suppression (leukopenia; thrombocytopenia), nausea, vomiting, and diarrhea, as host DNA synthesis can be damaged by flucytosine's actions, especially within rapidly dividing bone marrow and GI-tract epithelial cell progenitors.

Griseofulvin (inhibitor of fungal tubulin)
Griseofulvin is used orally only for dermatophytoses, including fungal infections of the nails, scalp, and skin when other antifungal topical agents have failed. (*e.g.*, ref. (Chen et al. 2016)) The drug binds to fungal tubulin, blocking the microtubule dynamics necessary for spindle formation, proper mitosis, and fungal growth.

Pharmacological Treatments for Helminthic, Parasitic, and Protozoan Infections

The anthelmintic (a.k.a. antihelminthic) benzimidazoles **albendazole**, **mebendazole**, **triclabendazole**, and **thiabendazole** (a.k.a. tiabendazole) are all thought to act by binding worm beta-tubulin (Table 3.3) and thereby disrupting worm-specific microtubule dynamics that are involved in both mitotic and movement processes. (Lacey 1990) **Thiabendazole/tiabendazole** may also directly inhibit the helminth-specific enzyme fumarate reductase. (*cf.* ref. (Zhou et al. 2011)) Other anthelmintic drugs share a common approach of paralyzing the worm to cause detachment and expulsion, including the neuromuscular junction depolarizing agent **pyrantel pamoate**, the glutamate-gated chloride channel agonist **ivermectin**, and the suspected calcium permeability modulating agent **praziquantel** (Table 3.3). **Niclosamide**, effective against tapeworms but not other worms like pinworms or roundworms, inhibits glucose uptake, oxidative phosphorylation, and anaerobic metabolism in its target. (Weinbach and Garbus 1969) **Diethylcarbamazine** is specifically used to treat filariasis and inhibits microfilarial arachidonic acid metabolism, making the microfilariae more susceptible to the host immune system (El-Shahawi et al. 2010). The antibacterial aminoglycoside **paromomycin** also treats several helminthic and parasitic infections, including tapeworm infections, amebiasis, giardiasis, and leishmaniasis. Similarly, the antibacterial **metronidazole** commonly used for anaerobic bacterial infections is also used in dracunculiasis, giardiasis, trichomoniasis, and amebiasis. **Permethrin** is an insecticide also used as a topical medication to treat scabies and lice, working by disrupting the function of neurons in lice and scabies mites.

African Trypanosomiasis is treated depending on the region and, hence, the prevailing infectious agent. *T. brucei gambiense* infection causes West African *chronic* sleeping sickness and is treated in its early stages (absent CNS involvement) with **pentamidine**, thought to interfere with both genomic and mitochondrial DNA of the *Trypanosoma* parasite. **Melarsoprol**, an extremely toxic, arsenic-containing medication, is effective on the CNS-resident parasite, and so reserved for more serious cases (Brun et al. 2001); when metabolized to melarsen oxide in the body, it irreversibly binds to sulfhydryl groups on the *Trypanosoma* pyruvate kinase, disrupting its energy production. *T. brucei rhodesiense* infection causes an East African *acute* sleeping sickness and is treated in its early stages (absent CNS involvement) with **suramin**, thought to combine with trypanosomal glycolytic enzymes, inhibiting energy metabolism. If CNS resident, *T. brucei rhodesiense* infection is treated with **nifurtimox-eflornithine** combination therapy (NECT), in which the **nifurtimox** (a nitrofuran) generates DNA-damaging nitro-anion radicals and **eflornithine** acts as a "suicide inhibitor" of trypanosomal ornithine decarboxylase that catalyzes the committed step in polyamine synthesis. Any relapse after NECT is treated with **melarsoprol.** American Trypanosomiasis ("Chagas disease" of the southwest USA and South and Central Americas, caused by *Trypanosoma cruzi* infection) is treated with the nitroimidazole **benznidazole**, which generates DNA-damaging nitro-anion radicals but is less toxic than **nifurtimox** (which, in turn, serves as a second agent against Chagas disease should benznidazole treatment fail).

Trichomoniasis, the sexually transmitted infection of *Trichomonas vaginalis* that inhabits the genitourinary tract causing vaginitis or urethritis, is treated with nitroimidazoles **metronidazole,** or **tinidazole**. Similarly, Giardiasis caused by drinking water contaminated with *Giardia duodenalis* or *Giardia lamblia* is also treated with these two nitroimidazoles. Drinking water can also be contaminated with the amoeba *Entamoeba histolytica* (Bosch and Siderovski 2013); when the infection of the intestinal lining is asymptomatic, only one of the following luminal agents (or "luminal amebicides") is used to treat the amebiasis: the antibacterial aminoglycoside **paromomycin**, or **diloxanide furoate**, or **iodoquinol.** *E. histolytica* amebiasis with mild to moderate symptoms of dysentery would also add **metronidazole** or **tinidazole** to the treatment regimen. **Diloxanide furoate** is a prodrug, metabolized in the GI tract to release diloxanide, which destroys *E. histolytica* trophozoites with an unknown mechanism. While diloxanide furoate has no serious adverse effects (except innocuous flatulence), it is not recommended in pregnancy. **Iodoquinol** also has an undetermined mechanism of action against *E. histolytica* trophozoites located within the intestinal lumen. However, it is known to chelate ferrous (Fe^{2+}) ions that are essential for metabolism and, fortunately, are poorly absorbed from the GI tract, thereby limiting its toxicity to the host. Iodoquinol must be used cautiously if the amebiasis patient has a comorbidity of optic neuropathy, renal, thyroid, or hepatic disease; discontinuation is warranted if iodoquinol treatment is seen to cause persistent diarrhea or iodine toxicity (dermatitis, urticaria, pruritis, fever). For this reason, iodoquinol is also contraindicated for those intolerant to iodine.

Primary amebic meningoencephalitis (PAM), caused by the rare but nearly always fatal "brain-eating amoeba" *Naegleria fowleri* (Bosch et al. 2022), is treated with a combination of drugs, often including **amphotericin B**, **azithromycin**, **fluconazole**, **rifampin**, and the steroid **dexamethasone** (the latter for its anti-inflammatory effects). A newer, phosphorylated fatty acid-like drug, **miltefosine**, appears effective against *N. fowleri in vitro* (Schuster et al. 2006) and in recent cases (Cope et al. 2016); in its use against *Leishmania*, miltefosine is seen to act on the promastigote and amastigote stages by interacting with lipids, inhibiting mitochondrial cytochrome c oxidase, and thereby causing apoptosis-like cellular death.

Pharmacology of Malarial Prophylaxis and Treatment

Prophylaxis - Dependent on the geographical location(Brunette and Nemhauser 2020), the female *Anopheles* mosquito injects into the bloodstream of its human victim one of five different protozoans that act in the human body as the etiology of malaria: namely, *Plasmodium falciparum* (a potentially life-threatening infection), *P. malariae*, *P. vivax*, *P. ovale*, or *P. knowlesi* (the latter having escaped its former simian-only restriction in its infectious target (Mohammad et al. 2022)). Travel to a region with endemic malaria generally necessitates prophylaxis with one of the following drugs:

Chloroquine – For the few areas left in the world with chloroquine-sensitive malarial protozoans (*e.g.*, Central America), **chloroquine** can still be used as a prophylaxis. Within the asexual phase of its lifecycle, the malarial protozoan degrades hemoglobin within erythrocytes to produce essential amino acids; this degradation produces a non-toxic heme biocrystal (*hemozoin*) within the digestive vacuoles of the parasite. Chloroquine accumulates in this digestive vacuole, prevents heme biocrystallization, and binds to the heme to form a highly toxic complex (*i.e.*, Fe(II)-protoporphyrin IX-chloroquine). Malarial protozoa that do not form hemozoin are resistant to chloroquine. (Lin et al. 2015)

Mefloquine – The quinine-related drug **mefloquine** is believed to bind the 80S ribosome of malarial protozoa and thereby inhibit plasmodial protein synthesis. (Wong et al. 2017) It is safe in pregnancy and with young children and has a long half-life allowing for weekly (rather than daily) dosing. Resistance is uncommon (except in regions of Southeast Asia). Extensive experience with mefloquine use by the world's military (*e.g.*, the Commonwealth realms of Australia and Canada) has led to the conclusion that this drug should be contraindicated with a patient history of psychiatric disorders, epilepsy, or arrhythmia/cardiac conduction defects.

Primaquine – **Primaquine** is used to prevent or treat malaria, and also to treat *Pneumocystis* pneumonia when in combination with clindamycin. While its mechanism of action is not fully understood, **primaquine** is lethal to liver-stage *P. vivax* and *P. ovale*, and to *P. vivax* in the blood stage. Primaquine should not be given to people with glucose-6-phosphate dehydrogenase (G6PD) deficiency due to the risk of hemolytic anemia (Brunette and Nemhauser 2020); given the fetus' uncertain G6PD status, primaquine is therefore also not recommended in pregnancy. Furthermore, in persons with cytochrome b5 reductase deficiency, primaquine causes methemoglobinemia – oxidation of hemoglobin from the ferrous (Fe^{2+}) to ferric (Fe^{3+}) state, eliminating oxygen-carriage capacity.

Tafenoquine – A newer drug, related to primaquine (Haston et al. 2019), **tafenoquine** is similarly used not only for prophylaxis but also for the radical cure (a.k.a. "anti-relapse therapy") of *P. vivax* and *P. ovale* malaria given its ability to eliminate the dormant liver-stage parasites ("hypnozoite" stage). Like primaquine, tafenoquine use is contraindicated in individuals with G6PD deficiency or unknown G6PD status.

Doxycycline – As first discussed in antibacterial pharmacology, the broad-spectrum tetracycline class-member **doxycycline** also has activity against Rickettsiae and other environmentally-borne infectious agents; coupled with its low cost and short time requirement for dosing (only 1-2 days before travel), doxycycline may be preferable for travelers with planned hiking, camping, and wading/swimming activities.

Atovaquone-Proguanil – **Atovaquone** selectively inhibits the malarial cytochrome bc_1 complex thereby collapsing the membrane potential across the Plasmodium mitochondrion, preventing proper energy/ATP production. If used alone, atovaquone will generally fail over the long term because Plasmodium species can evade by mutating their cytochrome bc_1 complex. **Proguanil** is therefore added as a "mitochondrial sensitizer", given that its metabolite cycloguanil inhibits plasmodial dihydrofolate reductase, similar to the action of trimethoprim discussed above. The combination of atovaquone and proguanil is generally well tolerated, and is safe for children with body weight above 5 kg; however, it is not advised in pregnancy, and use may result in a reversible elevation in liver enzymes (ALT/AST).

Treatment

The US Centers for Disease Control and Prevention (CDC) recommends that treatment decisions for malaria consider four main factors: the infecting Plasmodium species, the patient's clinical status, the anticipated drug susceptibility of the infecting protozoan as suspected from the geographical area of acquisition, and any prior use by the patient of antimalarial drugs including for prophylaxis. **Chloroquine** can be used if the Plasmodium species is chloroquine-sensitive. Otherwise, **artemisinin**-based combination therapy is recommended for malarial treatment. **Artemisinin** (a.k.a. the Chinese antipyretic *qinghaosu* (White et al. 2015)), and its analogs **artesunate** and **artemether**, are each rapidly metabolized to the active species dihydroartemisinin, which has a mechanism of action against the malarial protozoan of producing lethal free radicals in the food vacuole via iron-catalyzed cleavage. Monotherapy with a dihydroartemisinin pro-drug is strongly discouraged to prevent the selection of artemisinin-resistant malarial parasites; for example, the combination of **artemether-lumefantrine** is considered first-line therapy for uncomplicated *P. falciparum* malaria (and lumefantrine is only ever used in combination with artemether, so that the combination is sometimes called "co-artemether"). Artemisinin-containing combinations are allowed in second and third-trimester pregnancy, and intravenous artesunate is permitted at any stage of pregnancy for severe malaria. As previously mentioned, *P. vivax* or *P. ovale* infection also warrants adding **primaquine** or **tafenoquine** to ensure eradication of hepatic hypnozoites, but patients at risk of having glucose-6-phosphate dehydrogenase (G6PD) deficiency should be tested before their use.

Infectious Disease – Viruses – General Background

Viral organisms are ubiquitous throughout environments, similar to bacteria. They can be most easily thought about as genetic material, be it ribonucleic acids or deoxyribonucleic acids, surrounded by some kind of delivery system. These viral particles allow the introduction of viral genetic material into a host cell, which will use the host enzymes to produce viral proteins as part of the viral replicative process. Numerous viruses can infect humans, and their ability to infect and cause disease is termed virulence (discussed in the Bacterial section). Because viruses cannot survive individually and must infect a host cell to replicate, they are by definition not "alive." The capsid, or the covering of the genetic material, can be quite delicate depending on its composition. This can affect the virus's ability to survive outside of its host and its ability to spread from person to person. (Knipe 2022)

Some of the world's most famous viruses include human immunodeficiency virus (HIV), influenza virus, herpes virus, rhinovirus, and the hepatitis viruses HBV and HCV; the most recent pandemic has been caused by the coronavirus SARS-CoV-2 (a.k.a. COVID-19). Much of the naming of viruses has been determined based on how they were spread, what organs they affected, and even on their ability to be filtered. Unlike bacterial infections, certain viral infections can remain dormant inside the body and cause symptoms and disease later. Few options are available to treat these "dormant" infections, but the body can sometimes clear them over time (e.g., human papillomavirus or HPV). One way in which we have learned to prevent viral disease is through vaccination. Many vaccines are based on proteins expressed on the surface of viral particles. By exposing the immune system to these proteins in isolation (and oftimes with immune system boosting/activating agents), it can develop antibodies against them without having an actual viral infection. This allows the immune system to mount a more robust and quicker response to a real infection, sometimes completely preventing symptomatic infection. Given that certain viruses, such as HPV and hepatitis viruses, have been linked to the development of cancers, certain vaccines against these causative viruses offer a unique opportunity to eradicate these cancers. (Knipe 2022) The most recently developed vaccines against the COVID-19 coronavirus have gathered significant media attention and, thanks to the exhaustive effort and focus of scientists worldwide, have been some of the fastest ever to be developed. (Liang et al. 2022)

Diagnosis

Just as with bacterial infections, a thorough history and physical examination is the first step in diagnosing a viral infection. Unlike bacterial infections, cultures are significantly harder to obtain, and sensitivity can be low. Given how small viral molecules are, microscopic examination is not feasible. Electron microscopes do have the ability to visualize viruses, but they are not widely available. Molecular and serologic tests, such as PCR, are significantly more sensitive and can help provide a diagnosis significantly faster. Various immunoassays are also available, which are used for certain infections. How and when samples are obtained, from wherever viral shedding occurs, significantly affects the sensitivity and specificity of all types of tests. Rapid testing options are available for various viruses, such as influenza, and can help expedite the initiation of appropriate treatments. (Knipe 2022)

Central Nervous System Infections

Presentation
Many viruses can cause meningitis (infection and inflammation of the meninges) affecting patients of all ages and populations. Viral meningitis most commonly presents with the typical symptoms of meningitis, which include fever, headache, photophobia, neck stiffness, altered mental status, and nuchal rigidity. Enteroviruses are currently the most common cause of viral meningitis, affecting patients of all ages. This is a genus of the Picornaviridae family of viruses consisting of Coxsackie A and B, Echovirus, Poliovirus, and (more recently) enteroviruses designated by number. Enterovirus is a positive sense RNA virus that replicates using host transcription factors.

In affluent countries, the herpes simplex virus is currently the second most common cause in adults and adolescents of viral meningitis and viral encephalitis (infection and inflammation of the brain). Primary genital herpes can lead to complications, particularly when HSV-2 is present. Without pre-existing antibodies to HSV-1 or HSV-2, the first infection with either virus type is referred to as a primary herpes simplex infection, which is more associated with developing "*aseptic* meningitis" (brain meningeal inflammation that is negative in lab testing of CSF for bacterial infection). (Cassady and Whitley 2014) HSV-1, commonly known as oral herpes, classically presents as gingivostomatitis, keratoconjunctivitis, herpes labialis, herpetic whitlow on fingers, temporal lobe encephalitis, esophagitis, and erythema multiforme. It is essential to know that it affects the brain's temporal lobe. HSV-2, commonly known as genital herpes, classically presents as a vesicular rash on the genitals that can be painful or itchy, as well as small red bumps or tiny white blisters with ulcers on the genitalia. It is spread via sexual contact and perinatally. The virus remains latent in the sacral ganglia and correlates more to viral meningitis than HSV-1. It is also a common cause of neonatal infection. Herpes meningoencephalitis can present as headaches, fever, neck stiffness, photophobia, seizures, altered mental status, personality changes, hallucinations, and unusual behavior in patients. Varicella Zoster Virus (VZV) is another type of virus in the Herpes family that affects up to 30% of the US population at some point in their life. VZV can result in a variety of diseases that affect the central nervous system (CNS), such as cerebellar ataxia, arteritis, myelitis, meningitis, and encephalitis. (De La Blanchardiere et al. 2000) With primary or secondary reactivation of the virus, CNS infection might happen.

Epstein Barr Virus (EBV) is a double-stranded DNA virus that most commonly causes infectious mononucleosis. This disease can be asymptomatic but classically presents as pharyngitis, fatigue, fever, rash, cervical lymphadenopathy, and splenomegaly. Although rare, EBV has been seen to cause various CNS complications, including encephalitis, meningitis, cerebellitis, acute disseminated encephalomyelitis, transverse myelitis, and radiculopathy. (Jang and Lee 2011) Neurological complications of EBV infection occur in 1-18% of patients with infectious mononucleosis. (Hausler et al. 2002) The CNS complications that ensue closely resemble those seen in HSV encephalitis, with many similar symptoms. These symptoms include consciousness disturbance, decreased activity, bizarre behavior, gate disturbance, urine incontinence, and seizures.

Probably the most feared virus, HIV, can cause encephalitis and present in various ways. Increased deep tendon reflexes and muscle tone are frequently seen, associated with motor abnormalities such as tremors, irregular gait, and balance difficulties. Mini-Mental Status Examination (MMSE) results are compared to earlier results to look for any decline in cognitive function in subjects. (Nir et al. 2014) Encephalitis in HIV patients presents as a late manifestation of the disease. In contrast to progressive dementias, such as Alzheimer's, HIV-induced cognitive impairment has more of a waxing and waning presentation. Subcortical deficits such as psychomotor retardation, decreased concentration, and reduced attention are often the hallmarks of this disease's presentation. (Daliparty and Balasubramanya 2022)

Risk factors
In general, patients with any form of immunocompromise are at increased risk of being infected with a virus leading to meningitis. Children under 10 are most at risk of contracting enterovirus, with immunocompromised and pregnant patients being most at risk of developing complications. Regarding HSV infection, adolescence, education level, age of coitarche, and history of previous sexually transmitted disease all increase the risk of contracting the virus. HIV patients with CD4 counts less than 350 are at increased risk of encephalitis.

Pathophysiology
The pathophysiology of enteroviral meningitis has yet to be fully understood. However, it is believed that autophagy (degradation/recycling of cellular components) and apoptosis (programmed cell death) are two processes that enteroviruses aberrantly trigger to harm the central nervous system. (Messacar and Abzug 2023) The illness may also be influenced by the immunological response. HSV virus is spread via respiratory secretions and saliva. The virus most commonly remains latent in the trigeminal ganglia and is the most common cause of sporadic encephalitis. Varicella (chickenpox) is caused by a primary infection. But because it spreads and lays latent in the cranial, dorsal

root, or autonomic ganglia, the causative virus (VZV) never wholly leaves the body. EBV is spread via saliva and is commonly known as "the kissing disease". After invading B cells, EBV remains latent, which can potentially cause recurrent infection. The pathophysiology of HIV, most simply put, is via replication of the virus inside the host's CD4+ T-helper cells, subsequently leading to their death. These cells are essential for fighting off infections, and their loss ultimately causes a wholly compromised immune system if not treated.

Examination

Physical examination of a patient with suspected viral meningitis is critical in the diagnosis. There are several signs and tests that can be performed that can assist in ruling meningitis in or out of differential diagnoses. These examinations include nuchal rigidity, jolt accentuation, Kernig's sign, and Brudzinski's neck sign, discussed in the Bacterial section. These tests are relatively easy and can be performed when assessing for potential meningitis by general physicians who are not neurologists. Nuchal rigidity is considered positive if the patient has palpable resistance to passive neck flexion and is the most used maneuver. Jolt accentuation is one of the new techniques that is being used and involves the physician rotating the head of the patient 2-3 times per second and evaluating whether the patient's headache worsens. (Akaishi et al. 2019) The test can be done easily; however, the sensitivity is low, as seen in several studies. Brudzinski's neck sign is when there is a reflexive knee and hip flexion to passive flexion of the patient's neck (due to discomfort from meningeal stretch), while Kernig's sign is when there is an inability or patient discomfort with extending the leg when the hip is flexed (via the same meningeal stretch mechanism). Other physical examinations that should be done include hearing to assess for potential sensorineural hearing loss, a gait exam to evaluate for possible changes, and episodes of seizures should be monitored. In addition, an examination of the throat, the skin of the spine, and sometimes the genital region should be done to evaluate for primary infection.

Laboratory

Unlike in bacterial meningitis, abnormal laboratory values in blood tests may not be present for viral meningitis. Leukocytosis is neither sensitive nor specific in diagnosing a viral infection and therefore is not helpful in the diagnosis. On the other hand, cerebrospinal fluid (CSF) analysis via lumbar puncture is vital and can be used to ascertain a diagnosis of viral meningitis. It typically shows an elevated amount of white blood cells and elevated protein, but normal glucose levels. (Kohil et al. 2021) These results are helpful since glucose and protein values will differ if a bacteria or fungus causes the infection.

Imaging

Many times, when meningitis is suspected, a CT scan of the brain with and without contrast, as well as an MRI with gadolinium, will be obtained. In HSV, a brain CT scan classically shows the involvement of the bilateral medial temporal lobe, insular cortex, and gyrus; however, MRI is the imaging modality of choice and is abnormal in 90% of patients. (Ak and Mendez 2022) In VZV, on the other hand, a brain MRI may reveal high signal intensities in the basal ganglia, the most affected region. Radiology can also be used for HIV with CT and MRI typically showing cerebral atrophy, and multiple symmetric foci of hyperintense, non-enhancing lesions in a subcortical distribution. (Sharma et al. 2022)

Associated symptoms/conditions

Some associated symptoms that can be seen in enterovirus include mucocutaneous manifestations. These manifestations include vesicles on the hands, feet, and mouth and a generalized maculopapular rash. Malaise, gastrointestinal symptoms, and generalized lymphadenopathy can also be seen. (Logan and MacMahon 2008) As mentioned before, HSV-1 and HSV-2 initially present with oral or genital manifestations that are typically painful. Erythema multiforme is the specific cutaneous rash that can appear in patients with symmetrical, red, raised lesions anywhere on the body but is more noticeable on the fingers and toes. Secondary VZV skin eruption exhibits a typical unilateral, vesicular, painful cutaneous eruption ("zoster") that adheres to a distinctive dermatomal distribution. (Gnann Jr 2007) Increased excitability of central nociceptors in the spinal cord, which results in inflammation and disruption to the nerve cells and makes them more susceptible to painful stimuli, is what causes the classic pain pattern generated by the virus. Besides mononucleosis, EBV is associated with B cell lymphoma, Hodgkin's lymphoma, Burkitt's lymphoma, nasopharyngeal carcinoma (most commonly in Asians), and oral hairy leukoplakia.

Diagnosis

Diagnosis is confirmed via a lumbar puncture to assess cerebrospinal fluid. In viral meningitis, the CSF is most often clear, with glucose typically being normal with an elevated protein level. Other diagnostic tests include virus isolation, PCR, nucleic acid testing, and serological tests such as complement fixation, neutralization, and enzyme-linked immunosorbent assays (ELISA). Enterovirus replicates in the mucosa of the oropharynx and intestines; therefore, separate throat and rectal swabs can also be done to detect the virus. Older techniques such as a Tzank smear to detect HSV multinucleated giant cells can also be done but are not used as much. Viral cultures of serum, blood, and urine should all be obtained to rule out other causes and are one of the mainstays of identifying specific viral infections.

Treatment

Unfortunately, for many viruses that cause meningitis, no specific treatments or cures currently exist. Since many of these viruses remain latent in different ganglia in the body and commonly become reactivated, it is difficult to eradicate the virus from the body completely. However, certain antiviral agents do exist that are being used for a select few, including **acyclovir** and **valacyclovir,** that can be prescribed to prevent outbreaks of HSV. **Vidarabine** is another antiviral agent that has been used to treat herpes simplex encephalitis. These medications can lessen the severity and duration of symptoms in recurrent outbreaks and reduce the frequency of recurrence.

Management

Most cases of viral meningitis are typically self-limited and resolve within one to two weeks. However, in immunocompromised patients, the infection can be severe and lead to serious complications, including coma and death. The mainstay of management is symptomatic support, ensuring proper electrolyte balance, administering fluids, and consistently monitoring for complications. Current guidelines for managing VZV encephalitis include 10 mg/kg every 8 hours of IV **acyclovir** for seven days in immunocompetent patients and 10-14 days in immunosuppressed patients. (Gnann 2002) Higher doses of up to 12-15 mg/kg may be required for the immunosuppressed and severe cases. Acyclovir's oral prodrug **valacyclovir** has better pharmacokinetic properties and solves the drawback of poor bioavailability and, therefore, can also be used in treating VZV. Once an HIV diagnosis has been confirmed, the only thing that can be done in terms of management is to start the patient on Highly Active Anti-Retroviral Therapy (HAART). These medications can effectively reverse the pathologic damage caused by HIV, as seen both clinically and radiographically. (Lu et al. 2018)

Upper and Lower Respiratory Infections

Presentation

The most common disease-causing agents in humans are respiratory viruses, significantly impacting morbidity and mortality globally. An easy mechanism to distinguish between upper and lower respiratory viral infections is based on their anatomical location as well as the clinical presentation of the patient. Upper respiratory tract (URT) infections are most commonly caused by viruses, although many bacteria and fungi are also implicated. The URT consists of the nose/nostrils, nasal cavity, mouth, pharynx, epiglottis, and larynx. Therefore, when a virus invades one of these structures, it is known as a URT infection or "URI". The most common manifestations are sinusitis, common cold, pharyngitis, epiglottitis, and laryngotracheitis. The common cold is the most frequently encountered respiratory illness, accounting for most patient-doctor visits. This is caused mainly by Rhinovirus but can also be due to Coronavirus, Parainfluenza virus, Respiratory syncytial virus (RSV), and Adenovirus. Clinically, the classic common-cold symptoms of nasal discharge and blockage, sneezing, sore throat, and cough appear in adults and children after an incubation period of 48–72 hours. ([Internet] 2020) A headache and myalgia could also be present; however, very important to note, fever is uncommon. (Dasaraju and Liu 1996) Pharyngitis, commonly known as sore throat, occurs when there is inflammation of the mucus membranes of the oropharynx, either due to an underlying infection or allergies. In children, Type A Coxsackievirus is a common culprit of pharyngitis that presents with small blister-like bumps on the back of the throat or roof of the mouth that can ulcerate. (Wolford et al. 2022) EBV is a relatively common viral infection that affects adolescents and mainly causes infectious mononucleosis but can also present as pharyngitis and present in a similar fashion as cytomegalovirus. Adenovirus and Herpes Simplex Virus are other less prevalent causes. Clinically, patients with pharyngitis present with discomfort in their throat, causing dysphagia. Systemic symptoms such as fever, fatigue, headaches, and myalgias may also be present. Laryngotracheitis, commonly known as croup, is when there is inflammation of both the larynx and the trachea. This condition is frequently caused by the Parainfluenza virus and is most prominent in infants between six months and three years. Infants with croup can present with fever but classically have a barking cough and inspiratory stridor with hoarseness.

Bacteria more commonly cause lower respiratory tract (LRT) infections; however, there are several viral causes. The lower respiratory tract consists of the trachea, the bronchi, the bronchioles, and the alveoli. RSV commonly affects toddlers under the age of two and results in bronchiolitis. Infants with bronchiolitis typically have a cough with a runny nose that evolves into a deep, productive cough with the presence of fever, chest wall retractions, and grunting. (Hall et al. 1979) The most troublesome LRT infection is pneumonia, which several different viruses can cause. These include influenza, rhinoviruses, adenoviruses, cytomegalovirus, and (recently) COVID-19. The condition presents with chest pain, cough, fever, shortness of breath, and sputum production in some instances. Presentation can vary from asymptomatic to altered mental status, abdominal pain with vomiting, and diarrhea. A rapid high temperature, a sore throat, a headache, myalgias, and a general feeling of malaise are among the main symptoms of influenza. After two to four days of the fever, runny nose and coughing are typically seen. In children, gastrointestinal symptoms including nausea, upset stomach, and diarrhea may also be seen. Children experience neurological symptoms like spasms, consciousness difficulties, middle ear, and muscle inflammation more frequently than adults. The influenza virus in the elderly must be closely monitored due to the potential seriousness of the illness and the high mortality associated with developing a secondary infection, the most worrisome being superimposed bacterial pneumonia.

Risk factors

Patients with immunosuppression of any kind are at increased risk of contracting a respiratory virus. However, certain conditions have specific risk factors that make certain populations of patients more susceptible to catching one. For example, pharyngitis is more common in children and adolescents. It can be caused by smoking, not washing hands thoroughly or enough, and living or working in crowded places. Croup, caused by Parainfluenza or RSV, generally affects infants and toddlers due to their immature immune systems. Since respiratory tract infections are transmitted airborne or via respiratory droplets, they are easily spread from human to human. Pregnant women, residents of nursing homes, and obese patients with a BMI greater than 40 are also at increased risk. The fact that many patients can be asymptomatic and unaware they have been infected can potentially lead to pandemics of respiratory viruses, as was seen with COVID-19.

Pathophysiology

Most viral respiratory infections are transmitted via airborne secretions that are inhaled or saliva that is swallowed. Mucosa epithelial cells appear to be directly invaded by the viruses; however, depending on the particular organism, this may or may not result in cell death, sloughing, or loss of ciliary action. (*e.g.*, ref. (Lee et al. 2018)) Leukocyte infiltration and nasal secretions, including significant amounts of protein and immunoglobulin, both rise, suggesting that released cytokines and immunological processes may cause some of the symptoms. In pharyngitis, the nasopharynx and oral cavity's mucosal cells appear to be invaded by viral pathogens, causing edema and hyperemia of the tonsils and mucous membranes. The influenza virus contains specific enzymes that allow it to invade the respiratory tract of humans. Hemagglutinin, a viral surface glycoprotein, binds to sialic acid found in cell membranes of the upper respiratory tract. Once attached to sialic acid, another enzyme that the virus contains on its surface, neuraminidase, facilitates viral entry into host cells of the respiratory tract; neuraminidase activity also promotes the release of progeny virus after replication within these host cells. (Sriwilaijaroen et al. 2022; McAuley et al. 2019) Viral pneumonia has several different mechanisms by which it can arise. It can occur either through direct injection of the virus into a portion of the lung via inhalation, hematogenous spread from anatomically neighboring or distal infection, or contiguous spread. (Freeman and Leigh 2022)

Examination

Physical examination of patients with upper and lower respiratory viral infection will vary based on the affected site. Patients may initially present with a runny nose, nasal congestion, and cough, which can be vital in differentiating a viral cause of the illness from bacterial, as the profuse nasal discharge is typically absent in bacterial infection. Many patients may also only have a low-grade fever as opposed to bacterial cases of pneumonia that present with higher temperatures. In pharyngitis, the presence or absence of exudates and/or palatal vesicles can assist in differentiating between viral causes such as HSV and EBV. Cervical lymphadenopathy is seen in bacteria and viruses; however, palpating for splenomegaly and hepatomegaly can help physicians lean more toward a viral infection such as EBV.

Laboratory

Laboratory findings are not usually helpful when attempting to diagnose a viral infection. This is because of the varied values of labs in viral infection. A CBC with differential, when ordered, can show elevated, normal, or decreased WBC counts, all of which have been seen in viral respiratory infections. Chemistry panels are essential to assess the infection's severity on vital organs such as the kidneys. Inflammatory markers such as C-reactive protein are also commonly elevated in viral infections; however, such marker levels are not sensitive nor specific for them. Unfortunately, no definitive lab value can indicate a patient has a viral infection in the manner that procalcitonin (PCT) is associated with a bacterial infection.

Imaging

Chest X-ray remains the mainstay for the imaging of respiratory tract infections. In young infants with croup, tapering of the airway between the vocal cords is classically seen as a "steeple sign". Many coinciding features are seen in both bacterial and viral pneumonias. Some qualities that are most seen in viral infections are interstitial infiltrates, patchy distribution of interstitial infiltrates, and bilateral infiltrates. (Virkki et al. 2005) When influenza is suspected, the presence of focal infiltrates indicates superimposed bacterial pneumonia. (Dasaraju and Liu 1996) CT scans are also performed with patients with serious illnesses to look for consolidations, ground glass opacifications, and lung nodules. CT scans also commonly detect pneumonia with viral causes showing parenchymal defects.

Associated symptoms/conditions

Aside from the classic symptoms seen at the primary site of infection, several unique features can be apparent. As mentioned earlier, in cases of EBV, there is the presence of lymphadenopathy that can be generalized, as well as splenomegaly.

Diagnosis

Many viruses can be diagnosed clinically based on the patient's presenting symptoms. The common cold is an excellent example, as it has been proven difficult to isolate rhinovirus for a definitive diagnosis. With pharyngitis, a major cause is *Streptococcus pyogenes*; therefore, a Rapid Strep test is typically done to rule it out. Once excluded, serologic studies are more commonly used than performing viral cultures *per se*. In infants with bronchiolitis caused by RSV, nasopharyngeal specimens are collected for analysis via serologic testing, rapid diagnostic tests for antibody or viral antigens, or ELISA, which can confirm the diagnosis. Diagnostic testing for viral pneumonia generally utilizes the same strategies for URIs, including viral cultures to isolate the causative organism. (Freeman and Leigh 2022)

Treatment
In general, many viruses do not have definitive medications or treatments that can be utilized, and therefore a supportive and symptomatic treatment approach is taken. However certain specific viruses such as HSV have medications that can be used, mainly **acyclovir**, but only if clinically warranted or for immunosuppressed patients. In infants with bronchiolitis, a supportive and symptomatic treatment approach is taken (see management of croup below); however, in severe cases, **ribavirin** has been proven to improve a patient's condition. Certain antiviral agents have been seen to alleviate some symptoms of influenza, including **oseltamivir**, **peramivir**, and **baloxavir marboxil**. (Swierczynska et al. 2022) However, these medications are only beneficial if administered within two days of symptom onset.

Management
In toddlers with croup, the illness typically self-resolves. However, if it persists and it is severe, then racemic epinephrine is used, given its ability to constrict mucosal arterioles in the upper airway and alter capillary pressure leading to reduced airway edema and secretions.

Most patients with influenza recover within three days; however, if symptoms persist, it is compulsory to provide supportive treatment to these patients. In patients with viral pneumonia, oxygen therapy with noninvasive positive pressure ventilation or intubation may be done to ensure proper oxygenation. However, as mentioned before, symptomatic and supportive treatment is the mainstay of management.

Myocarditis/Viremia

Presentation
There are many different causes of myocarditis, including infectious and non-infectious causes. Regarding infectious causes, viruses remain the most common, with Coxsackievirus, Parvovirus B-19, Adenovirus, HIV, CMV, EBV, Influenzas A & B, human herpesvirus 6 (HHV-6), Rubella, Hepatitis B and C, and now COVID-19, frequently being implicated. Most patients with myocarditis typically have a prodrome period of flu-like sickness, including fever, fatigue, myalgias with vomiting, and diarrhea that can present anywhere from a few days to weeks before myocarditis ensues. (Kang and An 2022) The patient usually states that they had a respiratory or gastrointestinal infection in the preceding weeks. On presentation, the patient can have a wide range of symptoms, including chest pain, dyspnea, fatigue, palpitations, swelling of extremities, and syncope. On initial presentation, the illness may closely resemble the symptoms seen in Acute Coronary Syndrome, both physically and on an electrocardiogram (EKG). Depending on the stage at which the patient presents, they may have heart failure that is new onset, progressing, or in the chronic phase. In severe myocarditis, patients can develop cardiogenic shock and potentially life-threatening arrhythmias. (Sozzi et al. 2022) Infants and children are commonly affected by this illness and can have unique symptoms. In infants, severe respiratory distress or failure with hypoxia and cyanosis may lead to cardiac arrest. In children, difficulty breathing with grunting respirations and intercostal retractions may be seen along with loss of appetite.

Risk factors
In general, patients with immunosuppression of any kind are at increased risk of viral myocarditis. The illness is most commonly seen in young male adults, although women are also at risk. Patients with specific autoimmune diseases such as systemic lupus erythematosus (SLE) or conditions such as sarcoidosis are also at increased risk. Several medical interventions have been noted to cause myocarditis, including dialysis, implanted heart devices, radiation, and central venous lines.

Pathophysiology
Viruses cause myocarditis indirectly after initial infection: the virus is first exposed via direct inoculation to specific cell surface receptors at the primary site of infection, whether in the GI or respiratory tract or elsewhere. After entry and replication, the virus then seeds to other locations in the body, within and around the heart in this case, and begins to replicate there, leading to cell death of myocardial cells. The virus also directly activates the immune system, rapidly leading to inflammation of the myocardium. In subacute infection, heart autoantibodies and inflammatory proteins are produced as a result of increased autoimmune-mediated damage, activated T and B cells, and subsequent antibody production. (Kang and An 2022) The global enlargement of the heart and dilation of all chambers via sarcomeres eventually lead to dilated cardiomyopathy.

Examination
There are no findings on physical examination specific to myocarditis; however, certain signs and symptoms can be suspicious for myocarditis, indicating further workup is necessary. Depending on the severity of the illness, patients may or may not appear toxic. Assess carefully how the patient is breathing and note the presence of diaphoresis,

cyanosis, and paleness which are signs of a toxic patient. Visualization of rashes on the skin or erythema nodosum can indicate bacterial causes of myocarditis. Vital signs may show abnormalities, including hypotension, tachycardia, tachypnea, and fever. Depending on the stage and severity of the illness, the patient may present with symptoms of heart failure. This includes jugular venous distention, swelling of lower extremities, and a fluid wave in the abdomen indicative of ascites. Bilateral crackles may be heard during auscultation of the heart and lungs, representing pulmonary edema and an S3 gallop, a common finding in patients with heart failure. EKG should be done on all patients with chest pain or signs of cardiac dysfunction and can show ST segment changes.

Laboratory

Several laboratory values should be obtained when myocarditis is suspected. A basic metabolic panel (BMP), CBC with differential to assess for leukocytosis, inflammatory markers such as CRP, and cardiac enzymes including creatinine kinase, cardiac troponins, and BNP are all important to analyze. (*e.g.*, ref. (Mirna et al. 2022)) Additionally, liver function tests and rheumatologic screening to exclude systemic inflammatory diseases can assist in the diagnosis. Viral antibody titers are another significant lab value that can be used to detect the presence of a specific virus causing myocarditis. When warranted, a biopsy can be performed with the specimen displaying cardiomyocyte death and lymphocyte infiltration.

Imaging

Transthoracic Echocardiography (TTE) is the initial imaging test that should be performed when myocarditis is suspected. TTE is an ultrasound of the heart that can detect valve functionality and cardiac ejection fractions of the left and right ventricles, and can also show the degree of inflammation that may be present. Typically, patients with severe myocarditis will have a preserved left ventricular ejection fraction (LVEF) with global hypokinesis, although decreased LVEF may also be observed. (Kang and An 2022) It is also beneficial in excluding other causes of heart failure, such as amyloidosis, hemochromatosis, or congenital heart disease. Cardiac scintigraphy using radiolabeled antimyosin is another valuable imaging technique that can detect the severity of myocardial inflammation with high sensitivity. Due to the high mortality associated with coronary ischemia, a coronary angiogram may be indicated in patients with symptoms of new-onset heart failure. Increased diastolic pressures with decreased cardiac output are commonly viewed. Another imaging tool that may be used is contrast-enhanced MRI with gadolinium, which can also detect the degree of inflammation and edema present, although not very specific. Currently, the gold standard for diagnosis of myocarditis is an endomyocardial biopsy. However, due to inadequate sensitivity or specificity, it is only used after other imaging techniques have failed to diagnose patients whose condition worsens. (Angelini et al. 2000) Chest X-rays are not beneficial in diagnosing myocarditis, although it is commonly done and may show cardiomegaly.

Associated symptoms/conditions

Many of the symptoms of myocarditis are highly associated with clinical manifestations of heart failure and cardiac dysfunction. As mentioned before, the prodrome of flu-like illness is typically present in patients, including headaches, myalgias, fever or sore throat, and diarrhea or vomiting. The most dangerous complications are heart failure, arrhythmias that can be fatal, myocardial infarction, and sudden cardiac death. This is due to scar tissue that forms from the inflammation and damage caused by viral myocarditis. This makes it difficult for the heart to contract appropriately, leading to wall thickening and, eventually, ischemia. The pericardium can also be affected in some cases, leading to pericarditis. This can present with a pericardial friction rub on auscultation with patients complaining of chest pain that may improve when leaning forward.

Diagnosis

To diagnose viral myocarditis, antibody titers to specific viruses, including Coxsackie group B, HIV, CMV, EBV, Hepatitis, Influenza, and COVID-19, should be tested. In the initial stage of the disease, the titers can rise four-fold, with a progressive decline as the disease advances. As mentioned earlier, many cardiac imaging tools are utilized when diagnosing viral myocarditis. These include TTE, cardiac scintigraphy, MRI, and cardiac catheterization. Endomyocardial biopsy is currently the gold standard but is not very specific to the disease. An essential aspect of diagnosing myocarditis is excluding ischemic cardiomyopathy. Therefore, obtaining lab values for cardiac troponins and analyzing EKG for abnormalities is crucial.

Treatment

In many cases of viral myocarditis, the illness is self-limited within several months. The treatment of viral myocarditis involves supportive care with the replenishment of fluids and accompanying oxygen for patients with respiratory difficulty. Unfortunately, there are not any antiviral agents that are useful in the management of viral myocarditis and are not advised due to poor efficacy. Patients with symptoms of heart failure should be treated appropriately with medications such as ACE inhibitors, Beta-blockers (contraindicated in patients with signs of right-sided heart failure), and diuretics if needed (Albert et al. 2021). The ABCs of critical care should always be managed appropriately, as some patients may require intubation and placement on mechanical ventilators. Although NSAIDs are typically used in treating pericarditis, they are contraindicated in patients with myocarditis since they cause poor healing of the myocardium. Antiarrhythmics may be considered in certain patients; however, they should be used cautiously due to some causing decreased contractility. (Al-Akchar and Kiel 2022) In patients not showing clinical improvement with medication, surgical procedures such as intra-aortic balloon pump or ventricular assist device insertion can be beneficial. The last resort for treatment-refractory cases involves cardiac transplantation.

Management
Most cases are self-limited and resolve within several weeks or months. It is important to follow up with the patient and perform a repeat TTE to confirm the resolution of the infection. In cases of severe illness, admission to ICU may be required to ensure proper oxygenation and provide symptomatic treatment.

Intra-Abdominal Infections

Presentation
Intra-abdominal infections can range from asymptomatic to severe life-threatening sepsis. Although many bacteria and parasites are often implicated in abdominal infections, there are also several viral causes. Viral gastroenteritis is inflammation of the gastrointestinal tract most commonly caused by norovirus, rotavirus, astrovirus, and (occasionally) adenovirus. Patients present with loose, watery diarrhea, nausea, and non-bloody emesis. Painful abdominal cramps, loss of appetite, and systemic symptoms, including fever or chills with headaches, myalgias, and arthralgias, may also be seen. Rotavirus is primarily seen in infants and children but can infect patients of any age, whereas the other viruses are more present in adults. Symptoms can last from one day to several weeks, depending on the viral load. Cytomegalovirus (CMV) colitis is a more severe illness that presents as hematochezia, rectal bleeding, and diarrhea. (Azer and Limaiem 2022) The symptoms can imitate an acute episode of inflammatory bowel disease. Based on clinical presentation, it can be challenging to differentiate between CMV colitis and ulcerative colitis.

Risk factors
Viral gastroenteritis is an illness that can affect patients of all populations. Since it is highly contagious and can be transmitted via direct contact with an infected individual or contaminated objects, food, or drinks, it can be very easy to contract the virus. In particular, infants and young children are at increased risk of infection due to their immature immune systems and not following appropriate safety precautions such as proper hand washing. Individuals staying close to other people, such as in daycare centers, resorts, cruise ships, or other destinations, are at increased risk. The elderly, particularly those in nursing homes, are also at increased risk. With CMV colitis, immunosuppression of any kind vastly increases the risk of contracting the virus. Long-term corticosteroid use in patients with ulcerative colitis has also been associated with CMV colitis.

Pathophysiology
The mechanism by which these viruses cause illness is via infection of the enterocytes of the gastrointestinal tract. The virus exploits the enterocyte to proliferate, interfering with the development of the brush border and causing malabsorption and osmotic diarrhea as a result. Additionally, viral cytotoxins trigger enterocytes and intestinal villa to undergo direct damage and cell lysis, resulting in a fluid leak into the intestine. (Stuempfig and Seroy 2022) Loss of transporter functionality typically results from cell dysfunction and leads to electrolyte abnormalities and acid-base imbalance. The virus is then expelled through feces and, on rare occasions, vomit. CMV, in general, can be transmitted via respiratory droplets, saliva, blood, perinatally, and sexual contact. Infection is relatively common; however, immunocompetent individuals usually do not experience symptoms, so GI infection is underreported. Primary infection clears, but the virus remains latent in mononuclear cells. In immunocompromised patients, the reactivation of the virus can eventually cause colitis, among other manifestations.

Examination
Physical examination is an essential component when diagnosing abdominal infections. Inspection of the patient can clue the physician on the severity of the patient's illness based on their appearance. Palpation of the abdomen is required to assess for tenderness and potential peritonitis, the latter of which deserves immediate laparoscopy. Normal percussion of the epigastric region and upper midline reveals tympany, whereas it typically sounds dull over the liver. Therefore, percussing the patient in these regions is vital for evaluating any abnormalities. Auscultation is another critical element of physical examination that should be done to assess the quality of bowel sounds. Vitals may show increased temperature indicative of microbial infection. Mucous membranes should also be visualized to evaluate for signs of dehydration.

Laboratory
Obtaining a complete blood count with differential, testing for the presence of inflammatory markers, and also obtaining renal and liver function tests can be very beneficial when identifying a viral cause of an abdominal infection. Mild leukocytosis may be present, but the absence cannot exclude the diagnosis. Electrolyte imbalance may be seen due to dehydration from the excessive loss of fluids from diarrhea and vomiting. Measurement of alkaline phosphatase, amylase, lipase, GGT, total protein, and bilirubin levels can also assist in isolating the primary location of infection. An acute kidney injury may result from dehydration as well. These tests are only warranted for patients presenting with fever, abdominal pain, and extreme dehydration, as most cases of viral gastroenteritis are self-limited.

Imaging

Plain abdominal X-ray can help diagnose colitis (Bartram 1976); however, CT has become a prominent imaging resource. CT typically reveals thickening of the wall by more than 4 mm, infiltration of the pericolonic fat, and abnormal appearance or density of the colonic wall that may appear as a halo sign. (Delabrousse et al. 2013) It is beneficial in excluding specific causes of colitis, such as pseudomembranous colitis, which can show the accordion sign. Endoscopy is one of the mainstay procedures for diagnosing colitis which reveals irregular ulcers with rounded, well-circumscribed lesions with erythema and erosion. (Park et al. 2017) Ultrasonography may be initially used but requires expertise to visualize the sponginess of the colon wall. MRI is not effective and is not advised in diagnosing acute colitis.

Associated symptoms/conditions

Viral gastroenteritis is typically a self-limiting infection with no actual complications once resolved. However, one subsequent long-term effect seen in an average of 15% of cases is post-infectious IBS. (Card et al. 2018) CMV colitis can elicit several serious complications. It can cause severe hemorrhage, toxic megacolon, fulminant colitis, pseudomembrane formation, and colon perforation. (Park et al. 2017)

Diagnosis

There is currently no rapid testing for viral gastroenteritis, and it is, therefore, a clinical diagnosis. If the illness is severe, imaging and other laboratory tests should be performed to exclude other causes. In terms of CMV colitis, numerous diagnostic tests exist. These include anti-CMV IgG and IgM levels, blood CMV PCR, H&E staining (showing an "owl's-eye appearance" with cytoplasmic inclusions), and viral cultures. (Park et al. 2017) However, as mentioned before, endoscopy remains the mainstay for detecting CMV in colonic tissue with high specificity.

Treatment

Treating CMV colitis may include antivirals depending on the patient's immune system. Most immunocompetent patients will not require antiviral agents as the illness is typically self-limited, only requiring symptomatic treatment with fluid replacement. However, in immunosuppressed patients, **ganciclovir** can be used once CMV reactivation has been confirmed via endoscopy. (Azer and Limaiem 2022)

Management

Symptomatic and supportive therapy is the primary management for viral gastroenteritis. Most patients with viral gastroenteritis can be discharged the same day; however, admission can be warranted if the illness is severe with uncontrollable emesis and electrolyte disturbances. Fluid replacement, whether oral or IV in severe cases, is vital in these patients to avoid dehydration. Specifically, lactated ringers and saline have proven effective in managing dehydration caused by viral gastroenteritis. Antiemetics such as metoclopramide or ondansetron can help patients with nausea and vomiting. Anti-diarrheal agents are only used in patients with severe diarrhea whose electrolytes have been diminished at a rapid rate despite supplementation. In very severe infections, colectomy may be considered.

Skin, Soft Tissue, and Bone Infections

Presentation

Numerous viruses can cause skin and soft tissue infections in our world. Many of them present similarly; however, certain viruses have specific manifestations that are unique to them. In children, several viruses cause exanthems (reactive rashes) that accompany the primary symptoms associated with the infection. Chickenpox, caused by Varicella Zoster Virus (VZV), is one of the most common and well-known viruses expressing dermatologically. (Ayoade and Kumar 2022) It is a vastly contagious viral infection that initially presents as blistering, itchy red spots that transform into vesicles that then erupt and spread to different body areas. The rash is easy to identify since all lesions are at different stages of healing. While chickenpox from VZV is most common in children, shingles from VZV most commonly manifests in adults and the elderly. This presents as a tender, blistering rash that follows a dermatomal distribution. Affected patients may complain of a burning sensation and neuropathic pain lasting several months after the rash has resolved. Even the slightest touch of the region instigates the pain.
Molluscum contagiosum or "water warts", caused by a poxvirus, is another viral infection typically affecting children that presents as an exanthem. In this condition, singular (more common in sexually contracted cases) or groups (more common in children) of flesh-colored papules appear on the body. These papules are itchy and typically painless with a central umbilication. (Thandi and Whittam 2021) Also within the family of poxviruses, and now more relevant due to the number of growing cases, is Monkeypox. Initially, the skin manifestations of this virus exemplify themselves as mucosal lesions in the mouth, which quickly spread to the face and extremities. Firmly established lesions ranging from a few to potentially thousands can arise rapidly and are typically at the same age of evolution. (Moore et al. 2022)

Several infections can cause a maculopapular rash. Two significant and life-threatening causes that need to be identified quickly are measles and rubella. The accompanying symptoms make it easy to differentiate between the two. With both viruses, the rash begins on the face and spreads away from the medial portions of the body to the extremities and trunk. With rubella, the rash is accompanied by fever, lymphadenopathy (postauricular most commonly), and arthralgias. When congenitally contracted, the infant can have the classic "blueberry muffin" appearance. (Camejo Leonor and Mendez 2022) Measles, on the other hand, has the traditional presentation of cough, coryza, and conjunctivitis along with Koplik spots, which are bunched, white abrasions on the buccal mucosa and are typically present before the maculopapular rash and are pathognomonic for measles.

Another virus that has affected a vast amount of our population at one point or another is Herpes Simplex. The most common manifestation of this infection is gingivostomatitis, which results in mouth sores and ulcers on the inside of the mouth, gums, and lips (cold sores). The vesicles are typically painful and can affect any part of the body, including the genitalia, digits of the hands (herpetic whitlow), and other parts of the face (herpes gladiatorum). (Saleh et al. 2022) Warts are a common dermatologic condition seen in any age or demographic and are commonly caused by Human Papilloma Virus (HPV). Due to the various subtypes of this virus, several different types of skin presentations vary from cutaneous (verruca vulgaris, verruca plantaris) to anogenital warts (condyloma accuminata). These present as irregular exophytic growths in clusters or singularly, sometimes appearing like a cauliflower. (Luria and Cardoza-Favarato 2022) Bacteria most commonly cause soft tissue infections such as cellulitis, folliculitis, and impetigo; however, some outliers have been reported. Adenovirus and Varicella Zoster virus have both been seen to cause preseptal cellulitis that can quickly escalate to postseptal cellulitis, potentially causing serious concerns. It typically presents as a sudden onset of redness and swelling in unilateral or bilateral eyes, causing blurriness, photophobia, and tenderness around the orbits. (Bansal et al. 2020) Herpes Simplex Virus has been implicated as a rare cause of folliculitis, specifically folliculitis barbae, which presents as scaly, erythematous inflammation in the beard region.

Many viruses are implicated as causes of infectious arthritis. The most common are parvovirus, flaviviruses, hepatitis B, hepatitis C, rubella, Zika, and Chikungunya, with CMV, mumps, and herpes being rare causes. Parvovirus, also known as the Fifth disease, classically presents with a rash that appears as a "slapped cheek", most commonly in children. The joint manifestations are most similar to that seen in rheumatoid arthritis, with symmetrical and polyarticular symptoms including the proximal interphalangeal (PIP) and metacarpophalangeal (MCP) joints being involved. The flaviviruses Dengue and Zika have commonly affected individuals living in tropical regions. Hemorrhagic fever, thrombocytopenia leading to increased risk of bleeding, renal failure, and bone pain leading to the name "breakbone fever" are the most common manifestations of Dengue fever.

Risk factors

In general, patients that have immunosuppression of any kind are at increased risk of contracting a virus. However, certain conditions have specific risk factors that make certain populations of patients more susceptible to catching one; for example, in regards to VZV, Measles, and Rubella, the major at-risk group is the unvaccinated patient. Patients typically receive their first dose of the live-attenuated vaccine at one year of age, although there are many cases contracted congenitally. Although molluscum contagiosum is most commonly seen in children, adults can contract the virus via sexual contact. Patients with promiscuous sexual behavior have a heightened risk of being infected with Herpes Simplex, HPV, and Monkeypox. Also, since many of these viruses can be transmitted via skin contact, populations that live in close contact with each other, such as college dormitories or military camps, are at increased risk. Regarding viruses such as Chikungunya and Zika, individuals living in tropical regions are at an increased risk of being bitten by a mosquito transmitting the disease. Specific populations are at increased risk of contracting a virus leading to arthritis, including intravenous drug users and healthcare workers.

Pathophysiology

The pathophysiology of viral skin infections varies based on the specific virus. It can occur either via direct infection of the skin, or viral dissemination to other organs including the skin. With VZV chickenpox, the primary mechanism involves immunoglobulin production (IgG, IgM, and IgA), leading to a cell-mediated immune response after an individual contract the virus by either direct contact or inhalation of vapors from the fluid excreted from the vesicles. Shingles can subsequently develop via reactivation of the virus that remains latent in the dorsal ganglia. (Ayoade and Kumar 2022) Molluscum contagiosum, on the other hand, caused by the MCV poxvirus, directly infects skin cells and limits its spread solely to the epidermis, without causing disseminated disease. The spread of viruses, either hematogenous or through lymph nodes, is important in analyzing the progression of the disease. Once contracted via the oropharynx, nasopharynx, or an intradermal route, Monkeypox is an example of a virus that initially replicates at the primary entry point. It then proceeds to invade lymph nodes locally and eventually cause viremia that seeds into other organs. In general, most viruses invade local tissue at the transmission site via receptor-mediated endocytosis. The virus then replicates at the initial site and spreads to the regional lymphoid tissue, eventually leading to a viremic stage and causing disseminated infection. HPV has a specific pathophysiology involving the inactivation of particular host proteins, p53, and RB, leading to host cell cycle dysfunction. (Luria and Cardoza-Favarato 2022) Infected macrophages in the synovium are thought to be responsible for much of the pathology and inflammation seen in viral arthritis, through the release of pro-inflammatory cytokines and matrix metalloproteinases. (Tiwari and Bergman 2022)

Examination

Physical examination of patients with skin infections will vary based upon the particular virus the patient has. By performing a physical exam, one can visualize the rash, characterize it based on appearance, and monitor the progression of the rash. Although many of the exanthems may look similar, certain differences can make it simple to identify specific causes. Identifying the primary location of lesions, the presence of secondary lesions, and the appearance and color of the rash is the primary focus when dealing with rashes. The patient's general appearance can signal to the physician the severity of the illness the patient is experiencing. It is essential to perform a thorough physical exam to assess for oral, genital, or conjunctival lesions, as well as hepatosplenomegaly, nuchal rigidity, or neurologic dysfunction. (McKinnon and Howard 2000) In the instance that a patient presents with just a rash and no other symptoms, a patch test should be done to exclude dermatitis. Palpating the affected region in viral arthritis is necessary to assess for any tenderness or warmth.

Laboratory

Obtaining a complete blood count with differential, testing for the presence of inflammatory markers, and obtaining renal and liver function tests can be very beneficial when identifying a viral cause of a skin infection. Many specific laboratory tests exist, such as Tzanck smear for HSV, pap smears for HPV, and specific diagnostic tests that can be utilized to rule out common infections. CSF analysis should be performed in patients presenting with a rash and signs of altered mental status or change in behavior.

Imaging

In the typical sense, imaging has not been proven beneficial in diagnosing a viral skin infection. Microscopy is the mainstay of imaging when dealing with viral or other microbial skin infections. This includes entities such as colposcopy for visualization of "koilocytes" seen in HPV (*i.e.*, epithelial cells with hyperchromatic nuclei eccentrically displaced by perinuclear vacuoles). (Krawczyk et al. 2008)

Associated symptoms/conditions

As mentioned previously, many viruses that present with skin manifestations have other systemic findings associated with them. In disseminated viruses, fevers, general fatigue, anorexia, arthralgias/myalgias, tender lymphadenopathy, and altered mental status can be seen. HPV is a considerable risk factor for developing cervical cancer; therefore, any female, especially postmenopausal, that presents with normal vaginal bleeding should visit their OB/GYN and obtain further testing. In congenital rubella, the infant may present with a different type of exanthem that appears as a "blueberry muffin" rash, and other signs of infection, such as sensorineural hearing loss, patent ductus arteriosus, intellectual disabilities, and microcephaly.

Diagnosis

This diagnosis of many viral skin infections can be made clinically based on presentation. However, many diagnostic tests can be used to confirm the specific viral cause. Immunoglobulin testing is most widely used as initial testing for certain viruses such as measles and rubella. IgM antibodies are detected in patients that have newly developed the disease, whereas IgG represents immunity to the virus. Viral cultures and PCR are other testing tools that remain the mainstay of diagnosing many viral infections. Joint aspiration of the affected region is an essential component for diagnosing viral arthritis. It is also commonly clinically diagnosed, although detecting IgM antibodies can also be used to confirm.

Treatment

Unlike bacterial infections, where antibiotics are utilized to kill the causative agent, there are few widely used antivirals. Luckily, many viral skin infections are self-limiting and typically resolve in a few weeks. These include chickenpox, molluscum contagiosum, measles, and rubella. That said, treating the patient's symptoms with fever reducers, antibiotics in certain cases, and Vitamin A in the case of measles is important. (Huiming et al. 2005) Treatments for cutaneous and genital warts caused by HPV include salicylic acid, imiquimod, and trichloroacetic acid which have been proven to eliminate warts when applied topically. **Acyclovir** and **ganciclovir** can be used in cases of HSV and VZV, respectively. Shingles can be a painful and discomforting illness for many affected patients and should therefore be managed appropriately with medications such as gabapentin and duloxetine to provide comfort care. It is important to note that many of these viruses can be prevented with timely immunizations.

Management

As discussed previously, viral skin, bone, and joint infections are typically self-limited within 1-2 weeks. Therefore they are primarily managed with symptomatic treatment. In the majority of patients, there are no residual effects, and the illness is acute.

Anti-Viral Pharmacology

General Considerations

As previously mentioned, viruses can be considered packages of genetic material surrounded by a delivery system that injects "new instructions" into cells to subvert the host environment into producing new viral particles. As such, there are less obvious "viral Achilles' heels" to go after as anti-viral drug targets, given that much of the viral replication is being performed by host machinery that is ill-advised to perturb pharmacologically, lest such perturbation generates toxic side effects. Three central HIV targets that have proven successful in anti-viral drug development have been (i) the viral surface proteins that uniquely target host cells for binding and entry, (ii) the unique viral approaches to copying or reverse transcribing their tiny genomes, and (iii) unique viral proteases that process viral pro-proteins as faithfully translated by host machinery. In the case of the human immunodeficiency virus (HIV), the causative agent of the acquired immunodeficiency syndrome (AIDS) that exploded onto the world stage in the late 1980s, all three target classes have been successfully exploited (Broder 2010), and so HIV anti-viral agents are considered first. They are often used in combination with "High(ly) Active Anti-Retroviral Therapy" (HAART). (Lu et al. 2018; Arici et al. 2001)

Antivirals for HIV

Attachment / Fusion Inhibitors

The mature surface of HIV particles contains two virally-encoded "envelope" glycoproteins gp41 and gp120 that are directly involved in the binding to CD4 on target CD4+ T-helper lymphocytes and subsequent viral entry. **Fostemsavir** is a pro-drug dephosphorylated in the GI lumen to temsavir, an HIV attachment inhibitor that directly binds gp120 to prevent the binding of CD4. (Kozal et al. 2020) The monoclonal antibody **ibalizumab** binds CD4 directly (when it is already engaged by viral gp120) thereby serving as a post-attachment viral entry inhibitor. Beyond the key role played by the host CD4 cell-surface protein to HIV binding and entry, two chemokine receptors (CXCR4 and CCR5) also have roles as "viral entry co-receptors," and HIV is therefore subclassified into CXCR4-tropic and CCR5-tropic clades. The antiviral **maraviroc** works as a negative allosteric modulator of the CCR5 receptor, blocking its association with viral gp120. (Sayana and Khanlou 2009) An injectable polypeptide drug **enfuvirtide** also serves as a viral fusion inhibitor, but by binding directly to viral gp41 to prevent the conformational changes required for viral/host-cell fusion. Resistance to enfuvirtide can develop by mutation to the viral gp41 sequence. Its clinical use is generally restricted to patients with persistent HIV replication despite prior treatment with other antiviral regimens; adverse effects of enfuvirtide treatment include insomnia, headache, dizziness, and nausea.

Figure 3.9 Structure of the nucleoside reverse transcriptase inhibitor (NRTI) azidothymidine in comparison to thymidine (A), other anti-HIV NRTIs (B), and the tenofovir prodrug tenofovir disoproxil with its fumaric acid companion (C).

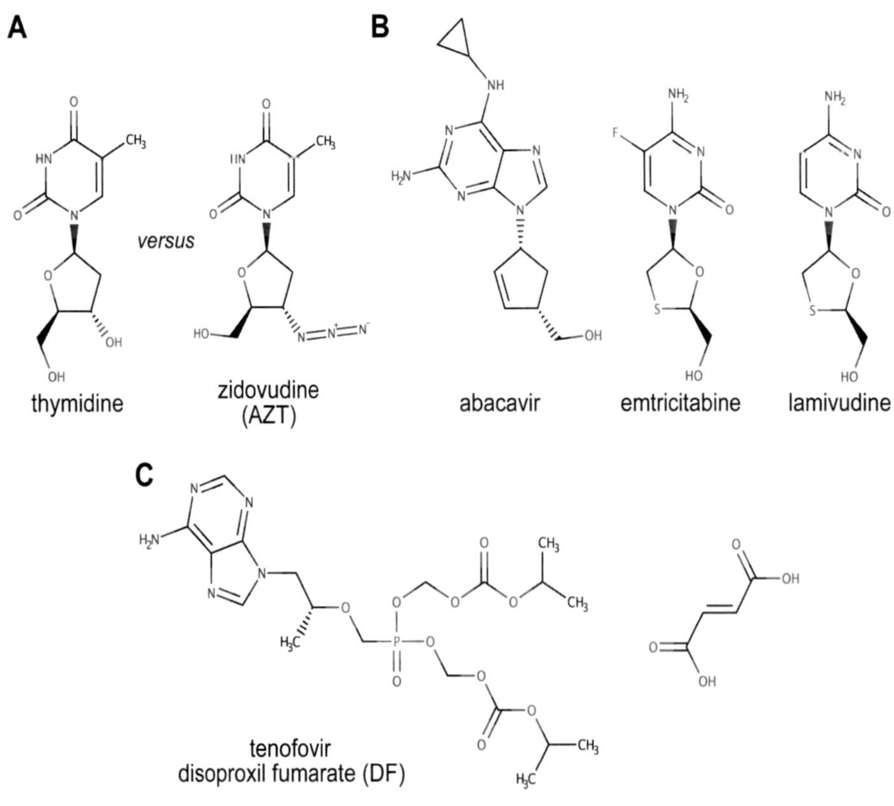

Nucleoside (Nucleotide) Reverse Transcriptase Inhibitors (NRTIs)

HIV is a retrovirus, meaning its genome is encoded by RNA. It thus requires the action of virally-encoded reverse transcriptase (RT) to convert its genome into double-stranded DNA once the viral particle has bound, fused with and entered its target host cell. One of the first HIV anti-viral agents identified, **azidothymidine** (a.k.a. zidovudine or AZT), appears very chemically similar to the normal nucleic acid building block thymidine (Figure 3.9A), but AZT selectively inhibits HIV's reverse transcriptase activity. Host cell enzymes convert AZT into a 5'-triphosphate ("nucleotide") form; at sufficiently high doses of AZT, its triphosphate form is also capable of inhibiting mitochondrial DNA polymerase, accounting for its observed toxic (but reversible) effects on cardiac and skeletal muscles. AZT has been used in pregnancy and HIV post-exposure prophylaxis. (Chappell and Cohn 2014) Other NRTIs include **abacavir**, the highly related **emtricitabine** and **lamivudine** (Figure 3.9B), and the prodrug **tenofovir DF** (Figure 3.9C). The latter can be used in pregnancy. Tenofovir can also be used with emtricitabine for HIV pre-exposure prophylaxis (Chou et al. 2019). These nucleoside-like NRTI drugs require three phosphate additions by cellular enzymes (two in the case of tenofovir; Figure 3.9C) in order to act as a "potential nucleic acid building block" by HIV reverse transcriptase and thereby competitively inhibit RT action and also terminate its growing chain of viral DNA if incorporated by mistake.

Non-nucleoside Reverse Transcription Inhibitors (NNRTIs)

As opposed to NRTIs, members of the class of non-nucleoside reverse transcription inhibitors (NNRTIs) act by allosteric inhibition of HIV RT enzymatic activity (*i.e.*, NNRTIs bind HIV RT at a site near, but distinct, from the NRTI binding site / active site of the enzyme). (Wang et al. 2019) In this way, these NNRTI drugs (*e.g.*, **doravirine**, **efavirenz**, **etravirine**, **nevirapine**, **rilpivirine**) do not compete with NRTIs, nor do they require cellular phosphorylation activity to become active inhibitors. **Nevirapine** is employed not only in treating HIV infection and its resultant acquired immunodeficiency syndrome but (like AZT) also used in the prevention of transmission of HIV from infected mothers to their newborns. Common adverse effects for all NNRTIs include nausea, headache, fever, and fatigue, with **nevirapine** also seen to cause relatively frequent (15–25%) hypersensitivity reactions (either skin rash or elevated liver enzymes) in the first three months after treatment initiation. (Notter et al. 2019)

Integrase Inhibitors ("-gravir" drugs)

Upon successful entry and reverse transcription of the HIV genome, the double-stranded DNA copy is integrated into the host cell's chromosomal DNA by the action of an HIV-encoded integrase enzyme. Five drugs, **bictegravir**, **cabotegravir**, **dolutegravir**, **elvitegravir**, and **raltegravir**, have a shared mechanism of action of inhibiting HIV integrase; HIV resistance can develop by mutation to that integrase. (Anstett et al. 2017) Integrase inhibitors are found in combination therapy for treating HIV infection; common adverse effects include headache, dizziness, nausea, diarrhea, and fatigue.

Protease Inhibitors ("-navir" drugs)

In later stages of HIV replication, HIV genome-encoded gag and gag-pol proteins require proteolytic maturation to form the new budding virion. So an HIV genome-encoded protease performs this vital maturation step. At least six drugs have clinical utility in inhibiting viral protease activity: **atazanavir**, **darunavir**, **fosamprenavir**, **ritonavir**, **saquinavir**, and **tipranavir**; HIV resistance can develop by mutation to that protease. (Ghosh et al. 2016) Of these protease-targeting drugs, ritonavir has found a unique pharmacological role. While **ritonavir** was initially developed as an inhibitor of HIV protease, it is rarely used for its own antiviral activity. Instead, it is widely used as a booster of the half-life of other protease inhibitors. More specifically, **ritonavir** is used to inhibit cytochrome P450-3A4 (CYP3A4), thereby enhancing other protease inhibitors' stability activity, reducing adverse effects, and generally improving the efficacy of HAART. However, given the general role of CYP3A4 in xenobiotic ("foreign compound") metabolism, ritonavir dosing also affects numerous other medications, compounding the challenge of prescribing multiple drugs concurrently.

Antivirals for Orthomyxoviruses (Influenza viruses)

Influenza viruses are members of the *Orthomyxoviridae* family, and influenza type A viruses are the primary infectious agents responsible for annual influenza epidemics and occasional influenza pandemics (Houser and Subbarao 2015). Both the influenza A viruses (IAVs) and type B viruses (IBVs) contain eight, negative-sense, single-stranded viral RNA (vRNA) gene segments that encode all essential and strain-specific viral proteins, including the viral surface proteins hemagglutinin (HA), neuraminidase (NA), and the M2 proton (ion) channel. The related antiviral drugs **amantadine** and **rimantadine** act to block the function of the M2 proton channel, which prevents viral endosomal escape (*i.e.*, the release of vRNA into the host cytoplasm). However, amantadine is no longer recommended for treating influenza A due to high amantadine resistance among currently circulating influenza A viruses. (Kumar et al. 2018) Similarly, samples tested from the 2009 pandemic and seasonal H3N2 flu have shown resistance to rimantadine, so it is no longer recommended as a flu treatment. (Fiore et al. 2011) Newer drugs **oseltamivir**, **peramivir**, and **zanamivir** share a different viral target: inhibiting viral neuraminidase activity to prevent the release of new virions from host cells; the actual clinical efficacy of these neuraminidase inhibitors, within either treatment or prophylaxis, has been actively debated in the literature. (*e.g.*, refs. (Swierczynska et al. 2022; Jefferson et al. 2014)) The newest drug, **baloxavir marboxil**, has a unique mechanism of action. When metabolized to baloxavir acid, it inhibits the virus' cap-dependent endonuclease activity critical to the "cap snatching" process by the viral polymerase during RNA transcription. (Noshi et al. 2018) It is widely acknowledged that these newer anti-influenza medications are only beneficial if administered within two days of the onset of influenza symptoms.

Antivirals for SARS-CoV-2 (COVID-19 virus)
Soon after the sudden emergence of the COVID-19 pandemic, the U.S. Food and Drug Administration approved the use of the injectable prodrug **remdesivir**, which was initially developed to treat hepatitis C (HCV; see below). Upon cellular conversion to the triphosphate-containing metabolite GS-441524, remdesivir becomes a ribonucleotide analogue, inhibiting the RNA polymerase of the COVID-19 virus (Gordon et al. 2020). A second approval was made for **nirmatrelvir** (Joyce et al. 2022), a protease inhibitor co-administered with the "booster" ritonavir (see above); early indications at the time of writing suggest that use of this nirmatrelvir/ritonavir combination can lead to a rebound of COVID-19 symptoms upon cessation of treatment. (Reis et al. 2022; Charness et al. 2022) A third approval was given to **molnupiravir**, which inhibits viral reproduction by promoting widespread mutations during COVID-19 viral RNA replication by its RNA-directed RNA polymerase (Painter et al. 2021). This approval was only narrowly given amid multiple concerns, including the potential mutagenic effects of this drug that could create new SARS-CoV-2 escape variants. (Thorlund et al. 2022; Kabinger et al. 2021)

Ribavirin – Broad spectrum antiviral drug
Ribavirin is an orally available, synthetic guanosine (nucleoside) analogue that is employed against a broad spectrum of RNA-genome and DNA-genome viruses, such as viral hemorrhagic fevers (*e.g.*, Lassa fever, Hantavirus), respiratory syncytial virus (RSV), and (in combination with other drugs) hepatitis C virus (HCV; see below). Its mechanism of action is not entirely clear but may include inhibiting viral RNA synthesis and mRNA capping. Adverse effects of ribavirin use include renal failure and anemia in the elderly; both sexes also need to use caution when on ribavirin and are sexually active, as congenital malformations can arise if ribavirin is taken during conception or pregnancy.

Table 3.4. Clinical utility, mechanisms of action, and adverse effects of four related *Herpes* virus drugs

Name & Route(s) of Administration	acyclovir (oral; i.v.) 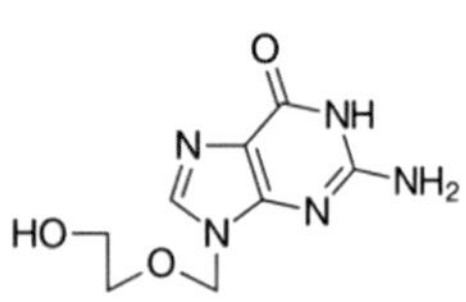	valacyclovir (oral) 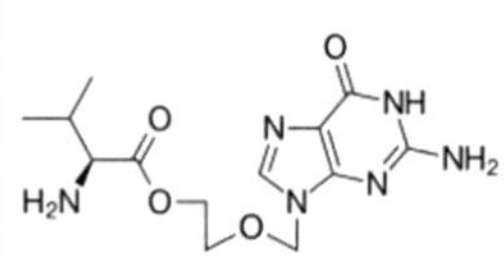	ganciclovir (ophthalmic; i.v.*) 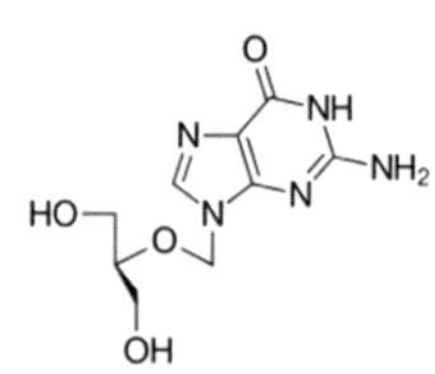	vidarabine (slow i.v. admin or topical) 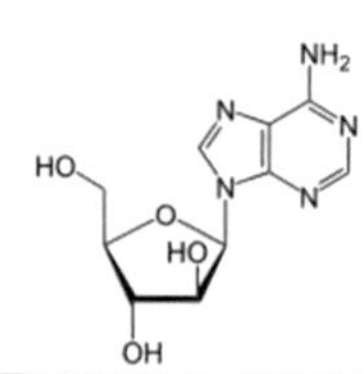
Mechanism of Action	Converted to the monophosphate by **viral thymidine kinase;** Monophosphate is converted to di- and triphosphate by mammalian kinases; Triphosphate inhibits viral DNA polymerase actions	L-valyl ester of acyclovir; almost completely metabolized to acyclovir. Triphosphate inhibits viral DNA polymerase actions	Converted to the monophosphate by CMV-specified protein kinase (UL97) Triphosphate inhibits viral DNA polymerase actions	Phosphorylated by cellular kinases to a triphosphate Triphosphate inhibits viral DNA polymerase actions
Mechanism of Resistance	Mutations in viral thymidine kinase and viral DNA polymerase	Similar to acyclovir	Due to a more common mutation in UL97	Changes in DNA polymerase
Adverse effects	Local inflammation during i.v. injection; Renal dysfunction if given i.v. too rapidly; Nausea and headache	Similar to acyclovir	Myelosuppression particularly after i.v. administration ***Increases AZT toxicity; thus, watch out for CMV retinitis in AIDS patients (switch away from AZT?)**	Nausea, vomiting, and diarrhea; Neurotoxicity late in therapy with high doses (reversible); Bone marrow disturbances reported
Clinical uses	Primarily used against HSV infections, chickenpox, and shingles. Other uses include prevention of CMV infections following transplant and severe complications of EBV infection	Similar to acyclovir (oral)	Similar to acyclovir	For HSV resistant to acyclovir

Antivirals for *Herpes* family DNA viruses (HSV, VZV, CMV)

As previously mentioned, herpes simplex virus-1 and -2 (HSV-1/2) causes genital herpes, varicella-zoster virus (VZV) causes chickenpox in children and can reinfect adults as shingles, and cytomegalovirus infection can cause various pathologies: colitis, retinitis, hepatitis, and pneumonitis being the most common. Four related nucleoside analogs, **acyclovir**, **valacyclovir**, **ganciclovir**, and **vidarabine**, are used for infections caused by one of these *Herpes* family viruses (Table 3.4). **Foscarnet** is a non-nucleoside inhibitor of viral DNA polymerase activity. It is used against acyclovir-resistant HSV infections and as a second-line drug for CMV eye infections in immunocompromised patients. Similar to the allosteric mechanism of action of anti-HIV NNRTIs, **foscarnet** (a pyrophosphate analogue) inhibits viral replication by binding to the pyrophosphate site of the Herpes virus' DNA polymerase (called pUL54 in the case of CMV); viral mutants can arise in the HSV and CMV genome to produce foscarnet resistance. Foscarnet has serious nephrotoxicity liability.

Antivirals for hepatitis viruses (HBV, HCV) (see Chapter 7 on Liver Disorders)

Hepatitis B

HBV infections have been treated with immune system modulatory drugs like the injectables **interferon α2b** and **peginterferon α2a**. These recombinant interferons induce host enzymes that inhibit the translation of HBV mRNAs and also are thought to help induce direct immune system attack of infected hepatocytes, including the activity of CD8+ T-lymphocytes. These injectable agents have many adverse effects, however, and can be toxic; side effects of use include fever, lassitude, headache, myalgia, acute/reversible hearing loss and/or tinnitus, bone marrow suppression, cardiovascular changes, rashes, alopecia, altered thyroid and renal functions, and exacerbations of existing autoimmune states (*e.g.*, thyroiditis). More recently, **lamivudine** and **tenofovir** have been used against HBV (*e.g.*, ref. (Kim et al. 2022)) (both drugs are mentioned in the anti-HIV section above).

Hepatitis C

The injectables **interferon α2b** and **peginterferon α2a**, in combination with **ribavirin**, were originally the drugs of choice for HCV infection, but have now been predominantly superseded by treatment with one or (usually) multiple "direct-acting agents" (DAAs) with specific HCV-encoded molecular targets from among its non-structural proteins. The viral NS5A protein functions in the replication, packaging, and assembly of the hepatitis C virus, and its inhibitors all end in the "-asvir" suffix (Table 3.5). The viral NS5B protein is the HCV's RNA-dependent RNA polymerase and also is involved in post-translational processing required for HCV replication; its inhibitors end in "-buvir" (Table 3.6). Finally, the inhibitors of HCV's NS3/4A protease activity all end in "-previr" (Table 3.7).

Table 3.5. Mechanisms of action and adverse effects of HCV NS5A inhibitors

NS5A Inhibitors ("-asvir")	**daclatasvir** Used as daclatasvir/ sofosbuvir	**elbasvir** Used as elbasvir/ grazoprevir	**ledipasvir** Used as ledipasvir/ sofosbuvir	**ombitasvir** Used with paritaprevir and ritonavir	**velpatasvir** Used as velpatasvir/sofosbuvir
Mechanisms of action	Inhibit functions of HCV-NS5A protein *Also*: an inhibitor of P-glycoprotein transporter (P-gp), organic anion transporting polypeptide (OATP) 1B1 and 1B3, and breast cancer resistance protein (BCRP)	Inhibit functions of HCV-NS5A protein	Inhibit functions of HCV-NS5A protein *Also*: an inhibitor of the drug transporters P-gp & BCRP	Inhibit functions of HCV-NS5A protein	Inhibit functions of HCV-NS5A protein *Also*: an inhibitor of the drug transporters P-gp & BCRP
Adverse effects	Headache and fatigue, usually mild to moderate Serious symptomatic bradycardia has been reported	Fatigue, headache, and nausea Elbasvir/grazoprevir should not be administered to patients with moderate or severe hepatic dysfunction	Fatigue, headache, and asthenia Serious symptomatic bradycardia in patients receiving ledipasvir/sofosbuvir with amiodarone	Nausea, pruritus, and insomnia Increased serum aminotransferases reported if using concomitant ethinyl estradiol-containing contraceptives	Headache and fatigue

Table 3.6. Mechanisms of action and adverse effects of HCV NS5B inhibitors

NS5B inhibitors ("-buvir")	**Sofosbuvir**	**Dasabuvir**
Mechanism of action	Nucleoside NS5B RNA polymerase chain terminator Rapidly converted to GS-331007 that is taken up by hepatocytes and converted by cellular kinases to active uridine analog 5'-triphosphate form GS-461203 Sofosbuvir is a substrate of drug transporter P-gp	Non-nucleoside NS5B RNA polymerase inhibitor
Adverse effects	Fatigue, headache, and asthenia in patients receiving sofosbuvir with ledipasvir Bradycardia in patients taking sofosbuvir and amiodarone in combination with another DAA, particularly in patients also receiving beta blockers, or with underlying cardiac problems	Nausea, pruritus, and insomnia. Increased serum aminotransferases if using concomitant ethinyl estradiol-containing contraceptives.
Clinical uses	Available in a fixed-dose combination with ledipasvir for the treatment of HCV genotypes 1, 4, 5, and 6 In combination with several other anti-HCV medications, including daclatasvir, simeprevir, peginterferon-alfa plus ribavirin, or ribavirin alone	Dasabuvir is available only as a fixed-dose combination with ombitasvir, paritaprevir, and ritonavir for the treatment of HCV genotype 1 Ritonavir functions as a pharmacologic booster to increase paritaprevir plasma concentrations

Table 3.7. Mechanisms of action and adverse effects of HCV NS3/4A protease inhibitors

NS3/4A protease inhibitors "-previr")	**Grazoprevir**	**Paritaprevir**	**Simeprevir**
Mechanism of action	NS3/4A protease inhibitor	NS3/4A protease inhibitor	Second-generation HCV protease inhibitor with enhanced binding affinity and specificity for NS3/4A
Adverse effects	Fatigue, headache, and nausea during therapy with elbasvir/grazoprevir Elevations in serum aminotransferases may occur	Nausea, pruritus, and insomnia. Increased serum aminotransferases if using concomitant ethinyl estradiol–containing contraceptives. Metabolism of paritaprevir, ritonavir, and dasabuvir by CYP3A cytochrome P450 system creates multiple potential drug-drug interactions	Photosensitivity, rash (occasionally severe); pruritus, or nausea. Transient, mild elevations in bilirubin Since simeprevir contains a sulfa group, caution should be used in patients with a history of sulfa allergy
Clinical uses	In combination with elbasvir for treatment of HCV genotypes 1 and 4	In combination with dasabuvir for HCV genotype 1 infection. In combination with ombitasvir and ritonavir for treatment of HCV genotype 4.	In combination with sofosbuvir, with or without ribavirin, for treatment of HCV. It may be administered in combination with peg-interferon-alfa and ribavirin

References

(CDC), C. f. D. C. a. P. 2019. Active Bacterial Core Surveillance Report, Emerging Infections Program Network, Streptococcus pneumoniae In https://www.cdc.gov/abcs/bact-facts-interactive-dashboard.html.

[Internet], I. o. *Common colds: Overview*. Institute for Quality and Efficiency in Health Care (IQWiG), October 8, 2020 2020 [cited. Available from https://www.ncbi.nlm.nih.gov/books/NBK279543/.

Aguirre Rivera, J., J. Larsson, I. L. Volkov, A. C. Seefeldt, S. Sanyal, and M. Johansson. 2021. Real-time measurements of aminoglycoside effects on protein synthesis in live cells. *Proc Natl Acad Sci U S A* 118 (9).

Ak, A. K., and M. D. Mendez. 2022. Herpes Simplex Encephalitis. *StatPearls*.

Akaishi, T., J. Kobayashi, M. Abe, K. Ishizawa, I. Nakashima, M. Aoki, and T. Ishii. 2019. Sensitivity and specificity of meningeal signs in patients with meningitis. *J Gen Fam Med* 20 (5):193-198.

Al-Akchar, M., and J. Kiel. 2022. Acute Myocarditis. *StatPearls*.

Albert, N. M., R. J. Tyson, C. L. Hill, A. D. DeVore, J. A. Spertus, C. Duffy, J. Butler, J. H. Patterson, A. F. Hernandez, F. B. Williams, L. Thomas, and G. C. Fonarow. 2021. Variation in use and dosing escalation of renin angiotensin system, mineralocorticoid receptor antagonist, angiotensin receptor neprilysin inhibitor and beta-blocker therapies in heart failure and reduced ejection fraction: Association of comorbidities. *Am Heart J* 235:82-96.

Alonzo, M. M., T. V. Lewis, and J. L. Miller. 2019. Disulfiram-like Reaction With Metronidazole: An Unsuspected Culprit. *J Pediatr Pharmacol Ther* 24 (5):445-449.

Anderson, N., A. Koshy, and K. Ross. 2022. Bacterial, Fungal and Parasitic Diseases of the Nervous System. In *Bradley and Daroff's neurology in clinical practice*, edited by J. Jankovic, J. C. Mazziotta, S. L. Pomeroy, N. J. Newman and W. G. Bradley. Edinburgh: Elsevier.

Angelini, A., V. Calzolari, F. Calabrese, G. M. Boffa, F. Maddalena, R. Chioin, and G. Thiene. 2000. Myocarditis mimicking acute myocardial infarction: role of endomyocardial biopsy in the differential diagnosis. *Heart* 84 (3):245-250.

Anstett, K., B. Brenner, T. Mesplede, and M. A. Wainberg. 2017. HIV drug resistance against strand transfer integrase inhibitors. *Retrovirology* 14 (1):36.

Arbiser, J. L., and S. L. Moschella. 1995. Clofazimine: a review of its medical uses and mechanisms of action. *J Am Acad Dermatol* 32 (2 Pt 1):241-247.

Arici, C., D. Ripamonti, V. Ravasio, F. Maggiolo, M. Rizzi, M. G. Finazzi, and F. Suter. 2001. Long-term clinical benefit after highly active antiretroviral therapy in advanced HIV-1 infection, even in patients without immune reconstitution. *Int J STD AIDS* 12 (9):573-581.

Ayoade, F., and S. Kumar. 2022. Varicella Zoster. *StatPearls*.

Azer, S. A., and F. Limaiem. 2022. Cytomegalovirus Colitis. *StatPearls*.

Bader, M. S., M. Loeb, D. Leto, and A. A. Brooks. 2020. Treatment of urinary tract infections in the era of antimicrobial resistance and new antimicrobial agents. *Postgrad Med* 132 (3):234-250.

Bansal, S., D. P. Nimmatoori, N. Singhania, R. C. Lin, C. M. Nukala, A. K. Singh, and G. Singhania. 2020. Severe nonbacterial preseptal cellulitis from adenovirus detected via pooled meta-genomic testing. *Clin Case Rep* 8 (12):3503-3506.

Barber, M., and M. Rozwadowska-Dowzenko. 1948. Infection by penicillin-resistant staphylococci. *Lancet* 2 (6530):641-644.

Barshak, M., and D. L. Kasper. 2022. Intraabdominal Infections and Abscesses. In *Harrison's principles of internal medicine*, edited by J. Loscalzo, A. S. Fauci, D. L. Kasper, S. L. Hauser, D. L. Longo and J. L. Jameson. New York: McGraw Hill.

Bartram, C. I. 1976. Plain abdominal X-ray in acute colitis. *Proc R Soc Med* 69 (8):617-618.

Beganovic, M., J. A. Cusumano, V. Lopes, K. L. LaPlante, and A. R. Caffrey. 2019. Comparative Effectiveness of Exclusive Exposure to Nafcillin or Oxacillin, Cefazolin, Piperacillin/Tazobactam, and Fluoroquinolones Among a National Cohort of Veterans With Methicillin-Susceptible Staphylococcus aureus Bloodstream Infection. *Open Forum Infect Dis* 6 (7):ofz270.

Besinger, B., and C. R. Stehman. 2020. Pancreatitis and Cholecystitis. In *Tintinalli's Emergency Medicine: A Comprehensive Study Guide, 9e*, edited by J. E. Tintinalli, O. J. Ma, D. M. Yealy, G. D. Meckler, J. S. Stapczynski, D. M. Cline and S. H. Thomas. New York, NY: McGraw-Hill Education.

Beutler, E. 1994. G6PD deficiency. *Blood* 84 (11):3613-3636.

Blair, H. A., and L. J. Scott. 2015. Delamanid: a review of its use in patients with multidrug-resistant tuberculosis. *Drugs* 75 (1):91-100.

Bosch, D. E., W. R. Jeck, and D. P. Siderovski. 2022. Self-activating G protein alpha subunits engage seven-transmembrane regulator of G protein signaling (RGS) proteins and a Rho guanine nucleotide exchange factor effector in the amoeba Naegleria fowleri. *J Biol Chem* 298 (8):102167.

Bosch, D. E., and D. P. Siderovski. 2013. G protein signaling in the parasite Entamoeba histolytica. *Exp Mol Med* 45:e15.

Broder, S. 2010. The development of antiretroviral therapy and its impact on the HIV-1/AIDS pandemic. *Antiviral Res* 85 (1):1-18.

Brun, R., R. Schumacher, C. Schmid, C. Kunz, and C. Burri. 2001. The phenomenon of treatment failures in Human African Trypanosomiasis. *Trop Med Int Health* 6 (11):906-914.

Brunette, G. W., and J. B. Nemhauser. 2020. *CDC Yellow Book: Health Information for International Travel*: Centers for Disease Control and Prevention (CDC).

Burnham, C.-A. D., and G. A. Storch. 2020. Diagnostic Microbiology. In *Nelson textbook of pediatrics*, edited by R. Kliegman, B. Stanton, J. W. St. Geme, III, N. F. Schor, R. E. Behrman and W. E. Nelson. Philadelphia, PA: Elsevier Inc., 1335-1341.e1331.

Bustos, J., I. Gonzales, H. Saavedra, S. Handali, H. H. Garcia, and P. Cysticercosis Working Group in. 2021. Neurocysticercosis. A frequent cause of seizures, epilepsy, and other neurological morbidity in most of the world. *J Neurol Sci* 427:117527.

Camejo Leonor, M., and M. D. Mendez. 2022. Rubella. *StatPearls*.

Card, T., P. Enck, G. Barbara, G. E. Boeckxstaens, J. Santos, F. Azpiroz, F. Mearin, Q. Aziz, J. Marshall, and R. Spiller. 2018. Post-infectious IBS: Defining its clinical features and prognosis using an internet-based survey. *United European Gastroenterol J* 6 (8):1245-1253.

Cassady, K. A., and R. J. Whitley. 2014. Pathogenesis and pathophysiology of viral infections of the central nervous system. In *Infections of the central nervous system*, edited by W. M. Scheld, R. J. Whitley, C. M. Marra, J. Goolsby, K. Oberle, D. Orzechowski and T. Mallon. Philadelphia: Wolters Kluwer Health, 49-64.

Cephalosporins. 2012. In *LiverTox: Clinical and Research Information on Drug-Induced Liver Injury*. Bethesda (MD). PMID: 31643977.

Chalmers, S. J., and M. E. Wylam. 2020. Methicillin-Resistant Staphylococcus aureus Infection and Treatment Options. *Methods Mol Biol* 2069:229-251.

Chambers, H. F. 1999. Penicillin-binding protein-mediated resistance in pneumococci and staphylococci. *J Infect Dis* 179 Suppl 2:S353-359.

Chang, Y. L., S. J. Yu, J. Heitman, M. Wellington, and Y. L. Chen. 2017. New facets of antifungal therapy. *Virulence* 8 (2):222-236.

Chappell, C. A., and S. E. Cohn. 2014. Prevention of perinatal transmission of human immunodeficiency virus. *Infect Dis Clin North Am* 28 (4):529-547.

Charness, M. E., K. Gupta, G. Stack, J. Strymish, E. Adams, D. C. Lindy, H. Mohri, and D. D. Ho. 2022. Rebound of SARS-CoV-2 Infection after Nirmatrelvir-Ritonavir Treatment. *N Engl J Med* 387 (11):1045-1047.

Chen, X., X. Jiang, M. Yang, U. Gonzalez, X. Lin, X. Hua, S. Xue, M. Zhang, and C. Bennett. 2016. Systemic antifungal therapy for tinea capitis in children. *Cochrane Database Syst Rev* (5):CD004685.

Chou, R., C. Evans, A. Hoverman, C. Sun, T. Dana, C. Bougatsos, S. Grusing, and P. T. Korthuis. 2019. Preexposure Prophylaxis for the Prevention of HIV Infection: Evidence Report and Systematic Review for the US Preventive Services Task Force. *JAMA* 321 (22):2214-2230.

Cohen-Poradosu, R., and D. Kasper. 2020. Anaerobic Infections: General Concepts. In *Mandell, Douglas, and Bennett's principles and practice of infectious diseases*, edited by J. E. Bennett, R. Dolin and M. J. Blaser. Philadelphia, PA: Elsevier, 2923-2932.

Cong, Y., S. Yang, and X. Rao. 2020. Vancomycin resistant Staphylococcus aureus infections: A review of case updating and clinical features. *J Adv Res* 21:169-176.

Cope, J. R., D. A. Conrad, N. Cohen, M. Cotilla, A. DaSilva, J. Jackson, and G. S. Visvesvara. 2016. Use of the Novel Therapeutic Agent Miltefosine for the Treatment of Primary Amebic Meningoencephalitis: Report of 1 Fatal and 1 Surviving Case. *Clin Infect Dis* 62 (6):774-776.

Crothers, K., W. Worodria, and L. Huang. 2022. Pulmonary Complications of HIV Infection. In *Murray & Nadel's textbook of respiratory medicine*, edited by V. C. Broaddus, J. D. Ernst, T. E. King, Jr., S. C. Lazarus, K. F. Sarmiento, L. M. Schnapp, R. D. Stapleton and M. B. Gotway. Philadelphia, PA: Elsevier, 1703-1727.

Cuenca-Estrella, M. 2004. Combinations of antifungal agents in therapy—what value are they? *J Antimicrob Chemother* 54 (5):854-869.

Curtis, S., K. Stobart, B. Vandermeer, D. L. Simel, and T. Klassen. 2010. Clinical features suggestive of meningitis in children: a systematic review of prospective data. *Pediatrics* 126 (5):952-960.

Daliparty, V. M., and R. Balasubramanya. 2022. HIV Encephalitis. *StatPearls*.

Das, S., N. K. Mohakud, M. Suar, and B. R. Sahu. 2018. Vaccine development for enteric bacterial pathogens: Where do we stand? *Pathog Dis* 76 (5).

Dasaraju, P. V., and C. Liu. 1996. Infections of the Respiratory System. In *Medical Microbiology.*, edited by S. Baron. Galveston (TX): University of Texas Medical Branch at Galveston.

Dash, C. H. 1975. Penicillin allergy and the cephalosporins. *J Antimicrob Chemother* 1 (3 Suppl):107-118.

De La Blanchardiere, A., F. Rozenberg, E. Caumes, O. Picard, F. Lionnet, J. Livartowski, J. Coste, D. Sicard, P. Lebon, and D. Salmon-Ceron. 2000. Neurological complications of varicella-zoster virus infection in adults with human immunodeficiency virus infection. *Scand J Infect Dis* 32 (3):263-269.

Delabrousse, E., F. Ferreira, N. Badet, M. Martin, and M. Zins. 2013. Coping with the problems of diagnosis of acute colitis. *Diagn Interv Imaging* 94 (7-8):793-804.

Diaz-Brochero, C., M. C. Valderrama-Rios, L. C. Nocua-Baez, and J. A. Cortes. 2022. First-generation cephalosporins for the treatment of complicated upper urinary tract infection in adults: A systematic literature review. *Int J Infect Dis* 116:403-410.

Diptyanusa, A., T. Ngamprasertchai, and W. Piyaphanee. 2018. A review of antibiotic prophylaxis for traveler's diarrhea: past to present. *Trop Dis Travel Med Vaccines* 4:14.
Dixit, D., R. P. Madduri, and R. Sharma. 2014. The role of tigecycline in the treatment of infections in light of the new black box warning. *Expert Rev Anti Infect Ther* 12 (4):397-400.
Doi, Y., J. I. Wachino, and Y. Arakawa. 2016. Aminoglycoside Resistance: The Emergence of Acquired 16S Ribosomal RNA Methyltransferases. *Infect Dis Clin North Am* 30 (2):523-537.
Duplessis, C., and N. F. Crum-Cianflone. 2011. Ceftaroline: A New Cephalosporin with Activity against Methicillin-Resistant Staphylococcus aureus (MRSA). *Clin Med Rev Ther* 3.
Edwards, D. I. 1980. Mechanisms of selective toxicity of metronidazole and other nitroimidazole drugs. *Br J Vener Dis* 56 (5):285-290.
El-Shahawi, G. A., M. Abdel-Latif, A. H. Saad, and M. Bahgat. 2010. Setaria equina: in vivo effect of diethylcarbamazine citrate on microfilariae in albino rats. *Exp Parasitol* 126 (4):603-610.
Falotico, J. M., and S. R. Lipner. 2022. Updated Perspectives on the Diagnosis and Management of Onychomycosis. *Clin Cosmet Investig Dermatol* 15:1933-1957.
Feklistov, A., V. Mekler, Q. Jiang, L. F. Westblade, H. Irschik, R. Jansen, A. Mustaev, S. A. Darst, and R. H. Ebright. 2008. Rifamycins do not function by allosteric modulation of binding of Mg2+ to the RNA polymerase active center. *Proc Natl Acad Sci U S A* 105 (39):14820-14825.
Ferrari, T. C., and P. R. Moreira. 2011. Neuroschistosomiasis: clinical symptoms and pathogenesis. *Lancet Neurol* 10 (9):853-864.
Fiore, A. E., A. Fry, D. Shay, L. Gubareva, J. S. Bresee, T. M. Uyeki, C. Centers for Disease, and Prevention. 2011. Antiviral agents for the treatment and chemoprophylaxis of influenza – recommendations of the Advisory Committee on Immunization Practices (ACIP). *MMWR Recomm Rep* 60 (1):1-24.
Fisher, M. C., A. Alastruey-Izquierdo, J. Berman, T. Bicanic, E. M. Bignell, P. Bowyer, M. Bromley, R. Bruggemann, G. Garber, O. A. Cornely, S. J. Gurr, T. S. Harrison, E. Kuijper, J. Rhodes, D. C. Sheppard, A. Warris, P. L. White, J. Xu, B. Zwaan, and P. E. Verweij. 2022. Tackling the emerging threat of antifungal resistance to human health. *Nat Rev Microbiol* 20 (9):557-571.
Frank, J. 2022. Syphilis. In *Conn's current therapy 2022*, edited by R. D. Kellerman, D. Rakel and H. F. Conn. Amsterdam: Elsevier, 1017-1020.
Freeman, A. M., and J. T. R. Leigh. 2022. Viral Pneumonia. *StatPearls*.
Gade, N. D., and M. S. Qazi. 2013. Fluoroquinolone Therapy in Staphylococcus aureus Infections: Where Do We Stand? *J Lab Physicians* 5 (2):109-112.
Ghosh, A. K., H. L. Osswald, and G. Prato. 2016. Recent Progress in the Development of HIV-1 Protease Inhibitors for the Treatment of HIV/AIDS. *J Med Chem* 59 (11):5172-5208.
Gnann Jr, J. W. 2007. Antiviral therapy of varicella-zoster virus infections. In *Human Herpesviruses: Biology, Therapy, and Immunoprophylaxis*, edited by A. Arvin, G. Campadelli-Fiume, E. Mocarski, P. S. Moore, B. Roizman, R. Whitley and K. Yamanishi. Cambridge.
Gnann, J. W., Jr. 2002. Varicella-zoster virus: atypical presentations and unusual complications. *J Infect Dis* 186 Suppl 1:S91-98.
Goldwater, P. N. 2005. Cefotaxime and ceftriaxone cerebrospinal fluid levels during treatment of bacterial meningitis in children. *Int J Antimicrob Agents* 26 (5):408-411.
Gopal, P., J. P. Sarathy, M. Yee, P. Ragunathan, J. Shin, S. Bhushan, J. Zhu, T. Akopian, O. Kandror, T. K. Lim, M. Gengenbacher, Q. Lin, E. J. Rubin, G. Gruber, and T. Dick. 2020. Pyrazinamide triggers degradation of its target aspartate decarboxylase. *Nat Commun* 11 (1):1661.
Gordon, C. J., E. P. Tchesnokov, E. Woolner, J. K. Perry, J. Y. Feng, D. P. Porter, and M. Gotte. 2020. Remdesivir is a direct-acting antiviral that inhibits RNA-dependent RNA polymerase from severe acute respiratory syndrome coronavirus 2 with high potency. *J Biol Chem* 295 (20):6785-6797.
Grossman, E. R., A. Walchek, and H. Freedman. 1971. Tetracyclines and permanent teeth: the relation between dose and tooth color. *Pediatrics* 47 (3):567-570.
Grossman, T. H. 2016. Tetracycline Antibiotics and Resistance. *Cold Spring Harb Perspect Med* 6 (4):a025387.
Gupta, A. K., and D. C. Lyons. 2015. The Rise and Fall of Oral Ketoconazole. *J Cutan Med Surg* 19 (4):352-357.
Gupta, K., and B. W. Trautner. 2022. Urinary Tract Infections, Pyelonephritis, and Prostatitis. In *Harrison's Principles of Internal Medicine, 21e*, edited by J. Loscalzo, A. Fauci, D. Kasper, S. Hauser, D. Longo and J. L. Jameson. New York, NY: McGraw-Hill Education.
Gurram, D. 2023. Diarrhea. In *Nelson pediatric symptom-based diagnosis : common diseases and their mimics*, edited by R. Kliegman, B. J. Bordini, H. Toth and D. Basel. Philadelphia, PA: Elsevier.
Hakenbeck, R., and J. Coyette. 1998. Resistant penicillin-binding proteins. *Cell Mol Life Sci* 54 (4):332-340.
Hall, C. B., W. J. Hall, and D. M. Speers. 1979. Clinical and physiological manifestations of bronchiolitis and pneumonia. Outcome of respiratory syncytial virus. *Am J Dis Child* 133 (8):798-802.
Hanlon, J. T., S. Perera, P. J. Drinka, C. J. Crnich, S. J. Schweon, M. Klein-Fedyshin, C. B. Wessel, S. Saracco, G. Anderson, M. Mulligan, and D. A. Nace. 2019. The IOU Consensus Recommendations for Empirical Therapy of Cystitis in Nursing Home Residents. *J Am Geriatr Soc* 67 (3):539-545.
Hannallah, R. S., K. A. Brown, and S. T. Verghese. 2019. Otorhinolaryngologic Procedures. In *A practice of anesthesia for infants and children*, edited by C. J. Coté, J. Lerman and B. J. Anderson. Philadelphia, PA: Elsevier.

Hasbun, R. 2022. Meningitis and Encephalitis. In *Youmans and Winn Neurological Surgery*: Elsevier, 432-432.e422.
Haston, J. C., J. Hwang, and K. R. Tan. 2019. Guidance for Using Tafenoquine for Prevention and Antirelapse Therapy for Malaria - United States, 2019. *MMWR Morb Mortal Wkly Rep* 68 (46):1062-1068.
Hausler, M., V. T. Ramaekers, M. Doenges, K. Schweizer, K. Ritter, and L. Schaade. 2002. Neurological complications of acute and persistent Epstein-Barr virus infection in paediatric patients. *J Med Virol* 68 (2):253-263.
Hawser, S., S. Lociuro, and K. Islam. 2006. Dihydrofolate reductase inhibitors as antibacterial agents. *Biochem Pharmacol* 71 (7):941-948.
Hilmarsdottir, I., S. Kidd, and A. Lau. 2023. Mycology. In *Tietz textbook of laboratory medicine*, edited by N. Rifai, R. W. K. Chiu, I. Young, C.-A. D. Burnham and C. Wittwer. St. Louis, Missouri: Elsevier, 1204.
Holland, T. L., A. S. Bayer, and V. G. Fowler. 2020. Endocarditis and Intravascular Infections. In *Mandell, Douglas, and Bennett's Principles and Practice of Infectious Diseases*, edited by J. E. Bennett, R. Dolin and M. J. Blaser: Elsevier, 1068-1108.
Hooper, D. C., and G. A. Jacoby. 2016. Topoisomerase Inhibitors: Fluoroquinolone Mechanisms of Action and Resistance. *Cold Spring Harb Perspect Med* 6 (9).
Houser, K., and K. Subbarao. 2015. Influenza vaccines: challenges and solutions. *Cell Host Microbe* 17 (3):295-300.
Huiming, Y., W. Chaomin, and M. Meng. 2005. Vitamin A for treating measles in children. *Cochrane Database Syst Rev* (4):CD001479.
Ierardi, E., G. Losurdo, R. F. Fortezza, M. Principi, M. Barone, and A. D. Leo. 2019. Optimizing proton pump inhibitors in Helicobacter pylori treatment: Old and new tricks to improve effectiveness. *World J Gastroenterol* 25 (34):5097-5104.
Jahan, N., T. Patton, and M. O'Keeffe. 2022. The Influence of Antibiotic Resistance on Innate Immune Responses to Staphylococcus aureus Infection. *Antibiotics (Basel)* 11 (5).
Jameson, J. L., A. S. Fauci, D. L. Kasper, S. L. Hauser, D. L. Longo, and J. Loscalzo. 2020. Pneumocystis Pneumonia, Candidiasis, and Other Fungal Infections. In *Harrison's Manual of Medicine, 20e*. New York, NY: McGraw-Hill Education.
Jancel, T., and V. Dudas. 2002. Management of uncomplicated urinary tract infections. *West J Med* 176 (1):51-55.
Jang, Y. Y., and K. H. Lee. 2011. Transient asymptomatic white matter lesions following Epstein-Barr virus encephalitis. *Korean J Pediatr* 54 (9):389-393.
Jefferson, T., M. A. Jones, P. Doshi, C. B. Del Mar, R. Hama, M. J. Thompson, E. A. Spencer, I. Onakpoya, K. R. Mahtani, D. Nunan, J. Howick, and C. J. Heneghan. 2014. Neuraminidase inhibitors for preventing and treating influenza in adults and children. *Cochrane Database Syst Rev* (4):CD008965.
Jorth, P., K. McLean, A. Ratjen, P. R. Secor, G. E. Bautista, S. Ravishankar, A. Rezayat, J. Garudathri, J. J. Harrison, R. A. Harwood, K. Penewit, A. Waalkes, P. K. Singh, and S. J. Salipante. 2017. Evolved Aztreonam Resistance Is Multifactorial and Can Produce Hypervirulence in Pseudomonas aeruginosa. *mBio* 8 (5).
Josefson, D. 2001. US fear of bioterrorism spreads as anthrax cases increase. *BMJ* 323 (7318):883.
Joyce, R. P., V. W. Hu, and J. Wang. 2022. The history, mechanism, and perspectives of nirmatrelvir (PF-07321332): an orally bioavailable main protease inhibitor used in combination with ritonavir to reduce COVID-19-related hospitalizations. *Med Chem Res* 31 (10):1637-1646.
Kabinger, F., C. Stiller, J. Schmitzova, C. Dienemann, G. Kokic, H. S. Hillen, C. Hobartner, and P. Cramer. 2021. Mechanism of molnupiravir-induced SARS-CoV-2 mutagenesis. *Nat Struct Mol Biol* 28 (9):740-746.
Kang, M., and J. An. 2022. Viral Myocarditis. *StatPearls*.
Kestler, B., and S. K. Tyler. 2022. Latent tuberculosis testing through the ages: the search for a sleeping killer. *Am J Physiol Lung Cell Mol Physiol* 322 (3):L412-L419.
Kim, J. H., J. H. Kim, W. H. Choe, S. Y. Kwon, B. C. Yoo, E. L. Yoon, and S. H. Kang. 2022. Switching from Tenofovir-Based Combination Therapy to Tenofovir Monotherapy in Multidrug-Experienced Chronic Hepatitis B Patients: a 5-Year Experience at Two Centers. *Antimicrob Agents Chemother* 66 (8):e0027522.
Kim, K., and L. Weiss. 2022. Parasitic Infections. In *Murray & Nadel's textbook of respiratory medicine*, edited by V. C. Broaddus, J. D. Ernst, T. E. King, Jr., S. C. Lazarus, K. F. Sarmiento, L. M. Schnapp, R. D. Stapleton and M. B. Gotway. Philadelphia, PA: Elsevier, 781-796.
Kisat, M., and A. Haider. 2020. Management of Intra-abdominal Infections. In *Current surgical therapy*, edited by J. L. Cameron and A. M. Cameron. Philadelphia, PA: Elsevier.
Knipe, D. M. 2022. Principles of Medical Virology. In *Harrison's Principles of Internal Medicine, 21e*, edited by J. Loscalzo, A. Fauci, D. Kasper, S. Hauser, D. Longo and J. L. Jameson. New York, NY: McGraw-Hill Education.
Kohil, A., S. Jemmieh, M. K. Smatti, and H. M. Yassine. 2021. Viral meningitis: an overview. *Arch Virol* 166 (2):335-345.
Kornhuber, J., M. Muehlbacher, S. Trapp, S. Pechmann, A. Friedl, M. Reichel, C. Muhle, L. Terfloth, T. W. Groemer, G. M. Spitzer, K. R. Liedl, E. Gulbins, and P. Tripal. 2011. Identification of novel functional inhibitors of acid sphingomyelinase. *PLoS One* 6 (8):e23852.
Koshy, A. 2021. Parasitic Infections of the Central Nervous System. In *Aminoff's neurology and general medicine*, edited by M. J. Aminoff and S. A. Josephson. London: Academic Press.

Kozal, M., J. Aberg, G. Pialoux, P. Cahn, M. Thompson, J. M. Molina, B. Grinsztejn, R. Diaz, A. Castagna, P. Kumar, G. Latiff, E. DeJesus, M. Gummel, M. Gartland, A. Pierce, P. Ackerman, C. Llamoso, M. Lataillade, and B. T. Team. 2020. Fostemsavir in Adults with Multidrug-Resistant HIV-1 Infection. *N Engl J Med* 382 (13):1232-1243.

Krawczyk, E., F. A. Suprynowicz, X. Liu, Y. Dai, D. P. Hartmann, J. Hanover, and R. Schlegel. 2008. Koilocytosis: a cooperative interaction between the human papillomavirus E5 and E6 oncoproteins. *Am J Pathol* 173 (3):682-688.

Kristich, C. J., L. B. Rice, and C. A. Arias. 2014. Enterococcal Infection-Treatment and Antibiotic Resistance. In *Enterococci: From Commensals to Leading Causes of Drug Resistant Infection*, edited by M. S. Gilmore, D. B. Clewell, Y. Ike and N. Shankar. Boston.

Kumar, B., K. Asha, M. Khanna, L. Ronsard, C. A. Meseko, and M. Sanicas. 2018. The emerging influenza virus threat: status and new prospects for its therapy and control. *Arch Virol* 163 (4):831-844.

Lacey, E. 1990. Mode of action of benzimidazoles. *Parasitol Today* 6 (4):112-115.

Landman, D., E. Babu, N. Shah, P. Kelly, O. Olawole, M. Backer, S. Bratu, and J. Quale. 2012. Transmission of carbapenem-resistant pathogens in New York City hospitals: progress and frustration. *J Antimicrob Chemother* 67 (6):1427-1431.

Lee, S., M. Hirohama, M. Noguchi, K. Nagata, and A. Kawaguchi. 2018. Influenza A Virus Infection Triggers Pyroptosis and Apoptosis of Respiratory Epithelial Cells through the Type I Interferon Signaling Pathway in a Mutually Exclusive Manner. *J Virol* 92 (14).

Lenaerts, A. J., V. Gruppo, K. S. Marietta, C. M. Johnson, D. K. Driscoll, N. M. Tompkins, J. D. Rose, R. C. Reynolds, and I. M. Orme. 2005. Preclinical testing of the nitroimidazopyran PA-824 for activity against Mycobacterium tuberculosis in a series of in vitro and in vivo models. *Antimicrob Agents Chemother* 49 (6):2294-2301.

Leukocytosis and Leukopenia. 2020. In *Harrison's Manual of Medicine*, edited by J. Jameson, A. S. Fauci, D. L. Kasper, S. L. Hauser, D. L. Longo and J. Loscalzo: McGraw Hill.

Leung, A. K. C., J. M. Lam, K. F. Leong, K. L. Hon, B. Barankin, A. A. M. Leung, and A. H. C. Wong. 2020. Onychomycosis: An Updated Review. *Recent Pat Inflamm Allergy Drug Discov* 14 (1):32-45.

Levinson, W., P. Chin-Hong, E. A. Joyce, J. Nussbaum, and B. Schwartz. 2022. Upper Respiratory Tract Infections. In *Review of Medical Microbiology & Immunology: A Guide to Clinical Infectious Diseases, 17e*. New York, NY: McGraw-Hill Education.

Lew, P. D., and F. S. Southwick. Skin and Soft Tissue Infections. In *Infectious Diseases: A Clinical Short Course, 4e*, edited by F. S. Southwick. New York, NY: McGraw-Hill Education.

Liang, H. Y., Y. Wu, V. Yau, H. X. Yin, S. Lowe, R. Bentley, M. A. Ahmed, W. Zhao, and C. Sun. 2022. SARS-CoV-2 Variants, Current Vaccines and Therapeutic Implications for COVID-19. *Vaccines (Basel)* 10 (9).

Lin, J. W., R. Spaccapelo, E. Schwarzer, M. Sajid, T. Annoura, K. Deroost, R. B. Ravelli, E. Aime, B. Capuccini, A. M. Mommaas-Kienhuis, T. O'Toole, F. Prins, B. M. Franke-Fayard, J. Ramesar, S. Chevalley-Maurel, H. Kroeze, A. J. Koster, H. J. Tanke, A. Crisanti, J. Langhorne, P. Arese, P. E. Van den Steen, C. J. Janse, and S. M. Khan. 2015. Replication of Plasmodium in reticulocytes can occur without hemozoin formation, resulting in chloroquine resistance. *J Exp Med* 212 (6):893-903.

Lionakis, M. S., and J. E. Edwards Jr. 2022. Pathogenesis, Diagnosis, and Treatment of Fungal Infections. In *Harrison's Principles of Internal Medicine, 21e*, edited by J. Loscalzo, A. Fauci, D. Kasper, S. Hauser, D. Longo and J. L. Jameson. New York, NY: McGraw-Hill Education.

Liu, C., A. Bayer, S. E. Cosgrove, R. S. Daum, S. K. Fridkin, R. J. Gorwitz, S. L. Kaplan, A. W. Karchmer, D. P. Levine, B. E. Murray, J. R. M, D. A. Talan, and H. F. Chambers. 2011. Clinical practice guidelines by the infectious diseases society of America for the treatment of methicillin-resistant Staphylococcus aureus infections in adults and children: executive summary. *Clin Infect Dis* 52 (3):285-292.

Logan, S. A., and E. MacMahon. 2008. Viral meningitis. *BMJ* 336 (7634):36-40.

Lu, D. Y., H. Y. Wu, N. S. Yarla, B. Xu, J. Ding, and T. R. Lu. 2018. HAART in HIV/AIDS Treatments: Future Trends. *Infect Disord Drug Targets* 18 (1):15-22.

Luria, L., and G. Cardoza-Favarato. 2022. Human Papillomavirus. In *StatPearls*. Treasure Island (FL).

Mahvi, D. A., and D. M. Mahvi. 2022. Stomach. In *Sabiston textbook of surgery: the biological basis of modern surgical practice*, edited by C. M. Townsend, Jr., R. D. Beauchamp, B. M. Evers, K. L. Mattox and D. C. Sabiston. St. Louis, Missouri: Elsevier, 1196-1239.

Marrazzo, J. M., and K. K. Holmes. 2022. Sexually Transmitted Infections: Overview and Clinical Approach. In *Harrison's Principles of Internal Medicine, 21e*, edited by J. Loscalzo, A. Fauci, D. Kasper, S. Hauser, D. Longo and J. L. Jameson. New York, NY: McGraw-Hill Education.

Martel, T. J., R. T. Jamil, and K. C. King. 2022. Vancomycin Flushing Syndrome. In *StatPearls*. Treasure Island (FL).

Mathison, B., and B. Pritt. 2022. Medical Parasitology. In *Henry's Clinical Diagnosis and Management by Laboratory Methods*, edited by R. A. McPherson and M. R. Pincus, 1290-1351.

Matteson, E., and D. Osmon. 2020. Infections of Bursae, Joints, and Bones. In *Goldman-Cecil Medicine*, edited by L. Goldman and A. I. Schafer: Elsevier, 1761-1767.

McAdam, A. J., and A. B. Onderdonk. 2018. Laboratory Diagnosis of Infectious Diseases. In *Harrison's Principles of Internal Medicine, 20e*, edited by J. L. Jameson, A. S. Fauci, D. L. Kasper, S. L. Hauser, D. L. Longo and J. Loscalzo. New York, NY: McGraw-Hill Education.

McAuley, J. L., B. P. Gilbertson, S. Trifkovic, L. E. Brown, and J. L. McKimm-Breschkin. 2019. Influenza Virus Neuraminidase Structure and Functions. *Front Microbiol* 10:39.

McGillicuddy, D. C., K. H. Shah, R. P. Friedberg, L. A. Nathanson, and J. A. Edlow. 2007. How sensitive is the synovial fluid white blood cell count in diagnosing septic arthritis? *The American Journal of Emergency Medicine* 25 (7):749-752.

McKinnon, H. D., Jr., and T. Howard. 2000. Evaluating the febrile patient with a rash. *Am Fam Physician* 62 (4):804-816.

Melander, R. J., D. V. Zurawski, and C. Melander. 2018. Narrow-Spectrum Antibacterial Agents. *Medchemcomm* 9:12-21.

Messacar, K., and M. J. Abzug. 2023. Enteroviruses and Parechoviruses. In *Principles and practice of pediatric infectious diseases*, edited by S. S. Long, C. G. Prober, M. Fischer and D. W. Kimberlin. Philadelphia, PA: Elsevier, 1228-1236.

Metlay, J. P., G. W. Waterer, A. C. Long, A. Anzueto, J. Brozek, K. Crothers, L. A. Cooley, N. C. Dean, M. J. Fine, S. A. Flanders, M. R. Griffin, M. L. Metersky, D. M. Musher, M. I. Restrepo, and C. G. Whitney. 2019. Diagnosis and Treatment of Adults with Community-acquired Pneumonia. An Official Clinical Practice Guideline of the American Thoracic Society and Infectious Diseases Society of America. *Am J Respir Crit Care Med* 200 (7):e45-e67.

Michaels, M., H. Chong, and M. Green. 2020. Chapter 205: Infections in Immunocompromised Persons. In *Nelson textbook of pediatrics*, edited by R. Kliegman, B. Stanton, J. W. St. Geme, III, N. F. Schor, R. E. Behrman and W. E. Nelson. Philadelphia, PA: Elsevier Inc., 1403-1410.

Miftahussurur, M., M. Cruz, P. Subsomwong, J. A. Jimenez Abreu, C. Hosking, H. Nagashima, J. Akada, and Y. Yamaoka. 2017. Clarithromycin-Based Triple Therapy is Still Useful as an Initial Treatment for Helicobacter pylori Infection in the Dominican Republic. *Am J Trop Med Hyg* 96 (5):1050-1059.

Mirna, M., L. Schmutzler, A. Topf, U. C. Hoppe, and M. Lichtenauer. 2022. Biological Sex and Its Impact on Clinical Characteristics in Patients Presenting with Myocarditis. *Med Princ Pract* 31 (1):74-82.

Mohammad, A. H., N. A. Naserrudin, S. S. Syed Abdul Rahim, J. Jelip, A. Atil, M. F. Sazali, A. J. Muyou, P. D. Kunasagran, N. Ahmad Kamarudin, Z. I. Azhar, R. Dapari, M. S. Jeffree, and M. R. Hassan. 2022. Narrative Review of the Control and Prevention of Knowlesi Malaria. *Trop Med Infect Dis* 7 (8).

Moore, M. J., B. Rathish, and F. Zahra. 2022. Monkeypox. *StatPearls*.

Morrison, N. E., and G. M. Marley. 1976. The mode of action of clofazimine DNA binding studies. *Int J Lepr Other Mycobact Dis* 44 (1-2):133-134.

Musher, D. M. 2020. Overview of Pneumonia. In *Goldman-Cecil Medicine*, edited by L. Goldman and A. I. Schafer: Elsevier, 592-603.

Nahid, P., S. R. Mase, G. B. Migliori, G. Sotgiu, G. H. Bothamley, J. L. Brozek, A. Cattamanchi, J. P. Cegielski, L. Chen, C. L. Daley, T. L. Dalton, R. Duarte, F. Fregonese, C. R. Horsburgh, Jr., F. Ahmad Khan, F. Kheir, Z. Lan, A. Lardizabal, M. Lauzardo, J. M. Mangan, S. M. Marks, L. McKenna, D. Menzies, C. D. Mitnick, D. M. Nilsen, F. Parvez, C. A. Peloquin, A. Raftery, H. S. Schaaf, N. S. Shah, J. R. Starke, J. W. Wilson, J. M. Wortham, T. Chorba, and B. Seaworth. 2019. Treatment of Drug-Resistant Tuberculosis. An Official ATS/CDC/ERS/IDSA Clinical Practice Guideline. *Am J Respir Crit Care Med* 200 (10):e93-e142.

Nayak, S. U., R. Talwani, B. Gilliam, G. Taylor, and M. Ghosh. 2011. Cryptococcal Meningitis in an HIV-Positive Pregnant Woman. *J Int Assoc Physicians AIDS Care (Chic)* 10 (2):79-82.

Nir, T. M., N. Jahanshad, E. Busovaca, L. Wendelken, K. Nicolas, P. M. Thompson, and V. G. Valcour. 2014. Mapping white matter integrity in elderly people with HIV. *Hum Brain Mapp* 35 (3):975-992.

Nosanchuk, J., and G. Thompson. 2022. Fungal Infections: Endemic. In *Murray & Nadel's textbook of respiratory medicine*, edited by V. C. Broaddus, J. D. Ernst, T. E. King, Jr., S. C. Lazarus, K. F. Sarmiento, L. M. Schnapp, R. D. Stapleton and M. B. Gotway. Philadelphia, PA: Elsevier, 748-762.

Noshi, T., M. Kitano, K. Taniguchi, A. Yamamoto, S. Omoto, K. Baba, T. Hashimoto, K. Ishida, Y. Kushima, K. Hattori, M. Kawai, R. Yoshida, M. Kobayashi, T. Yoshinaga, A. Sato, M. Okamatsu, Y. Sakoda, H. Kida, T. Shishido, and A. Naito. 2018. In vitro characterization of baloxavir acid, a first-in-class cap-dependent endonuclease inhibitor of the influenza virus polymerase PA subunit. *Antiviral Res* 160:109-117.

Notter, J., A. Bregenzer, P. Vernazza, and C. R. Kahlert. 2019. Nevirapine in HIV maintenance therapy - can "old drugs" survive in current HIV management? *Swiss Med Wkly* 149:w20053.

Oliphant, C. M., and G. M. Green. 2002. Quinolones: a comprehensive review. *Am Fam Physician* 65 (3):455-464.

Ostrosky-Zeichner, L., and M. Al-Obaidi. 2019. Antifungal and Antiviral Therapy. In *Critical care medicine : principles of diagnosis and management in the adult*, edited by J. E. Parrillo and R. P. Dellinger. Philadelphia, PA.: Elsevier, 807-821.

Painter, W. P., W. Holman, J. A. Bush, F. Almazedi, H. Malik, N. Eraut, M. J. Morin, L. J. Szewczyk, and G. R. Painter. 2021. Human Safety, Tolerability, and Pharmacokinetics of Molnupiravir, a Novel Broad-Spectrum Oral Antiviral Agent with Activity Against SARS-CoV-2. *Antimicrob Agents Chemother*.

Paludan, S. R. 1998. Interleukin-4 and interferon-gamma: the quintessence of a mutual antagonistic relationship. *Scand J Immunol* 48 (5):459-468.

Papp-Wallace, K. M., A. R. Mack, M. A. Taracila, and R. A. Bonomo. 2020. Resistance to Novel beta-Lactam-beta-Lactamase Inhibitor Combinations: The "Price of Progress". *Infect Dis Clin North Am* 34 (4):773-819.

Park, S. C., Y. M. Jeen, and Y. T. Jeen. 2017. Approach to cytomegalovirus infections in patients with ulcerative colitis. *Korean J Intern Med* 32 (3):383-392.

Perfect, J. 2021. Fungal Infections of the Central Nervous System. In *Aminoff's neurology and general medicine*, edited by M. J. Aminoff and S. A. Josephson. London: Academic Press, 803-819.

Pichichero, M. E. 2006. Cephalosporins can be prescribed safely for penicillin-allergic patients. *J Fam Pract* 55 (2):106-112.

Playe, S. J. 2007. Quinolones for Kids? The Good News Is the Bad News. *Emergency Medicine News* 29 (3):14.

Powell, D. A., and M. C. Nahata. 1982. Chloramphenicol: new perspectives on an old drug. *Drug Intell Clin Pharm* 16 (4):295-300.

Prosser, G. A., and L. P. de Carvalho. 2013. Kinetic mechanism and inhibition of Mycobacterium tuberculosis D-alanine:D-alanine ligase by the antibiotic D-cycloserine. *FEBS J* 280 (4):1150-1166.

Queller, J. N., and N. Bhatia. 2015. The Dermatologist's Approach to Onychomycosis. *J Fungi (Basel)* 1 (2):173-184.

Rahal, J. J., Jr., and M. S. Simberkoff. 1979. Bactericidal and bacteriostatic action of chloramphenicol against meningeal pathogens. *Antimicrob Agents Chemother* 16 (1):13-18.

Rajagopalan, S. 2016. Parasitic Infections. In *Taylor and Kelly's Dermatology for Skin of Color, 2e*, edited by A. P. Kelly, S. C. Taylor, H. W. Lim and A. M. A. Serrano. New York, NY: McGraw-Hill Education.

Ramakrishnan, K. 2022. Necrotizing Skin and Soft-Tissue Infections. In *Conn's current therapy 2022*, edited by R. D. Kellerman, D. Rakel and H. F. Conn. Amsterdam: Elsevier.

Reis, S., M. I. Metzendorf, R. Kuehn, M. Popp, I. Gagyor, P. Kranke, P. Meybohm, N. Skoetz, and S. Weibel. 2022. Nirmatrelvir combined with ritonavir for preventing and treating COVID-19. *Cochrane Database Syst Rev* 9:CD015395.

Romano, A., F. Gaeta, R. L. Valluzzi, M. Maggioletti, C. Caruso, and D. Quaratino. 2016. Cross-reactivity and tolerability of aztreonam and cephalosporins in subjects with a T cell-mediated hypersensitivity to penicillins. *J Allergy Clin Immunol* 138 (1):179-186.

Ropp, P. A., M. Hu, M. Olesky, and R. A. Nicholas. 2002. Mutations in ponA, the gene encoding penicillin-binding protein 1, and a novel locus, penC, are required for high-level chromosomally mediated penicillin resistance in Neisseria gonorrhoeae. *Antimicrob Agents Chemother* 46 (3):769-777.

Rosenberg, G. 2022. Brain Edema and Disorders of Cerebrospinal Fluid Circulation. In *Bradley and Daroff's Neurology in Clinical Practice*: Elsevier, 1327-1344.

Ryan, K. J. 2022. Infectious Diseases: Syndromes and Etiologies. In *Sherris & Ryan's Medical Microbiology, 8e*. New York, NY: McGraw-Hill Education.

Saleh, D., S. N. S. Yarrarapu, and S. Sharma. 2022. Herpes Simplex Type 1. *StatPearls*.

Sarkar, M., R. E. Polk, P. S. Guzelian, C. Hunt, and H. T. Karnes. 1990. In vitro effect of fluoroquinolones on theophylline metabolism in human liver microsomes. *Antimicrob Agents Chemother* 34 (4):594-599.

Saullo, J., and B. Alexander. 2022. Fungal Infections: Opportunistic. In *Murray & Nadel's textbook of respiratory medicine*, edited by V. C. Broaddus, J. D. Ernst, T. E. King, Jr., S. C. Lazarus, K. F. Sarmiento, L. M. Schnapp, R. D. Stapleton and M. B. Gotway. Philadelphia, PA: Elsevier, 763-780.

Sayana, S., and H. Khanlou. 2009. Maraviroc: a new CCR5 antagonist. *Expert Rev Anti Infect Ther* 7 (1):9-19.

Schneider, T., and H. G. Sahl. 2010. Lipid II and other bactoprenol-bound cell wall precursors as drug targets. *Curr Opin Investig Drugs* 11 (2):157-164.

Schuster, F. L., B. J. Guglielmo, and G. S. Visvesvara. 2006. In-vitro activity of miltefosine and voriconazole on clinical isolates of free-living amebas: Balamuthia mandrillaris, Acanthamoeba spp., and Naegleria fowleri. *J Eukaryot Microbiol* 53 (2):121-126.

Schwarz, S., C. Kehrenberg, B. Doublet, and A. Cloeckaert. 2004. Molecular basis of bacterial resistance to chloramphenicol and florfenicol. *FEMS Microbiol Rev* 28 (5):519-542.

Sharma, R., S. Sekhon, and M. Cascella. 2022. White Matter Lesions. *StatPearls*.

Shea, J., T. A. Halse, D. Kohlerschmidt, P. Lapierre, H. A. Modestil, C. H. Kearns, F. F. Dworkin, J. L. Rakeman, V. Escuyer, and K. A. Musser. 2021. Low-Level Rifampin Resistance and rpoB Mutations in Mycobacterium tuberculosis: an Analysis of Whole-Genome Sequencing and Drug Susceptibility Test Data in New York. *J Clin Microbiol* 59 (4).

Shirasawa, H., and K. Nagino. 2005. [Voriconazole-medical needs, evidence, potential for the future]. *Nihon Ishinkin Gakkai Zasshi* 46 (4):223-228.

Shuclick, R., and I. Ibrahim-zada. 2020. Management of Echinococcal Cyst Disease of the Liver. In *Current surgical therapy*, edited by J. L. Cameron and A. M. Cameron. Philadelphia, PA: Elsevier, 361-365.

Sidcrovski, S. II. 2006. *Tularemia*. Philadelphia: Chelsea House Publishers.

Sifri, C., and L. Madoff. 2020. Infections of the Liver and Biliary System (Liver Abscess, Cholangitis, Cholecystitis). In *Mandell, Douglas, and Bennett's principles and practice of infectious diseases*, edited by J. E. Bennett, R. Dolin and M. J. Blaser. Philadelphia, PA: Elsevier, 1037-1045.

Smith, C. F. 2022. Infestations and Bites. In *Clinical Dermatology: Diagnosis and Management of Common Disorders, 2e*, edited by C. Soutor and M. K. Hordinsky. New York, NY: McGraw-Hill Education.

Southwick, F. S. 2020. Cardiovascular Infections. In *Infectious Diseases: A Clinical Short Course, 4e*, edited by F. S. Southwick. New York, NY: McGraw-Hill Education.

Sozzi, F. B., E. Gherbesi, A. Faggiano, E. Gnan, A. Maruccio, M. Schiavone, L. Iacuzio, and S. Carugo. 2022. Viral Myocarditis: Classification, Diagnosis, and Clinical Implications. *Front Cardiovasc Med* 9:908663.

Sriwilaijaroen, N., C. J. Vavricka, H. Kiyota, and Y. Suzuki. 2022. Influenza A Virus Neuraminidase Inhibitors. *Methods Mol Biol* 2556:321-353.

Staecker, H. 2021. Re-evaluating aminoglycoside ototoxicity. *J Cyst Fibros* 20 (1):5.

Stevens, D. L., and A. E. Bryant. 2022. Infections of the Skin, Muscles, and Soft Tissues. In *Harrison's Principles of Internal Medicine, 21e*, edited by J. Loscalzo, A. Fauci, D. Kasper, S. Hauser, D. Longo and J. L. Jameson. New York, NY: McGraw-Hill Education.

Stone, K. J., and J. L. Strominger. 1971. Mechanism of action of bacitracin: complexation with metal ion and C 55 -isoprenyl pyrophosphate. *Proc Natl Acad Sci U S A* 68 (12):3223-3227.

Stuempfig, N. D., and J. Seroy. 2022. Viral Gastroenteritis. *StatPearls*.

Sulfonamides and Vitamin K Deficiency. 1945. *Nutrition Reviews* 3 (2):35-36.

Swierczynska, M., D. M. Mirowska-Guzel, and E. Pindelska. 2022. Antiviral Drugs in Influenza. *Int J Environ Res Public Health* 19 (5).

Takesue, Y., S. Kusachi, H. Mikamo, J. Sato, A. Watanabe, H. Kiyota, S. Iwata, M. Kaku, H. Hanaki, Y. Sumiyama, Y. Kitagawa, K. Nakajima, T. Ueda, M. Uchino, T. Mizuguchi, Y. Ambo, M. Konosu, K. Ishibashi, A. Matsuda, K. Hase, Y. Harihara, K. Okabayashi, S. Seki, T. Hara, K. Matsui, Y. Matsuo, M. Kobayashi, S. Kubo, K. Uchiyama, J. Shimizu, R. Kawabata, H. Ohge, S. Akagi, M. Oka, T. Wakatsuki, K. Suzuki, K. Okamoto, and K. Yanagihara. 2018. Antimicrobial susceptibility of common pathogens isolated from postoperative intra-abdominal infections in Japan. *J Infect Chemother* 24 (5):330-340.

Tamma, P. D., S. E. Cosgrove, and L. L. Maragakis. 2012. Combination therapy for treatment of infections with gram-negative bacteria. *Clin Microbiol Rev* 25 (3):450-470.

Taqi, S. A., S. A. Zaki, A. R. Nilofer, and L. B. Sami. 2012. Trimethoprim-sulfamethoxazole-induced Steven Johnson syndrome in an HIV-infected patient. *Indian J Pharmacol* 44 (4):533-535.

Tenover, F. C., D. P. Nicolau, and C. M. Gill. 2022. Carbapenemase-producing Pseudomonas aeruginosa -an emerging challenge. *Emerg Microbes Infect* 11 (1):811-814.

Thandi, C. S., and L. Whittam. 2021. Diagnosis and management of common viral skin infections. *Prescriber* 32 (4):10-14.

Thomas, K. E., R. Hasbun, J. Jekel, and V. J. Quagliarello. 2002. The diagnostic accuracy of Kernig's sign, Brudzinski's sign, and nuchal rigidity in adults with suspected meningitis. *Clin Infect Dis* 35 (1):46-52.

Thorlund, K., K. Sheldrick, G. Meyerowitz-Katz, S. Singh, and A. Hill. 2022. Making Statistical Sense of the Molnupiravir MOVe-OUT Clinical Trial. *Am J Trop Med Hyg*.

Tiwari, V., and M. J. Bergman. 2022. Viral Arthritis. *StatPearls*.

Tosi, M. F. 2019. Normal and impaired immunologic responses to infection. In *Feigin and Cherry's Textbook of Pediatric Infectious Diseases*, edited by J. D. Cherry, G. J. Harrison, S. L. Kaplan, W. J. Steinbach and P. J. Hotez: Elsevier, 15-40.

van de Beek, D., J. de Gans, L. Spanjaard, M. Weisfelt, J. B. Reitsma, and M. Vermeulen. 2004. Clinical features and prognostic factors in adults with bacterial meningitis. *N Engl J Med* 351 (18):1849-1859.

Vazquez-Laslop, N., and A. S. Mankin. 2018. How Macrolide Antibiotics Work. *Trends Biochem Sci* 43 (9):668-684.

Virkki, R., T. Juven, J. Mertsola, and O. Ruuskanen. 2005. Radiographic follow-up of pneumonia in children. *Pediatr Pulmonol* 40 (3):223-227.

Walker, A. C., D. F. Gaieski, and N. J. Johnson. 2020. How do I manage central nervous system infections (meningitis/encephalitis)? In *Evidence-based practice of critical care*, edited by C. Deutschman and P. Neligan: Elsevier, 313-318.

Wang, Y., E. De Clercq, and G. Li. 2019. Current and emerging non-nucleoside reverse transcriptase inhibitors (NNRTIs) for HIV-1 treatment. *Expert Opin Drug Metab Toxicol* 15 (10):813-829.

Weinbach, E. C., and J. Garbus. 1969. Mechanism of action of reagents that uncouple oxidative phosphorylation. *Nature* 221 (5185):1016-1018.

White, N. J., T. T. Hien, and F. H. Nosten. 2015. A Brief History of Qinghaosu. *Trends Parasitol* 31 (12):607-610.

Willems, L., R. van der Geest, and K. de Beule. 2001. Itraconazole oral solution and intravenous formulations: a review of pharmacokinetics and pharmacodynamics. *J Clin Pharm Ther* 26 (3):159-169.

Winstanley, T. G., and R. C. Spencer. 1986. Moraxella catarrhalis: antibiotic susceptibility with special reference to trimethoprim. *J Antimicrob Chemother* 18 (3):425-426.

Wittler, R. 2022. Tickborne Rickettsial Diseases (Rocky Mountain Spotted Fever and Other Spotted Fever Group Rickettsioses, Ehrlichioses, and Anaplasmosis). In *Conn's current therapy 2022*, edited by R. D. Kellerman, D. Rakel and H. F. Conn. Amsterdam: Elsevier, 676-680.

Wolford, R. W., A. Goyal, S. Y. Belgam Syed, and T. J. Schaefer. 2022. Pharyngitis. *StatPearls*.

Wong, W., X. C. Bai, B. E. Sleebs, T. Triglia, A. Brown, J. K. Thompson, K. E. Jackson, E. Hanssen, D. S. Marapana, I. S. Fernandez, S. A. Ralph, A. F. Cowman, S. H. W. Scheres, and J. Baum. 2017. Mefloquine targets the Plasmodium falciparum 80S ribosome to inhibit protein synthesis. *Nat Microbiol* 2:17031.

Yahav, D., A. Lador, M. Paul, and L. Leibovici. 2011. Efficacy and safety of tigecycline: a systematic review and meta-analysis. *J Antimicrob Chemother* 66 (9):1963-1971.

Zagari, R. M., L. Frazzoni, G. Marasco, L. Fuccio, and F. Bazzoli. 2021. Treatment of Helicobacter pylori infection: a clinical practice update. *Minerva Med* 112 (2):281-287.

Zapun, A., C. Contreras-Martel, and T. Vernet. 2008. Penicillin-binding proteins and beta-lactam resistance. *FEMS Microbiol Rev* 32 (2):361-385.

Zhanel, G., I. Critchley, L. Y. Lin, and N. Alvandi. 2019. Microbiological Profile of Sarecycline, a Novel Targeted Spectrum Tetracycline for the Treatment of Acne Vulgaris. *Antimicrob Agents Chemother* 63 (1).

Zhang, J., L. Li, Q. Lv, L. Yan, Y. Wang, and Y. Jiang. 2019. The Fungal CYP51s: Their Functions, Structures, Related Drug Resistance, and Inhibitors. *Front Microbiol* 10:691.

Zhou, Q., Y. Zhai, J. Lou, M. Liu, X. Pang, and F. Sun. 2011. Thiabendazole inhibits ubiquinone reduction activity of mitochondrial respiratory complex II via a water molecule mediated binding feature. *Protein Cell* 2 (7):531-542.

Zimmerli, W. 2022. Osteomyelitis. In *Harrison's Principles of Internal Medicine, 21e*, edited by J. Loscalzo, A. Fauci, D. Kasper, S. Hauser, D. Longo and J. L. Jameson. New York, NY: McGraw-Hill Education.

Zou, M., L. Tang, S. Zhao, Z. Zhao, L. Chen, P. Chen, Z. Huang, J. Li, L. Chen, and X. Fan. 2012. Systematic review and meta-analysis of detecting galactomannan in bronchoalveolar lavage fluid for diagnosing invasive aspergillosis. *PLoS One* 7 (8):e43347.

Case Study Questions

Case Study

A 70-year-old patient presents to their family physician complaining of a four-day history of cough and fever, progressing in the last 24 hours to increasing malaise and shaking chills. They live alone at home and have a thirty-pack-year history of cigarette smoking. They developed an increasingly severe productive cough with clear sputum for the past eight months. Today, prior to arrival at the physicians' clinic, their cough produced an orange-red sputum. In the clinic, their respiration rate was 20 breaths per minute and their forehead temperature was 102.5 °F.

A chest X-ray is performed and reveals lobar pneumonia. While this normally would trigger an empirical prescription of one (or more) antibiotics, the patient, in this case, study has also provided a sputum sample for Gram staining and culture; it is positive for *Streptococcus pneumoniae* (Gram-positive diplococci). What would be an ideal drug regimen for this patient, assuming they have no drug allergies?

Quiz Questions

1a. A 21-year-old male with no medical history presents to the emergency department via ambulance after his fraternity brothers called 911. Over the last 24 hours, he has complained of a headache that has not improved with either acetaminophen or ibuprofen by mouth. He is in notable distress and rates his headache 10 out of 10. Vital signs obtained during triage reveal a heart rate of 134, respiratory rate of 20, blood pressure of 128/78, and temperature of 103.2 °F. On physical examination, he is a well-developed, well-nourished young man in acute distress, tachycardic and tachypneic, but the heart and lung sounds are normal otherwise. When examining his neck, he complains of discomfort and you notice he brings his legs up slightly as soon as you try to flex his neck. Aside from obtaining a thorough laboratory workup and ordering appropriate treatment, what is the next best step in the management of this patient?

A. Computed Tomography of the brain
B. Magnetic resonance imaging of the brain
C. Lumbar puncture
D. Neurosurgical consultation

1b. Which of the following drugs is the most appropriate to apply to this meningitis case?

A. amphotericin B (AmB)
B. albendazole
C. artemisinin
D. abacavir
E. atazanavir
F. ceftriaxone

2a. A 62-year-old female with a medical history of IV heroin abuse presents to the emergency department with complaints of subjective fevers and night sweats. The patient admits that she has been feeling ill for a few days now, but otherwise appears to be a poor historian. Vital signs include a heart rate of 122, respiratory rate of 18, blood pressure of 102/64, and a temperature of 100.6 °F. On examination, she is a cachectic, toxic-appearing female, appears older than the stated age, has a grade III/VI holosystolic murmur at the left sternal border, and you note purple-pink nodules on her hands that she says are tender. Which of the following additional findings would give her a diagnosis of definitive infectious endocarditis (IE) using Duke criteria?

A. Leukocytosis >12,000 and findings of glomerulonephritis
B. Transthoracic echocardiogram showing mitral valve prolapse
C. Two blood cultures drawn on the same day growing *Staphylococcus epidermidis*
D. One blood culture out of two growing *Coxiella burnetii*

2b. Which of the following drugs is the most appropriate to apply to this IE case?

A. acyclovir
B. baloxavir marboxil
C. clotrimazole
D. doxycycline
E. emtricitabine
F. fluconazole
G. griseofulvin

3a. A 48-year-old female with a past medical history of hypertension and diabetes mellitus type 2 presents to the office as a walk-in for complaints of body aches, fever, malaise, and dry cough for the last five days. The patient states that there may be something going around in her home as both her children and her husband have had similar symptoms over the last week. Her physical exam is nonfocal. She is afebrile in the office. What is the next best step in the management of this patient?

A. Urgently send the patient for a chest X-ray
B. Recommend symptomatic management including over-the-counter analgesics
C. Prescribe course of amoxicillin
D. Prescribe course of oseltamivir

3b. Had the 48-year-old female presented earlier to the clinic, which antiviral agent would most likely have been prescribed?

A. azidothymidine
B. bictegravir
C. zanamivir
D. dasabuvir
E. efavirenz
F. foscarnet
G. grazoprevir

4a. A 24-year-old male with a medical history of cystic fibrosis requiring bilateral lung transplantation nine months ago presents with complaints of worsening hemoptysis. It first began as a few drops, but in the last 24 hours, he has coughed up more than 2 cups of bright red blood. He is intubated for airway protection and undergoes an urgent bronchoscopy to identify the bleeding. No specific source is found, but BAL is sent for an array of testing and returns positive for galactomannan. CT of the chest reveals various nodular opacities and a reversed halo sign. Which of the following is the next best step in the management of this patient?

A. Begin itraconazole
B. Begin fluconazole
C. Begin amphotericin B
D. Begin voriconazole

4b. The 24-year-old male with cystic fibrosis presenting with worsening hemoptysis is provided with the appropriate antibiotic. Which of the following is the most likely complaint that might make the patient return to your care?

A. Transient vision aberrations
B. Thrush
C. Stevens-Johnson syndrome

5a. A 50-year-old male with a past medical history of HIV is brought by his family for concerns about changes in his behavior over the last two weeks. His partner is concerned because he has become increasingly confused, recently leaving a stove top on and almost starting a fire. His partner states that he is usually good about taking his medications but he is unsure if he has been taking his antiretrovirals. A more thorough history reveals that they have three cats at home. Laboratory findings are normal except for a CD4 count of 25. On exam, he is notably encephalopathic. MRI of the brain is performed and reveals multiple ring-enhancing lesions. Which of the following is the best treatment to begin for this diagnosis?

A. Artesunate
B. Pyrimethamine and sulfadiazine
C. Vancomycin, cefepime and ampicillin
D. Albendazole and corticosteroids

5b. The reason for combining pyrimethamine and sulfadiazine together as antimicrobial therapy is:

A. The two drugs work on two different biosynthetic pathways.
B. Sulfadiazine is a "booster" that inhibits CYP3A4 to protect pyrimethamine from metabolism.
C. The two drugs work on two parts of the same biosynthetic pathway.
D. Pyrimethamine inhibits P-glycoprotein (P-gp) to prevent sulfadiazine efflux.

Case Study Answers

A macrolide with a cephalosporin, or a fluoroquinolone.
The American Thoracic Society has recommended (Metlay et al. 2019) the following antibacterial drug regimens as initial treatment strategies for community-acquired pneumonia (CAP) (see lists in Table 3.8). The 70-year-old patient has CAP caused by *Streptococcus pneumoniae*. In the United States in 2019, there were over 30,000 cases, and over 3,000 deaths, from *Strep. pneumoniae*; moreover, an estimated 30% or more of these cases were resistant to one or more antibiotics, with resistance to the macrolide erythromycin being the most prevalent in 2019 case report analyses ((CDC) 2019). For this reason, combining a macrolide with a cephalosporin is a good first approach (to mitigate against possible macrolide resistance). If the patient presents with a history of penicillin-allergic response(s), it is advisable to avoid cephalosporin treatment (as they share the β-lactam ring core structure, and hence the potential for eliciting allergy, with the penicillins; see above). A fluoroquinolone might therefore be a first choice in the face of penicillin allergy potential with this patient.

Table 3.8. American Thoracic Society recommended (Metlay et al. 2019) **initial treatment strategies for community-acquired pneumonia (CAP) in out-patients**

Status of Presenting Patient	Recommended Regimen
With a co-morbidity (*e.g.*, chronic heart, lung, or renal disease; or alcoholism/liver disease; or diabetes mellitus; or cancer; or asplenia)	A combination of: (Amoxicillin/clavulanate *OR* a cephalosporin) *AND* (a macroline *OR* Doxycycline) *OR* Monotherapy with a fluoroquinolone
Without a co-morbidity *AND* **Without** risk factors for having methicillin-resistant *Staph. aureus* (MRSA) or *Pseudomonas aeruginosa*	Amoxicillin, *OR* Doxycycline, *OR* a macrolide (if local pneumococcal resistance is <25%)

Quiz Answers

1a. C. The above patient has bacterial meningitis. He is of college age and appears to live in a fraternity house, a dormitory setting creating close living quarters with others. He has the triad of headache, fever, and neck stiffness. On exam, he has a clear Brudzinski's sign causing him to flex his hips and legs with neck flexion. A lumbar puncture for cerebrospinal fluid analysis is the next best step in his management. While imaging can be obtained, it is not necessary to make the diagnosis and will only delay sampling. If the patient had focal neurologic deficits, concern for cerebral abscess would have warranted obtaining CT imaging first and likely subsequent neurosurgical evaluation. MRI of the brain can be helpful for cases of suspected viral meningitis, particularly if there are findings like temporal enhancement which can suggest herpes virus encephalitis. Our patient, however, is not encephalopathic.

1b. F. The third-generation cephalosporin ceftriaxone is the only antibacterial agent in the list of possible answers for this case of bacterial meningitis (common causes include *Neisseria meningitidis, Streptococcus pneumoniae, Haemophilus influenzae,* group B *Streptococcus*, and *Listeria monocytogenes*). Amphotericin B is an anti-fungal agent but this is not a case of fungal meningitis, so answer A is incorrect. Albendazole is an anthelmintic benzimidazole often given with corticosteroids for neurocysticercosis, so answer B is incorrect. Artemisinin is given within anti-malarial therapy, so answer C is incorrect. Abacavir and atazanavir are anti-viral agents, so answers D and E are incorrect.

2a. D. The above patient has infectious endocarditis, likely secondary to Staphylococcus in the setting of her IV drug abuse. She presents with three minor criteria, including known IV drug abuse, fever, and immunologic phenomena (the tender purple-pink nodules are Osler nodes). This places her in the possible IE category. For her to have definitive IE by clinical criteria, she needs either two major criteria, one major and three minor criteria, or fiver minor criteria. Leukocytosis is not in any criteria and glomerulonephritis is another immunologic phenomenon, so A is incorrect. Echocardiographic evidence, needed as a major criterion, includes vegetations, oscillating intracardiac mass on a valve or supporting structure without anatomical explanation, new partial dehiscence of a prosthetic valve, or new valve regurgitation. Mitral valve prolapse is relatively common in the population and is not a new regurgitation, so B is incorrect. Major criteria with blood culture criteria include two separate blood cultures showing typical bacteria, of which *Staphylococcus epidermidis* is not one, so C is incorrect.

2b. D. The American Centers for Disease Control and Prevention (CDC.gov) recommends the tetracycline-class antibiotic doxycycline as first-line treatment for non-pregnant adults with Q fever (*Coxiella burnetii* infection); adults with endocarditis caused by *C. burnetii* are recommended to receive 100 mg of doxycycline every 12 hours (along with hydroxychloroquine: 200 mg every 8 hours) for at least 18 months. Acyclovir, baloxavir marboxil, emtricitabine, and griseofulvin are all antiviral agents, so answers A, B, E, and G are all incorrect. Clotrimazole and fluconazole are anti-fungal agents, so answers C and F are also incorrect.

3a. B. This patient likely has influenza. Given that the patient has mild symptoms without shortness of breath or concern for bacterial superinfection, a chest x-ray is not warranted, so A is incorrect. After five days and without a productive cough or other signs of bacterial pneumonia, treatment with amoxicillin is also not warranted given the information that was provided, so C is incorrect. Similarly, oseltamivir would be indicated for influenza, but it should be given within two days of symptom onset, so D is incorrect. At this stage of her illness, symptomatic management is the best choice.

3b. C. Similar to oseltamivir, zanamivir is an effective drug against the influenza virus when given early (within two days of symptom onset). Azidothymidine (AZT), bictegravir, and efavirenz are anti-HIV therapeutics, so answers A, B, and E are incorrect. Dasabuvir and grazoprevir are anti-HCV therapeutics, so answers D and G are incorrect. Foscarnet is primarily used to treat viral infections involving the *Herpesviridae* family, so F is incorrect.

4a. D. This patient suffers from invasive pulmonary aspergillosis and should be started on voriconazole. Isavuconazole is also a first-line anti-fungal medication but was not given as an answer choice. This patient has a significant risk factor: immunosuppression from a solid organ transplant. Hemoptysis can occur with invasive aspergillosis and should be suspected in immunocompromised patients. Although serum galactomannan can have a limited utility, BAL galactomannan has a very high sensitivity and specificity for invasive aspergillosis. Itraconazole would be the treatment of Histoplasmosis, which the history did not suggest given no history of endemic travel nor any mediastinal and/or hilar lymphadenopathy. Severe disease can also be managed with amphotericin. Fluconazole would be appropriate for speciated Candidal pneumonia, but echinocandins like caspofungin are preferred due to concern for possible resistant species. Mucormycosis could have similar findings and presentation and would be treated with amphotericin B; however, mucormycosis would not test positive for galactomannan.

4b. A. This patient is being treated with voriconazole (established in previous question #4a), which has a common adverse effect of transient vision aberrations such as blurred vision, vision color changes, visual disturbances, and/or enhanced visual perception. Thrush is usually caused by Candida species, and voriconazole is an effective agent against even fluconazole-resistant Candida species, so B is incorrect. Voriconazole is not a sulfa drug (the latter being a common inducer of Steven-Johnson syndrome), so C is incorrect.

5a. B. This patient is suffering from toxoplasmosis. He is immunocompromised and should begin treatment immediately. Toxoplasmosis can initially present with changes in personality and progress to encephalopathy. Having cats can be a risk factor, particularly as he is immunocompromised. The ring-enhancing lesions on MRI are characteristic and taken together with the history point towards this diagnosis. Artesunate is the treatment for cerebral malaria, for which the question stem did not provide risk factors such as endemic travel. Vancomycin, cefepime, and ampicillin can be used empirically for the management of suspected meningitis, but this patient is encephalopathic without meningeal signs. Finally, albendazole and corticosteroids are used for the management of neurocysticercosis, which could have ring-enhancing lesions of MRI of the brain, but this patient should have more focal findings with this disease and not global encephalopathy.

5b. C. Pyrimethamine and sulfadiazine are "folate antagonists" that inhibit dihydropteroate synthase and dihydrofolate reductase, respectively (Figure 3.4 in this chapter); this combination therapy is usually given with folic acid supplements to reduce the incidence of thrombocytopenia. Answer A is incorrect because both drugs work on the same tetrahydrofolate-generating synthetic pathway. Ritonavir (not sulfadiazine) is often used as a CYP3A4 inhibitor to boost the efficacy of other medications, so B is incorrect. Three HCV NS5A inhibitors are known to act to inhibit P-gp (Table 3.5), but not pyrimethamine, so D is incorrect.

CHAPTER 4

ALLERGIC RHINITIS AND DIFFICULTY BREATHING

KAREN WOODFORK, PHD

West Virginia University, Morgantown, West Virginia, USA

Symptoms: Immuno-Infectious
Cardio-Renal-Respiratory

DRUG LIST FOR ALLERGIC RHINITIS

H1 Antihistamines	
Azelastine	Second-generation antihistamine and mast cell stabilizer, nasal spray
Brompheniramine	First-generation antihistamine, PO
Carbinoxamine	First-generation antihistamine, PO
Cetirizine	Second-generation antihistamine, PO
Chlorcyclizine	First-generation antihistamine, PO
Chlorpheniramine	First-generation antihistamine, PO
Clemastine	First-generation antihistamine, PO
Cyproheptadine	First-generation antihistamine, PO
Desloratadine	Second-generation antihistamine, PO
Dexbrompheniramine	First-generation antihistamine, PO
Dexchlorpheniramine	First-generation antihistamine, PO
Diphenhydramine	First-generation antihistamine, PO; IM/IV for severe allergic reactions
Doxylamine	First-generation antihistamine, PO
Fexofenadine	Second-generation antihistamine, PO
Hydroxyzine	First-generation antihistamine, PO
Levocetirizine	Second-generation antihistamine, PO
Loratadine	Second-generation antihistamine, PO
Olopatadine	Second-generation antihistamine and mast cell stabilizer, nasal spray
Promethazine	First-generation antihistamine, PO, rectal, IM, IV
Pyrilamine	First-generation antihistamine, PO
Triprolidine	First-generation antihistamine, PO

Corticosteroids	
Beclomethasone	Glucocorticoid, nasal spray
Betamethasone	Glucocorticoid, IM for severe allergic reactions
Budesonide	Glucocorticoid, nasal spray
Ciclesonide	Glucocorticoid, nasal spray
Cortisone	Glucocorticoid, PO
Dexamethasone	Glucocorticoid, PO; IM/IV for severe allergic reactions
Flunisolide	Glucocorticoid, nasal spray
Fluticasone	Glucocorticoid, nasal spray
Hydrocortisone	Glucocorticoid, PO; IV for severe allergic reactions
Methylprednisolone	Glucocorticoid, PO; IM/IV for severe allergic reactions
Mometasone	Glucocorticoid, nasal spray
Prednisolone	Glucocorticoid, PO
Prednisone	Glucocorticoid, PO
Triamcinolone	Glucocorticoid, nasal spray; IM for severe allergic reactions

Anti-Leukotriene Drugs	
Montelukast	Leukotriene receptor antagonist, PO
Zafirlukast	Leukotriene receptor antagonist, PO

Mast Cell Stabilizers

Cromolyn	Mast cell stabilizer, nasal spray

Short-acting Muscarinic Agonists

Ipratropium	Short-acting muscarinic agonist, nasal spray

Nasal Decongestants

Pseudoephedrine	Sympathomimetic, PO
Phenylephrine	Sympathomimetic, nasal drops, nasal spray, PO
Oxymetazoline	Sympathomimetic, nasal spray

General Background

Allergic rhinitis (AR) is a common atopic condition that is characterized by rhinorrhea, nasal congestion, postnasal drip, sneezing, and/or itching of the nose and palate. AR may be episodic (caused by exposure to specific allergens), seasonal (caused by exposure to environmental allergens that are present only during certain seasons), or chronic (perennial). AR may coexist with allergic conjunctivitis, asthma, and/or chronic sinusitis. Although AR is not life-threatening in and of itself, it can cause a significant negative impact on sleep, school or work performance, and quality of life. It may also be accompanied by life-threatening conditions such as severe asthma or anaphylaxis.

Diagnosis

The diagnosis of allergic rhinitis is largely based on a thorough history and physical exam consistent with the features below.

Presentation

Persons with AR present with one or more of the following symptoms: rhinorrhea with clear discharge, postnasal drip, nasal congestion, anosmia, cough, fatigue, malaise, and itching of the nose, palate, and/or inner ear. Allergic rhinoconjunctivitis (ARC) involves symptoms of AR along with those of allergic conjunctivitis (tearing, red, itchy, and/or swollen eyes). Symptoms of sinusitis and otitis media (earache, itching ears, and/or headache) may also be present.

Risk Factors

The presence of asthma is associated with an increased incidence of AR; approximately 30 to 40 % of individuals who have AR develop asthma, and up to 85% of those with asthma also have AR. Other atopic conditions, such as eczema, also positively correlate with AR. Environmental factors, such as exposure to passive cigarette smoke and mold, have been associated with AR. A family history of atopic disease is a risk factor for AR, and polymorphisms in genes encoding inflammatory mediators have been correlated with an increased occurrence of AR. Although individual risk factors, such as dietary composition and obesity, have been studied in the context of AR, no conclusive association has been shown.

Pathophysiology

AR involves inflammation of the mucous membranes of the nose and may also involve the eyes, sinuses, pharynx, eustachian tubes, and middle ear. It is a type I hypersensitivity process involving an immunoglobin E (IgE)-mediated response to an extrinsic protein, or allergen. Sensitization to an allergen occurs when antigen-presenting cells activate T lymphocytes in the draining lymph nodes. Concurrently, epithelial cells release cytokines such as interleukin-25 (IL-25) and IL-33 which stimulate a T_H2 cell response, resulting in the release of additional pro-inflammatory cytokines (IL-4, IL-13) and ultimately, the conversion of B lymphocytes into plasma cells that produce allergen-specific IgE antibodies.

Within minutes of re-exposure to the allergen, the mast cells and basophils in the nasal mucosa that are coated with allergen-specific IgE generate an early-phase response that involves the release of pre-formed inflammatory mediators (e.g., as histamine, tryptase, chymase, heparin, chondroitin sulfate, and tumor necrosis factor-α (TNF-α)). Shortly thereafter, these cells synthesize other inflammatory mediators including leukotrienes (LT) and prostaglandin D_2 (PGD_2). The result of the early response is vasodilatation, increased vascular permeability, edema, mucus secretion, and a mild cellular infiltrate of mostly granulocytes. Pruritis and sneezing result from the stimulation of sensory neurons by histamine, and mucus hypersecretion results from the stimulation of parasympathetic cholinergic neurons.

A late-phase response may occur around 2 – 4 hours after an early-phase response, or it may appear as an isolated event. Symptoms include mucus secretion, erythema, heat, burning, itching, and induration of the mucous membrane. During the late-phase response, all of the mediators of the early-phase response, except for PGD_2, reappear. Since PGD_2 is exclusively produced by mast cells, and other mediators of the early-phase response are produced by basophils, it is likely that basophils, not mast cells, are important mediators of the late-phase response. During the late-phase response, there is an influx of eosinophils and mononuclear cells, and a later infiltration of activated T cells which produce T_H2 cytokines. The recruitment of these inflammatory cells to the mucosa is mediated by chemokines (e.g., RANTES, MCP-1) and surface adhesion molecules (e.g., integrins, selectins), which in turn are upregulated by inflammatory mediators such as IL-1 and TNF-α. Eosinophils are believed to be key mediators of the pathophysiology of AR; they are commonly found in the nasal secretions of patients with AR, and they are also seen in the sputum of those who have asthma. Late-phase inflammation can induce a state of airway hyperresponsiveness to allergens and irritants, which is consistent with a relationship between allergic rhinitis and asthma.

Examination
The patient's history and physical examination will reveal the manifestations of AR, such as nasal watery rhinorrhea, nasal congestion, sneezing, nasal itching, and mouth breathing. Adults regularly blow their noses or clear their throats, whereas younger children may frequently sniffle, snort, or cough to expel mucus, and they may exhibit a transverse supra-tip nasal crease from frequent nose wiping or rubbing. Palatal clicking can be heard from rubbing an itchy palate with the tongue. Chronic inflammation in the nasal mucosa can cause venous stasis in the periorbital region, resulting in dark shadows below the eyes (allergic shiners). Anterior rhinoscopy may show the nasal mucous membranes to have a bluish "mother of pearl" coloration due to chronic nasal obstruction. If children become obligate mouth-breathers, they may exhibit physical signs such as long facies, narrow maxillae, flattened malar eminences, overbites, and high-arched palates.

Laboratory
Skin testing involves the injection of specific antigens beneath the skin. In skin prick testing, multiple antigens are injected into the epidermis, whereas in intradermal testing, the antigens are injected into the dermis. In an individual who is sensitized to a specific allergen, injection of that specific substance elicits a positive wheal-and-flare response. Skin testing is an indirect measure of the presence of allergen-specific IgE on tissue mast cells and basophils. A direct assay of allergen-specific IgE in the serum, known as serum-specific IgE (SSIge), can be used in individuals who are unable to undergo skin testing due to extensive dermatitis, immune deficiency, or other comorbidities, or when their use of antihistamines would produce assay interference.

Imaging
Imaging is generally not utilized in the diagnosis of allergic rhinitis.

Associated Symptoms/Conditions
As stated previously, there is a strong association between AR and asthma. AR may exacerbate asthma if postnasal drip irritates the lower respiratory tract, or if obligate mouth breathing results in inhalation of cold, dry air. Nasal stimulation may initiate bronchoconstriction via the vagal-mediated rhinobronchial reflex. Additional atopic conditions, such as atopic dermatitis and allergic conjunctivitis, are also associated with AR.

Nasal mucous membrane swelling and secretion can lead to eustachian tube obstruction, which can lead to serous otitis media. This can lead to hearing loss, and chronic hearing loss in children may lead to delayed speech development. Obstructed nasal passages can also predispose one to the development of bacterial sinusitis. Although it is not a primary cause of obstructive sleep apnea, AR is associated with sleep-disordered breathing, decreased sleep quality, and daytime fatigue.

Diagnosis
A history of typical allergy systems is the basis for the diagnosis of AR. A clinical diagnosis can be made if a patient presents with one or more of the classic AR symptoms (rhinorrhea, sneezing, nasal congestion, and itching) in a pattern consistent with an allergic cause. Triggers should be identified via history, skin testing, or SSIge, and these may be used to identify the specific causative allergen(s) when there is an inadequate response to empiric treatment, when the diagnosis is uncertain, or when knowledge of the causative allergen is needed to target therapy. Rhinoscopy is useful for determining the presence of a nasal polyp or deviated septum, both of which can cause airflow obstruction that patients may perceive as nasal congestion. Clinicians should assess patients with a clinical diagnosis of AR for associated conditions such as asthma, conjunctivitis, rhinosinusitis, otitis media, atopic dermatitis, and sleep-disordered breathing.

AR symptoms are classified by severity (mild, moderate, or severe), and by duration (intermittent, persistent). Mild symptoms are not troublesome to the patient and do not interfere with sleep, work, or daily activities; moderate to severe symptoms are troublesome to the patient and do interfere with sleep, work, and/or daily activities. Symptoms are classified as intermittent if they occur for less than 6 weeks and persistent if they occur for 6 weeks or more.

Treatment
Drugs commonly used in the treatment of AR include intranasal corticosteroids (i.e., glucocorticoids or "steroids"), oral antihistamines, intranasal antihistamines, oral leukotriene receptor antagonists, and for specific symptoms, intranasal short-acting muscarinic agonists, antitussives, expectorants, and sympathomimetics.

Management
In addition to pharmaceutical treatments, clinicians may recommend avoidance of the known allergen(s) when possible or suggest environmental controls (e.g., air filters, mattress and pillow covers, keeping pets out of the bedroom). Individuals who have an inadequate response to pharmaceuticals may elect to have allergen-specific immunotherapy, which involves repeated dosing of the allergen to induce immune tolerance to it.

General Treatment Strategies

Antihistamines are an option for monotherapy in mild disease and may be used in combination therapy for moderate to severe disease. They are usually administered orally but are also available in intranasal formulations. Intranasal corticosteroids are the mainstay of preventive treatment of AR in persons with moderate to severe, persistent symptoms. Oral corticosteroids are used only as short-term, add-on treatments for severe AR flare-ups. Oral leukotriene receptor antagonists can be taken daily to prevent AR symptoms. Specific residual symptoms may be addressed with other drugs; for example, rhinorrhea may be treated with intranasal short-acting muscarinic agonists, cough may be treated with antitussives and expectorants, and nasal congestion may be addressed with sympathomimetics.

H_1 Antihistamines

Background
The H_1 antihistamines are classified as either first- or second-generation compounds. Second-generation antihistamines produce much less sedation than first-generation drugs and are classified as minimally sedating (**loratadine**, **desloratadine**, **fexofenadine**, and **azelastine**) or low-sedation drugs (**cetirizine** and **levocetirizine**).

Most antihistamines that are used in the management of AR are administered orally; however, azelastine, a second-generation drug with mast cell-stabilizing activity, is used as a nasal spray. The antihistamines are most effective if given before allergen exposure; this prevents the activation of H_1 receptors by newly released histamine. Second-generation drugs are preferred for oral administration because they produce less sedation than first-generation drugs. In addition to their use in the treatment of allergic rhinitis, the H_1 antihistamines are used to decrease nasal secretions associated with the common cold, sinusitis, influenza, or other upper respiratory infections. These drugs are also used for the relief of allergic conjunctivitis and urticaria. The first-generation H_1 antihistamines have utility in the management of certain non-allergic conditions such as motion sickness, anxiety, insomnia, and nausea/vomiting. Certain H_1 antihistamines may also be employed as adjunctive treatment of anaphylaxis in combination with epinephrine and glucocorticoids.

Pharmacokinetics
The first-generation antihistamines are lipophilic and well absorbed after oral administration, with peak blood levels occurring within 2 to 3 hours and a duration of action usually between 4 to 6 hours. Most first-generation drugs are substrates of hepatic cytochrome P450 (CYP) 2D6, and some are also metabolized by other CYPs. The metabolites and a small amount of the parent compound are excreted in the urine. The first-generation antihistamines are not substrates of the p-glycoprotein drug efflux pump.

The second-generation antihistamines are also rapidly absorbed, with peak plasma concentrations occurring within 1 to 3 hours, but they have longer durations of action from 12 to 24 hours. As compared to first-generation antihistamines, second-generation drugs are less lipophilic, and they have ionization profiles that make them less able to cross the blood-brain barrier. Like first-generation drugs, loratadine and desloratadine are metabolized by CYP2D6, but they are also metabolized by CYP3A4, resulting in potential drug interactions with CYP3A4 inducers and inhibitors. Cetirizine, levocetirizine, and fexofenadine are mainly eliminated unchanged. The second-generation antihistamines are substrates of p-glycoprotein, and their transport by p-glycoprotein in the vascular endothelium of the CNS is believed to be a major reason for their relative exclusion from this site and minimal sedating activity.

Mechanism of Action
H_1 antihistamine drugs are inverse agonists of H_1 receptors, shifting the dynamic balance toward the inactive conformation of the receptor. The effectiveness of these drugs against allergy symptoms arises from their capacity to block histamine-mediated vasoconstriction, microvascular permeability enhancement, and sensory nerve terminal stimulation. Many antihistamines have additional effects that are not mediated by H_1 receptors. The first-generation H_1 blockers have varying degrees of antimuscarinic activity that contribute to their ability to produce sedation, combat motion sickness, inhibit nausea and vomiting, and decrease motor symptoms such as tremor and dystonia. This activity also causes the antimuscarinic side effects described below. In addition to antimuscarinic activity, several first-generation antihistamines have other pharmacological effects which expand or enhance their therapeutic utility. Promethazine, for example, has limited indications in breathing-related conditions and is used only as an adjunct in the

treatment of anaphylactic shock. However, its ability to block NMDA glutamate receptors and α adrenoceptors provides it with additional efficacy in its use as a sedative, and its antagonism of D_2 dopamine receptors in the chemoreceptor trigger zone provides it with antiemetic and anti-motion sickness effects beyond those produced by muscarinic blockade. Cyproheptadine is an antagonist at $5HT_{2A}$ serotonin receptors, thus it is sometimes used to counteract certain side effects of the selective serotonin reuptake inhibitor antidepressants. Diphenhydramine, pyrilamine, and promethazine have local anesthetic activity and are occasionally used to produce anesthesia in persons who are allergic to standard agents. Certain second-generation antihistamines such as cetirizine, as well as intranasal antihistamines such as azelastine and olopatadine, act to inhibit the release of inflammatory substances by mast cells in addition to their antihistaminic activity.

Adverse Effects, Contraindications, Drug Interactions
The most frequent adverse effect of first-generation antihistamines is sedation, which is produced by the blockade of H_1 and muscarinic receptors in the CNS and is additive with the sedating effects of alcohol or other CNS depressants. Paradoxical excitation can be seen at normal doses, more commonly in children than adults, and it frequently occurs when toxic dosages are ingested. The first-generation antihistamines also produce antimuscarinic effects, resulting in potential adverse effects of dry mouth and respiratory passages, blurred vision, sedation, cognitive impairment, urinary retention, and constipation. Promethazine's additional α adrenoceptor- and D_2 dopamine receptor-blocking activities may produce adverse effects of orthostatic hypotension and extrapyramidal side effects, respectively. Tolerance to certain antihistamines may develop after prolonged administration.

The effects of toxic doses of first-generation antihistamines are similar to those of atropine and include excitement, hallucinations, dry mouth, dilated pupils, flushing, convulsions, urinary retention, sinus tachycardia, coma, and death. Hydroxyzine is contraindicated in pregnancy due to animal studies showing teratogenicity and a lack of human data. Other first-generation antihistamines lack evidence of teratogenicity in animals, but they also lack human safety data. The American College of Obstetricians and Gynecologists (ACOG) and the American College of Allergy, Asthma, and Immunology consider loratadine an acceptable alternative in pregnancy, preferably after the first trimester, in individuals who are unable to take first-generation antihistamines.

In contrast, the second-generation H_1 antihistamines lack antimuscarinic activity and are minimally able to cross the blood-brain barrier, so their side effects are less prominent. Cetirizine is the most sedating of the second-generation antihistamines, but its L-enantiomer, levocetirizine, may be less sedating. Loratadine and desloratadine are minimally sedating, but doses above the normal therapeutic range can cause sleepiness. In contrast, fexofenadine is unlikely to produce sedation even at high therapeutic doses.

Corticosteroids

Background
Corticosteroids can be classified as having glucocorticoid effects (e.g., suppression of immune function and inflammation, stimulation of catabolism of muscle, bone, and fat) and/or mineralocorticoid effects (e.g., sodium retention). Drugs with structures that maximize glucocorticoid effects while minimizing mineralocorticoid effects are known as glucocorticoids, anti-inflammatory steroids, or steroidal anti-inflammatory drugs (SAIDs), and it is these which are used in the treatment of AR. SAIDs are most commonly administered by nasal inhalation, on a daily basis, to prevent the development of symptoms. Oral or parenteral drugs are sometimes used on an acute basis to control a severe flare-up.

Pharmacokinetics
Once absorbed into the blood plasma, glucocorticoids become highly bound to the proteins transcortin (corticosteroid-binding globulin, CBG) and albumin. The binding of these drugs to CBG is high affinity and low capacity, whereas binding to albumin is low affinity and high capacity. Only the unbound drug is available to enter the cell and produce effects. Cortisone and prednisone must be bioactivated via enzymatic reduction by 11β-hydroxysteroid dehydrogenase in order to exert activity. This enzyme is primarily found in the liver but is also present in the eye, skin, bone, and adipocytes. In situations where this enzymatic activity is impaired (e.g., severe liver failure) or in circumstances where the drug is administered at its site of action (e.g., inhalation), a drug that does not require bioactivation should be used. The glucocorticoids or their bioactivated metabolites are eliminated at hepatic and non-hepatic sites, generally via CYP3A4. The reduced, inactive metabolites are then conjugated with sulfate or glucuronide and eliminated in the urine. Some glucocorticoids are known CYP inducers; for example, prednisone increases hepatic production of CYP2C19, and dexamethasone induces CYP3A4 and CYP2D6. Many glucocorticoids, including dexamethasone, prednisone, and methylprednisolone, are substrates of p-glycoprotein. Corticosteroids act at the level of the genome, and because of this, their biological half-lives are longer than their physical half-lives. Cortisone and hydrocortisone are classified as short-acting glucocorticoids, with biological half-lives of less than 12 hours. Beclomethasone, methylprednisolone, prednisone, prednisolone, and triamcinolone are intermediate-acting glucocorticoids that have biological half-lives between 12 – 36 hours. Long-acting glucocorticoids such as betamethasone and dexamethasone have biological half-lives of 36 hours or longer. Glucocorticoids can also be classified by their affinity for the

glucocorticoid receptor (GR). For example, fluticasone and mometasone, and the active metabolites of beclomethasone and ciclesonide, have a high affinity for the GR, whereas budesonide, triamcinolone, and flunisolide have a moderate affinity, and dexamethasone, prednisone, and hydrocortisone have a lower affinity.

Mechanism of Action

Glucocorticoids exert their immune suppressive effect by binding to the intracellular GR, which initiates pathways that modulate the transcription of inflammatory and anti-inflammatory genes. The classical steroid pathway begins with the binding of an agonist to the GR, followed by translocation of the GR complex to the nucleus, entry through the nuclear pore, dimerization with another glucocorticoid-bound GR, and binding to cis-elements (glucocorticoid response elements, GREs) of genes that are regulated by glucocorticoids. The binding of GR dimers to GREs increases the transcription of anti-inflammatory genes such as I-κB and annexin A1 (lipocortin). Increased production of I-κB results in the sequestration of NF-κB in the cytoplasm, making it unable to move to the nucleus and promote inflammatory gene transcription. Annexin A1 is an inhibitor of phospholipase A2; therefore, glucocorticoid-stimulated increases in annexin A1 expression result in decreased eicosanoid production. Annexin A1 also down-regulates numerous aspects of lymphocyte function such as adhesion and chemotaxis.

In addition to inducing the expression of anti-inflammatory genes, ligand-bound GR can inhibit the transcription of other genes; this inhibition is believed to be responsible for the ability of glucocorticoids to cause thinning of the skin and impaired wound healing. Glucocorticoids also affect inflammatory gene transcription via additional pathways that involve histone acetylation. In one pathway, ligand-bound GR monomers inhibit the activity of the NF-κB-histone acetyltransferase (HAT) complex, leading to decreased histone acetylation in regions of pro-inflammatory genes (e.g., COX-2, cytokines) and, subsequently, decreased transcription of these genes. Ligand-bound GR can also bind to and activate histone deacetylase 2 (HDAC2), an enzyme that removes acetyl groups from histones. The deacetylation of histones causes the chromatin in that area to condense, resulting in decreased inflammatory gene transcription.

Adverse Effects, Contraindications, Drug Interactions

The adverse effects produced by glucocorticoids are dependent upon the route of administration and the duration of treatment. Topical or inhalational routes of administration produce fewer and less significant adverse effects than systemic routes, and short-term administration (less than 10 – 14 days) is less problematic than long-term. When inhaled through the nose or mouth, adverse effects are generally localized to the site of administration. For example, glucocorticoid particles can deposit on the mucus membranes, resulting in localized immune suppression that usually manifests as infection with *Candida* spp. (candidiasis or thrush). Bacterial and viral infections may also occur. Glucocorticoids inhaled into the lung can also cause irritation and cough. Systemic adverse effects of inhaled glucocorticoids are generally minimal; however, prolonged use of a high-dose inhaled form may produce systemic effects.

Glucocorticoids administered via oral and parenteral routes can produce adverse effects on a variety of organ systems. Short-term glucocorticoid use can produce CNS stimulation manifesting as insomnia, restlessness, euphoria, anxiety, hypomania, or rarely, psychosis. Appetite stimulation may occur; conversely, some people can experience nausea or vomiting. There is a slight increase in the risk of infection with short-term glucocorticoid administration, but this is not as significant as that produced by long-term use.

The use of systemic glucocorticoid therapy for longer than two weeks is associated with a dose-dependent increased risk of severe adverse effects, which limits the utility of these drugs for the long-term management of disease. For example, chronic immune suppression results in a significantly elevated risk of infection ranging from mild (e.g., colds) to severe (e.g., sepsis, reactivation of latent tuberculosis). In addition, the overt signs and symptoms of an infection can be attenuated or masked by the use of glucocorticoids. The risk of CNS events such as insomnia, depression, hypomania, psychosis, and seizures, is increased as well.

Chronic exposure to high-dose, usually systemic, glucocorticoids causes suppression of the hypothalamus-pituitary-adrenal (HPA) axis. This results from the ability of glucocorticoids to produce feedback inhibition of the hypothalamus, decreasing its ability to release corticotropin-releasing factor (CRF). Glucocorticoids also cause feedback inhibition of the release of adrenocorticotropic hormone (ACTH) by the anterior pituitary. This results in a down-regulation of the adrenals' ability to produce cortisol. Therefore, if a situation arises in which endogenous cortisol production must be increased in order to maintain homeostasis (e.g., physical injury, surgery, psychological stress), the HPA axis will not be able to respond by producing an adequate amount of cortisol. An adrenal crisis can occur as a result, manifesting as weakness, hypotension, fainting, and potentially cardiovascular collapse and death. In clinical situations in which HPA axis suppression is likely (e.g., long-term use of high-dose glucocorticoids), supplemental glucocorticoids may be given if an additional cortisol need is anticipated; for example, before surgery or following an accident. Adrenal crisis can also develop if glucocorticoids are discontinued abruptly; therefore, following long-term use, the dose of these drugs should be tapered before discontinuation.

Chronic use of systemic glucocorticoids can produce several metabolic effects that are often referred to as iatrogenic Cushing's syndrome, which manifests similarly to Cushing's resulting from cortisol hypersecretion. The signs and symptoms of Cushing's syndrome include facial puffiness ("moon facies") and fat redistribution from the extremities to the trunk, back of the neck ("buffalo hump"), and supraclavicular fossae; growth of fine hair on the face, thighs, and trunk; acne; thinning of the skin, with development of striae (parallel streaks of red, glossy skin that become whitish over time), bruising, and impaired wound healing; muscle wasting and myopathy; hyperglycemia, with potential for weight gain, visceral fat deposition, and type 2 diabetes; hypocalcemia, with potential for osteoporosis in adults and growth retardation in children; increased risk of posterior subcapsular cataracts; elevated intraocular pressure and glaucoma; and menstrual irregularities and impaired sperm production. For glucocorticoids with significant mineralocorticoid potency (e.g., hydrocortisone), sodium retention, potassium wasting, and hypertension can occur.

Contraindications for glucocorticoids include abrupt discontinuation after prolonged, systemic dosing, and use during some types of severe infection. Caution is warranted in disease states that can be worsened by glucocorticoids (e.g., diabetes, osteoporosis, cataracts). The risks vs. benefits should be measured carefully when considering the use of these drugs during pregnancy.

Interactions can occur when glucocorticoids are given in conjunction with other drugs that share their adverse effects, and therapeutic failure may result when certain glucocorticoid adverse effects (e.g., hypoglycemia) counteract the intended effect of another drug (e.g., oral hypoglycemic agents). Interactions that impact drug elimination can occur when glucocorticoids that are metabolized by CYP3A4 are given in conjunction with drugs that induce or inhibit this enzyme. Dexamethasone is a CYP3A4 inducer and may decrease concentrations of other drugs that are metabolized by this enzyme. Blood levels of glucocorticoids that are p-glycoprotein substrates, such as prednisone and dexamethasone, may be elevated if p-glycoprotein inhibitors are given simultaneously. Individuals who are immunocompromised as a result of their use of glucocorticoids may generate an inadequate response to vaccination, and they may require more frequent boosters.

Leukotriene Receptor Antagonists

Background

The orally administered leukotriene receptor antagonists, montelukast and zafirlukast, are used as a prophylactic treatment in the management of asthma. These drugs are similarly used in the prophylaxis of allergic rhinitis; however, they are not first-line and are only recommended for persons who are intolerant of, or whose disease is not adequately controlled by oral or intranasal antihistamines or intranasal glucocorticoids. This is because they tend to be less effective than glucocorticoid nasal sprays, are similar in efficacy to oral antihistamines, and carry a potential risk of neuropsychiatric events such as behavior/mood changes and suicidal ideation.

Pharmacokinetics

The leukotriene receptor antagonists are rapidly absorbed after oral administration, with peak blood concentrations seen after 3 – 4 hours. Animal studies suggest these drugs are minimally able to cross the blood-brain barrier. Elimination of montelukast results primarily from metabolism by CYP2C8, as well as some metabolism by CYP2C9 and CYP3A4. Montelukast and its metabolites are secreted into the bile; urinary excretion is negligible. Zafirlukast is extensively metabolized by CYP2C8, and the parent drug and its metabolites are primarily eliminated via biliary secretion. In vitro data suggest that the leukotriene receptor antagonists are potent CYP2C8 inhibitors, but in vivo studies have failed to demonstrate clinically relevant interactions with CYP2C8 substrates. However, there is in vivo evidence of the ability of zafirlukast to inhibit the metabolism of drugs by CYP2C9 and CYP3A4. Both leukotriene receptor antagonists may be weak inducers of CYP1A2.

Mechanism of Action

The leukotriene receptor antagonists block the ability of the cysteinyl leukotrienes (LTC_4, LTD_4, and LTE_4) to interact with the $CysLT_1$ receptor. The cysteinyl leukotrienes are arachidonic acid metabolites that are released by mast cells and eosinophils in response to allergens. They interact with two types of cysteinyl leukotriene receptors ($CysLT_1$ and $CysLT_2$) which are found on cells such as macrophages and smooth muscle, and they are important mediators of the pathophysiological processes seen in allergic rhinitis and asthma. The binding of an agonist to the $CysLT_1$ receptor produces bronchoconstriction, increased mucus secretion, increased vascular permeability (edema, congestion), and inflammatory cytokine production in the airways. The $CysLT_2$ receptor initiates many of the same actions as the $CysLT_1$ receptor, but it is less well-studied and is not a target for currently available drugs.

Elevations of LTC_4 are seen in allergic rhinitis during early- and late-phase reactions, producing symptoms of nasal congestion (most prominently), sneezing, and nasal itching. The leukotriene receptor antagonists prevent the signs and symptoms of allergic rhinitis by blocking the binding of LTC_4 to the $CysLT_1$ receptor.

Adverse Effects, Contraindications, Drug Interactions

Most adverse effects of the leukotriene receptor antagonists are mild (e.g., headache, fatigue, gastrointestinal upset), but certain rare adverse effects are dangerous. Suicidal thoughts and behavior are the most concerning, but other neuropsychiatric events such as anxiety, depression, agitation, attention and memory impairment, sleep abnormalities, seizures, paresthesia, and hypoesthesia have been reported. Some patients treated with leukotriene receptor antagonists for asthma have developed eosinophilia and vasculitis consistent with Churg-Strauss syndrome (eosinophilic granulomatosis with polyangiitis (EGPA)). This event occurs more frequently in people who were able to either decrease or eliminate an oral corticosteroid because they began leukotriene receptor antagonist therapy. Zafirlukast has been associated with symptomatic and asymptomatic elevations in hepatic enzyme levels, which usually resolve upon discontinuation but rarely culminate in a need for hepatic transplant or death. Persons who have developed hepatic toxicity from zafirlukast should not receive it in the future.

Because the leukotriene receptor antagonists are weak inducers of CYP1A2, they may produce a clinically significant depression of blood levels of drugs that are highly metabolized by this isoform and have small therapeutic indexes (e.g., warfarin). Zafirlukast is a weak CYP3A4 inhibitor, so it may produce significant interactions with drugs that are major substrates of CYP3A4 and have low therapeutic indexes (doxorubicin, vincristine).

Mast Cell Stabilizers

Background

Cromolyn sodium is the only pure mast cell stabilizing drug currently available in the US, and it is available in a nasal spray for the treatment of allergic rhinitis. Certain H_1 antihistamines, such as cetirizine, azelastine, and olopatadine, also have mast cell-stabilizing effects. Cromolyn is generally believed to be less effective than glucocorticoid nasal sprays or antihistamines. It is most commonly used in children with mild or episodic AR because of its excellent safety profile. It can be used before a predictable exposure or on a regular basis.

Pharmacokinetics

Cromolyn is minimally absorbed following inhalation. It is rapidly eliminated ($t_{1/2}$ = 80 - 90 minutes), and the majority absorbed drug is excreted, unchanged, in the feces. For prolonged protection against AR symptoms, it must be administered three to six times each day.

Mechanism of Action

Cromolyn inhibits the release of histamine and leukotrienes (degranulation) by allergen-sensitized mast cells, but the specific mechanism by which it produces this effect is unclear. Its action blocks the early- and late-phase responses.

Adverse Effects, Contraindications, Drug Interactions

Because inhaled cromolyn is minimally absorbed, its adverse effects via this route of administration are limited to the nasal mucosa (sneezing, itching, congestion). There are no drug interactions reported for cromolyn.

Short-Acting Muscarinic Agonists

Background

Ipratropium bromide nasal spray is indicated for symptomatic treatment of rhinorrhea resulting from intermittent or persistent AR, and from the common cold. It is less effective than glucocorticoid nasal sprays for itching, sneezing, and nasal congestion, so it is not used as a first-line drug in AR.

Pharmacokinetics

Following administration as a nasal spray, less than 20% of a dose of ipratropium is systemically absorbed. Around 50% of the absorbed drug is excreted unchanged in the urine. The half-life of ipratropium is approximately 2 hours.

Mechanism of Action

Stimulation of M_3 muscarinic receptors by acetylcholine increases watery secretion by the nasal mucosa. Ipratropium blocks the effect of parasympathetic tone in the nasal mucosa, and it also blocks the parasympathetic activity which is initiated by histamine, bradykinin, and certain eicosanoids. Its action is particularly marked in circumstances of excessive secretion.

Adverse Effects, Contraindications, Drug Interactions

Local effects of ipratropium on the nasopharynx include nasal dryness, epistaxis, and xerostomia. A reduction of mucociliary clearance can result in result in the development of mucus plugs. Although there is minimal systemic absorption of ipratropium following nasal inhalation, there is potential for systemic anticholinergic adverse effects at high levels of use. Similarly, ipratropium may have additive effects with drugs that also carry significant anticholinergic activity (e.g., atropine, oxybutynin).

Nasal Decongestants

Background

Nasal decongestant sprays such as phenylephrine and oxymetazoline are not recommended as a long-term monotherapy for AR, but they are highly effective at decreasing nasal congestion and can be used alone or in combination, on a temporary basis for intermittent AR, or as part of a drug regimen for persistent AR. Pseudoephedrine is a nasal decongestant that is available only for oral administration, and phenylephrine is available in oral formulations and nasal sprays for nasal congestion and in parenteral formulations that are used in the treatment of hypotension and shock. Systemically administered nasal decongestants carry certain adverse effects that are different from those produced when these drugs are administered via the intranasal route.

Pharmacokinetics

Following intranasal administration of phenylephrine, absorption is rapid, but less than 20% of the drug is systemically absorbed. Following oral administration, approximately 38% is absorbed, with an onset of action of 15 – 30 minutes. The primary route of elimination for phenylephrine is hepatic and intestinal metabolism by monoamine oxidase. The duration of action of inhaled phenylephrine ranges from 30 minutes to 4 hours; systemically administered phenylephrine has an elimination half-life of 2.1 – 3.4 hours. Pseudoephedrine, administered orally, has an onset of action of about 30 minutes and an elimination half-life of 9 – 16 hours; elimination is accelerated by urinary acidification and slowed by alkalinization of the urine. Pharmacokinetic data for oxymetazoline nasal spray are limited, but one study showed low systemic bioavailability (2.3%) and slow absorption (half-time approximately 1 hour). The route of elimination for oxymetazoline is unknown, but its duration of action is longer than that of the other nasal decongestant sprays, requiring only twice daily administration as compared to every 4 hours for phenylephrine.

Mechanism of Action

Stimulation of α_1 adrenoceptors directly causes constriction of the veins, venules, and venous sinusoids. All nasal decongestants act as agonists of α_1 adrenoceptors, so they cause significant vasoconstriction in the venous circulation of the nasal mucosa. This reduced blood flow decreases edema and congestion in the nasal passages, and this increases nasal airway patency and drainage of sinus secretions.

Adverse Effects, Contraindications, Drug Interactions

Two adverse effects of nasally administered decongestants are of greatest concern: rhinitis medicamentosa (also known as rebound congestion) and the potential for systemic adverse effects. Rhinitis medicamentosa is the development of rhinorrhea, postnasal drip, or sneezing after more than 3 days of use of a nasal decongestant. It is associated with chronic use of a nasal decongestant spray, and it is more common with phenylephrine than oxymetazoline. Rhinitis medicamentosa occurs when prolonged exposure to an agonist causes the downregulation of α_1 adrenoreceptors, resulting in decreased drug efficacy. If the drug is discontinued after tolerance develops, congestion returns, potentially at a higher intensity. These symptoms may be relieved by repeat administration of the drug, which results in escalating use and dependency. It is for this reason that monotherapy with nasal decongestant sprays is not recommended for long-term therapy. However, when combined with a glucocorticoid nasal spray, the ability of inhaled nasal decongestants to produce rhinitis medicamentosa is minimal, suggesting that inflammation is involved in this condition. Rhinitis medicamentosa is not caused by orally administered decongestants.

Cardiovascular stimulation can be caused by orally administered decongestants, or it may occur if high or supratherapeutic doses of nasal sprays are used. Agonism of α_1 adrenoceptors results in vasoconstriction, which contributes to an increase in blood pressure. Pseudoephedrine, due to its weak agonism of β_1 adrenoceptors, may also cause increased heart rate and contractility, increasing systolic blood pressure beyond what is seen with α_1 adrenoceptor agonists. Hypertension, tachycardia, reflex sinus bradycardia, arrhythmia, and myocardial ischemia may occur with oral decongestants or high-dose exposure to inhaled formulations. Geriatric patients and those with pre-existing cardiovascular disease are more susceptible to cardiovascular effects, and oral decongestants should be used cautiously in these populations. Additional systemic effects from sympathomimetic action include increased intraocular pressure, urinary retention, nausea/vomiting, and ischemic colitis due to splanchnic arterial vasoconstriction.

Nasal decongestants, particularly when administered orally, can participate in additive or antagonistic interactions with drugs that have similar or opposite physiological effects. Pseudoephedrine and oral phenylephrine should not be combined with MAO inhibitors to avoid causing a hypertensive crisis, and nasal inhalation of oxymetazoline or phenylephrine should be used cautiously, if at all, in this situation.

References

Bousquet J, Schünemann HJ, Togias A, et al., Allergic Rhinitis and Its Impact on Asthma Working Group. Next-generation Allergic Rhinitis and Its Impact on Asthma (ARIA) guidelines for allergic rhinitis based on Grading of Recommendations Assessment, Development and Evaluation (GRADE) and real-world evidence. J Allergy Clin Immunol. 2020 Jan;145(1):70-80.e3. doi: 10.1016/j.jaci.2019.06.049. Epub 2019 Oct 15. Erratum in: J Allergy Clin Immunol. 2022 Jun;149(6):2180. PMID: 31627910.

Choi BY, Han M, Kwak JW, Kim TH. Genetics and Epigenetics in Allergic Rhinitis. *Genes*. 2021; 12(12):2004. https://doi.org/10.3390/genes12122004.

Hoyte FCL, Nelson HS. Recent advances in allergic rhinitis. F1000Res. 2018 Aug 23;7:F1000 Faculty Rev-1333. doi: 10.12688/f1000research.15367.1. PMID: 30210782; PMCID: PMC6107993.

Kawauchi H, Yanai K, Wang DY, Itahashi K, Okubo K. Antihistamines for Allergic Rhinitis Treatment from the Viewpoint of Nonsedative Properties. Int J Mol Sci. 2019 Jan 8;20(1):213. doi: 10.3390/ijms20010213. PMID: 30626077; PMCID: PMC6337346.

Schuler Iv CF, Montejo JM. Allergic Rhinitis in Children and Adolescents. Pediatr Clin North Am. 2019 Oct;66(5):981-993. doi: 10.1016/j.pcl.2019.06.004. Epub 2019 Aug 5. PMID: 31466686.

Testa D, DI Bari M, Nunziata M, Cristofaro G, Massaro G, Marcuccio G, Motta G. Allergic rhinitis and asthma assessment of risk factors in pediatric patients: A systematic review. Int J Pediatr Otorhinolaryngol. 2020 Feb;129:109759. doi: 10.1016/j.ijporl.2019.109759. Epub 2019 Oct 31. PMID: 31734564.

Wahid NWB, Shermetaro C. Rhinitis Medicamentosa. 2022 Sep 5. In: StatPearls [Internet]. Treasure Island (FL): StatPearls Publishing; 2022 Jan–. PMID: 30855902.

Quiz Questions

1. A 19-year-old man initiates therapy with loratadine for seasonal allergies. He notes that, although this drug is marketed as non-sedating, he is experiencing significant sleepiness while taking it. Which of the following could account for this?

A Taking his medication with milk
B Taking his medication with apple juice
C Concomitant use of ketoconazole
D Concomitant use of phenytoin
E H_2 receptor variant with increased affinity for loratadine

2. A 78-year-old woman went to the emergency department with abdominal bloating and an inability to void her bladder; she had been unable to urinate for 16 hours. A urinary catheter was inserted and 2.5 L of urine was withdrawn. Subsequent testing revealed no calculi or masses in the bladder, urethra, ureters, or kidneys. The woman's medical records indicated that she was being treated with oxybutynin for an overactive bladder. She reported no significant side effects as a result of this treatment. For two days prior to admission to the hospital, she reported having had a cold and taking the maximum over-the-counter dose of diphenhydramine every 6 to 8 hours since her cold symptoms began. What is a possible explanation for the sudden onset of her inability to void her bladder?

A Inhibition of p-glycoprotein by oxybutynin increased her diphenhydramine blood level
B Additive antimuscarinic effects of oxybutynin and diphenhydramine caused urinary retention
C Inhibition of CYP3A4 by diphenhydramine increased her oxybutynin blood level
D Diphenhydramine's antimuscarinic effect antagonized the therapeutic effect of oxybutynin
E Diphenhydramine has agonist actions at α_1 adrenoceptors, which causes urinary retention

3. Two identical culture dishes of human T lymphocytes are used in an experiment. Dish 1 is treated with a therapeutic concentration of budesonide, and dish 2 is treated with the vehicle in which the budesonide is dissolved (control). After allowing sufficient time for the effects of budesonide to occur, a pro-inflammatory cytokine is added to each dish of T lymphocytes. How will the response of the T lymphocytes in dish 1 compare to those in dish 2?

A Dish 1 will contain a lower level of annexin-A1
B Dish 1 will contain a higher level of TNF-α
C Dish 1 will contain a larger amount of NF-κB in the nucleus
D Dish 1 will contain fewer GR bound to GRE
E Dish 1 will contain a larger amount of I-κB in the cytoplasm

4. A 27-year-old man has developed severe allergic rhinitis after moving from the desert back home to a hot, humid region filled with pollen and mold. He is currently using loratadine PO and a fluticasone nasal spray, but his symptoms are not well controlled. Which of the man's comorbidities would cause his physician to avoid prescribing a drug that acts as an antagonist of the CysLT1 receptor?

A He does not want to use an additional nasal inhaler
B His most prominent allergy symptom is congestion
C He is beginning to develop posterior subcapsular cataracts
D He has poorly controlled depression, with suicidality
E He has a moderate degree of renal impairment

5. Identical twin sisters, age 41, have episodic AR, mainly associated with exposure to cat dander. They travel across the country to their aunt's house for a family emergency, and upon arrival, they discover that the aunt has eight cats, so they rush to the local drugstore to buy something to help with the symptoms they expect. Sister #1 buys pseudoephedrine, and Sister #2 buys phenylephrine nasal spray. The sisters stay with their aunt for two weeks and regularly use their respective medications. After returning home, they thoroughly wash their laundry and then discontinue their drugs. What is expected to occur?

A Sister 1 will experience rebound congestion; Sister 2 will not experience rebound congestion
B Sister 2 will experience rebound congestion; Sister 1 will not experience rebound congestion
C Sister 1 will experience rebound hypertension; Sister 2 will not experience rebound hypertension
D Sister 2 will experience rebound hypertension; Sister 1 will not experience rebound hypertension
E Both sisters will experience rebound hypertension and rebound congestion

Quiz Answers

1. C. Ketoconazole is a potent inhibitor of CYP3A4, one of the enzymes responsible for the metabolism of second-generation antihistamines such as loratadine. Inhibition of loratadine metabolism has led to higher blood levels of this drug, resulting in somnolence. Milk (calcium) does not interfere with loratadine absorption. Apple juice contains compounds that inhibit the OATP, a transporter responsible for the intestinal uptake of fexofenadine, not loratadine. Phenytoin induces CYP3A4, which would result in decreased loratadine efficacy. Finally, if this patient exhibited an H_2 receptor polymorphism that caused it to have a high affinity for loratadine, the effects would not be seen in the brain, as H_2 receptor actions are most prominent in the GI tract.

2. B. Oxybutynin is an antispasmodic drug that acts as a direct-acting smooth muscle relaxant, and it also has nonselective muscarinic receptor antagonist effects. It is used to treat neurogenic bladder/overactive bladder. Although the patient had not complained of anticholinergic effects prior to beginning treatment with diphenhydramine, the additive antimuscarinic effects of oxybutynin and diphenhydramine likely resulted in urinary retention. Diphenhydramine, like other first-generation antihistamines, is predominantly metabolized by CYP2D6, and it is also metabolized to a minor extent by other CYPs. Diphenhydramine is not a CYP3A4 inhibitor nor is it eliminated by p-glycoprotein, and oxybutynin is not a p-glycoprotein inhibitor. Diphenhydramine is not an agonist of α_1 adrenoceptors; however, agonism of α_1 adrenoceptors would potentially cause urinary retention.

3. E. When a glucocorticoid molecule binds to GR, it translocates to the nucleus and binds to another glucocorticoid-bound GR. This dimer binds to glucocorticoid response elements, which increases the transcription of anti-inflammatory genes such as I-κB and annexin A1. Increased production of I-κB sequesters NF-κB in the cytoplasm, preventing it from moving to the nucleus and increasing inflammatory gene transcription. Answer choices A, B, C, and D are the opposite of the correct answer.

4. D. The leukotriene receptor antagonists, montelukast and zafirlukast, are not considered first-line drugs not only because they tend to be less effective than glucocorticoid nasal sprays, are similar in efficacy to the oral antihistamines, and are associated with an increased risk of neuropsychiatric effects, including mood changes and suicidal ideation. Since this man already has depression with suicidal thoughts, adding another drug that also carries this risk would be undesirable. However, the leukotriene receptor agonists are orally administered, they are effective against LTC_4-mediated nasal congestion, they do not cause posterior subcapsular cataracts as the glucocorticoids may do, and they are primarily eliminated by hepatic CYP metabolism, not renal excretion of the parent compound.

5. B. Rhinitis medicamentosa, or rebound congestion, occurs after more than three days of use of a nasal spray decongestant. It is not associated with orally administered decongestants; since pseudoephedrine is only given PO, it cannot be the cause of this condition. In contrast, phenylephrine can be administered PO or via nasal spray. Rhinitis medicamentosa is more common with phenylephrine than with oxymetazoline nasal spray. Although orally administered nasal decongestants or high doses of nasal sprays can cause hypertension, a person does not develop rebound hypertension (return of previously suppressed hypertension) when the drugs are discontinued.

CHAPTER 5

ASTHMA AND CHRONIC OBSTRUCTIVE PULMONARY DISEASE (COPD)

KAREN WOODFORK, PHD

West Virginia University, Morgantown, West Virginia, USA

Symptoms: Immuno-Infectious
Cardio-Renal-Respiratory

DRUG LIST FOR ASTHMA AND COPD*

Short-Acting β_2-adrenoceptor Agonists (SABAs)
Albuterol (inhaled) [A, C]
Levalbuterol (inhaled) [A, C]
Terbutaline (PO, SC, IV) [A, C]

Long-Acting β_2-adrenoceptor Agonists (LABAs)
Arformoterol (inhaled) [C]
Formoterol (inhaled) [A, C]
Indacaterol (inhaled) [C]
Olodaterol (inhaled) [C]
Salmeterol (inhaled) [A, C]
Vilanterol (inhaled) [A, C]

Short-Acting Muscarinic Antagonists (SAMAs)
Ipratropium (inhaled) [A, C]

Long-Acting Muscarinic Antagonists (LAMAs)
Aclidinium (inhaled) [C]
Glycopyrrolate (inhaled) [C]
Revefenacin (inhaled) [C]
Tiotropium (inhaled) [A, C]
Umeclidinium (inhaled) [A, C]

Inhaled Corticosteroids (ICS)
Beclomethasone [A, C]
Budesonide [A, C]
Ciclesonide [A]
Fluticasone [A, C]
Mometasone [A]

Systemic Corticosteroids
Betamethasone (IM) [A]
Cortisone (PO) [A]
Dexamethasone (PO, IM, IV) [A, C]
Hydrocortisone (PO, IM, IV) [A, C]
Methylprednisolone (PO, IM, IV) [A, C]
Prednisolone (PO) [A, C]
Prednisone (PO) [A, C]
Triamcinolone (IM) [A]

Anti-Leukotriene Drugs
Leukotriene Receptor Antagonists (LTRAs)
Montelukast (PO) [A]
Zafirlukast (PO) [A]

Leukotriene Synthesis Inhibitor
Zileuton (PO) [A]

Mast Cell Stabilizers
Cromolyn (inhaled) [A]

Anti-IgE Antibodies
Omalizumab (SC) [A]

Anti-IL-5 Antibodies
Benralizumab (SC) [A]
Mepolizumab (SC) [A]
Reslizumab (IV) [A]

IL-4 Receptor Antagonist
Dupilumab (SC) [A]

Anti-Thymic Stromal Lymphopoietin (TSLP) Antibody
Tezepelumab (SC) [A]

Methylxanthines
Aminophylline (IV) [A, C]
Theophylline (PO) [A, C]

Phosphodiesterase 4 (PDE4) Inhibitors
Roflumilast (PO) [C]

ICS + LABA Combinations
Budesonide; formoterol [A, C]
Fluticasone; salmeterol [A, C]
Fluticasone; vilanterol [A, C]
Formoterol; mometasone [A, C]

ICS + LAMA + LABA Combination
Fluticasone; umeclidinium; vilanterol [A, C]
Budesonide; glycopyrrolate; formoterol [C]

LAMA + LABA Combination
Aclidinium; formoterol [C]
Glycopyrrolate; formoterol [C]
Tiotropium; olodaterol [C]
Umeclidinium; vilanterol [C]

SABA + SAMA Combination
Ipratropium; albuterol [A, C]

* Drugs marked with an "A" or "C" carry an FDA-approved indication or are commonly used off-label for asthma or COPD, respectively.

Asthma

General Background
Asthma is a common, chronic condition that is characterized by episodes of airway obstruction that result from inflammation, mucus hypersecretion, and bronchoconstriction. Although the changes seen in the airways are initially fully reversible, irreversible changes may occur as the disease progresses. Asthma most commonly presents in childhood, but it may also present in adults. Up to three-quarters of school-aged children with asthma outgrow this condition by mid-adulthood.

Diagnosis
Although asthma is characterized by a classic set of signs and symptoms, distinguishing it from other chronic respiratory conditions can be difficult. A history and physical examination will demonstrate symptoms that are consistent with asthma (wheezing, cough, dyspnea, chest tightness) and are relieved by bronchodilator medications.

Pulmonary function testing will demonstrate variable expiratory airflow obstruction. Laboratory studies may also be useful in the diagnosis of some cases of asthma.

One way that asthma has been classified is according to the frequency and severity of symptoms, with distinctions made between mild intermittent, mild persistent, moderate persistent, and severe persistent asthma. In addition, asthma has been classified by phenotype, i.e., a recognizable cluster of demographic, clinical, and/or physiological characteristics. The common phenotypes described by the Global Initiative for Asthma (GINA) are the following:

- Allergic asthma: This type of asthma is associated with a personal or family history of atopic disease, and its onset is usually during childhood. Sputum eosinophilia is characteristic of this condition. Therapy with inhaled corticosteroids (ICS) usually produces a good response.
- Non-allergic asthma: In this condition, asthma is not associated with allergies. Individuals may show neutrophilia, eosinophilia, or only a small number of inflammatory cells in the sputum. Non-allergic asthma is less responsive to ICS.
- Adult-onset (late-onset) asthma: This form of asthma begins in adulthood, and it is seen more often in female patients. It is usually non-allergic and may require higher doses of ICS or be relatively refractory to ICS treatment. In persons with adult-onset asthma, the possibility of occupational asthma should be investigated. Occupational asthma stems from workplace exposure to certain sensitizing chemicals and/or plant or animal dusts. Symptoms are decreased before beginning the work week and are exacerbated following exposure at work.
- Asthma with persistent airflow limitation: With this phenotype, patients with long-term asthma experience airway remodeling which results in obstruction that is persistent or incompletely reversible.
- Asthma with obesity: In some individuals who have obesity, a state of chronic inflammation produces effects in the airways that are consistent with asthma. Sleep-disordered breathing may also be present.

Presentation

Individuals with asthma will present with a history of episodic wheezing or coughing, resulting in dyspnea or respiratory distress. In children, chronic coughing is frequently the sole presenting complaint. Symptoms may be more prominent at night and are worsened by triggers such as allergens (e.g., dust mites, mold, animal dander, cockroaches, pollen), cold exposure, exercise, viral infections, chemical irritants or sensitizers, or in some cases, aspirin or other cyclooxygenase-1 inhibitors.

During an acute exacerbation, individuals will present with wheezing and/or coughing resulting in respiratory distress, and they may report chest tightness or pressure. Chest pain is rarely a symptom of asthma. Patients may appear completely healthy when they are not experiencing an acute exacerbation.

Status asthmaticus is an acute, life-threatening asthma exacerbation that is characterized by hypoxemia, hypercarbia, and secondary respiratory failure. Symptoms are unresponsive to initial bronchodilator treatment, and aggressive therapy must be utilized to avoid the death of the patient.

Risk Factors

Asthma affects between 15 – 20 % of people in high-income countries and 2 – 4% of those in lower-income countries. It is more commonly seen in children than adults, with most cases diagnosed before the age of 18. Many children experience remission at the time of puberty, but asthma symptoms may return during adulthood for some of these individuals. Childhood asthma is more common in males than females in adulthood, asthma is more prevalent in females.

Genetics plays a role in the development of asthma in children. A personal or family history of atopic disease (allergic rhinitis, eczema, and asthma) is associated with an increased risk of developing asthma; however, inheritance of asthma does not follow simple Mendelian genetics.

Prenatal exposure to maternal tobacco smoking is associated with an increased risk of asthma in the offspring, even if the parent(s) stop smoking after the child is born. Some studies have implicated maternal vitamin D deficiency and excessive omega-6 fatty acid consumption as factors that increase the risk of asthma in the offspring.

In children, the risk of developing asthma is associated with exposure to air pollutants such as tobacco smoke, particulates, and gases (e.g., NO_2), and with exposure to allergens such as dust mites, cockroaches, and fungi. Exposure to farm animals in early life is inversely related to the risk of developing asthma; however, studies of the effect of household animal (dog, cat) exposure on the development of asthma have shown mixed results. Obesity is associated with an increased prevalence of asthma in children and with more severe symptoms.

Viral and bacterial respiratory infections can trigger asthma exacerbations in children and adults; however, their role in the causation of asthma is unclear.

In adolescents and adults, risk factors include obesity, exposure to tobacco smoke, presence of allergic or non-allergic rhinitis, eosinophilia, post-menopausal hormone replacement therapy, and occupational exposure to certain animal substances (e.g., dander and dust mite proteins), plant substances (e.g., grain or cotton dust), metals (e.g., chromium, nickel), and other chemicals used in a variety of industrial processes.

Asthma is also influenced by many social determinants of health. In the US, the incidence of asthma is associated with income below the poverty level, poor quality housing, mold and rodent exposure, and high indoor and outdoor air pollution. Barriers to healthcare access negatively influence outcomes for individuals with asthma.

Pathophysiology

Asthma is a chronic inflammatory disease of the airways. The innate and adaptive immune systems become activated by stimuli such as allergens, infections, or chemicals to produce a state of chronic airway inflammation. This produces airway edema, mucus hypersecretion, and bronchial hyperreactivity. Airway remodeling may result in permanent structural changes such as increased smooth muscle mass, mucous gland hyperplasia, angiogenesis, thickening of the sub-basement membrane, and subepithelial fibrosis.

Activation of Th1, Th2, and Th17 lymphocytes is an intrinsic part of the mechanism by which asthma triggers produce the pathological changes characteristic of the disease. Th1 cells are activated in response to infections, particularly with viruses, and they produce interferon (IFN)-γ and interleukin (IL)-27, which eliminate viruses but also cause airway inflammation.

The Th2 pathway is initiated when dendritic cells present allergens to naïve T cells, which then differentiate into Th2 cells that release cytokines that play important roles in the pathological processes of asthma (Il-4, IL-5, IL-9, IL-13). For example, IL-4 and IL-13 up-regulate inducible nitric oxide synthase (iNOS) in bronchial epithelial cells, resulting in increased production of nitric oxide (NO). While NO is beneficial because it stimulates bronchodilation, it also increases mucus secretion and extravasation of leukocytes, and it promotes cellular injury. The fraction of exhaled NO (FeNO) is used as a biomarker of asthma, with increased levels seen in allergic forms. IL-4 and IL-13 also contribute to asthma pathophysiology by stimulating the production of periostin by eosinophils, fibroblasts, and epithelial cells. Periostin is an extracellular matrix protein that stimulates NF-κB expression in fibroblasts and epithelial cells, resulting in fibrosis and airway remodeling. IL-5 is a pro-eosinophilic cytokine that promotes eosinophilic airway inflammation. IL-4, IL-9, and IL-13 stimulate B lymphocytes to release immunoglobin (Ig)E, which, when bound to an antigen, stimulates mast cells to release histamine, prostaglandins, and leukotrienes. Histamine initiates bronchoconstriction, increases bronchial mucus secretion, and produces edema by increasing vascular permeability. Certain prostaglandins ($PGF_{2\alpha}$) and leukotrienes (LTC_4, LTD_4, and LTE_4) cause bronchoconstriction. In addition, LTC_4, LTD_4, and LTE_4 increase vascular permeability, resulting in edema.

Finally, activation of Th17 cells produces two cytokines, IL-17 and IL-22, which contribute to airway remodeling. IL-17 induces an epithelial-to-mesenchymal transition in the airways and promotes infiltration of neutrophils, and IL-22 increases smooth muscle growth.

A limitation of the phenotypic classification of asthma is that phenotypes are defined by observable characteristics and not by underlying disease processes. Classification of asthma into pathophysiological endotypes may be more useful in guiding the use of certain asthma medications. Some of the more well-known asthma endotypes are listed below:

- Allergic asthma: This endotype is characterized by a Th2 response and elevations in eosinophils, IgE, periostin, FeNO, and LTE_4.
- Infection-induced asthma: Th1 and Th2 responses are implicated in this endotype, which is characterized by elevations in neutrophils and LTE_4. Viral infection can damage the airway epithelium, allowing allergens to penetrate further into subepithelial tissues.
- Aspirin-sensitive asthma: In this form of asthma, aspirin and nonsteroidal anti-inflammatory drugs (NSAIDs; Chapter 9) elicit bronchoconstriction. Chronic rhinosinusitis and nasal polyps are characteristic of this endotype. A Th2 response is apparent, and elevations in eosinophils, periostin, FeNO, and LTE_4 are seen.
- Airflow obstruction caused by obesity: This endotype is characterized by an enhanced Th2 response and high levels of circulating proinflammatory cytokines, resulting in systemic inflammation and oxidative stress.
- Exercise-induced asthma: Here, symptoms develop 5 – 15 minutes after a brief period of exertion or about 15 minutes into a prolonged exercise session, and they resolve after 30 – 60 minutes of rest. Symptoms are worsened when exercise is done in the cold. A Th2 response is evident, and elevated levels of neutrophils are seen.
- Neutrophilic asthma: This form is associated with exposure to tobacco smoke and diesel exhaust particles. A Th17 response and elevation of neutrophils are characteristic of this endotype.
- Severe steroid-dependent asthma: This endotype is likely a combination of Th1, Th2, and Th17 responses.

Examination

Wheezing is a prominent physical finding during an asthma exacerbation, but it is likely not present at other times. Asthmatic wheezes are characterized as "musical" – they are of a high, variable pitch, and they start and stop at varying points in the respiratory cycle. In contrast, a monophonic wheeze is characteristic of bronchial narrowing due to an aspirated foreign body or bronchogenic cancer. A low-pitch wheeze that clears with coughing is a sign of excess airway secretion that is characteristic of bronchitis or bronchiectasis. Asthmatic wheezes are more likely to be heard on expiration, and an inspiratory wheeze often suggests a different etiology. The cough that is characteristic of asthma is dry and hacking, but a productive cough, with clear or whitish sputum, may be seen.

The presence or absence of wheezing is not an accurate indicator of asthma severity. Symptoms of severe airway obstruction include tachypnea, tachycardia, prolonged expiration, and adopting a "tripod position" in which the individual uses extended arms to support the upper chest. During a severe asthma attack, a person may use the accessory muscles of breathing during inspiration, and systolic blood pressure may decrease during inspiration to a significant degree (i.e., pulsus paradoxus). If respiratory arrest is imminent, the patient will appear exhausted, drowsy, or confused. Air will not be able to enter or leave the lungs well, so a "silent chest" will be noted, along with cyanosis and other signs of hypoxia. Pulse oximetry can be used to assess the severity of an asthma attack, but oxygen saturation may not decrease significantly until the asthma attack is severe.

Many patients with allergic asthma also have allergic rhinitis (Chapter 4) and will display the pale nasal membranes and cobblestone posterior pharynx that are characteristic of this condition. Additionally, allergic asthma patients may also display signs of atopic dermatitis. Nasal polyps are common in individuals with aspirin/NSAID-sensitive asthma.

Spirometry is the method of choice for diagnosing asthma, although it is often not possible to perform in children under the age of five. This procedure requires the patient to inhale as much air as possible, then exhale rapidly, forcefully, and completely into a spirometer. The spirometer measures the forced expiratory volume in one second (FEV_1) and the total amount of air exhaled, which is known as the forced vital capacity (FVC). A reduction in the FEV_1/FVC ratio indicates that airway obstruction is present. The flow-volume curve that is generated by the spirometer exhibits a characteristic shape in asthma and can also help to distinguish it from other respiratory diseases. It is of note that spirometry may appear normal if the patient is not experiencing asthma symptoms at the time of measurement and in individuals who have cough-variant asthma.

The ability of a short-acting bronchodilator to acutely reverse airflow obstruction can be tested by performing spirometry measurements, then administering the nebulized bronchodilator, then repeating the spirometry 10 – 15 minutes later. Most individuals with asthma exhibit a bronchodilator response; however, a bronchodilator response can also be seen in some individuals with other pulmonary diseases (e.g., COPD and cystic fibrosis). The bronchodilator response in asthma is generally much larger (approximately 15 – 20% response) than that seen in other conditions.

Bronchoprovocation testing can be used to diagnose asthma in individuals who have normal baseline airflow or cough-variant asthma. Patients are exposed to a stimulus such as inhaled methacholine, inhaled mannitol, exercise, or dry air. Individuals with asthma exhibit a greater degree of bronchoconstriction in response to these stimuli than those without disease; however, a small percentage of non-asthmatic persons will also display hyperresponsiveness to such stimuli. Individuals with COPD, allergic rhinitis, or cystic fibrosis may experience a false positive bronchoprovocation result.

Peak expiratory flow (PEF) can be measured by the patient at home using an inexpensive device. PEF measurement can be used to confirm reversible airway obstruction in patients whose initial spirometry measurement is normal. It is also used to monitor patients who have been diagnosed with asthma to assess the effectiveness of treatments or the removal of triggers.

Laboratory

There are no definitive blood tests for diagnosing asthma; however, measurement of certain biomarkers may be useful in distinguishing asthma endotypes and selecting the most effective types of therapy for them. For example, the presence of eosinophilia in the sputum or blood is characteristic of allergic asthma. Tests for sensitivity to specific allergens can help in identifying triggers that patients should avoid. Eosinophilia in the context of severe asthma suggests that anti-IL5 antibodies may be useful as an add-on therapy. The presence of high levels of IgE can be helpful in deciding whether a patient should be treated with an anti-IgE antibody.

Measurement of FeNO can help to confirm a diagnosis of asthma, but it is not a definitive test. While elevated levels are seen in most individuals with allergic and some other endotypes of asthma, a normal level may be seen in some with allergic asthma and in those with certain endotypes. Elevated FeNO may be seen in non-asthmatic individuals who have conditions such as allergic rhinitis and eosinophilic bronchitis.

Imaging
A chest radiograph is recommended for persons presenting with atypical features such as chronic purulent sputum production, fever, clubbing of the fingernails, inspiratory crackles, hemoptysis, significant hypoxemia in the absence of an acute attack, lack of reversal by bronchodilators, weight loss, or localized wheezing. It is also used in individuals over age 40 who present with new-onset moderate-severe asthma symptoms to rule out other conditions (e.g., heart failure). High-resolution computed tomography (HRCT) can be used if abnormalities are seen on chest radiography.

Associated Symptoms/Conditions
The presence of atopic disease is associated with asthma. Allergic rhinitis (Chapter 4) is seen in most patients who have allergic asthma and in 60% of those who have non-allergic asthma. Chronic rhinosinusitis is often seen in patients with severe asthma. Although gastroesophageal reflux disease (GERD; Chapter 20) can produce a cough that can mimic asthma, it is also commonly associated with asthma itself. Obesity can produce a pattern of dyspnea that can mimic asthma; however, it is also a risk factor for the development of asthma and is associated with more severe asthma symptoms. Persons with asthma have an increased risk of developing COPD.

Diagnosis
The diagnosis of asthma is made on the basis of classical symptoms (e.g., episodic musical wheezing) and physical findings, in conjunction with the demonstration of variable airway obstruction, preferably by spirometry. A diagnosis of asthma is confirmed by the presence of an obstructive spirometry pattern that completely or significantly (> 15% increase in FEV1) reverses following administration of a bronchodilator. In a patient who experiences a cough without wheezing, the presence of reversible airway obstruction would also result in an asthma diagnosis. Although some individuals with asthma do not display reversibility in their airway obstruction, a lack of reversibility should cause the physician to investigate alternate diagnoses.

The presence of a normal spirometry pattern does not exclude a diagnosis of asthma in patients who are asymptomatic at the time of measurement. For these individuals, spirometry can be repeated when they are symptomatic, or they may be given a device to measure PEF at home under asymptomatic and symptomatic conditions and after bronchodilator administration. Bronchoprovocation testing may be used to confirm asthma in patients with normal spirometry and in those with atypical symptoms. This method is not used in the routine diagnosis of asthma because it is expensive and requires a pulmonary function laboratory staffed with individuals who are experts in its application.

In some circumstances in which spirometry cannot be performed (e.g., infants and young children), a presumptive diagnosis of asthma is made when symptoms and examinations are typical of asthma and a trial of a bronchodilator produces a positive result. If the diagnosis of asthma is not clear-cut, or if spirometry cannot be performed, measurement of FeNO can aid in the diagnosis of individuals aged five and older, although this is not a definitive test for asthma.

When making a diagnosis of asthma, it is important to exclude other diagnoses that can cause similar symptoms. Acute onset of wheezing and dyspnea in conjunction with a history of recent allergen exposure suggests the possibility of anaphylaxis, which characteristically manifests with cutaneous flushing, urticaria, itching, and hypotension. Wheezing sounds may also be produced by the narrowing of non-bronchial respiratory passages; for example, stridor is an inspiratory wheeze that is usually caused by an obstruction in the upper airways and is often seen in infectious childhood illnesses such as croup, or in foreign body aspiration. Vocal cord dysfunction may also produce wheezing, particularly on expiration; this is more commonly seen in adults and adolescents.

Cough may be a symptom of pneumonia, bronchitis, bronchiolitis, bronchiectasis, neoplastic processes, or other pulmonary conditions. Cough may also result from a variety of non-pulmonary conditions such as allergic rhinitis (Chapter 4) or GERD (Chapter 20), and it is a common side effect of angiotensin-converting enzyme (ACE) inhibitors. Dyspnea is seen in conditions such as heart failure, pulmonary embolism, and interstitial lung disease. COPD can manifest with dyspnea and cough. Although it is thought of as an irreversible obstructive condition, its symptoms may be worsened by factors such as exercise and may be partially reversible with bronchodilators.

Treatment
The inhaled, fast-acting "rescue" medications have long been a mainstay for the treatment of acute asthma attacks. These include the short-acting β_2-adrenoceptor agonists (SABAs), and, to a lesser extent, the short-acting muscarinic antagonists (SAMAs), which are only used in conjunction with a SABA. Preventive or "control" medications include inhaled corticosteroids (ICS), inhaled long-acting β_2-adrenoceptor agonists (LABAs), and inhaled long-acting muscarinic antagonists (LAMAs). Inhaled mast cell stabilizers (e.g., cromolyn) can be used as preventives, but only in certain scenarios. Orally administered anti-leukotriene drugs are useful as adjunctive therapy and as monotherapy in specific circumstances. Oral methylxanthines are seldom used today. Injectable biologics are used in severe asthma; these include antibodies against IgE, IL4 and IL-13, and IL-5. Status asthmaticus is treated aggressively with continuous inhalation of albuterol (a SABA), along with the continuous infusion of corticosteroids. Inhaled

ipratropium (a SAMA) can also be of benefit, as can intravenous magnesium sulfate, which relaxes bronchial smooth muscle. Intubation and ventilation may be necessary in certain cases.

Management

Asthma management involves optimizing the control of existing asthma symptoms and minimizing the risk of future exacerbations and pulmonary function decline. In addition to drug therapy, avoidance of triggers is an important part of asthma management. Allergen testing can be used to determine potential triggers for asthma attacks. For individuals with specific allergies, exposure to these allergens should be eliminated or reduced by environmental controls such as air filters, pest management, etc. Workplace exposures to potential triggers should be investigated and minimized where possible. Subcutaneous immunotherapy (SCIT), in which an allergen is administered subcutaneously, is used as an adjunct treatment for individuals with allergic asthma.

Patient education has been shown to improve asthma management in many studies; this education may include strategies for controlling trigger exposure, optimizing medication adherence, and rapidly identifying exacerbations of asthma.

General Treatment Strategies

In its 2020 Focused Update to Asthma Management Guidelines, the US Expert Panel Working Group of the National Heart, Lung, and Blood Institute (NHLBI) and National Asthma Education and Prevention Program Coordinating Committee (NAEPPCC) recommended a stepwise approach to the treatment of asthma (Table 5.1). The step is chosen based on the severity of the patient's symptoms and the response to previous therapies. The physician may move to a higher step (more medications, higher doses) if the patient's asthma is worsening, or the physician may deescalate to a lower step (fewer medications, lower doses) if the patient's symptoms have been well controlled for at least three months. If the patient is on an alternate therapy and their symptoms are not adequately controlled, the preferred therapy at that step should be implemented before moving to a higher step.

The NHLBI/NAEPPCC guidelines incorporate the use of "SMART" (single maintenance and reliever therapy), a protocol that uses a combination product containing an ICS + formoterol, as both a daily control medication and a rescue inhaler. Although formoterol is classified as a LABA, and LABAs are generally not used as rescue medications, it has a rapid onset of action which allows it to be used in this manner. Unlike the other LABAs, formoterol may be administered more than twice a day without significant adverse effects.

Age (yrs.)	Treatment	Step 1	Step 2	Step 3	Step 4	Step 5	Step 6
< 5	Preferred	PRN SABA; Add short course of ICS in respiratory infection	PRN SABA & daily low-dose ICS	PRN SABA & daily medium-dose ICS	PRN SABA & daily [LABA + medium-dose ICS]	PRN SABA & daily [LABA + high-dose ICS]	PRN SABA & daily [LABA + high-dose ICS] & oral systemic corticosteroid
	Alternate		PRN SABA & daily: • cromolyn, or • montelukast		PRN SABA & daily medium-dose ICS & montelukast	PRN SABA & daily high-dose ICS & montelukast	PRN SABA & daily high-dose ICS & montelukast & oral systemic corticosteroid
5 – 11	Preferred	PRN SABA	PRN SABA & daily low-dose ICS	Daily & PRN use of [formoterol + low-dose ICS]	Daily & PRN use of [formoterol + medium-dose ICS]	PRN SABA & daily [LABA + high-dose ICS]	PRN SABA & daily [LABA + high-dose ICS] & oral systemic corticosteroid

	Alternate		PRN SABA & daily:
			• LTRA, or
			• cromolyn, or
			• nedocromil, or
			• theophylline
				PRN SABA & daily:
				• medium-dose ICS, or
				• [LABA + low-dose ICS], or
				• low-dose ICS &:
				  • LTRA, or
				  • theophylline
					PRN SABA & daily:
					• [LABA + medium-dose ICS], or
					• medium-dose ICS &
					  • LTRA, or
					  • theophylline
						PRN SABA & daily high dose ICS &:
						• LTRA, or
						• theophylline
							PRN SABA & daily high-dose ICS & oral systemic corticosteroid &:
							• LTRA, or
							• theophylline

12 +	Preferred	PRN SABA	• PRN SABA & daily low-dose ICS, or • PRN [SABA + ICS]	Daily & PRN use of [formoterol + low-dose ICS]	Daily & PRN use of [formoterol + medium-dose ICS]	PRN SABA & daily [LABA + medium – high-dose ICS] & LAMA	PRN SABA & daily [LABA + high-dose ICS] & oral systemic corticosteroid

	Alternate		PRN SABA & daily:
			• LTRA, or
			• cromolyn, or
			• nedocromil, or
			• zileuton, or
			• theophylline
				PRN SABA & daily:
				• medium-dose ICS, or
				• low-dose ICS &:
				  • LABA, or
				  • LAMA, or
				  • LTRA, or
				  • theophylline, or
				  • zileuton
					PRN SABA & daily:
					• [LABA + medium-dose ICS], or
					• [LAMA + medium-dose ICS], or
					• medium-dose ICS &:
					  • LTRA, or
					  • theophylline,
					  • or zileuton
						PRN SABA & daily:
						• [LABA + medium-high dose ICS], or
						• LTRA & high-dose ICS	

Table 5.1. Stepwise Approach for Management of Asthma, adapted from the 2020 Focused Update to Asthma Management Guidelines, the US Expert Panel Working Group of the National Heart, Lung, and Blood Institute (NHLBI) and National Asthma Education and Prevention Program Coordinating Committee (NAEPPCC). Step 1 applies to the treatment of intermittent asthma; Steps 2 – 6 apply to individuals with persistent asthma. Combination products are indicated by drugs inside of brackets, separated by a plus sign, e.g., [Drug 1 + Drug 2]. Choices amongst multiple drugs or combinations are indicated by bullet points, indicating that one of these can be selected. Note that nedocromil is only available as an ophthalmic preparation in the US.

Chronic Obstructive Pulmonary Disease (COPD)

General Background

According to the Global Initiative for Chronic Obstructive Lung Disease (GOLD), a project initiated by the National Heart, Lung, and Blood Institute (NHLBI) and the World Health Organization (WHO), COPD is defined as a "heterogeneous lung condition characterized by chronic respiratory symptoms (dyspnea, cough, sputum production, exacerbation) due to abnormalities of the airway (bronchitis, bronchiolitis) and/or alveoli (emphysema) that cause persistent, often progressive, airflow obstruction." The classical definition of COPD includes three forms: chronic bronchitis, emphysema, and obstructive asthma. Chronic bronchitis is defined as a chronic productive cough over a defined period (three months in each of two successive years) in a patient for whom other causes of cough have been excluded. Emphysema describes structural changes in which the pulmonary acini become enlarged or destroyed.

The current definition recognizes that COPD manifestations exist on a spectrum, and most patients exhibit some degree of chronic bronchitis, emphysema, and/or obstructive asthma. A separate condition, asthma-COPD overlap syndrome (ACOS), has been defined, encompassing features of both diseases.

Diagnosis

The diagnosis of COPD requires a thorough history, including symptoms, the pattern of onset, and exposure to smoke, fumes, chemicals, and dusts. Spirometry is used to evaluate lung function, and imaging may be used to elucidate the diagnosis. No laboratory tests are diagnostic for COPD, but certain tests may be conducted to identify conditions in individuals with atypical presentations and to exclude diagnoses that can present similarly.

Presentation

The characteristic symptoms of COPD are chronic cough, sputum production, and dyspnea. The intensity of these symptoms may vary over the course of hours, days, or weeks. Symptoms are generally worst in the mornings because sputum has not been expectorated during the night.

Patients often first present with complaints of chronic cough and exertional dyspnea. However, sedentary individuals may not notice exertional dyspnea, and because the progression of symptoms is gradual, individuals often unknowingly adjust their activity level to avoid feeling shortness of breath. Severe disease presents with dyspnea at rest. Wheezing is a less common chronic manifestation of COPD; a small number of individuals experience feelings of chest tightness.

Patients may report episodes of increased cough and dyspnea along with purulent sputum and potentially wheezing and/or fever. These exacerbations of COPD may become more frequent and severe with disease progression.

Risk Factors

In high-income countries, the most prominent risk factor for COPD is tobacco smoking, accounting for over 70% of cases. Passive smoke exposure and cannabis smoking can also contribute to COPD development. The number of pack-years of smoking correlates positively with the incidence of COPD; however, less than half of heavy smokers eventually develop COPD, and some lifelong non-smokers develop this condition. Maternal smoking is associated with reduced lung function in the offspring; this may predispose an individual to develop COPD from other exposures.

Electronic nicotine delivery systems (i.e., e-cigarettes, vaping) can expose the user to harmful substances, as evidenced by the outbreak of vaping-associated lung injury in the US in 2019.

In low to middle-income countries, tobacco smoking accounts for only 30 – 40% of cases. Over 85% of COPD cases worldwide are seen in these countries, so on a global basis, non-smoking risk factors are responsible for over 50% of the total burden of COPD. Air pollution represents the greatest non-smoking risk factor for COPD, and it also increases the risk of COPD exacerbations, hospitalization, and mortality.

Outdoor air can contain a spectrum of pollutants resulting from the burning of fossil fuels and wood/biomass, industrial emissions, and natural events (e.g., forest fires and volcanic eruptions). Pollutants such as particulates, ozone, NO_2, SO_2, volatile organic compounds (VOCs), and heavy metals can produce oxidative stress and stimulate inflammatory processes seen in COPD. Living in an urban area has a positive association with COPD.

Indoor air pollution is also a risk factor for the development of COPD. In low to middle-income countries, many households burn biomass (wood, animal dung, crop residues) or coal in poorly vented stoves or open fires for cooking and heating. This exposes household members, predominantly the individuals cooking or tending the fire, to a high concentration of particulates and other inflammatory pollutants. Buildings in high-income countries can also suffer from indoor air pollution. These structures are often tightly sealed; building materials and furniture may outgas VOCs and other contaminants, resulting in indoor air that can contain a higher concentration of certain air pollutants than is seen outdoors.

Occupational exposure to vapors, gases, dusts, or fumes (VGDF) is another risk factor for COPD in smokers and never-smokers. The variable nature of different workplace exposures makes it difficult to characterize the relationship between specific exposures and COPD. However, certain occupations, such as foundry work and machining, and certain occupational exposures, such as disinfectants and pesticides, have shown statistically significant associations with COPD.

Age is a risk factor for the development of COPD, with most cases presenting in mid-life. The onset of COPD in early adulthood suggests the presence of α-1 antitrypsin deficiency (AATD). In this disorder, mutation of the *SERPINA1* gene results in a non-functional version of AAT, which is a serine protease that inhibits neutrophil elastase. In the absence of adequate levels of functional AAT, neutrophil elastase breaks down the elastin of the alveoli and causes emphysema. Current research involves genome-wide association studies. Multiple associations have been identified, but the mechanistic significance of these variants is yet to be elucidated.

Atopic disease, asthma, and increased airway responsiveness are risk factors for COPD. Female patients tend to develop COPD at a lower number of pack-years of smoking than male patients. A history of pulmonary infections, particularly tuberculosis, is associated with an elevated risk of COPD. Host factors, such as impaired lung development and accelerated lung aging, may also increase the risk of COPD.

Diet has recently been studied with respect to risk and outcome in COPD. High intake of foods rich in antioxidants (e.g., fruits and vegetables) is inversely correlated with COPD incidence and disease severity. It is not clear how much of this relationship is causative and how much is the result of disease (e.g., dyspnea impairing eating). There is currently little data from dietary intervention trials.

Persons with low socioeconomic status can experience multiple COPD risk factors, such as indoor and outdoor air pollution, occupational exposure, smoke exposure, infections, and poor diet. These, combined with limited access to health care and screening, increase the risk of negative outcomes from COPD.

Pathophysiology

COPD is a chronic condition that affects the airways, the lung parenchyma, and the pulmonary vasculature. It is characterized by chronic inflammation and remodeling of the small airways, resulting in obstructive airway disease that is irreversible or minimally reversible with bronchodilators. Changes in the airway epithelium result in symptoms of chronic bronchitis, and destruction of the pulmonary acini produces the characteristic histology of emphysema.

The pathophysiology of COPD is evident in the small airways (< 2mm) early in the disease process. The epithelium of the small airways contains a characteristic mixture of cell types. These include ciliated epithelial cells, which push foreign material away from the alveoli and toward the large airways; basal cells, which replenish the epithelium after injury; and club cells (formerly called Clara cells), which are the major secretory cell of the small airways. Club cells secrete surfactants and other proteins of the pulmonary fluid that aid in the immune response; they also function as stem cells, and they metabolize xenobiotics via cytochrome P450 (CYP450). Mucus-secreting goblet cells, which are prominent in the larger airways, are less common in the small airways. The small airways terminate in the pulmonary acini, each of which is a unit consisting of a respiratory bronchiole and its associated alveolar ducts, alveolar sacs, and alveoli.

Exposure to inhaled oxidants initiates a reprogramming of the cells of the small airway epithelium, resulting in the development of features similar to those seen in the upper airways. The changes occur, even in the absence of inflammation, in most individuals who smoke. One important change involves a loss of club cells and ciliated cells, with replacement by squamous epithelium. This results in decreased production of protective pulmonary fluid and impaired mucociliary clearance. An increase in the number of goblet cells is also seen; this causes the pathological production of mucus in the small airways.

As COPD becomes more advanced, additional pathology becomes apparent. Neutrophils, macrophages, and lymphocytes get recruited to the airways and lung parenchyma. These cells and others release inflammatory mediators, resulting in chronic inflammation. Matrix metalloproteinases produced by macrophages and elastase produced by neutrophils are implicated in the destruction of the lung parenchyma that is characteristic of emphysema. While it seems paradoxical that an increased risk of infection could occur in an inflammatory state, in COPD, the epithelial barrier becomes less functional, the airway microbiome becomes disrupted, and an epithelium-specific immune suppression develops at least in part because the macrophages that have been recruited to the airways exhibit defective phagocytosis.

Small airway remodeling results from a decrease in the production of elastin and an increase in the production of disordered collagen; this produces narrower, stiffer airways with less elastic recoil. Within the pulmonary vasculature, intimal and smooth muscle hyperplasia can be seen.

Emphysema can be characterized by the location of damage to the pulmonary acini. In proximal acinar (centriacinar) emphysema, the respiratory bronchioles are dilated or destroyed, and damage occurs preferentially in the upper parts of the lung. This form of emphysema is more commonly seen with cigarette smoking and can also be seen in coal workers' pneumoconiosis. In panacinar emphysema, all parts of the acinus are dilated or destroyed, and the lung bases are more commonly involved. This form is most frequently seen in individuals with α-1 antitrypsin deficiency but may occur along with proximal acinar emphysema in smokers. In distal acinar (paraseptal) emphysema, the alveolar ducts are affected, and small subpleural collections of gas are seen in the periphery of the secondary pulmonary lobule. Distal acinar emphysema may be seen in association with other types of emphysema, or it may occur alone, usually with spontaneous pneumothorax in a young adult.

As with asthma, different forms of COPD may exhibit a prevalence of different inflammatory responses. Th1 responses are associated with viral infection, Th2 responses are associated with allergy and are believed to be involved in ACOS, and Th17 responses are associated with emphysema.

Exacerbations of COPD are periods of acute worsening characterized by FEV_1 reduction, airway neutrophilia, peripheral blood leukocytosis, and the presence of viral and/or bacterial pathogens. COPD exacerbations can be classified as having either a pro-inflammatory endotype, which is associated with bacterial infection, a Th1 inflammatory endotype, which is associated with viral infection, a Th2 inflammatory endotype, which is associated with eosinophilia, and a pauci-inflammatory endotype, in which there are low concentrations of airway biomarkers.

Examination

The physical exam of a person with early COPD may be normal, or the patient may exhibit minor symptoms such as prolonged expiration (decreased FEV_1) or wheezing upon forced exhalation. In more severe disease, hyperinflation of the lungs will be evidenced by increased resonance in response to percussion. An increased anteroposterior chest diameter ("barrel chest") may be seen; this larger lung volume provides increased recoil upon expiration to help open the obstructed airways. Auscultation of the chest may reveal decreased breath sounds due to lessened air movement, distant heart sounds because the lungs are enlarged, crackles at the lung bases due to alveolar destruction, and/or wheezes caused by air movement through collapsing airways.

In severe disease, the patient may use pursed lip breathing with slow exhalation to produce a build-up of pressure in order to open the more distal airways. The patient may adopt postures (e.g., the tripod position) to relieve dyspnea and may need to use the accessory muscles of the neck and shoulders to aid in respiration. Neck veins may be distended due to increased intrathoracic pressure, especially during expiration. Right-sided heart failure may result in an enlarged, tender liver. The patient may also exhibit Hoover's sign, a paradoxical inward movement of the lower rib cage during inspiration that results from the contraction of a diaphragm which is flat at the beginning of inspiration. In situations of respiratory failure, the patient may exhibit cyanosis and hypercapnia, and asterixis (flapping tremor) may be seen.

Spirometry is the primary tool used for the diagnosis of COPD. The presence of an obstructive spirometry pattern that is not fully reversible following bronchodilator administration indicates the presence of COPD. Individuals with COPD may show an improvement in FEV_1 from bronchodilator administration, but a post-bronchodilation FEV_1/FVC

< 0.7 will confirm the diagnosis of COPD. The severity of COPD can be staged according to the GOLD grades, which are based on post-bronchodilation FEV_1 (see Table 5.2).

Grade	Severity	Criterion
GOLD 1	Mild	$FEV_1 \geq 80\%$ of predicted
GOLD 2	Moderate	$50\% \leq FEV_1 < 80\%$ of predicted
GOLD 3	Severe	$30\% \leq FEV_1 < 50\%$ of predicted
GOLD 4	Very Severe	$FEV_1 < 30\%$ of predicted

Table 5.2. GOLD Grades in Patients Diagnosed with COPD ($FEV_1/FVC < 0.7$) Adapted from the Pocket Guide to COPD Diagnosis, Management, and Prevention, A Guide for Health Care Professionals, 2023 Edition.

Some individuals exhibit structural features (e.g., emphysema) or functional abnormalities (hyperinflation of the lungs, low FEV_1) that are characteristic of COPD, but they do not meet the criteria for COPD because their post-bronchodilation FEV_1/FVC is ≥ 0.7. These individuals are classified as pre-COPD or PRISm (preserved ratio impaired spirometry) and are at elevated risk of developing airway obstruction in the future.

The severity of the patient's symptoms is assessed using a validated questionnaire, such as the modified British Medical Research Council (mMRC) questionnaire or the COPD Assessment Test (CAT). A 6-minute walk test can be used to assess a patient's functional capacity.

Laboratory

Pulse oximetry is a simple, non-invasive way to measure blood oxygen saturation (SpO_2). Arterial blood gas measurement is performed only under specific circumstances, such as in an acute exacerbation of COPD when the $FEV_1 < 50\%$ of predicted, or the $SpO_2 < 92\%$. It may also be used if the patient is experiencing depressed consciousness, or if they have severe airflow obstruction and require assessment for hypercapnia. Elevated serum bicarbonate will also contribute to the diagnosis of hypercapnia.

Testing for AAT deficiency should be done in individuals with irreversible obstructive spirometry, particularly if they developed this condition at 45 years of age or younger, are a nonsmoker, or have a family history of emphysema.

Additional tests may be run to rule out conditions such as heart failure, which manifests with dyspnea on exertion, or GERD, which can produce chronic cough.

Imaging

Although chest radiography has poor sensitivity for detecting COPD, it is routinely performed as part of its evaluation to exclude the many conditions in the differential diagnosis of dyspnea, e.g., benign or malignant lung tumors, bronchiectasis, pneumothorax, pneumonia, tuberculosis, pulmonary embolism, bronchiolitis obliterans (constrictive bronchiolitis), interstitial lung disease, lymphangioleiomyomatosis, and diffuse panbronchiolitis.

The characteristic findings of COPD on chest radiography are most often seen in advanced disease. A flat diaphragmatic contour and increased retrosternal airspace indicate hyperinflation of the lungs. Bullae, which are radiolucent areas larger than 1 cm in diameter, are indicative of areas of severe disease in which the parenchyma has been destroyed. Enlargement of the right ventricle and pulmonary artery may be seen in circumstances where COPD has resulted in pulmonary hypertension and cor pulmonale.

A CT scan may be done to evaluate any abnormalities seen on the chest radiograph and to better detect and classify emphysema. CT is also used to screen for lung cancer and to diagnose pulmonary embolism.

Associated Symptoms/Conditions

Asthma and atopic disorders are risk factors for the development of COPD, as are infections with tuberculosis and other respiratory pathogens. Smoking is a prominent risk factor for COPD, and individuals with COPD who smoke are at risk of developing the pathologies that arise from smoking, e.g., lung and other cancers, cardiovascular disease, periodontal disease, infertility, impaired sexual function, premature and low birth weight babies, miscarriages, certain birth defects, impaired immunity, osteoporosis, type 2 diabetes, cataracts and macular degeneration, slow wound healing, and premature aging of the skin.

Sleep apnea, GERD, hypertension, ischemic heart disease, heart failure, atrial fibrillation, obesity, metabolic syndrome, diabetes, anxiety, and depression show associations with COPD. Conditions arising from COPD include pulmonary hypertension, right-sided heart failure/cor pulmonale, weight loss, and muscle wasting. Acute exacerbations of COPD are associated with bacterial infections (e.g., *H. influenzae*, *S. pneumoniae*, *M. catarrhalis*) and pulmonary emboli.

Diagnosis
The diagnosis of COPD begins with a history and examination demonstrating the symptoms of COPD (chronic cough, dyspnea, sputum production, exacerbations). Factors supporting a COPD diagnosis include chronic tobacco smoke exposure, indoor biomass burning, family history of COPD, and occupational exposures to vapors, gases, dusts, or fumes. Spirometric testing is required for a definitive diagnosis of COPD. The presence of an obstructive spirometry pattern that is not fully reversible following bronchodilator administration, as demonstrated by a post-bronchodilation $FEV_1/FVC < 0.7$, confirms the diagnosis of COPD. Chest radiography can be used to exclude alternate diagnoses, but the radiographic features characteristic of COPD are usually not seen unless the disease is severe. A CT scan can be used to exclude certain alternate diagnoses and assess the extent and type of emphysema that may be present.

Treatment
Pharmacotherapy is used to reduce COPD symptoms, improve exercise tolerance and health status, and decrease the frequency and severity of exacerbations. Bronchodilators are a mainstay of COPD treatment; these include the SABAs, LABAs, SAMAs, and LAMAs. Bronchodilators relax airway smooth muscle, and they increase the FEV_1 by widening the airways, not by increasing lung elastic recoil. Bronchodilators also decrease dynamic hyperinflation at rest and during exercise, so they increase exercise capacity. SABAs and SAMAs are used on an as-needed basis; combinations of SABA + SAMA have shown superiority to monotherapy. LABAs and LAMAs are used on a daily basis to prevent or reduce symptoms, and combinations of LABA + LAMA have shown superiority over monotherapy as well.

ICSs are added to bronchodilator therapy to reduce exacerbations in patients with moderate to very severe COPD and may have a mortality benefit when used in this manner. Therapy with LABA + LAMA + ICS has shown benefits over LABA + LAMA alone. The magnitude with which a patient responds to ICS is related to blood eosinophil count; patients with values ≥ 300 cells/μL are most likely to benefit, and ICS should be avoided in those with eosinophils $<$ 100 cells/μL, or a history of repeated pneumonia or mycobacterial infection. Monotherapy with ICS is not recommended. Systemic glucocorticoids are not used as maintenance therapy, but a short course can improve lung function in severe exacerbations.

Methylxanthines are occasionally used in combination with other bronchodilators, but their adverse effects are limiting. Mucolytic agents can be helpful adjuncts to bronchodilator and ICS therapy. Chronic therapy with azithromycin or erythromycin can decrease the risk of exacerbations. The addition of a phosphodiesterase 4 (PDE_4) inhibitor can be beneficial in patients who have severe to very severe COPD and a history of exacerbations. Emphysema in individuals with AATD may be slowed by α1-antitrypsin augmentation therapy.

Long-term oxygen therapy is indicated in patients with hypoxemia, with or without hypercapnia. Non-invasive positive pressure ventilation (NIPPV) is a standard of care for decreasing morbidity and mortality in patients hospitalized with COPD exacerbations, and it has shown benefits in decreasing exacerbations in patients with stable COPD. In patients with very severe COPD, lung volume reduction surgery has shown a survival benefit in select populations. Lung transplantation may improve the quality of life and prolong survival in certain individuals.

Management
Identification and reduction of exposure to risk factors is a cornerstone of COPD management. For individuals who smoke, smoking cessation is a key intervention in reducing the progression of the disease; these individuals should be offered smoking cessation medications and counseling. Reducing household air pollution and occupational exposures is also recommended. Patient education on self-management is important, and pulmonary rehabilitation is indicated in patients with symptoms and/or a high risk of exacerbation. Regular exercise has shown benefits in improving physical capacity in COPD patients. Adherence to the regionally relevant vaccination schedule is also recommended to decrease the risk of infection.

General Treatment Strategies
Initial pharmacological treatment of COPD is determined by the severity of the patient's symptoms and the risk of exacerbation. Symptoms are monitored on a regular basis, and pharmacological therapy may be escalated or de-escalated. The 2023 GOLD guidelines recommend initial maintenance treatment as follows:

In patients who have had one or no moderate exacerbations (i.e., not leading to hospitalization):

- For those with an mMRC score of 0 – 1 or CAT score < 10, SABA, LABA, SAMA, or LAMA (long-acting preferred except in patients with very occasional symptoms).
- For those with an mMRC score of ≥ 2 or CAT score ≥ 10, LABA + LAMA.

In patients who have had two or more moderate exacerbations, or one or more exacerbations leading to hospitalization:

- LABA + LAMA; if blood eosinophils are ≥ 300 cells/μL, consider also adding an ICS.

For all patients, short-acting bronchodilators (SABAs and SAMAs) are used on an as-needed basis to manage episodic symptoms.

Follow-up treatment guidelines are based on the persistence of dyspnea and the occurrence of exacerbations. The provider should also note the patient's adherence, inhaler technique, and the impact of any comorbidities on their response to therapy. The 2023 GOLD report provides guidelines for the following persisting symptoms:

Dyspnea:

- Escalate to LABA + LAMA.
- If dyspnea is still problematic, consider:
    - Switching the inhaler drug(s) or inhaler device.
    - Implementing or escalating non-pharmacological treatments.
    - Investigating and treating other causes of dyspnea.

Exacerbations:

For patients with blood eosinophils < 300 cells/μL

- Escalate to LABA + LAMA.
- If there is an inadequate response to LABA + LAMA,
    - For patients with blood eosinophils < 100 cells/μL, initiate
        - ✓ Roflumilast in patients with FEV_1 < 50% of predicted and chronic bronchitis.
        - ✓ Azithromycin; best evidence is in current non-smokers.
    - For patients with blood eosinophils ≥ 100 cells/μL
        - Escalate from a single bronchodilator to LABA + LAMA + ICS.
        - If symptoms are not adequately controlled by LABA + LAMA + ICS, initiate
            - ✓ Roflumilast in patients with FEV_1 < 50% of predicted and chronic bronchitis.
            - ✓ Azithromycin; best evidence is in current non-smokers.

For patients with blood eosinophils ≥ 300 cells/μL

- Escalate to LABA + LAMA + ICS.
- If there is an inadequate response to LABA + LAMA + ICS, initiate
    - ✓ Roflumilast in patients with FEV_1 < 50% of predicted and chronic bronchitis.
    - ✓ Azithromycin; best evidence is in current non-smokers.

GOLD guidelines indicate that combination inhalers may be more convenient and effective than multiple drug therapy, and they suggest considering de-escalation of ICS if pneumonia or considerable adverse effects occur.

Drugs for Management of Asthma and COPD

The following drug classes, with few exceptions, are used in the treatment of asthma and COPD. The biologics are only indicated in the treatment of asthma, and roflumilast is only indicated in COPD.

β_2-adrenoceptor Agonists

Background

Inhaled short-acting β_2-adrenoceptor agonists (SABAs) are used to provide rapid relief of symptoms resulting from acute bronchoconstriction and are used as rescue medications within the context of asthma and COPD. Continuous inhalation of albuterol is used to treat status asthmaticus. Albuterol inhalation 15 – 30 minutes prior to exercise is indicated as prophylaxis for exercise-induced asthma. An epinephrine inhaler is available over-the-counter in the US for relief of mild intermittent asthma episodes in persons aged 12 years or older. Although this represents a cost-effective alternative to a physician visit and prescription drugs, self-management of asthma may result in inadequate symptom control and delayed treatment of exacerbations.

Inhaled long-acting β_2-adrenoceptor agonists (LABAs) are used as preventive/control medications for asthma and COPD. They are an add-on therapy for asthma that is not adequately controlled by ICS, but they are not used without a preventive medication (e.g., ICS) because this strategy is associated with an increased risk of asthma-related hospitalization and death. However, LABAs, alone or with LAMAs ± ICS, can be used as control therapy for COPD at all stages.

LABAs are not used as rescue medications for episodes of acute bronchoconstriction because their onset of action is often too slow, and their duration of action is too long. Formoterol, however, is an exception to this rule. A combination of formoterol + ICS (e.g., budesonide), used daily and on an as-needed basis, is the foundation of SMART therapy for asthma.

Pharmacokinetics
The SABAs produce relief of bronchoconstriction within 5 – 10 minutes. Following inhalation of albuterol aerosol, effects peak in 30 minutes – 2 hours and last for 2 – 6 hours. It is estimated that 90% of a dose from an albuterol aerosol inhaler is swallowed and absorbed via the GI tract, but less than 20% of a dose administered via a nebulizer is absorbed. For oral inhalation of levalbuterol, effects peak within 1.3 hours and last for 3 – 6 hours. Nebulized levalbuterol has a similar onset of action and time-to-peak effect, but the duration may be longer, from 5 – 8 hours.

The LABAs have varying onsets of action following inhalation, ranging from that of formoterol (1 – 3 minutes) and indacaterol (5 minutes) to that of olodaterol (20 minutes). All of the LABAs have longer half-lives than the SABAs. Very long-acting drugs, like indacaterol and olodaterol, have half-lives between 45-126 hours. Salmeterol and formoterol are dosed twice daily, and the other LABAs are given once a day.

Formoterol, which has the shortest half-life of the LABAs (10 hours), may be used in a combination product with an ICS as both preventive and rescue therapy (SMART). It can be used as a rescue drug because it has an onset of action at least as rapid as the SABAs, and its duration of action is shorter than that of the other LABAs. Various formulations of formoterol + ICS can be used up to 8 times/day for children aged 4 – 11, and 12 times/day for individuals aged 12 and older. Although indacaterol has a short onset of action which is comparable to that of albuterol, it is not used in SMART because of its long half-life.

Mechanism of Action
The SABAs and LABAs are moderately selective agonists of β_2-adrenoceptors. The binding of agonists to these receptors acts via the G_s protein to stimulate the activity of adenylyl cyclase, which converts ATP to cAMP, which in turn activates protein kinase A (PKA). PKA inactivates myosin light chain kinase by phosphorylation, resulting in less cross-bridging of myosin and actin, and therefore relaxation of the bronchial smooth muscle.

β_2-adrenoceptor agonists may also exert anti-inflammatory effects such as inhibition of mast cell degranulation, reduction of microvascular permeability, and stimulation of mucociliary function. These effects are not robust enough to allow LABAs to be used alone as asthma preventive/control medications. Concomitant use of an ICS is necessary for individuals with asthma, but not for those with COPD.

Adverse Effects, Contraindications, Drug Interactions
The adverse effects of the β_2-adrenoceptor agonists, when administered by inhalation, are much less severe than what is seen when drugs of this class are administered systemically. This is because the drug is delivered directly to the site of action, so the dose required is lower than would be needed if given via systemic administration. In addition, only a fraction of the inhaled drug is absorbed. With aerosol inhalers, most drug absorption is due to the drug being deposited in the mouth and swallowed, so the use of proper inhalation technique, a spacer chamber, and rinsing the mouth after drug dosing can minimize systemic absorption. However, because their selectivity for the β_2-adrenoceptor is not absolute, SABAs and LABAs can produce cardiovascular, nervous system, and metabolic adverse effects, particularly at higher doses. SABAs and LABAs can cause nervousness, tremor, tachycardia, QT interval prolongation, hyperglycemia, and hypokalemia.

LABAs are contraindicated as monotherapy for asthma. Caution should be used when β_2-adrenoceptor agonists are used in individuals who have conditions that may be worsened by their systemic effects (e.g., cardiac arrhythmia, diabetes). Although SABAs and LABAs can be used together, these drugs should not be used in conjunction with other drugs of the same class.

Muscarinic Antagonists
Background
Short-acting muscarinic antagonists (SAMAs) and long-acting muscarinic antagonists (LAMAs) are bronchodilators used in the treatment of asthma and COPD. In asthma, muscarinic antagonists are less effective as bronchodilators than are the β_2-adrenoceptor agonists. In COPD, muscarinic antagonists are as or more effective than β_2-adrenoceptor agonists.

One inhaled SAMA, ipratropium, is available in the US. Ipratropium carries an FDA-approved indication for the treatment of bronchospasm due to COPD. It is used off-label as a rescue inhaler for asthma in individuals who cannot tolerate SABAs, and as prophylaxis for exercise-induced asthma. A combination of ipratropium and albuterol can be used in COPD if additional symptom control is needed. This combination is used off-label for emergency management of asthma exacerbations.

LAMAs are commonly used as control medications for COPD. They may also be used as control medications in steps 3 – 5 of the NHLBI guidelines for the management of asthma; for this indication, they are used in combination with ICS or with ICS + LABA.

Pharmacokinetics
The onset of action of ipratropium is 15 – 30 minutes, and the time to peak effect is 1 – 2 hours. Ipratropium's onset of action is considerably slower than that of the SABAs, so it is not a preferred choice as a rescue inhaler for asthma. Ipratropium is minimally absorbed from the lung and the GI tract, so little systemic exposure occurs following oral inhalation. The duration of action of ipratropium is 4 – 5 hours.

All of the LAMAs, with the exception of aclidinium and glycopyrrolate, have durations of action that allow once-daily dosing. Aclidinium and glycopyrrolate are dosed twice a day. Glycopyrrolate is approximately 40% absorbed following inhalation; the other LAMAs are minimally absorbed from the lung and GI tract.

Mechanism of Action
The binding of ACh to M_3 receptors in the lung stimulates signaling via the G_q-PLC-IP_3-Ca^{2+} pathway, which culminates in the contraction of bronchial smooth muscle and stimulation of tracheobronchial mucus secretion. ACh is released by parasympathetic neurons, which regulate bronchomotor tone, but it is also secreted by airway epithelial cells, and this process is up-regulated under conditions of inflammation.

The SAMAs and LAMAs have traditionally been classified as competitive antagonists of muscarinic receptors; however, many have been found to be inverse agonists. Their beneficial effect on the lung stems from their ability to block the effect of ACh on M_3 receptors. Inverse agonists also reverse the effect of constitutive M_3 activation. In addition to blocking M_3 receptors, ipratropium has some ability to block neuronal M_2 receptors, which function as inhibitory autoreceptors on cholinergic nerves. Because of this, ipratropium can potentially enhance ACh release from the vagal nerve endings of the lung, counteracting its bronchodilator effect. The LAMAs exhibit higher selectivity for M_3 receptors and are not subject to this concern.

Adverse Effects, Contraindications, Drug Interactions
Because the muscarinic antagonists are administered by inhalation, and because all except glycopyrrolate are minimally absorbed, adverse effects are usually localized. Dry mouth results from the deposition of drug particles in the mouth and subsequent blockade of M_3 receptors on the salivary glands. Pharyngeal irritation/cough results from drug particle deposition in the throat. If the drug deposits on the cornea during nebulizer use, an increase in intraocular pressure can occur. Urinary retention has occasionally been reported, particularly in high-dose administration and in elderly patients.

LAMAs should not be used as rescue drugs. Muscarinic antagonists should be used cautiously or avoided in individuals who have conditions that may be worsened by them (e.g., glaucoma, bladder obstruction).

Because systemic exposure to inhaled muscarinic antagonists is low, drug interactions are unlikely. The use of multiple LAMAs should be avoided. Systemically administered anticholinergic drugs may worsen SAMA and LAMA adverse effects such as xerostomia.

Corticosteroids
Background
ICS are the cornerstone of anti-inflammatory management in asthma and COPD. They are drugs of choice for use as control medications in all stages of persistent asthma, and they are used in conjunction with a LABA and a LAMA to decrease the risk of exacerbations in individuals with corticosteroid-sensitive COPD. Most studies have shown that an ICS alone does not significantly slow disease progression in COPD. It is of note that ICS use in COPD is associated with an increased risk of pneumonia. In individuals who experience this effect, de-escalating or deprescribing ICS should be considered.

Systemically administered corticosteroids are used as a short-term treatment in patients experiencing severe asthma or COPD exacerbations. Oral corticosteroids are used in the management of severe persistent asthma (step 6) but are to be avoided if possible due to their significant adverse effects.

The pharmacokinetics, mechanism of action, adverse effects, contraindications, and interactions of the corticosteroids are described in Chapter 4.

Anti-Leukotriene Drugs: Leukotriene Receptor Antagonists (LTRAs) and Leukotriene Synthesis Inhibitors
Background
The binding of cysteinyl leukotrienes to CysLT receptors has been associated with asthma pathophysiology, including chemoattraction of eosinophils, stimulation of inflammatory mediators, increased endothelial membrane permeability leading to airway edema, smooth muscle contraction, and enhanced secretion of thick, viscous mucus. Antileukotriene drugs diminish the signs and symptoms of asthma by inhibiting the physiologic actions resulting from the binding of

LTD_4 to the $CysLT_1$ receptor. Clinically, the drug has been shown to inhibit early- and late-phase bronchoconstriction due to antigen challenge.

LTRAs are an alternate preventive/control medication for asthma; zileuton, a leukotriene synthesis inhibitor, is indicated for individuals aged 12 and older. LTRAs and zileuton are also used as prophylaxis for exercise-induced asthma. For this indication, they are given at least two hours prior to exercise.

The pharmacokinetics, mechanism of action, and adverse effects of the LTRAs are described in Chapter 4. The corresponding information below pertains to zileuton.

Pharmacokinetics
Following oral administration, absorption of zileuton is rapid, and first-pass metabolism via dihydroxylation to an inactive metabolite occurs in the intestine. Zileuton is a substrate and inhibitor of hepatic CYP1A2. Zileuton is a substrate of CYP3A4 and may compete with other CYP3A4 substrates to inhibit their metabolism. Zileuton is highly bound to plasma protein. Excretion is mainly renal, as the glucuronide.

Mechanism of Action
Zileuton is a selective inhibitor of 5-lipoxygenase, which catalyzes the conversion of arachidonic acid to 5-HPETE, the first compound in the leukotriene synthesis pathway. Administration of zileuton results in reduced levels of leukotrienes.

Adverse Effects, Contraindications, Drug Interactions
Most adverse effects of zileuton are mild and self-limited; however, an increase in liver enzymes can be seen up to approximately five times more frequently than in control patients. Liver enzymes usually return to baseline within a month of discontinuation. Cases of severe liver injury, including life-threatening liver injury and death, have been reported in post-marketing use of the drug. Liver function tests should be performed prior to initiating zileuton therapy and then monthly for three months, every two to three months for the remainder of the year, and periodically thereafter. Zileuton should be discontinued if the patient experiences hepatic transaminase elevations greater than 5 times the upper limit of normal or if signs of liver dysfunction (jaundice, etc.) develop. Zileuton is contraindicated in active liver disease or with persistent hepatic transaminase elevations 3 or more times the upper limit of normal.

Zileuton, like the LTRAs, is associated with neuropsychiatric events, including suicidal thoughts and behaviors, and should be avoided in people with these conditions.

Mast Cell Stabilizers
Mast cell stabilizers, also known as chromones or cromones, are an alternative choice as a preventive/control medication for asthma. Their safety profile makes them a reasonable choice for use in children who demonstrate a response to them. Cromolyn sodium is the only pure mast cell stabilizing drug currently available in the US, where it is available as a solution for nebulization. The pharmacokinetics, mechanism of action, and adverse effects of cromolyn are described in Chapter 4.

Anti-IgE Antibodies
Background
Allergic asthma is characterized by high levels of circulating IgE directed against the allergens that the patient is sensitized to. Omalizumab is a humanized murine monoclonal antibody (IgG) directed against human IgE; it is the only drug of this class available in the US. It is indicated as an add-on preventive therapy for patients 6 years of age or older who have moderate to severe persistent allergic asthma that is not well-controlled with an ICS, and in whom testing has revealed positive reactivity to a perennial aeroallergen. It has been shown to reduce the frequency and severity of asthma exacerbations and to allow for a reduction in corticosteroid dose.

IgE binds to the high-affinity IgE Fc receptor (FcεRI), which is found on mast cells and basophils, and the low-affinity IgE Fc receptor (FcεRII, CD23), which is found on monocytes, macrophages, eosinophils, dendritic cells, epithelial cells, platelets, and others. The binding of IgE to FcεRI on mast cells is the first step in allergic/immune responses. Antigen binding/cross-linking of two membrane-bound IgE molecules activates the mast cells, resulting in the release of histamine and other inflammatory mediators (degranulation).

Pharmacokinetics
Omalizumab is administered by subcutaneous injection once every four weeks. Once injected, it enters the bloodstream and forms complexes with IgE molecules. Omalizumab and omalizumab-IgE complexes are cleared by mechanisms that clear IgG, e.g., degradation by the hepatic reticuloendothelial system (RES). The serum elimination half-life of omalizumab averages 26 days.

Mechanism of Action
Omalizumab is a monoclonal antibody directed against IgE. Complexes of omalizumab-IgE are rapidly eliminated from the bloodstream, reducing free serum IgE levels by more than 90%. A decrease in IgE binding to the FcεRI on mast cells inhibits the early phase of the allergic response. Importantly, omalizumab does not cross-link IgE that is already bound to its receptor, so it does not stimulate mast cell degranulation.

Omalizumab inhibits the late phase of the allergic response by displacing IgE from FcεRII on monocytes, eosinophils, dendritic cells, epithelial cells, and platelets, so the release of inflammatory mediators and cytokines by these cells is diminished. Over time, a lack of IgE bound to the Fc receptors causes these receptors to be internalized and degraded.

Adverse Effects, Contraindications, Drug Interactions
The most serious adverse effect noted with omalizumab is the potential for anaphylaxis. This can occur immediately following the first dose or after multiple doses. Approximately 60 – 70% of cases of anaphylaxis occur within the first three doses, and symptoms can develop more than 2 hours after drug administration. Because of this, it is recommended that omalizumab is administered in a healthcare setting that is equipped to treat anaphylaxis.

Injection site reactions are common and sometimes severe. There have been post-marketing reports of a serum sickness-like reaction occurring within 1 – 5 days of drug administration. Symptoms include rash or hives, fever, arthralgia, and lymphadenopathy. Initiation of omalizumab while decreasing the dose of an oral corticosteroid can precipitate Churg-Strauss syndrome.

Omalizumab should not be used in patients who experienced a hypersensitivity reaction to it, and it should be used cautiously in patients allergic to hamster proteins, as it is produced in Chinese hamster ovary cells. Corticosteroid therapy should not be abruptly discontinued when omalizumab is initiated. Individuals who live in areas where helminth infections are common should be treated for existing infections and monitored for new infections since IgE is an essential part of helminth defense. Although the risk is low, patients should be monitored for the development of malignancies, and it should be used cautiously in patients with existing malignancies. Individuals who are taking omalizumab may have a diminished response to vaccination.

Anti-IL-5 Antibodies
Background
Th2 inflammatory profiles are seen in most people who have severe asthma. IL-5 is one of the cytokines released by Th2 cells; it stimulates eosinophil recruitment, proliferation, maturation, and survival, resulting in eosinophilic inflammation in the airways. Mepolizumab and reslizumab are humanized monoclonal antibodies directed against IL-5, and benralizumab is a humanized antibody directed against the IL-5 receptor found on eosinophils, IL-5Rα. Each of these drugs is indicated as an add-on control therapy for individuals with severe eosinophilic asthma. These drugs have been shown to decrease the frequency of asthma exacerbations and reduce corticosteroid requirements. Mepolizumab has additional indications for the treatment of Churg-Strauss syndrome and hypereosinophilic syndrome.

Mepolizumab is indicated for use in individuals aged 6 or older, benralizumab in individuals 12 and older, and reslizumab in adults only. Reslizumab is not approved for use in individuals under the age of 18 because its initial clinical trial showed a 2-fold increase in the asthma exacerbation rate in that population.

Pharmacokinetics
Benralizumab is given SC every 4 weeks for the first three doses, then every 8 weeks thereafter. Mepolizumab is given SC every 4 weeks., and reslizumab is administered by IV infusion every 4 weeks.

The anti-IL-5 antibodies are eliminated by proteolytic enzymes in the liver and throughout the body. The half-life is 16 – 22 days for mepolizumab, 15.5 days for benralizumab, and 24 hours for reslizumab.

Mechanism of Action
Mepolizumab and reslizumab bind circulating IL-5 and prevent its interaction with its receptors. Benralizumab binds the IL-5Rα, preventing its interaction with IL-5. These actions prevent eosinophil recruitment, proliferation, maturation, and survival.

Adverse Effects, Contraindications, Drug Interactions
The most common adverse effects of the anti-IL5 antibodies are injection site reactions. Hypersensitivity reactions and antibody formation to the drug have been documented with all three anti-IL-5 agents. Anaphylaxis has been seen at a high enough frequency with reslizumab that it is recommended to be administered in a healthcare setting that is equipped to treat this emergency. An increase in new primary malignancy was noted in clinical trials of reslizumab. Herpes zoster and other opportunistic infections have been seen in patients taking mepolizumab.

Each anti-IL-5 antibody is contraindicated in individuals who have experienced a hypersensitivity response to it. Caution should be used with mepolizumab and benralizumab in people who are sensitive to hamster proteins. Corticosteroid therapy should not be abruptly discontinued when an anti-IL-5 antibody is initiated. Individuals who live in areas where helminth infections are common should be treated for existing infections and monitored for new infections. If a new helminth infection develops, the anti-IL-5 agent should be discontinued until the infection is treated and resolved. Individuals who are taking anti-IL-5 antibodies may have a diminished response to vaccination.

IL-4 Receptor Antagonists

Background

IL-4 and IL-13 are cytokines involved in pathological processes of asthma and other atopic diseases. IL-4 is produced by Th2 cells and basophils. It activates macrophages and eosinophils and causes B lymphocytes to undergo isotype switching to IgE synthesis. IL-13 promotes goblet cell hyperplasia and mucus hypersecretion; it also stimulates smooth muscle cell and fibroblast proliferation, resulting in airway remodeling.

Dupilumab is a monoclonal antibody directed against the IL-4Rα subunit that is a component of the IL-4 and IL-13 receptors. It is indicated as an add-on control therapy for individuals over age 12 who have severe eosinophilic asthma. It has been shown to reduce the incidence of exacerbations and improve lung function in these individuals. It is also used to treat moderate to severe atopic dermatitis, chronic rhinosinusitis with nasal polyps, eosinophilic esophagitis, and prurigo nodularis.

Pharmacokinetics

Dupilumab is administered SC every other week. It exhibits nonlinear target-mediated pharmacokinetics and is believed to be eliminated via similar proteolytic pathways as IgG.

Mechanism of Action

Dupilumab is a human monoclonal IgG4 antibody directed against the IL-4Rα subunit of the IL-4 and IL-13 receptors. It blocks the binding of IL-4 and IL-13 to their respective receptors and prevents the inflammatory responses that they produce.

Adverse Effects, Contraindications, Drug Interactions

Injection site reaction is the most common adverse effect of dupilumab. Serious hypersensitivity reactions, including anaphylaxis, and the development of anti-drug antibodies, have been reported. Conjunctivitis and eosinophilia have been seen in a small percentage of patients treated with the drug. Eosinophilic granulomatosis with polyangiitis has been reported in asthmatic patients treated with dupilumab.

Patients who have experienced hypersensitivity to dupilumab should discontinue treatment. Caution should be used in people who have hypersensitivity to hamster proteins. Individuals who live in areas where helminth infections are common should be treated for existing infections and monitored for new infections. If a new helminth infection develops and fails to respond to treatment, dupilumab should be discontinued until the infection resolves.

Anti-Thymic Stromal Lymphopoietin (TSLP) Antibodies

Background

TSLP is a pleotropic cytokine secreted by epithelial cells. In the lung, it is released by bronchial epithelial cells in response to allergens and infectious, chemical, and physical insults. It is an upstream regulator that acts on a broad range of immune cells, such as dendritic cells, B cells, eosinophils, basophils, mast cells, innate type II cells, $CD4^+$ T cells, $CD8^+$ T cells, and natural killer T cells. It also acts on smooth muscle cells. TSLP is associated with the Th2 response. Elevated levels of this protein are found in the lungs of people with asthma, and its levels correlate with disease severity.

The high-affinity TSLP receptor is a heterodimer consisting of the IL-7Rα chain paired with a TSLP-specific receptor component, TSLPR. Activation of this receptor initiates a JAK-STAT pathway that results in pro-inflammatory signaling. Tezepelumab is a human monoclonal IgG2λ that binds TSLP and prevents its interaction with its receptors. It is indicated as an add-on control medication for individuals over age 12 who have severe asthma of any endotype. Patients treated with tezepelumab show a decreased incidence of asthma exacerbation as compared to control patients.

Pharmacokinetics

Tezepelumab is administered SC every 4 weeks. It is eliminated by proteolytic degradation in the liver and throughout the body, with an elimination half-life of 26 days.

Mechanism of Action

Tezepelumab binds to TSLP and prevents its interaction with its receptor. This blocks the wide variety of downstream processes that are associated with inflammatory responses in asthma. Decreases in blood and airway eosinophils, IgE, FeNO, IL-5, and IL-13 are seen following the administration of tezepelumab.

Adverse Effects, Contraindications, Drug Interactions
Hypersensitivity reactions have occurred in response to tezepelumab. Other adverse effects include pharyngitis, arthralgia, and back pain. Antibodies to the drug have been noted in some patients.

Tezepelumab is contraindicated in patients who have experienced hypersensitivity to it. It should be used cautiously in individuals with hamster protein hypersensitivity. Corticosteroids should not be abruptly discontinued upon initiation of tezepelumab. Patients with pre-existing helminth infections should be treated before initiating tezepelumab. If a helminth infection does not respond to treatment, tezepelumab should be discontinued until the infection is resolved. It is recommended that patients should not receive live attenuated virus vaccines during treatment with tezepelumab.

Methylxanthines
Background
Theophylline and aminophylline are seldom-used control medications for asthma and COPD. This is because their effectiveness is lower than that of currently recommended drugs (e.g., ICS, LABAs, LAMAs), and their safety profile is undesirable. Occasionally these drugs are used in patients whose disease is not controlled by first-line therapy.

Pharmacokinetics
Theophylline is given PO, and aminophylline, a prodrug salt of theophylline, is given IV. Since 100 mg of aminophylline is equivalent to 80 mg of theophylline, errors in dosing are possible when switching between the forms. Theophylline is metabolized mainly by CYP1A2, and secondarily by CYP2E1 and CYP3A4. Its half-life varies according to patient variables such as age, hepatic function, smoking status, and drug interactions. The half-life of theophylline in nonsmoking adults is 6.5—10.5 hours. The elimination of theophylline is usually first-order, but zero-order elimination has been seen in some individuals.

Mechanism of Action
Theophylline demonstrates bronchodilator, anti-inflammatory, and immunomodulatory actions, but the mechanisms by which it produces these effects are not completely clear. While it was initially believed that theophylline acts as a PDE4 inhibitor, resulting in inhibition of the breakdown of cAMP, this effect is not seen at usual serum concentrations. The antagonism of adenosine receptors has been proposed as a mechanism by which theophylline produces bronchodilation, but some evidence contradicts this hypothesis. The CNS stimulatory effects of theophylline may be explained by adenosine receptor antagonism.

Adverse Effects, Contraindications, Drug Interactions
The therapeutic window of the methylxanthines is small; adverse effects are significant at high therapeutic doses. It is recommended that physicians should monitor theophylline levels in patients who are taking this drug to maintain peak levels between 10 – 15 mcg/mL. Common adverse effects of theophylline include nausea/vomiting, diarrhea, anxiety, insomnia, tremors, and headaches; at high serum concentrations, rhabdomyolysis, tachycardia, cardiac arrhythmia, hypokalemia, hyperglycemia, seizures, and death can occur. Theophylline toxicity occurs at lower serum concentrations when it has been taken chronically than in a situation of acute overdose.

Theophylline should be used cautiously in any condition that could be worsened by its adverse effects, e.g., cardiovascular disease and GI disease. There are many physiological interactions that can occur between theophylline and other drugs that produce one or more of its adverse effects. Given its narrow therapeutic window, the potential for CYP-mediated interactions should also be noted.

Roflumilast
Background
Roflumilast is a PDE4 inhibitor that is approved as an add-on control medication for patients with severe COPD involving chronic bronchitis, who have a history of exacerbations. It has been shown to modestly improve lung function and reduce the number of exacerbations. A topical formulation of roflumilast is used in the treatment of plaque psoriasis.

Pharmacokinetics
Following oral administration, roflumilast is highly bound to plasma protein. It undergoes metabolism by CYP3A4 and CYP1A2 to produce an N-oxide metabolite with 1/3 the activity of the parent drug, but with a longer half-life (30 hours) than the parent drug (17 hours). Most of the parent drug and its metabolite are excreted in the urine.

Mechanism of Action
Roflumilast and its N-oxide metabolite are selective inhibitors of PDE4, an enzyme that hydrolyzes and inactivates cAMP; inhibition of PDE4 results in an intracellular accumulation of cAMP. The mechanisms by which roflumilast may counteract the pathophysiology of COPD include inhibiting the release of reactive oxygen species from

neutrophils and eosinophils, blocking the epithelial to mesenchymal transition (inhibiting fibrosis), improving mucociliary function, and reducing the secretion of pro-inflammatory cytokines such as IL-8, IL-17, and TNF-α.

Adverse Effects, Contraindications, Drug Interactions

Psychiatric adverse effects, such as anxiety, insomnia, depression, and suicidal ideation are sometimes seen in roflumilast-treated patients. GI adverse effects such as nausea, anorexia, and diarrhea are common, and weight loss has been reported in up to 20% of patients. A patient's weight should be monitored while taking roflumilast, and the drug discontinued in cases of loss of more than 10% of body weight.

Roflumilast is contraindicated in patients with moderate to severe hepatic disease. It should be used cautiously, if at all, in individuals with psychiatric diseases that may be worsened by it. Drug interactions may occur if roflumilast is given with inducers or inhibitors of CYP3A4 or CYP1A2.

References

Bisgaard H, Bønnelykke K. Long-term studies of the natural history of asthma in childhood. J Allergy Clin Immunol. 2010 Aug;126(2):187-97; quiz 198-9. doi: 10.1016/j.jaci.2010.07.011. PMID: 20688204.

Christenson SA, Smith BM, Bafadhel M, Putcha N. Chronic obstructive pulmonary disease. Lancet. 2022 Jun 11;399(10342):2227-2242. doi: 10.1016/S0140-6736(22)00470-6. Epub 2022 May 6. PMID: 35533707.

Duffy SP, Criner GJ. Chronic Obstructive Pulmonary Disease: Evaluation and Management. Med Clin North Am. 2019 May;103(3):453-461. doi: 10.1016/j.mcna.2018.12.005. Epub 2019 Mar 14. PMID: 30955513.

Expert Panel Working Group of the National Heart, Lung, and Blood Institute (NHLBI) administered and coordinated National Asthma Education and Prevention Program Coordinating Committee (NAEPPCC). 2020 Focused Updates to the Asthma Management Guidelines: A Report from the National Asthma Education and Prevention Program Coordinating Committee Expert Panel Working Group. J Allergy Clin Immunol. 2020 Dec;146(6):1217-1270. doi: 10.1016/j.jaci.2020.10.003. Erratum in: J Allergy Clin Immunol. 2021 Apr;147(4):1528-1530. PMID: 33280709; PMCID: PMC7924476.

Gans MD, Gavrilova T. Understanding the immunology of asthma: Pathophysiology, biomarkers, and treatments for asthma endotypes. Paediatr Respir Rev. 2020 Nov;36:118-127. doi: 10.1016/j.prrv.2019.08.002. Epub 2019 Oct 9. PMID: 31678040.

Global Initiative for Asthma (GINA). 2022 GINA Report, Global Strategy for Asthma Management and Prevention. Available at: https://ginasthma.org/wp-content/uploads/2022/07/GINA-Main-Report-2022-FINAL-22-07-01-WMS.pdf.

Global Initiative for Chronic Obstructive Lung Disease (GOLD). Global Strategy for the Diagnosis, Management and Prevention of Chronic Obstructive Pulmonary Disease: 2023. Available at: https://goldcopd.org/wp-content/uploads/2022/12/GOLD-2023-ver-1.1-2Dec2022_WMV.pdf.

Global Initiative for Chronic Obstructive Lung Disease (GOLD). Pocket Guide to COPD Diagnosis, Management, and Prevention, A Guide for Health Care Professionals, 2023 Edition. Available at: https://goldcopd.org/wp-content/uploads/2022/12/POCKET-GUIDE-GOLD-2023-ver-1.1-2Dec2022_WMV.pdf.

Kraïm-Leleu M, Lesage FX, Drame M, Lebargy F, Deschamps F. Occupational Risk Factors for COPD: A Case-Control Study. PLoS One. 2016 Aug 3;11(8):e0158719. doi: 10.1371/journal.pone.0158719. PMID: 27487078; PMCID: PMC4972406.

Silverman EK. Genetics of COPD. Annu Rev Physiol. 2020 Feb 10;82:413-431. doi: 10.1146/annurev-physiol-021317-121224. Epub 2019 Nov 15. PMID: 31730394; PMCID: PMC7193187.

Yang IA, Jenkins CR, Salvi SS. Chronic obstructive pulmonary disease in never-smokers: risk factors, pathogenesis, and implications for prevention and treatment. Lancet Respir Med. 2022 May;10(5):497-511. doi: 10.1016/S2213-2600(21)00506-3. Epub 2022 Apr 12. PMID: 35427530.

Quiz Questions

1. A 14-year-old boy has persistent asthma that has not been well controlled with daily inhaled medium-dose budesonide and as-needed (PRN) albuterol. His physician wants to change his therapy to a formoterol + budesonide combination inhaler to be used once daily, and any time the boy feels an episode of bronchoconstriction beginning. The boy's mother, a pharmacy technician, recognizes that formoterol belongs to the same class of drugs as the inhaler her father uses for COPD, indacaterol. She asks the physician why the boy can't use budesonide and indacaterol inhalers together whenever he experiences acute bronchoconstriction. What should the physician tell her?

A While indacaterol acts as rapidly as other rescue drugs, its duration of action is too long to be used for this purpose
B While indacaterol has a short duration of action similar to other rescue drugs, its onset of action is too slow
C Indacaterol is actually used in this manner, but it is not available in a convenient combination inhaler
D Indacaterol should not be used with budesonide because they have the same mechanism of action
E Indacaterol inhibits long bone growth and should not be used until an individual's adult size is reached

2. A 65-year-old man who has COPD experiences frequent exacerbations of his chronic bronchitis despite adherence to a protocol of daily LABA + LAMA, plus a rescue inhaler when needed. The man's FEV_1 is 45% of that predicted for his age, he is a current 1 pack/day smoker, and his blood eosinophil count is 85 cells/μL. A drug with what mechanism of action would be the most reasonable choice to decrease his exacerbations?

A Short-acting antagonism of muscarinic receptors
B Inhibition of phosphodiesterase 4 (PDE4)
C Short-acting agonism of β_2 adrenoceptors
D Agonism of the glucocorticoid receptor (GR)
E Inhibition of binding of IL-4 and IL-13 to their receptors

3. A 21-year-old warehouse worker has asthma. He has been self-medicating with an over-the-counter epinephrine inhaler, but he has run out of it and does not have money to buy another. The next time he has an asthma attack, he uses his roommate's fluticasone inhaler as a regular rescue inhaler. What is expected to occur?

A He will experience relief of bronchospasm, but likely after 15 minutes rather than 5
B He will be likely to develop oral candidiasis but will experience rapid relief
C He will experience drug-induced worsening of his bronchospastic episode
D He will experience a faster and more complete relief of bronchospasm
E He will continue to experience bronchospasm despite his use of the drug

4. A 25-year-old man complains of chest tightness and difficulty breathing whenever he exercises. His physical exam and spirometry are normal at rest, but upon exercise challenge, he experiences a decrease in the FEV_1/FVC ratio which is completely reversed by the administration of inhaled albuterol. Which of the following drugs would be most useful to control his respiratory symptoms if it is to be administered 15 – 30 minutes before exercise?

A Omalizumab
B Montelukast
C Albuterol
D Salmeterol
E Fluticasone

5. A 29-year-old sheep farmer has been suffering from severe eosinophilic asthma since the age of eight. She has been hospitalized for asthma exacerbations four times in the past two years, and she needs to use her albuterol inhaler several times per day. In order to alleviate the severity and symptoms of her asthma, the farmer's pulmonologist prescribes a drug that is a monoclonal antibody directed against IL-5. What counseling should the farmer receive?

A Wear sunscreen or a hat/long sleeves/pants to prevent photosensitivity from the drug
B Get regular screening for infections with worms, which this drug and your occupation put you at risk of
C Return for regular checkups on your heart rate and rhythm because this drug can affect them
D Liver function tests will need to be performed monthly for the first three months you are on this drug
E You are likely to produce excessive levels of antibodies from any vaccines that you receive

Quiz Answers

1. A. Indacaterol has an onset of action of 1 – 3 minutes, so that does not prevent it from being used as a rescue drug; however, it has a very long half-life (days), so it cannot be dosed multiple times per day on an as-needed basis. It only holds FDA approval for the treatment of COPD, not asthma, and it is not commonly used off-label for asthma. B is incorrect because indacaterol's onset of action is fast, and its duration is long. C is incorrect because indacaterol is not used in SMART protocols for the reasons above. D is incorrect because indacaterol is a LABA, and budesonide is an ICS. E is incorrect because indacaterol does not inhibit long bone growth.

2. B. Roflumilast is a PDE4 inhibitor that is indicated for COPD patients who have chronic bronchitis and experience exacerbations despite appropriate initial therapy. A is incorrect because that is the mechanism of SAMAs, which are rescue medications used in COPD, not control medications to reduce exacerbations. C describes the mechanism of action of SABAs, which are rescue medications. D describes the mechanism of action of corticosteroids. This choice is incorrect because this patient has a blood eosinophil count of less than 100 cells/μL, so he is not likely to benefit from ICS. E is incorrect because it is the mechanism of action of dupilumab, a drug that is indicated as an add-on control medication for decreasing exacerbations in people with severe eosinophilic asthma.

3. E. Fluticasone is an ICS and is to be used only as a control or preventive drug, not as a rescue medication. It does not act as a bronchodilator and will not relieve his symptoms. A would be more characteristic if the man used a LABA such as salmeterol as a rescue medication. It would produce bronchodilation, but much slower than albuterol or epinephrine. B is incorrect because candidiasis develops after multiple dosing of an ICS, and the ICS will not cause immediate relief. C is incorrect because although the ICS would not help, it is not likely to cause bronchospasm. D is incorrect because the ICS will not produce rapid relief of bronchospasm.

4. C is correct. Albuterol can be administered via inhalation 15 – 30 minutes before exercise as prophylaxis for exercise-induced asthma. A is incorrect because omalizumab is an add-on control therapy for moderate to severe allergic asthma. B is incorrect because although montelukast can be used as prophylaxis for exercise-induced asthma, it is orally administered and must be taken at least 2 hours before exercise. D is incorrect because salmeterol is a LABA, so it is indicated as a control medication for asthma. E is incorrect because fluticasone is indicated as control medication, and is administered on a daily basis for this indication, not as acute prophylaxis 15 – 30 minutes before exercise.

5. B is the correct answer. The anti-IL-5 antibodies, benralizumab, mepolizumab, and reslizumab inhibit IgE production. Since IgE is the major protective mechanism against helminths, and this woman's job as a livestock farmer potentially exposes her to helminth infection, she should be monitored for infections with worms. A is incorrect because the anti-IL-5 antibodies do not cause photosensitivity. C is an adverse effect of the methylxanthines, which can cause tachycardia and other arrhythmias. D is an adverse effect of zileuton, which can cause elevations in liver transaminases and hepatic damage. Zafirlukast, an LTRA described in Chapter 4, can also cause transaminase elevations. E is incorrect because a diminished response to vaccination, not an excessive response, may result from the use of the anti-IL-5 antibodies.

CHAPTER 6

COUGH AND EXCESSIVE MUCUS

LEAH HAMMER, PHD AND KAREN WOODFORK, PHD

West Virginia University, Morgantown, West Virginia, USA

Symptoms: Immuno-Infectious
Cardio-Renal-Respiratory

The authors dedicate this chapter to the late Dr. Elizabeth E. Davis. Dr. Davis was a friend, mentor, and *de facto* family to Dr. Hammer. To both authors, she was a dedicated pharmacology educator and colleague. With every word that we write, she is remembered.

DRUG LIST FOR COUGH AND EXCESSIVE MUCUS

Antitussives

Benzonatate	Antitussive, non-opioid, PO
Chlophedianol	Antitussive, non-opioid, PO
Codeine	Antitussive, opioid, PO
Dextromethorphan	Antitussive, non-opioid, PO
Dihydrocodeine	Antitussive, opioid, PO
Diphenhydramine	H_1 antihistamine, first generation, PO
Hydrocodone	Antitussive, opioid, PO

Expectorants

Guaifenesin	Mucoactive agent, expectorant, PO
Hypertonic saline	Mucoactive agent, expectorant, inhalation
Mannitol	Mucoactive agent, expectorant, inhalation

Mucolytics

N-acetylcysteine	Mucoactive agent, mucolytic, inhalation, PO, IV
Dornase alpha	Mucoactive agent, mucolytic, inhalation

Cystic Fibrosis Transmembrane Conductance Regulator (CFTR) Modulators

Elexacaftor	CFTR corrector (only available in combination with ivacaftor and tezacaftor), PO
Ivacaftor	CFTR potentiator, PO
Lumacaftor	CFTR corrector (only available in combination with ivacaftor), PO
Tezacaftor	CFTR corrector (only available in combination with ivacaftor, or with elexacaftor and ivacaftor), PO

Pulmonary Surfactants

Beractant	Pulmonary surfactant (bovine), intratracheal
Calfactant	Pulmonary surfactant (bovine), intratracheal
Lucinactant	Pulmonary surfactant (synthetic), intratracheal
Poractant alpha	Pulmonary surfactant (porcine), intratracheal

General Background

Cough and excessive respiratory mucus (sputum) production are symptoms of a wide variety of conditions ranging from relatively mild infections like the common cold, to potentially life-threatening disorders such as cystic fibrosis (CF), severe infections, and cancer. When assessing cough, it is important to investigate the underlying cause and exclude serious conditions which require acute management rather than simply control of cough and mucus production.

Diagnosis

The diagnostic criteria for the many conditions that can produce a cough are too extensive to completely document in a single chapter; instead, an overview of the most common conditions will be presented.

Presentation
Cough can be classified as acute (less than 3 weeks duration), subacute (between 3 – 8 weeks), and chronic (greater than 8 weeks duration). The most common causes of acute cough are acute viral upper respiratory infection (URI, the common cold) and acute bronchitis, which is most often viral but can be bacterial in about 10% of cases. Other infectious causes of acute cough include acute rhinosinusitis, pneumonia, and pertussis. Non-infectious causes of acute cough include asthma (Chapter 5), acute exacerbations of chronic obstructive pulmonary disorder (COPD; Chapter 5), allergic rhinitis (Chapter 4), congestive heart failure (Chapter 11), pulmonary embolism, and aspiration.

When acute cough is caused by infection (Chapter 3), it will likely be accompanied by additional symptoms such as fever, malaise, and/or myalgia. Acute rhinosinusitis may present with a cough that occurs in response to increased nasal mucus production and postnasal drip. It is generally considered to be viral in origin if it has been present for less than 10 days but is more likely to be bacterial if present for more than 10 days. Pneumonia may be viral or bacterial in origin (Chapter 3). Viral pneumonia generally presents with a gradual onset of symptoms, a lower fever, a lack of purulent sputum, and may have a prodrome of viral URI. In contrast, bacterial pneumonia tends to have a more sudden onset, a higher fever, and significant production of mucus and purulent secretions. Pertussis (whooping cough) is characterized by bloody, purulent sputum and episodes of coughing lasting for up to several minutes, followed by a loud gasp for air. Pertussis lasts up to six weeks and consists of three phases, the catarrhal phase (low fever, sneezing, nasal congestion), the paroxysmal phase (classic coughing episodes followed by vomiting), and the convalescent phase (chronic cough).

When an acute cough is non-infectious in nature, symptoms stem from the pathophysiology of the disease. Asthma involves airway inflammation and hyperreactivity resulting in episodes of bronchoconstriction, causing wheezing. Cough is initiated by increased mucus and edema of the airways. COPD involves two conditions: chronic bronchitis, which is characterized by mucus hypersecretion and small airway obstruction, and emphysema, which involves the destruction of the alveolar septa and reduced surface area for gas exchange. Acute exacerbations of COPD most commonly result from acute bronchitis or bacterial pneumonia, but they can also develop following exposure to allergens, air pollutants, or other irritants. In an acute exacerbation of COPD, the patient experiences increased pulmonary inflammation and airway hyperresponsiveness, resulting in bronchoconstriction and accumulation of purulent, thick mucus in the bronchioles and alveoli, which initiates cough. In allergic rhinitis, cough is initiated by increased nasal mucus secretion and post-nasal drip, resulting in airway irritation. Cough in the context of acute congestive heart failure results when left ventricular failure causes blood to back up in the pulmonary vasculature, resulting in pulmonary edema, which stimulates cough. Other symptoms of left ventricular failure include shortness of breath (often on exertion), orthopnea, peripheral and/or abdominal edema (ascites), and right upper quadrant pain due to hepatic congestion. An embolus lodged in a pulmonary artery will produce cough in a manner similar to that of left ventricular failure, but in this case, pulmonary edema results from blood backing up in the vessels proximal to the embolus. Aspiration of food or liquid into the airways causes irritation, resulting in cough, and may also initiate infection (aspiration pneumonia).

Subacute cough is most commonly a post-infectious process in which inflammation from one of the infectious processes described above is still present. Subacute cough is generally self-limiting and disappears as the illness resolves.

Chronic cough can result from a variety of conditions. Upper airway cough syndrome is a common cause of chronic cough. Here, chronic postnasal drip, usually resulting from allergic or non-allergic rhinitis, rhinosinusitis, or sinusitis irritates the upper airways and causes cough. Another common cause of chronic cough is gastroesophageal reflux disease (GERD; Chapter 20); in this disorder, reflux of acidic gastric contents irritates the pharynx and larynx, and aspiration of small amounts of acid may occur. Cough associated with GERD is worsened by lying down, which increases the reflux of gastric contents.

Some infections, such as tuberculosis, produce a cough that is classified as chronic. Post-infectious cough can become chronic and is generally the result of epithelial damage. Angiotensin-converting enzyme (ACE) inhibitors are drugs that are well-known to produce a chronic, non-productive cough.

Chronic bronchitis involves mucus hypersecretion and airway inflammation, both of which can trigger a cough. Cough-variant asthma is a form of asthma in which the only symptom is a non-productive cough that occurs throughout the day and night. Non-asthmatic eosinophilic bronchitis involves the infiltration of eosinophils into the respiratory epithelia. These eosinophils release inflammatory cytokines which activate sensory nerves that initiate coughing. Obstructive sleep apnea is characterized by transient upper airway obstruction during sleep which triggers a reflexive cough to open the airways.

Interstitial lung disease is a collection of disorders involving progressive pulmonary inflammation and fibrosis; chronic cough results from the effects of inflammatory mediators on sensory neurons. Idiopathic interstitial pneumonia is the most common form of interstitial lung disease; other forms can result from exposure to environmental agents or certain drugs, or from autoimmune disease.

Cough is also a symptom of CF, a disease that results from inactivating mutations in the gene encoding the CF transmembrane conductance regulator (CFTR) protein. The CFTR is a channel that carries Cl^- and water across cell membranes and regulates the function of other channels involved in mucociliary clearance. CFTR channels are also involved in the production of non-respiratory mucus, sweat, digestive enzymes, tears, and saliva. The mutations causing CF are divided into categories (class 1 – 5) which reflect their effects on the production, trafficking, function, and stability of the CFTR protein. These mutations result in decreased Cl^- secretion and increased Na^+ and water resorption, resulting in thick mucus secretions in the lung and other organs. This thick mucus obstructs the airways, is irritating, and provides an environment that promotes infections. In healthy individuals, the main component of mucus is the glycoprotein mucin, but in individuals with CF, respiratory secretions contain very little mucin, instead comprised predominantly of dead inflammatory and epithelial cells, and the polymerized DNA and filamentous actin derived from them.

Tumors in the lung can cause a mass effect that directly stimulates stretch receptors. They may also cause physical obstruction, resulting in mucus accumulation and an increased risk of infection. Neurogenic cough is the result of sensory neuropathy, most often idiopathic in nature.

Risk Factors

Risk factors for infectious causes of cough include exposure to the causative organism(s) and conditions that impair host immunity. Asthma and allergic rhinitis/rhinosinusitis are associated with exposure to environmental factors such as cigarette smoke, as well as a personal or family history of atopic disease. Heart failure is associated with advanced age, hypertension, smoking, prior myocardial infarction, atrial fibrillation, and other cardiovascular conditions. Pulmonary emboli most often occur in individuals who have deep vein thrombosis; the vascular damage, hypercoagulable state, and venous stasis seen in this condition are more commonly found with advanced age, obesity, smoking, metabolic syndrome, and chronic inflammatory disease. Aspiration of food or drink is more common in the elderly and in persons with neurological disorders.

Risk factors for conditions producing chronic cough also are varied. GERD is more common in persons with obesity, hiatal hernia, esophageal dysmotility, impaired tone of the lower esophageal sphincter, or delayed gastric emptying. Smoking is the primary risk factor for the development of COPD. Obstructive sleep apnea is associated with anatomical variants (e.g., tonsillar hypertrophy), obesity, advanced age, pregnancy, smoking, and alcohol use. Interstitial lung disease and lung cancers are associated with exposure to a wide variety of toxicants and carcinogens.

Pathophysiology

Epithelial cells of the airways are separated from the air space by a thin layer of liquid comprised of water and mucus. This layer, known as airway surface liquid (ASL) is important for the optimal functioning of the airways. ASL is made up of two layers, the periciliary layer and the mucus layer. The mucus layer is a gel-like layer comprised of water, gel-forming mucin glycoproteins, and small amounts of other constituents including cellular debris. Mucus is secreted by goblet cells that are interspersed between epithelial cells, and submucosal glands. In healthy airways, ciliated epithelial cells continuously remove mucus by propelling it toward the mouth, where it can be swallowed. Irritation of the airways, whether due to infection, inflammation, or irritants, usually results in increased secretion of mucus and a change in the composition of mucus. In severe disease states, mucus can be too thick. Thick mucus that is not readily removed from the airways is susceptible to colonization by pathogens, increasing the risk of respiratory tract infections. It can also block airways, reducing oxygen exchange. Conversely, sometimes cough is dry because mucus is not present in sufficient amounts to facilitate the expulsion of debris.

A typical cough consists of three respiratory phases: (1) a brief inspiratory phase, (2) a compression phase in which the expiratory muscles contract while the glottis is closed, and (3) an expiratory phase in which the glottis opens and air is expelled at high velocity. The cough reflex is initiated by stimulation of sensory nerves in the pharynx, trachea, main carina, branching points of the large airways, and distal smaller airways. Vagal sensory neurons that arise from the nodose ganglion and jugular ganglion are distributed throughout the airways and are responsible for detecting the stimuli that cause cough. These neurons can be classified on the basis of the speed of conduction of their action potentials (C-fibers, Aδ-fibers, Aβ-fibers), and on their sensitivity to chemical (nociceptors) vs. mechanical (stretch receptors) stimuli. A variety of airway nociceptors are found on C-fibers and Aδ-fibers, while stretch receptors are found on Aδ-fibers or Aβ-fibers.

The receptors that respond to cough-evoking stimuli include ionotropic receptors of the transient receptor potential (TRP) family and metabotropic receptors, including G protein-coupled receptors (GPCRs) and receptors that signal via the Janus kinase-signal transducer and activator of transcription proteins (JAK-STAT) pathway. The most studied ionotropic receptor involved in cough is the TRP vanilloid 1 (TRPV1) receptor. The TRPV1 receptor is a nonselective cation channel that, when activated by heat, capsaicin, acids, or certain GPCRs, initiates the influx of sodium and calcium ions. Neurons that express TRPV1 frequently also express TRP subfamily A member 1 (TRPA1) and TRP subfamily M member 8 (TRPM8) receptors. TRPA1 receptors are activated by allyl isothiocyanate (found in horseradish and wasabi) and acrolein (a byproduct of combustion), and cough results from this process. TRPM8 receptors are activated by menthol and cool temperatures; their activation causes cough suppression. Acidic substances, in addition to activating TRPV1 receptors, can initiate cough by binding the acid-sensing ion channels (ASIC) ASIC1, ASIC2, and ASIC3 on nodose Aδ-fibers. Adenosine triphosphate (ATP), which is released by airway epithelial cells, binds to purinergic receptors (P2X), which aggregate in homotrimeric (P2X3) or heterotrimeric (P2X2/3) configurations to function as cation channels and trigger a cough.

GPCRs involved in cough include the bradykinin BK2 receptor, the prostaglandin EP_3 receptor, and the leukotriene $CysLT_1$ receptor. Receptors for interferon-α (IFN-α), IFN-β, and IFN-γ are expressed on vagal C-fiber neurons. IFN-α and IFN-β are agonists of the IFN-α/β receptor (IFNAR), and IFN-γ is an agonist of the IFN-γ receptor (IFNGR). IFNAR and IFNGR initiate signaling via the JAK-STAT pathway. Large amounts of IFNs are produced during airway infections, and these are believed to play an important role in the cough produced by respiratory pathogens.

Once the cough reflex has been initiated by stimulation of vagal sensory neurons, impulses travel to the nucleus tractus solitarius in the brainstem, and from there, they project to the respiratory centers of the brain within the upper brain stem, medulla, and pons. Certain vagal afferent neurons release glutamate, which activates N-methyl-D-aspartate (NMDA) receptors on post-synaptic neurons. Others release substance P, which activates neurokinin-1 (NK-1) receptors on post-synaptic neurons. Both NMDA and NK-1 receptor stimulation increases action potential firing in these post-synaptic neurons. Post-synaptic neurons also express μ opioid receptors, which, when stimulated, decreases their action potential firing. Similarly, γ-aminobutyric acid (GABA), via GABA-A and GABA-B receptors, and agonists of the orphan σ1 receptor, also depress action potentials.

Examination

A detailed history and physical exam are necessary to elucidate the diagnosis of a cough. The patient should be questioned regarding the cough's characteristics and duration, as well as the presence of fever, malaise, myalgia, fatigue, shortness of breath, sputum (note color), hemoptysis, prodromal URI, and weight loss. Any diurnal variation in the cough, as well as factors that aggravate or relieve it, should be noted. The patient's occupational and environmental exposures, smoking/vaping history, comorbidities (e.g., GERD, heart failure, asthma, etc.), as well as the use of ACE inhibitors, are important clues in the diagnosis of the condition underlying cough.

Physical examinations commonly performed in the diagnosis of cough include vital signs, auscultation of the lung and heart, otoscopic and oropharyngeal examination, anterior rhinoscopy, transillumination of the sinuses, and examination of the abdomen and extremities.

Laboratory

When an infectious etiology is suspected, diagnostic tests may be used to detect the infectious organism (e.g., influenza, SARS-CoV2, respiratory syncytial virus (RSV), cytomegalovirus (CMV), tuberculosis, etc.). A CBC with differential may be helpful in distinguishing viral from bacterial pneumonia. Certain non-infectious causes of chronic cough may also warrant disease-specific laboratory tests. For example, if heart failure is suspected, a basic metabolic panel and levels of brain natriuretic peptide and troponin T may be useful; if CF is suspected, measurement of sweat chloride and DNA testing are indicated.

Imaging

Most cases of mild to moderate acute or subacute cough do not require imaging, but if acute cough is severe, or in high-risk individuals, a chest X-ray can be used to elucidate the diagnosis. In cases of chronic cough, a chest X-ray is usually indicated unless an alternate cause (e.g., ACE inhibitor use) is apparent. Certain causes of chronic cough (e.g., neoplasia) warrant further imaging such as CT scan, PET scan, sinus imaging, etc.

Associated Symptoms/Conditions

Viruses are the most common causative organisms for URI; these include members of the rhinovirus, adenovirus, coronavirus, enterovirus, influenza virus, and RSV groups. SARS-CoV2 is a cause of both URI and viral lower respiratory infections. The most common cause of bacterial URIs is Group A streptococci.

Viruses are the most common cause of lower respiratory tract infections. Acute bronchitis is associated with influenza virus A and B, parainfluenza, rhinovirus, and RSV. Bacteria such as *Streptococcus pneumonia* and *Staphylococcus aureus* are less common causes of acute bronchitis.

Pneumonia may be of viral or bacterial etiology (Chapter 3), or a coinfection may be present. Common viral causes of pneumonia include influenza types A/B/C; RSV, which is the most common cause of viral pneumonia in infants and young children; and parainfluenza viruses type 1/2/3/4, which are associated with a seasonal pneumonia-like illness in young children. SARS-CoV2 is also a cause of viral pneumonia. Other less common causes of viral pneumonia include rhinovirus, adenovirus, enteroviruses, varicella-zoster virus, hantavirus, Epstein-Barr virus, herpes simplex virus, CMV, and measles. These tend to be more common in individuals who have immune-compromising conditions (e.g., immunosuppressant drugs, cancer chemotherapy, HIV).

Bacterial pneumonia is classified by the context in which is acquired. Community-acquired pneumonia is most commonly caused by *S. pneumoniae*, followed by *Klebsiella pneumoniae*, *Haemophilus influenzae*, and *Pseudomonas aeruginosa*. Hospital-acquired and healthcare-associated pneumonias are most often caused by methicillin-resistant *Staphylococcus aureus* (MRSA) and *Pseudomonas aeruginosa*. Ventilator-associated pneumonia is caused by non-multi-drug resistant organisms (*S. pneumoniae* and other *Streptococcus* spp., *H. influenzae*, and methicillin-sensitive *Staphylococcus aureus* (MSSA)) and multi-drug resistant organisms (*P. aeruginosa*, MRSA, *Acinetobacter* spp., and antibiotic-resistant *Enterobacteriaceae*). Prior antibiotic treatment and increased length of hospitalization are associated with increased risk of drug-resistant pneumonia. Atypical pneumonia is most often caused by *Legionella*, *Mycoplasma pneumoniae*, *Chlamydia pneumoniae*, and *Chlamydia psittaci*.

Diagnosis

Most cases of acute and subacute cough do not require any specific diagnostic tests and are treated symptomatically unless there is suspicion of severe underlying pathology. Chronic cough generally requires imaging (above) and often requires pulmonary function testing via one or more of the following: spirometry, bronchoprovocation testing, a six-minute walk test, and measurement of lung volumes, diffusion capacity, and/or respiratory muscle pressure. Bronchoscopy may be required to assess for any masses in the trachea or vocal cords, and biopsy or bronchoalveolar lavage may be needed if certain infectious or neoplastic conditions are believed to be possible causes of the patient's cough. Disease-specific tests are useful in certain circumstances, e.g., electrocardiography and echocardiography for heart failure, upper endoscopy and gastroduodenoscopy for GERD, or a sleep study for obstructive sleep apnea.

Treatment

Infections or other underlying conditions that are producing a patient's cough must be managed appropriately. Often, the resolution of these conditions will resolve the cough. In some conditions (e.g., certain bacterial lung infections), it may be inadvisable to suppress a cough because this may counteract the body's defense mechanisms. The treatment of the multitude of conditions potentially underlying cough is beyond the scope of this chapter; instead, we will focus on addressing the symptoms of cough and sputum production. Cough is managed pharmacologically using antitussive drugs, and symptoms related to airway mucus production are treated with mucoactive agents. This class of drugs includes expectorants, which help to clear mucus from the airways, and mucolytics, which disrupt the structure of the mucus and decrease its viscosity. For patients who have CF, specific expectorants as well as the CFTR modulators are used to increase the amount of water in the pulmonary mucus and decrease its viscosity. Pulmonary surfactants are used in situations of neonatal respiratory distress and pediatric acute respiratory distress syndrome. Although they are neither antitussives nor mucoactive agents, they reduce the surface tension of the alveoli, preventing their collapse.

Management

Management of cough includes treatment of any underlying conditions that are producing the cough and pharmacotherapy with antitussives and/or mucoactive agents. Avoidance of triggers of cough (e.g., allergens, dry air, cold air), and use of soothing preparations (throat lozenges, honey tea, salt water gargle) is also helpful. Some individuals experience a chronic cough that is very difficult to control with conventional antitussives but which may respond to neuromodulators such as gabapentin or amitriptyline.

General Treatment Strategies

Antitussive drugs act at the level of the central nervous system to inhibit the cough reflex. Over-the-counter (OTC) drugs are commonly used by patients to self-manage their cough and sputum production. In the US, dextromethorphan is the only strictly antitussive drug that is available OTC; diphenhydramine, an antihistamine with antitussive qualities, is also available OTC. Benzonatate, available by prescription in the US, is used for mild to moderate cough, with opioid antitussives being reserved for more severe cough.

Guaifenesin is the only expectorant available for OTC use in the US. Hypertonic saline nasal spray is available, but the inhaled formulation is accessible by prescription only and predominantly used for CF. Inhaled mannitol is also indicated only for CF.

The mucolytic drugs are reserved for specific conditions. N-acetylcysteine is administered by inhalation or intratracheal instillation for severe pulmonary conditions such as pneumonia, CF, and atelectasis. Dornase alfa is primarily used in patients with CF, as are all of the CFTR modulators. Pulmonary surfactants are primarily used for prophylaxis and treatment of neonatal respiratory distress syndrome in premature infants.

The use of OTC cough and cold medicines in children has recently come under scrutiny in the US. *OTC antitussives, expectorants, decongestants, and antihistamines are not recommended for use in children under the age of 6 years.* Children under the age of 2 years appear to be at the greatest risk, and all cough medicines are labeled to reflect this risk. Whether children are more sensitive to the CNS effects of these drugs remains to be determined. Dosing errors are implicated as a major contributing factor in cases where children have been harmed by these drugs.

Antitussives

Consumers in the US have many choices for drugs to treat cough, and most do not require a prescription. Despite the wide use of antitussive drugs, data supporting their efficacy at recommended doses is sparse, and there is very little interest in drug development in this field.

Benzonatate

Background
Benzonatate is a non-opioid antitussive drug that is available only by prescription in the US. It belongs to the ester-type local anesthetic class of drugs and is believed to work by anesthetizing vagal afferent fibers of the airways.

Pharmacokinetics
Benzonatate is a mixture of polyethoxy esters of 4-(butylamino) benzoic acid which have varying degrees of hydrophobicity. It is administered orally, with an onset of action of 15 – 20 minutes and a duration of action of 3 – 8 hours. Once absorbed into the bloodstream, as with other ester local anesthetics, benzonatate undergoes hydrolysis in the plasma, predominantly by plasma pseudocholinesterase. This produces benzonatate's major metabolite, 4-(butylamino) benzoic acid, and methylated polyethylene glycol, both of which are eliminated in the urine and feces.

Mechanism of Action
Benzonatate is a local anesthetic agent. Once absorbed into the bloodstream, it acts by anesthetizing the stretch receptor fibers of the pulmonary vagal afferent nerves. Benzonatate may also have a similar action at the medulla. Similar to the local anesthetics, benzonatate is a reversible inhibitor of the Nav1.7 subtype of voltage-gated Na^+ channel. Benzonatate has greater effects on the Na^+ channel in its inactivated state, and it also produces a greater effect at depolarized potentials, where channels are more likely to be in the inactivated state.

Adverse Effects, Contraindications, Drug Interactions
Benzonatate is supplied in liquid-filled capsules. If the patient chews the capsule or dissolves it in the mouth, it will cause local anesthesia in the oropharyngeal cavity, potentially resulting in laryngospasm, bronchospasm, dysphagia, or choking. At recommended doses, benzonatate is generally well tolerated, with typical adverse effects being sedation, dizziness, and nausea. It becomes dangerous in overdose, with effects including confusion, hallucinations, CNS stimulation followed by CNS depression, and cardiovascular and/or respiratory collapse.

Because benzonatate is an ester-type local anesthetic, its metabolism to compounds related to para-aminobenzoic acid (PABA) results in a similar potential to cause allergic reactions. Benzonatate should not be used in individuals who have hypersensitivity to ester local anesthetics because of the possibility of severe allergic reactions and anaphylaxis. Benzonatate formulations also contain methyl- and propylparaben and can cause hypersensitivity reactions in those who are allergic to parabens.

Benzonatate is not known to participate in any drug interactions.

Chlophedianol (clophedianol)

Background
Chlorphedianol is a non-opioid, centrally acting antitussive that is available OTC in combination with an antihistamine (dexbrompheniramine), expectorant (guaifenesin), and/or decongestant (phenylephrine, pseudoephedrine) in some countries. It is not available in the US.

Pharmacokinetics
Chlophedianol is absorbed following oral administration and is metabolized in the liver and excreted via the kidneys. The exact routes of metabolism have not been identified.

Mechanism of Action
Chlophedianol has a depressant effect on the cough centers of the medulla, but a specific target has not been identified. It may also exert local anesthetic and anticholinergic effects.

Adverse Effects, Contraindications, Drug Interactions
Because chlophedianol is available only in combination products, little information on the adverse effects or interactions of this drug in isolation is available. Combination products can elicit adverse effects such as sedation, paradoxical CNS stimulation, and anticholinergic effects, which are at least in part due to the antihistamine component.

Dextromethorphan
Background
Dextromethorphan is a centrally-acting antitussive drug that is widely available throughout the world without a prescription. Although it is chemically related to the opioid analgesic, levorphanol, the inability of naloxone, an opioid receptor antagonist, to block the antitussive effect of dextromethorphan suggests that it suppresses cough via alternative mechanisms (discussed below). Currently, the only indication for dextromethorphan as a single agent in the US is cough, but it is commonly found in OTC combination products including decongestants such as phenylephrine, antihistamines such as diphenhydramine, and/or expectorants such as guaifenesin. It is also a component of two prescription formulations: dextromethorphan with quinidine is approved in the US to treat pseudobulbar affect, and dextromethorphan with bupropion is approved for the treatment of major depressive disorder. These formulations have been investigated for use in the treatment of several neurological disorders including agitation due to Alzheimer's disease, diabetic neuropathic pain, chorea, bipolar disorder, brain injury, and smoking cessation.

Pharmacokinetics
Dextromethorphan is a substrate of CYP2D6, which is a polymorphic enzyme conferring different degrees of activity. Approximately 90% of individuals are extensive metabolizers in whom CYP2D6 is the major metabolic pathway for dextromethorphan, resulting in its rapid first-pass metabolism to an active metabolite, dextrorphan. Dextrorphan may then be metabolized by UDP-glucuronosyltransferase to form dextrorphan-o-glucuronide, or via CYP3A4/A5 to produce 3-hydoxymorphinan, which also undergoes glucuronidation. Dextrorphan-o-glucuronide is the major metabolite found in the plasma; it is permanently charged and is relatively unable to cross the blood-brain barrier. In individuals who lack (poor metabolizers) or express low levels (intermediate metabolizers) of CYP2D6, dextromethorphan follows what is usually a minor metabolic pathway via CYP3A4. This results in the production of 3-methoxymorphinan, and the synthesis of dextrorphan is completely or partially bypassed. 3-methoxymorphinan is converted to 3-hydoxymorphinan, which undergoes glucuronidation as stated above. The glucuronide conjugates are rapidly excreted by the kidneys.

Dextromethorphan's extensive first-pass metabolism causes it to have a low oral bioavailability (1 – 2%). Its antitussive effects appear within 15 – 30 minutes of oral administration and last for 3 to 6 hours. Poor or intermediate CYP2D6 metabolizers have a prolonged duration of action of dextromethorphan and an increased risk of adverse effects as compared to wild-type (extensive) metabolizers. In contrast, ultrarapid metabolizers have higher levels of dextrorphan and may be more likely to experience its psychoactive effects.

The addition of quinidine or bupropion to dextromethorphan takes advantage of the inhibitory effect of these drugs on CYP2D6. By blocking the major route of first-pass metabolism of dextromethorphan, they minimize the production of dextrorphan and maximize the amount of dextromethorphan that is available to distribute to the CNS.

Mechanism of Action
Dextromethorphan and dextrorphan have multiple receptor-binding activities. Although structurally similar to opioids, neither dextromethorphan nor dextrorphan binds to opioid receptors. Both compounds act as low-affinity, noncompetitive antagonists of NMDA receptors. This mechanism may allow them to interfere with the cough reflex by blocking the effect of glutamate released by the vagal afferents that carry cough-stimulatory signals. At high doses, the ability of dextromethorphan and dextrorphan to antagonize NMDA receptors is thought to be responsible for the neurobehavioral adverse effects listed below.

Dextromethorphan also acts as a high- to moderate-affinity agonist of σ_1 receptors in the brain. These receptors are found on the neurons that are synapsed upon by the vagal afferents from the lung, and their stimulation down-regulates the activity of these afferent neurons. Additional actions of dextromethorphan include antagonism of nicotinic receptors, α_1- and α_2-adrenoceptors, and H_1 histamine receptors; inhibition of the transporters for serotonin (SERT) and norepinephrine (NET); and blockade of L-type calcium channels.

Adverse Effects, Contraindications, Drug Interactions
Dextromethorphan is associated with several adverse effects when taken at recommended doses. These include dry mouth, tachycardia, nausea, and dizziness, which may be mediated by antagonism of central muscarinic receptors. It may also cause confusion, nervousness, and irritability. Dextromethorphan should be used with caution in children as described previously.

Because it is devoid of opioid receptor affinity, dextromethorphan has been claimed to have no abuse liability. However, higher doses can produce a dissociative state similar to that produced by NMDA receptor antagonists like ketamine and phencyclidine, and the incidence of substance misuse disorder involving dextromethorphan has increased in recent decades, particularly among teenagers. Individuals taking high doses (> 4 mg/kg) of dextromethorphan report feelings of euphoria or drunkenness, visual hallucinations, dissociation, agitation, and delusions. This phenomenon is termed "robo-tripping" or "robo-ing" by some, a nickname derived from a popular brand name for dextromethorphan cough syrup. Misusing high doses of dextromethorphan that is formulated with other drugs such as acetaminophen and antihistamines is also dangerous.

Dextromethorphan has been associated with serotonin syndrome. Although this is usually due to the co-administration of dextromethorphan with other serotonergic drugs or supratherapeutic doses of dextromethorphan, there have been reports of serotonin syndrome following normal antitussive doses of dextromethorphan. Since dextromethorphan is metabolized by the polymorphic CYP2D6 enzyme, it is likely that genetics play a role in susceptibility to serotonin syndrome.

The most serious interactions associated with dextromethorphan use are those involving concomitant administration with other drugs that increase synaptic serotonin levels, resulting in an increased risk of serotonin syndrome. Drugs that inhibit the metabolism of dextromethorphan (especially via inhibition of CYP2D6) increase its plasma concentration and may increase the risk of adverse effects.

Opioids

Background

In the US and other parts of the world, codeine is the main opioid agonist used in cough medicines; others include dihydrocodeine and hydrocodone. The opioid antitussives are usually formulated with an antihistamine, mucolytic, decongestant, and/or antipyretic. The dose thought to suppress cough may be lower than that used for analgesia, although, as with the OTC antitussives, there is little research supporting its antitussive effect, especially in children. Codeine is a controlled substance in the US, but the low doses used in cough mixtures fall under schedule V; in some US states, these cough mixtures may be available legally without a prescription from a doctor. However, many pharmacies will not dispense schedule V opioids without a legitimate prescription because of the abuse liability associated with this drug class. Combination products containing hydrocodone or dihydrocodeine are prescription only.

Pharmacokinetics

The opioid antitussives are administered orally. Codeine is well absorbed, and its maximal plasma level is seen approximately one hour after administration. Approximately 70 – 80% of codeine is metabolized via UDP-glucuronosyltransferase to codeine-6-glucuronide. Around 5 – 10% is converted by CYP2D6 to morphine, and around 10% is converted via CYP3A4 to norcodeine. Genetic polymorphisms in CYP2D6 can result in differences in efficacy and adverse effects of codeine. Codeine and its metabolites are excreted in the urine. Its half-life is approximately 2 – 4 hours.

Dihydrocodeine undergoes significant first-pass metabolism. Approximately 43% of a dose is converted to dihydromorphine via CYP2D6. It also undergoes conversion to nordihydrocodeine and dihydrocodeine-6-glucuronide. Dihydrocodeine and its metabolites are excreted by the kidneys, and the half-life of dihydrocodeine is 3.3 – 4.5 hours.

Hydrocodone's major route of elimination is CYP3A4-mediated conversion to norhydrocodone. CYP2D6-mediated conversion to hydromorphone also occurs to a lesser extent. Hydrocodone and its metabolites undergo renal excretion. The half-life of hydrocodone is approximately 4 hours.

Mechanism of Action

Codeine, dihydrocodeine, and hydrocodone are agonists of μ opioid receptors, with a potency less than that of morphine. The antitussive effect of these opioids may be related to the presence of μ opioid receptors on the nerve terminals which the vagal afferents synapse upon. The binding of an agonist to these receptors decreases action potential firing and may suppress the cough reflex. They may also have an action on cough receptors in the proximal airways.

Adverse Effects, Contraindications, Drug Interactions

Respiratory depression is the most serious adverse effect of opioids; however, at the recommended doses used in combination products for cough, it is of greatest concern in children less than 12 years of age, and in situations of overdose. Because of this, in the US, the FDA requires labeling of opioid cough suppressants stating that they are not indicated for individuals under the age of 18.

Dependence and potential for misuse are also significant concerns, so OTC preparations are sold in small volumes, with purchase limits, to decrease this risk. Codeine/promethazine cough syrup has become a recreational drug among teens and young adults.

Even in the low doses used in cough preparations, opioids can cause constipation and a decrease in mental acuity. Other adverse effects of the opioid component of these combination products include nausea and vomiting, miosis, alterations in accommodation, drowsiness, and dizziness.

Because the opioids are used in combination with other drugs, care should be taken to avoid the co-administration of other opioid-containing products (e.g., for analgesia). Caution should be used when administered with drugs that induce or inhibit CYP2D6 or CYP3A4, and the patient should be monitored for drug efficacy and adverse effects. Opioids should not be used with monoamine oxidase inhibitors due to the risk of promoting serotonin syndrome.

Diphenhydramine

Background

Diphenhydramine is an H_1 antihistamine that is used alone or in combination products for cough associated with allergic rhinitis or URI. As with the other antitussives, only a few studies have examined its efficacy in cough.

Pharmacokinetics

Diphenhydramine is well absorbed following oral administration, with an onset of action of 15 – 30 minutes, and a duration of action from 4 – 6 hours. Its major route of metabolism is via CYP2D6, for which it is a substrate and inhibitor. It is metabolized by CYP1A2, CYP2C9, and CYP2C19 to a lesser extent.

Mechanism of Action

Diphenhydramine is a first-generation H_1 antihistamine. As such, it is an inverse agonist of the H_1 receptor and also possesses antimuscarinic and local anesthetic (Na^+ channel blocking) effects. The antihistamine and antimuscarinic effect of diphenhydramine can decrease the postnasal drip that stimulates cough. Limited evidence suggests that diphenhydramine decreases cough reflex sensitivity, but the mechanism of action of this effect remains unclear. Histamine does not appear to increase the sensitivity to capsaicin-induced cough, and unlike some other antihistamines (e.g., chlorpheniramine), diphenhydramine does not inhibit the TRPV1 receptor that is activated by capsaicin, acid, and other cough stimuli.

Adverse Effects, Contraindications, Drug Interactions

The most frequent adverse effect of diphenhydramine is sedation, which is produced by the blockade of H_1 and muscarinic receptors in the CNS and is additive with the sedating effects of alcohol or other CNS depressants. Paradoxical excitation can be seen at normal doses, more commonly in children than adults, and it frequently occurs when toxic dosages are ingested. Diphenhydramine also produces antimuscarinic effects, resulting in dry mouth and respiratory passages, blurred vision, sedation, cognitive impairment, urinary retention, and constipation. The effects of toxic doses are similar to those of atropine, including excitement, hallucinations, dry mouth, dilated pupils, flushing, convulsions, urinary retention, sinus tachycardia, coma, and death.

Because it is an inhibitor of CYP2D6, diphenhydramine has the potential to increase blood levels of drugs that are primarily eliminated by this enzyme.

Expectorants

Expectorants are used to help clear mucus from the airways. Expectorants are not cough suppressants; instead, they hydrate and increase the secretion of pulmonary mucus, which increases the efficiency of the airway cilia and helps soothe irritated airways. Drug therapy with expectorants is not always necessary for minor coughs and upper respiratory tract infections. Increasing fluid intake and humidifying room air both are effective ways to hydrate mucus. As with antitussives, evidence for the efficacy of OTC expectorants is not strong, yet they are found in many cough preparations.

Expectorants are also used in the management of CF to decrease the viscosity of pulmonary mucus and promote expectoration. Some women use expectorants to increase vaginal secretions while attempting to become pregnant; however, this is an off-label use.

Guaifenesin

Background

Guaifenesin, also known as guaiphenesin or glyceryl guaiacoloate, is the most commonly used expectorant in OTC medicines. It is available in many oral formulations including single agents, combination products (especially with dextromethorphan), and extended-release formulations. A prescription formulation with hydrocodone, with or without pseudoephedrine, is also available.

Guaifenesin is used for a dry, non-productive cough in which there is thick mucus or mucus plugs. It should not be used in cases of cough in which excessive secretions are present (e.g., asthma, chronic bronchitis) without a doctor's supervision, and it should not be used for cough due to heart failure or ACE inhibitors. Guaifenesin is not indicated for children under 2 years of age due to safety and efficacy concerns.

Pharmacokinetics
The pharmacokinetic properties of guaifenesin are not well described, although it is known that the drug is recovered entirely as metabolites in the urine. At least one metabolite, beta-(2-methoxyphenoxy)-lactic acid, is active.

Mechanism of Action
Guaifenesin is believed to decrease the viscosity of bronchial secretions by increasing the incorporation of water into the sputum. This facilitates the removal of mucus by ciliary clearance and by coughing. Some evidence also suggests that guaifenesin may decrease cough reflex sensitivity in individuals who have URI, but not in healthy subjects.

Adverse Effects, Contraindications, Drug Interactions
Guaifenesin is generally well tolerated at recommended doses. Headache, drowsiness, and dizziness are rare adverse effects. At higher doses, nausea, vomiting, abdominal pain, and diarrhea may occur. High doses or excessive use of guaifenesin may result in nephrolithiasis. The kidney stones of some high-dose users of guaifenesin have been found to contain the beta-(2-methoxyphenoxy)-lactic acid metabolite.

There are no known interactions with guaifenesin.

Hypertonic Saline
Background
Inhaled hypertonic saline (7%) is commonly used to increase mucociliary clearance and improve lung function in individuals with CF. Hypertonic saline for oral inhalation is not available OTC.

Pharmacokinetics
When administered systemically, sodium chloride (NaCl) distributes to the plasma and interstitial fluid. Concentration within the cell is maintained at a constant level by the action of the Na^+/K^+ ATPase. NaCl is excreted mainly in the urine, but it is also found in the feces and sweat. In individuals with CF, the sodium content of the sweat is higher than normal.

The pharmacokinetics of inhaled hypertonic saline have not been specifically described. In the context of inhalation administration, the plasma concentration of NaCl is expected to be lower than that resulting from parenteral administration for indications such as hypovolemic shock. This is because a lower dose is used: 4 mL of 7% NaCl for CF (280 mg) vs. 1 L IV bolus of 0.9% NaCl (9 g) for shock. Also, some of the NaCl would be expected to remain in the mucus and be eliminated from the body when the sputum is coughed up.

Mechanism of Action
When NaCl is applied to the respiratory epithelium, it causes water to move from the interstitial fluid of the epithelium into the periciliary fluid on its surface. This decreases the viscosity of the airway mucus, which enhances mucociliary clearance and promotes expectoration.

Hypertonic saline appears to have several other mucoactive mechanisms that are particularly important in the context of CF. The high-molecular-weight glycoproteins (mucins) that comprise the mucus gel exist in a tangled web of heavily glycosylated dimers, formed by disulfide bonds. Cross-linking between the mucin strands adds to the integrity of the mucus gel. Hypertonic saline may disrupt the ionic bonds between the tangled mucin dimers, reducing cross-linking. In purulent mucus, as seen in diseases such as CF, necrotic neutrophils release DNA, filamentous actin, and proinflammatory mediators into the mucus gel. Hypertonic saline is thought to play a role in liberating this DNA from the mucus gel, rendering the gel more susceptible to breakdown by endogenous lytic enzymes.

Adverse Effects, Contraindications, Drug Interactions
Systemic adverse effects are not common with inhaled hypertonic saline, although it does have an unpleasant taste, may narrow the airways, and stimulates cough. Cough may be considered a beneficial effect since it aids the clearance of mucus from the airways.

There are no listed interactions for inhaled hypertonic saline. The amount of NaCl administered by inhalation is so low that it is not likely that clinically significant interactions exist.

Mannitol
Background
Inhaled mannitol is indicated as an add-on maintenance treatment for adults with CF. It is supplied as capsules containing mannitol powder and dosed twice daily via a relatively complicated process. An inhaled short-acting bronchodilator is administered 5 – 15 minutes prior to each dose. A capsule of mannitol is placed in a handheld inhaler,

and the powder is released by a press of two buttons. The patient inhales the powder through a steady, deep inhalation. This process is repeated for each of the 10 capsules comprising a single dose. Inhaled mannitol has been shown to significantly improve pulmonary function parameters, but its cost in the US is nearly 175 times that of hypertonic saline. No studies to date have done a direct comparison of inhaled mannitol to hypertonic saline.

Pharmacokinetics
The bioavailability of mannitol, when administered by inhalation, is 59%, and the mean time to peak plasma concentration is 1.5 hours. Approximately 55% of absorbed mannitol is excreted in the urine as the unchanged drug; the remainder undergoes dehydrogenation to produce fructose. The half-life of inhaled mannitol is 4.7 hours.

Mechanism of Action
Similar to hypertonic saline, mannitol acts as an osmotic agent to promote the movement of water into the periciliary fluid and increase the hydration of mucus. This improves mucociliary function and eases the expectoration of mucus during cough. Like hypertonic saline, inhaled mannitol is a bronchial irritant, which causes cough, which also increases the clearance of mucus.

Adverse Effects, Contraindications, Drug Interactions
Inhaled mannitol powder can cause severe bronchoconstriction, and it is for this reason that a short-acting bronchodilator should be administered 5 – 15 minutes before each dose. Prior to initiating treatment with inhaled mannitol, patients should undergo a mannitol tolerance test in a facility equipped to handle acute bronchospasm. Those who experience bronchospasm, or a decrease in oxygen saturation or FEV_1, should not be treated with inhaled mannitol.

Additional adverse effects seen with inhaled mannitol include pharyngolaryngeal pain, throat irritation, hemoptysis, rhinorrhea, lower respiratory tract infection, and CF exacerbation. Inhaled mannitol is contraindicated in individuals with mannitol or gelatin sensitivity, in those who fail the mannitol tolerance test, and in those for whom the mannitol tolerance test is contraindicated (e.g., aortic or cerebral aneurism, stroke, recent myocardial infarction).

Although there are many potential interactions when mannitol is administered systemically, for example in the treatment of acute renal failure or cerebral edema, there is little knowledge of any interactions that occur with inhaled mannitol. As with inhaled hypertonic saline, the amount of mannitol administered via inhalation is much smaller than the amount given systemically (400 mg for inhalation vs. up to 140 g/dose for cerebral edema), so interactions are not likely to be clinically significant.

Mucolytics

Mucolytics are drugs that change the biophysical properties of mucus, decreasing its viscosity by "lysing" the mucus. Typically, mucolytics are divided into "classic" mucolytics that disrupt the disulfide bonds, thus breaking down the long strands of mucin, and "peptide" mucolytics which disrupt mucus via other mechanisms.

N-acetylcysteine

Background
N-acetylcysteine (NAC) is a classic mucolytic that is available for inhaled, intravenous or oral administration and is used in the management of COPD and other respiratory diseases. Like many mucoactive drugs, its effectiveness has been questioned. Inhaled NAC does not appear to be any more effective than simple hydration for clearing mucus. Oral NAC may improve pulmonary function in select patients (including COPD patients), but this effect may be due to its reported antioxidant properties rather than an effect on mucus viscosity. Intravenous NAC is used for the prevention of hepatotoxicity in acetaminophen overdose. Oral forms of NAC are available OTC as dietary supplements in the US.

Pharmacokinetics
When administered by inhalation, only a small fraction of NAC is absorbed. When given via the oral route, NAC is rapidly absorbed, but its bioavailability is low (9%). Once in circulation, NAC is deacetylated by the liver and within most tissues, producing cysteine and disulfides.

Mechanism of Action
NAC contains free sulfhydryl groups which are thought to disrupt the disulfide bonds between mucin strands in bronchial secretions. This decreases the viscosity of the mucus and assists in expectoration and drainage. Acetylcysteine has no effect on cellular debris (fibrin, DNA). When administered orally, very little NAC distributes to the airway mucus. It is deacetylated to cysteine, which contains a thiol group that is thought to confer the antioxidant properties of the drug.

Adverse Effects, Contraindications, Drug Interactions
Although IV NAC used in the context of acetaminophen overdose has been reported to cause anaphylactoid reactions, it is rare with inhaled or oral acetylcysteine. Bronchospasm can occur following inhalation of NAC; pretreatment with an inhaled short-acting bronchodilator may prevent bronchospasm in susceptible individuals. Inhaled NAC should be used cautiously in individuals with asthma. All formulations of NAC are associated with nausea and vomiting, in part due to its strong, unpleasant sulfuric odor and taste. Drowsiness, clamminess, and fever have been reported from inhaled NAC.

There are no reported interactions for inhaled NAC.

Dornase Alfa
Background
Dornase alfa is a peptide mucolytic that is widely used as part of the management of CF. It is a recombinant human deoxyribonuclease produced by genetically engineered Chinese hamster ovary cells. It has been shown to improve pulmonary function tests and to decrease the occurrence of acute exacerbations and lower respiratory infections in individuals with CF.

Pharmacokinetics
Dornase alfa is administered via inhalation, and very little is absorbed systemically in adults, but small amounts are detectable in the blood of children who receive adult doses. Rapid degradation by proteases in the blood renders the small amount of absorbed drug inactive. The half-life following IV administration is 3 – 4 hours.

Mechanism of Action
The pulmonary secretions of individuals with CF contain large amounts of DNA and filamentous actin released from necrotic neutrophils and other cells. Dornase alfa hydrolyzes the extracellular DNA found in these secretions, rendering them less viscous and more easily cleared from the airways. Patients report a decreased frequency of cough, dyspnea, and chest congestion.

Adverse Effects, Contraindications, Drug Interactions
Mild to moderate adverse effects associated with dornase alfa use include hoarseness/voice alteration, pharyngitis, chest pain, dyspnea, and less frequently, conjunctivitis and laryngitis. This drug is contraindicated in patients who are known to be hypersensitive to hamster proteins. There are no known drug interactions for dornase alfa.

Cystic Fibrosis Transmembrane Conductance Regulator (CFTR) Modulators

The CFTR modulators are relatively new additions to the limited pool of drugs to manage CF. Unlike other available treatments, these orally administered drugs target the defective proteins that underlie the symptoms of CF, including life-threatening pulmonary symptoms. It is of note that the CFTR modulators, as single drugs, are only effective in individuals with specific mutations in the *CFTR* gene. The most common *CFTR* mutation is *ΔF508*, which confers deletion of phenylalanine at position 508 of the CFTR protein and is seen in approximately 45-50% of individuals who have CF worldwide. *ΔF508* results in abnormal folding of newly formed CFTR protein, causing it to be retained and degraded at the endoplasmic reticulum prior to reaching the cell surface. Other mutations in the *CFTR* gene cause the production of ion channels that do not open properly in response to intracellular stimuli (e.g., *G551D*), or in the production of less protein (*A455E*) or less stable protein (*A1412X*), or in the complete absence of the CFTR protein (*G542X*). The CFTR modulators compensate for *CFTR* mutations in one of two ways: by increasing the probability that the CFTR channel will be in its open state (CFTR potentiators), or by enhancing the processing and trafficking of normal and select mutant forms of the CFTR, which increases their delivery to the cell surface (CFTR correctors). There is currently only one FDA-approved CFTR potentiator, ivacaftor. Ivacaftor is available alone or in combination with one or more CFTR correctors, which are not available as single drug products.

The CFTR potentiator and corrector combination products are effective in a larger number of patients than ivacaftor alone. However, these combinations do not restore adequate function in patients who have both a single *ΔF508* mutation and one minimal-function mutation (i.e., produces either no CFTR protein or a CFTR protein that does not respond to ivacaftor). Individuals who are homozygous for mutations resulting in no CFTR protein currently also have no drugs available to address their underlying dysfunctions.

CFTR Potentiators
Background
Ivacaftor, as a monotherapy, is indicated for individuals who have an ivacaftor-responsive mutation in the *CFTR* gene. It is a component of the CFTR potentiator and corrector combinations: with lumacaftor, with tezacaftor, and with elexacaftor and tezacaftor.

Pharmacokinetics
Following oral administration, ivacaftor is extensively bound to plasma albumin and α_1-acid glycoprotein. It is metabolized, mainly by CYP3A, to an inactive metabolite and to an active metabolite (M1) that is one-sixth as potent as the parent drug. Metabolites are mainly excreted in the feces. Ivacaftor has a half-life of approximately 12 hours. Ivacaftor and its M1 metabolite are weak inhibitors of CYP3A, CYP2C9, and p-glycoprotein.

Mechanism of Action
Ivacaftor specifically targets CFTR proteins that contain a mutation at *G551D* or other locations that cause the CFTR proteins to respond inadequately to intracellular stimuli. The binding of ivacaftor to a mutant CFTR protein opens its chloride channel, resulting in a more functional protein. Because ivacaftor only targets certain specific mutations that control CFTR channel opening, it is ineffective in CF patients who possess mutations that interfere with the trafficking of the CFTR to the plasma membrane, such as *ΔF508*, and in those in whom no CFTR protein is produced.

Adverse Effects, Contraindications, Drug Interactions
Elevated liver enzymes have been seen in up to 15% of patients taking ivacaftor, so liver function tests are recommended prior to initiating therapy and regularly throughout treatment (every three months during the first year of treatment and then once a year). Dosage reduction may be necessary for patients who have liver dysfunction. Other common adverse effects associated with ivacaftor use include diarrhea, abdominal pain, oropharyngeal pain/pharyngitis, URI, and headache. These effects are usually mild. Cataracts and lens opacities have been reported in children and adolescents taking ivacaftor, so routine eye exams are recommended.

Because ivacaftor's main route of elimination is metabolism via CYP3A, and the parent drug and M1 also function as weak inhibitors of CYP3A isoforms, dosage adjustments may be needed if ivacaftor is co-administered with CYP3A substrates, inducers, or inhibitors. In addition, ivacaftor and its M1 metabolite are weak inhibitors of CYP2C9 and p-glycoprotein, so dosage adjustments may be necessary for drugs that are eliminated through these pathways.

CFTR Correctors
Background
CFTR correctors function to counteract mutations in the CFTR gene which impair the trafficking of the CFTR protein to the plasma membrane. The most common CF mutation, *ΔF508*, falls into this category, and individuals who are homozygous for *ΔF508* produce misfolded CFTR protein that is degraded before it can reach the cell surface. The small amount of ΔF508 CFTR protein that reaches the plasma membrane is less stable and has a lower probability of being in the channel-open state than does the wild-type CFTR. CFTR correctors are always formulated in combination with ivacaftor; this is done so that the CFTR proteins that are moved to the cell surface by the action of the CFTR corrector are then stimulated to open by ivacaftor. CFTR potentiator and corrector combinations are all orally administered and include ivacaftor + lumacaftor, ivacaftor + tezacaftor, and ivacaftor + elexacaftor + tezacaftor.

Pharmacokinetics
Following absorption, lumacaftor is extensively bound to plasma albumin. Approximately 51% of the drug is excreted in the feces unchanged, and it is also metabolized via oxidation and glucuronidation. Lumacaftor is an inducer and inhibitor of p-glycoprotein. There is minimal elimination of lumacaftor in the urine; its average half-life is 26 hours.

Tezacaftor is highly bound to plasma albumin. It is extensively metabolized, mainly via CYP3A, to a metabolite with similar potency to the parent drug (M1), a metabolite that is much less potent (M2), and an inactive metabolite (M5). Tezacaftor is a mild inducer of CYP3A. Approximately 72% of the drug is excreted in the feces unchanged, and a minor amount is eliminated in the urine. The half-life of tezacaftor averages 15 hours.

After absorption, elexacaftor is highly bound to plasma albumin. It is metabolized, mainly via CYP3A, to an active metabolite, M23-ELX, which has a potency similar to the parent drug. Elexacaftor has the potential to inhibit certain organic anion transporters involved in specific drugs' transport. Nearly 90% of a dose of elexacaftor is excreted in the feces unchanged, and it has an average half-life of approximately 30 hours.

Mechanism of Action
The CFTR correctors improve cellular processing and trafficking of the ΔF508 CFTR and other mutant CFTR proteins which do not translocate properly to the cell surface. The action of the CFTR correctors results in an increase in the amount of protein found on the plasma membrane. Lumacaftor and tezacaftor are classified as type I correctors: they stabilize the interface between the membrane-spanning domain and the nucleotide-binding domain of the CFTR protein. Elexacaftor is classified as a type III corrector. It acts by stabilizing the CFTR's nucleotide-binding domain 1, and it has recently been shown to have co-potentiator activity with ivacaftor for *ΔF508* and certain other gating mutants.

Adverse Effects, Contraindications, Drug Interactions
The adverse effects and interactions of the CFTR potentiators are relevant in the context of the combination products in which they are found. Because all combination products contain ivacaftor, the potential for elevated liver enzymes and cataracts or lens opacities in children is present. Adverse effects seen with the ivacaftor + lumacaftor combination include chest discomfort, dyspnea, and elevated blood pressure; hepatic encephalopathy is a severe effect that is rarely seen. The ivacaftor + tezacaftor combination is associated with headache, dizziness, nasal congestion, and nausea. Adverse effects seen in patients taking the ivacaftor, tezacaftor, and elexacaftor combination include upper respiratory tract infection, influenza, abdominal pain, diarrhea, elevated bilirubin, and rash.

Drug interactions with the CFTR potentiator and corrector combinations result from the ability of the individual components to interact with various CYPs, organic anion transporters, and/or p-glycoprotein, as described above.

Pulmonary Surfactants

Background
Pulmonary surfactant is a complex substance comprised of phospholipids and surfactant proteins that are secreted by the lungs. This substance lowers the surface tension of fluid in the alveoli, allowing the lungs to expand on intake of breath, and preventing the collapse of the alveoli at the end of an exhalation. In utero, the fetus begins to make surfactant between 24 and 28 weeks of gestation. Most babies have enough surfactant by 35 weeks of gestation to be able to breathe air if they are born before full term. However, premature babies, especially those born before 30 weeks of gestational age, are at the greatest risk of developing respiratory distress syndrome (RDS), a direct result of surfactant deficiency. The standard of care is to administer corticosteroids to pregnant women who are at high risk of preterm delivery. This results in increased production of fetal surfactant.

Premature neonates who require further treatment to prevent complications of RDS may, under specific circumstances, receive exogenous surfactants by intratracheal administration. Intratracheal administration requires an experienced practitioner with intubation skills to avoid causing damage to the newborn lung. In previous years, pulmonary surfactant was routinely administered to preterm babies because it improved survival, but this is no longer the case. Currently, continuous positive airway pressure (CPAP) therapy is initiated soon after birth for preterm infants at risk of RDS, and corticosteroids may also be given. Exogenous surfactants are now reserved for infants showing signs of RDS or who require intubation for stabilization. These drugs are most effective when administered within the first 30-60 minutes of life.

Three of the four available pulmonary surfactants are derived from animal tissue: beractant (cattle), calfactant (cattle), and poractant alfa (pigs). These are referred to as natural surfactants, and all appear to be equally effective. Lucinactant was the first synthetic version of a human surfactant approved in the US. It is a proprietary peptide that mimics human surfactant protein B (SP-B), and it appears to be as safe and effective as the natural surfactants.

Pharmacokinetics
Because the pulmonary surfactants are administered intratracheally, directly to their site of action, only a small amount (approximately 5%) reaches the systemic circulation. Clearance of surfactant is believed to involve type II alveolar cells. Human pharmacokinetic studies of the pulmonary surfactants have not been done, but animal studies indicate that less than 30% of a calfactant dose is present in the lungs 24 hours after administration. Poractant appears to be cleared more slowly, with 20% and 45% cleared from the lungs of newborn and adult animals, respectively, within 24 hours. No data for beractant or lucinactant are available.

Mechanism of Action
All of the pulmonary surfactants replace the pulmonary surfactant that is deficient in some premature neonates. Surfactant lowers the surface tension of the air-liquid interface of the alveolar surfaces and stabilizes the alveoli against collapse.

Adverse Effects, Contraindications, Drug Interactions
It is difficult to distinguish between the adverse effects of the pulmonary surfactants and the adverse events that can result from preterm birth. Clinical trials with preterm infants indicate that pulmonary surfactants can produce bradycardia, decreased oxygen saturation, hypoxia, and endotracheal tube reflux. Administration of pulmonary surfactant can cause lung function to rapidly return, and if O_2 ventilation is not adjusted accordingly, hyperoxia and hypocarbia can occur. Close monitoring of arterial blood gases is required during surfactant treatment, and the ventilator settings must be adjusted to prevent these abnormalities.

Interactions can occur between pulmonary surfactants and antimicrobial drugs that are administered via inhalation to certain neonates with RDS. The activity of the following antimicrobials may be reduced if they are administered at the same time as surfactant: amikacin, amphotericin B, gentamicin, kanamycin, neomycin, paromomycin, streptomycin, tobramycin, and vancomycin.

References

Chung KF, McGarvey L, Song WJ, Chang AB, Lai K, Canning BJ, Birring SS, Smith JA, Mazzone SB. Cough hypersensitivity and chronic cough. Nat Rev Dis Primers. 2022 Jun 30;8(1):45. doi: 10.1038/s41572-022-00370-w. PMID: 35773287; PMCID: PMC9244241.

Evans MS, Maglinger GB, Fletcher AM, Johnson SR. Benzonatate inhibition of voltage-gated sodium currents. Neuropharmacology. 2016 Feb;101:179-87. doi: 10.1016/j.neuropharm.2015.09.020. Epub 2015 Sep 16. PMID: 26386152.

Mazzone SB, McGarvey L. Mechanisms and Rationale for Targeted Therapies in Refractory and Unexplained Chronic Cough. Clin Pharmacol Ther. 2021 Mar;109(3):619-636. doi: 10.1002/cpt.2003. Epub 2020 Aug 28. PMID: 32748976; PMCID: PMC7983941.

Naqvi KF, Mazzone SB, Shiloh MU. Infectious and Inflammatory Pathways to Cough. Annu Rev Physiol. 2022 Sep 28. doi: 10.1146/annurev-physiol-031422-092315. Epub ahead of print. PMID: 36170660.

Silva AR, Dinis-Oliveira RJ. Pharmacokinetics and pharmacodynamics of dextromethorphan: clinical and forensic aspects. Drug Metab Rev. 2020 May;52(2):258-282. doi: 10.1080/03602532.2020.1758712. Epub 2020 May 12. PMID: 32393072.

Sweet DG, Carnielli V, Greisen G, Hallman M, Ozek E, Te Pas A, Plavka R, Roehr CC, Saugstad OD, Simeoni U, Speer CP, Vento M, Visser GHA, Halliday HL. European Consensus Guidelines on the Management of Respiratory Distress Syndrome - 2019 Update. Neonatology. 2019;115(4):432-450. doi: 10.1159/000499361. Epub 2019 Apr 11. PMID: 30974433; PMCID: PMC6604659.

Taylor CP, Traynelis SF, Siffert J, Pope LE, Matsumoto RR. Pharmacology of dextromethorphan: Relevance to dextromethorphan/quinidine (Nuedexta®) clinical use. Pharmacol Ther. 2016 Aug;164:170-82. doi: 10.1016/j.pharmthera.2016.04.010. Epub 2016 Apr 29. PMID: 27139517.

Terlizzi V, Masi E, Francalanci M, Taccetti G, Innocenti D. Hypertonic saline in people with cystic fibrosis: review of comparative studies and clinical practice. Ital J Pediatr. 2021 Aug 6;47(1):168. doi: 10.1186/s13052-021-01117-1. PMID: 34362426; PMCID: PMC8343926.

Quiz Questions

1. A 3-year-old girl is diagnosed with cystic fibrosis, and it is determined that her disease results from a mutation that causes her CFTR proteins to respond inadequately to intracellular signaling, opening minimally. She will be started on a single drug that helps restore function to her CFTR protein, increasing the likelihood that the Cl^- channels will remain open. Which of the following will be necessary for this patient as a result?

A Annual liver function tests
B Liver function tests once every three months for the first year of therapy, followed by annual testing
C Annual ECG
D ECG once every three months for the first year of therapy, followed by annual testing
E Annual BUN and creatinine clearance
F BUN and creatinine clearance once every three months for the first year of therapy, followed by annual testing

2. A 31-year-old woman who has been trying to conceive for the past two years is diagnosed with kidney stones after being rushed to the hospital with acute abdominal pain. Her husband tells the ED doctor that she is taking no medicines except for an OTC cough syrup which she started taking after reading about it on an online discussion board for women who are trying to conceive. What drug is she most likely taking?

A Dextromethorphan
B Codeine
C Guaifenesin
D Diphenhydramine
E Benzonatate

3. A 3-month-old boy is brought to a healthcare clinic because he has experienced recurrent respiratory infections and is not growing as rapidly as his siblings did. The boy was born at home, and his mother did not receive prenatal care. He is diagnosed with a condition that results from being homozygous for a mutation of the *CFTR* gene, resulting in decreased stability of the CFTR protein and impairment of its transport to the plasma membrane. By what mechanism will dornase alfa be beneficial to this boy?

A It hydrolyzes DNA in bronchial secretions
B It disrupts disulfide bonds between mucin molecules in bronchial secretions
C It hydrates bronchial secretions by drawing water to the perciliary layer
D It corrects misfolding of CFTR proteins
E His mutation makes it unlikely that this medication will have any benefit

4. Which drug is used to relieve cough and exerts its effect primarily via an effect on peripheral afferent nerves, rather than a central mechanism?

A Dextromethorphan
B Codeine
C Diphenhydramine
D Loratadine
E Benzonatate

5. A 25-year-old woman is suffering from viral bronchitis, so she decides to take an OTC antitussive drug that acts as an antagonist of NMDA receptors and an agonist of σ_1 receptors. She takes this drug at its recommended dose, but after three appropriately-timed doses, she notices that she has been feeling increasingly drunk, and she has started experiencing minor hallucinations that are unrelated to fever. Suspecting this is a drug side effect, she stops taking the drug. Several months later, the woman takes a home genetic test, which reveals a polymorphism that would likely have accounted for her experience with the OTC antitussive. What is the drug that caused her side effect, and what genetic polymorphism caused it?

A Benzonatate, CYP3A4 ultra-rapid metabolizer
B Benzonatate, CYP2D6 poor metabolizer
C Codeine, CYP3A4 ultra-rapid metabolizer
D Codeine, CYP2D6 poor metabolizer
E Dextromethorphan, CYP3A4 ultra-rapid metabolizer
F Dextromethorphan, CYP2D6 poor metabolizer

Quiz Answers

1. B. Ivacaftor is the drug in question. It is a CFTR potentiator, and it increases the likelihood of the open state for the CFTR Cl^- channel. It is only indicated for persons who have one mutation that produces a CFTR protein that is responsive to ivacaftor (e.g., *G551D*). Elevations in liver enzymes can be caused by ivacaftor. The recommended monitoring protocol is to perform liver function tests once every three months for the first year of therapy, followed by annual testing.

2. C. Expectorants are being used off-label by women who are trying to conceive. The only expectorant listed is guaifenesin, which can cause nephrolithiasis. Expectorants are thought to increase vaginal secretions, making it more likely that sperm will survive transit to the egg. Dextromethorphan and codeine are antitussives, not expectorants, and diphenhydramine is an antihistamine with anticholinergic activity. It is likely to dry vaginal secretions rather than increase them. Benzonatate is an ester-type local anesthetic antitussive drug that is available only by prescription in the US. It does not cause nephrolithiasis.

3. A. The airway mucus of patients with cystic fibrosis contains large amounts of DNA and other components from necrotic neutrophils. By hydrolyzing the DNA in mucus, dornase alfa helps "thin" the mucus, making it easier to expectorate. N-acetylcysteine disrupts disulfide bonds, expectorants such as hypertonic saline can hydrate the mucus, and the CFTR correctors correct the conformational instability of chloride channels due to misfolding of the CFTR transmembrane proteins in CF patients. There are currently no drugs that act via the CFTR protein that can treat individuals who are homozygous for mutations resulting in class I dysfunction (no CFTR protein is made).

4. E. Benzonatate is a local anesthetic and is thought to anesthetize vagal afferent fibers of the airways. Loratadine is a second-generation antihistamine and is not used as an antitussive. All of the other drugs in the list are centrally acting.

5. F. Dextromethorphan is the only drug listed which, at high blood levels, can cause a feeling of drunkenness and hallucinations, and it is an NMDA receptor antagonist and σ_1 receptor agonist. Dextromethorphan is metabolized by CYP2D6, to dextrorphan, a metabolite that is also active. Dextrorphan undergoes glucuronidation, or CYP3A4/A5-mediated metabolism to another compound which is then glucuronidated. Individuals who are poor CYP2D6 metabolizers have an increased risk of adverse effects and a prolonged action of dextromethorphan. Dextromethorphan, in high doses, can cause euphoria, feelings of drunkenness, visual hallucinations, dissociation, agitation, and delusions. While benzonatate can cause hallucinations in overdose, it is a local anesthetic that acts by anesthetizing stretch receptor fibers in the vagal afferents from the lungs. Codeine may be available OTC in certain combination products in some US states and in some countries outside of the US, but its action is believed to stem from its agonism of μ opioid receptors, and it is not known for causing hallucinations.

CHAPTER 7

LIVER DISORDERS

MONTE TROUTMAN, DO[1], AND VICTOR V. UTESHEV, PHD[2]

[1] University of North Texas Health Science Center, Fort Worth, Texas, USA
[2] Epigen Biosciences Inc., San Diego, California, USA

Symptoms: Immuno-Infectious
Endo-Repro-Gastrointestinal

DRUG LIST FOR Hepatitis B (HBV):
pegylated interferon (PEG-IFNa)
adefovir (dipivoxil)
lamivudine
telbivudine
tenofovir (disoproxil fumarate)
entecavir

DRUG LIST FOR Hepatitis C (HCV):
daclatasvir+sofosbuvir
ombitasvir+paritaprevir+dasabuvir+ritonavir
sofosbuvir+ledipasvir
sofosbuvir+velpatasvir+voxilaprevir

General Background (see also Chapter 3)

The liver is the second largest organ in the body after the skin. It is composed of two major systems: the hepatocellular and biliary systems. The liver has a multitude of functions. It also produces bile that is transported through the biliary system with the gallbladder functioning as a storage depot between meals. The liver is involved in many major functions including protein synthesis (albumin and coagulation factors) and degradation, nutrient metabolism of carbohydrates, and lipids. It also has the unique capacity to regenerate after injury. The number of disorders of the liver is innumerable. The various presentations of liver disorders are also wide-ranging. Liver disorders present in a variety of manners. These include symptoms, abnormal liver chemistries, jaundice, or abnormal imaging. Symptoms are often vague and minimal unless they are the result of gallstone-related disorders. These symptoms include fatigue, pruritis, vague right upper quadrant pain, dark urine, and light-colored stools. Some symptoms of liver disease are indicative of more advanced liver disease including cirrhosis. These symptoms would include edema, ascites, and GI bleeding including acute upper GI bleeding.

Diagnosis

Imaging: Imaging plays a major role in the assessment of liver disorders. The most used are ultrasound of the liver, gallbladder, and abdomen for ascites. CT scan of the abdomen is used for better details of the liver, pancreas, and abdomen cavity for ascites, and biliary tract inspection (gallbladder, biliary tree). MRI/MRCP is used specifically for more details of the biliary tree and assessment of the liver for liver masses, especially for hepatocellular carcinoma.

Laboratory results: Often the initial abnormality found in liver disorders is abnormal liver chemistries or enzymes formerly referred to as abnormal liver function tests (LFTs). Since these lab tests do not generally measure liver function, they are not called LFTs anymore. The exception to tests that measure liver function is serum albumin and INR (prothrombin time). However, low serum albumin and prolonged INR occur with more advanced liver disease. When a patient has abnormal liver function, a stepwise approach is used to pursue the cause or a differential diagnosis. The first step is to determine if the reason is acute, chronic, or acute-on-chronic. If someone has increased liver chemistries with no history of liver disease, no family history of liver disease with normal imaging, and no risk factors then an acute cause is plausible. A chronic condition usually is considered when abnormal liver chemistries are present for 6 months or more. Patient history, review of previous chemistries, review of previous imaging, and physical examination aid in the determination of chronicity. Some physical findings more indicative of chronic disease are ascites, edema, palmar erythema, testicular atrophy, painful gynecomastia, hepatic encephalopathy, Dupuytren's contracture, Terri's nails, caput medusa, and digital clubbing. Imaging may demonstrate findings more indicative of chronic disease. An acute-on-chronic disorder would be a sudden increase in liver enzymes in the setting of chronic liver disease. The most common lab tests for liver disorders are AST (Aspartate transaminase), ALT (Alanine transaminase), serum alkaline phosphatase, serum bilirubin, serum albumin, and INR. With more advanced liver disease serum sodium and serum creatinine are useful. The platelet count should also be considered in the assessment. The next step is to classify the disorder into hepatocellular, cholestatic, or mixed. This classification will help narrow the broad differential of abnormal liver enzymes into categories. Hepatocellular disease is when the transaminases are the predominantly elevated enzymes. Aminotransaminases are the AST and ALT enzymes contained in hepatocytes and become elevated with damage or necrosis of the hepatocytes. The cholestatic classification occurs with an elevation of the serum alkaline phosphatase liver enzyme. Elevation of this enzyme implies inflammation of the cells of the biliary tree known as cholangiocytes. This enzyme can also be of bone origin. When there is no clear-cut indication of why this enzyme is elevated then the gamma-glutamyl transferase (GGTP) will elevate and indicate liver origin. In some instances, both sets of enzymes (hepatocellular and cholestatic) are elevated and there is no predominate pattern. This is called a mixed pattern. When this occurs using the R factor will help delineate the pattern to help classify which category is predominating. If it does not fit into cholestatic or hepatocellular then it is called mixed. The R factor can be found on MDcalc. If the factor is less than 2 the disorder is cholestatic, if greater than 5 the disorder is hepatocellular. If the factor is 2 to 5 then it is called mixed. This mixed pattern is often caused by drug-induced liver injury (DILI). When assessing elevated transaminases (AST and ALT) it is important to note that females occupy the lower half of the range of normal. Therefore, for females with AST and/or ALT elevated in the upper half of the range of normal, this should be considered elevated enzymes. Several scoring systems exist to assess the severity of liver disease especially if cirrhosis has developed. The Child-Pugh Score is calculated using serum albumin, serum total bilirubin, INR, grade of ascites, and grade of encephalopathy. While a more up-to-date score is the NaMELD which includes the serum sodium, serum creatinine, INR, and serum total bilirubin. These scores assess the severity and prognosis of liver disease especially when cirrhosis has developed. Both can be found at MDCalc.

Common Types of Liver Disease

The most common disorders causing **hepatocellular disorders** are:

- Viral hepatitis with hepatitis A, B, C, D, and E being the most common.
- All can cause acute infections with B and C being the most common cause of chronic hepatitis in the USA.
- Alcohol-related liver disease is both acute and chronic.
- Drug-induced liver Injury (DILI).
- Autoimmune hepatitis.
- Metabolic dysfunction-associated steatotic liver disease (MASLD; formerly known as non-alcoholic liver disease, NAFLD).
- Hemochromatosis.
- Alpha-1 anti-trypsin deficiency.
- Wilson Disease.

The most common disorders causing **cholestatic disorders** are:

- Primary Biliary Cholangitis (PBC).
- Primary Sclerosing Cholangitis (PSC).
- Hepatic Space Occupying lesions such as primary and metastatic tumors, cysts, and abscesses.
- Infiltrative disorders such as lymphomas and amyloidosis.
- Granulomatous disorders such as sarcoidosis, tuberculosis, and medications.
- Drug-induced liver injury (DILI).

Severe elevation of AST and ALT (over 1000 IUs) are usually limited to:

- Acute viral hepatitis.
- Drugs and toxins with acetaminophen are the most common.
- Ischemic hepatitis in the setting of hypotensive or hypovolemic situations.
- Acute flare of autoimmune hepatitis.

Another rule is that alcoholic liver disease does not raise the AST and ALT over 300 IUs and has an AST/ALT ratio of over 2/1.

Hepatitis A (HAV)

Presentation: The course of the disease is 2-6 months, with sudden onset of fever, loss of appetite, nausea & vomiting, fatigue, and abdominal pain.

Risk Factors: Fecal oral transmission.

Pathophysiology: RNA virus with 2-to-4-week incubation. Damage is secondary to inflammation-driven liver cell death. (Lemon et al. 2017; Dienstag 2022) Not a chronic progressive disease.

Examination: Jaundiced, enlarged tender liver, dark urine.

Laboratory: Elevated AST and ALT, often over 1000 IUs, and elevated total bilirubin over 5 mg/dl.

Imaging: Rarely needed but usually a liver ultrasound is done.

Associated symptoms/conditions: Symptoms of all acute viral hepatitis are usually fatigue, jaundice, fever, loss of appetite, and nausea. Chronic viral hepatitis symptoms are similar.

*Diagnosis: S*erum Anti-HAV with IgM lasting for months and IgG indefinitely.

Treatment: Symptomatic no antivirals.

Management: The course of the disease is 2-6 months. Excellent prognosis.

Hepatitis B (HBV)

Presentation: Acute phase similar to hepatitis A (above), though can have a chronic asymptomatic phase or progress to cirrhosis and hepatocellular carcinoma.

Risk Factors: Underdiagnosed in the USA. Risky behavior (Men who have sex with men; IV drug use; Blood transfusion; Exposure to sex workers; Incarceration; Piercing; Tattoos; Multiple sex partners; Unprotected sex; Vertical transmission; Positive for HIV). Increased risk if born in countries with > 2% carrier rate (South/Central America; Western Africa; SE Asia; Middle East). Children from high carrier rate via vertical transmission. Susceptible healthcare workers who receive a needle stick contaminated with blood from an HBV-infected patient have a 6-30% risk of contracting the disease.

Pathophysiology: DNA virus with an incubation period in the range of 70-80 days.

Examination: Similar to hepatitis A in the acute phase. In the chronic phase, can be normal or present with signs of chronic liver disease (ascites and edema, encephalopathy, firm liver, jaundice, spider angiomas). (de Bruyn and Graviss 2001)

Laboratory: serology includes HBsAg, HBeAg, Anti HBs, Anti HBe, and Anti HBc.

Imaging: Rarely needed acutely but liver ultrasound is frequently done. Ultrasound surveillance is recommended every 6 months for all HbSAg-positive patients to screen for the development of hepatocellular carcinoma. (Terrault et al. 2018)

Associated symptoms/conditions: About 5% of adults infected with hepatitis B will go on to develop an infection, and 5% of those will go on to develop cirrhosis annually. About 10-15% with chronic infection and cirrhosis go on to develop hepatocellular carcinoma (over 5 years). Hepatitis B has been associated with a number of conditions, including glomerulonephritis, polyarteritis nodosa, and cryoglobulinemia, among others. (Iloeje et al. 2006; Varbobitis and Papatheodoridis 2016; Kappus and Sterling 2013)

Diagnosis: Low chronicity. Serology includes HBsAg, HBeAg, Anti HBs, Anti HBe, and Anti HBc.

Treatment: Pre- and post-exposure vaccination prophylaxis is available. Numerous and complicated strategies for treating HBV with a variety of antiviral agents exist and are beyond the scope of this text.

Management: Screening for hepatocellular carcinoma is recommended with ultrasound every 6 months in those positive for HBsAg and with cirrhosis. Avoid alcohol and use caution with medications known to be liver toxic. Vaccinate against Hepatitis A.

Hepatitis C (HCV)

Presentation: Acute infection presents similarly to the other viral hepatitides. Chronic infection with progression to cirrhosis and hepatocellular carcinoma is possible, similar to hepatitis B. Of those with acute infection, about 70% go on to develop chronic infection, and of those, untreated, about 15-30% will go on to develop cirrhosis.

Risk Factors: Bloodborne transmission. Risky behavior (Men who have sex with men; IV drug use; Blood transfusion; Exposure to sex workers; Incarceration; Piercing; Tattoos; Multiple sex partners; Unprotected sex; Vertical transmission; Positive for HIV). The risk for healthcare workers sustaining a needlestick from a Hepatitis C positive patient is approximately 2%.

Pathophysiology: RNA virus. 6 genotypes. Incubation is 2 weeks to 6 months.

Examination: Similar to other hepatitides in the acute phase. The chronic phase may be normal or with stigmata of chronic liver disease (ascites and edema, encephalopathy, firm liver, jaundice, spider angiomas). (de Bruyn and Graviss 2001)

Laboratory: Serology anti-HCV. Increased AST and ALT. Detection during acute infection is unusual due to mild to minimal symptoms.

Imaging: Usually not needed but liver ultrasound is frequently done.

Associated symptoms/conditions: Can progress to cirrhosis and hepatocellular carcinoma. Extrahepatic manifestations include autoimmune anemia and thrombocytopenia, the skin condition porphyria cutanea tarda, autoimmune hypothyroidism, peripheral neuropathy, and lymphoma, among others. (Cacoub and Saadoun 2021)

Diagnosis: Serology for anti-HCV. High rate of chronicity. Increased AST and ALT. RNA levels if anti-HCV positive.

Treatment: Unlikely Hepatitis B, there is no vaccine for hepatitis C. There are a number of complicated strategies for the treatment of hepatitis C utilizing antivirals, the details of which are beyond the scope of this text.

Management: Avoid alcohol, vaccinate against Hepatitis A and B. Monitoring for esophageal varices with endoscopy every 3 years is suggested in patients with cirrhosis. Ultrasound surveillance for hepatocellular carcinoma every 6 months in patients with HCV and cirrhosis. (Cacoub and Saadoun 2021; Younossi et al. 2021)

Hepatitis Delta (HDV)

Presentation: Only presents if the patient has Hepatitis B. Increasing occurrence in the USA.

Risk Factors: Bloodborne and vertical transmission.

Pathophysiology: RNA virus.

Examination: Incubation 90 days.

Laboratory: Transaminitis in chronic Hepatitis B is an alarm for testing for HDV.

Imaging: Usually not needed.

Associated symptoms/conditions: Symptoms of all acute viral hepatitis are usually fatigue, jaundice, fever, loss of appetite, and nausea. Chronic viral hepatitis symptoms are similar.

Diagnosis: Transaminitis in chronic Hepatitis B is an alarm for testing for HDV.

Treatment: Treatment is available but suboptimal.

Management: No vaccine.

Hepatitis E (HEV)

Presentation: Rare chronic disease. Most severe with pregnancy.

Risk Factors: Highest in developing countries. Fecal oral and vertical transmission.

Pathophysiology: RNA virus. Incubation 2-9 weeks.

Examination: Enlarged tender liver, jaundiced, can progress to liver failure.

Laboratory: Markedly elevated AST and ALT over 1000 IUs, bilirubin elevated over 5 mg%.

Imaging: Ultrasound of the liver is rarely done.

Associated symptoms/conditions: Symptoms of all acute viral hepatitis are usually fatigue, jaundice, fever, loss of appetite, and nausea. Chronic viral hepatitis symptoms are similar.

Diagnosis: Serology of anti-HEV and HEV RNA titers.

Treatment: None available and care is supportive.

Management: Recombinant vaccine available.

Metabolic Dysfunction-Associated Steatotic Liver Disease (MASLD) formerly known as Non-Alcoholic Liver Disease (NAFLD)

Presentation: MASLD/NAFLD (will be referred to hereafter as MASLD) is fast becoming the most common cause of chronic liver disease in the USA. It is now the second most common reason for liver transplantation.

Risk Factors: Conditions that predispose to MASLD are obesity, metabolic syndrome, diabetes, and genetic predisposition.

Pathophysiology: MASLD constitutes a spectrum of illness starting with fatty infiltration of liver cells (steatosis) then, progressing to steatosis with inflammation (Non-Alcoholic Steatohepatitis or NASH) with increasing fibrosis that culminates in a late-stage fibrotic liver known as cirrhosis. (Martin et al. 2021; Kudaravalli and John 2022)

Examination: Physical findings are few until the progression to cirrhosis when findings of chronic liver disease and associated portal hypertension may be evident.

Laboratory: It can present with elevated transaminases and will have a negative serologic workup for other hepatic disorders. Monitoring of MASLD is based on fibrotic scoring that can be done with specialized imagery techniques as well as serologic fibrotic scoring (FIB-4 and ELF).

Imaging: Often liver imaging for other reasons can detect MASLD. Liver elastography is a method to measure liver "stiffness" and infer fibrosis. It's useful for monitoring the progression of the disease. (Gherlan 2015)

Associated symptoms/conditions: Usually associated with obesity and or metabolic syndrome but can have a hereditary component.

Diagnosis: Made based on establishing hepatic steatosis in the absence of significant alcohol use and exclusion of other causes. (Chalasani et al. 2018)

Treatment: The development of specific treatment modalities are in process. Current recommendations include weight loss, increased physical activity, dietary changes, Vitamin E (in non-diabetics), and coffee consumption. Pioglitazone can be considered in patients with biopsy-proven NASH.

Management: Avoid alcohol. Vaccinate for Hep A and B. Attention to weight loss, diet, and exercise. Screening for HCC and esophageal varices in patients with cirrhosis is advised. (Garcia-Tsao et al. 2017; Heimbach et al. 2018; Chalasani et al. 2018; Weiss 1993) There is concern that MASLD has an increased risk of hepatocellular carcinoma prior to the development of cirrhosis but screening guidelines are in development.

Wilson Disease

Presentation: Rare genetic disorder with a highly variable presentation, with onset from childhood to middle adulthood. It should be suspected when there is a combined liver, neurologic (movement disorder), and psychiatric presentation.

Risk Factors: Genetic disease with the autosomal recessive inheritance pattern.

Pathophysiology: Copper accumulation in the liver, brain, kidney, and cornea leading to progressive neurologic dysfunction with cirrhosis.

Examination: Ocular exam may reveal a Kayser-Fleischer ring, a dark ring around the iris, in 50-90% of affected individuals

Laboratory: Labs reveal hepatocellular damage pattern.

Imaging: Imaging of the liver is sometimes performed to assess disease severity.

Associated symptoms/conditions: In addition to liver disease, there are well-known neurologic, psychiatric, and ocular manifestations. As noted earlier, Keyser-Fleischer rings are common and, when present, are pathognomonic for the condition. The neurologic disease typically presents with movement disorders that range from hyperkinetic (chorea, choreoathetosis, tremors) to rigidity. Psychiatric symptoms include depression, emotional lability, and cognitive disturbances; however, psychosis is not common.

Diagnosis: Lab testing of serum ceruloplasmin (low), serum copper and urinary copper (elevated), and copper dry weight via biopsy are hallmarks.

Treatment: Agents that remove (chelate) and/or inhibit the absorption of copper from the body (e.g., zinc).

Management: Attention should be paid to the development of copper deficiency. Wilson's can cause cirrhosis, and so the previously discussed management of cirrhosis applies here (e.g., vaccinations, avoid alcohol, observe for HCC or varices).

Hemochromatosis

Presentation: Iron overload syndrome is most commonly inherited though with some less common secondary causes such as oral intake or multiple blood transfusions. Hereditary hemochromatosis presents with diabetes mellitus, skin bronzing/hyperpigmentation, advanced liver disease, cardiomyopathy, and arthropathy (classically of the metacarpophalangeal joints). (Barton and Edwards 1993)

Risk Factors: Autosomal recessive inheritance; excessive iron absorption.

Pathophysiology: Iron overload can cause functional changes leading to cellular damage.

Examination: Hepatomegaly or findings of cirrhosis and portal hypertension, increased skin pigmentation.

Laboratory: Lab testing relies on elevated ferritin levels, increased iron saturation, iron overload on biopsy tissue, all in the setting of elevated AST and ALT.

Imaging: MRI can help identify iron levels in the liver.

Associated symptoms/conditions: Can see hypogonadism and testicular atrophy. Chondrocalcinosis (accumulation of calcium in the cartilage of joints) may be seen. (Bacon et al. 2011)

Diagnosis: Patents have elevated AST and ALT. Elevated ferritin and iron saturation will prompt genetic testing of HFE and C282Y labs. A liver biopsy with iron levels is the hallmark of diagnosis.

Treatment: Avoid alcohol, Vitamin C, raw seafood, and iron supplements. Monitored phlebotomies. If can't tolerate phlebotomies then chelating agents.

Management: Monitor ferritin levels during treatment and consider genetic counseling of relatives. Monitoring for liver cancer.

Autoimmune Hepatitis (AIH)

Presentation: Requires exclusion of other causes of hepatocellular disease.

Risk Factors: Increased risk in females.

Pathophysiology: Autoimmune disorder with autoantibodies and elevated gamma globulins.

Examination: Interface necrosis on histology from the liver biopsy is required.

Laboratory: AST, ALT, and gamma globulin elevation are predominate lab abnormalities.

Imaging: Not usually helpful but liver ultrasound is usually done.

Associated symptoms/conditions: Other autoimmune conditions are possible.

Diagnosis: Interface necrosis on histology from the liver biopsy is required.

Diagnosis centers on elevated anti-nuclear antibodies (ANA), anti-smooth muscle antibodies (ASMA), and other less common markers if ANA and ASMA are not diagnostic.

Treatment: Steroids and immunomodulators.

Management: Monitor for side effects of treatment and advancement of the disease.

Alcoholic Liver Disease

Presentation: Progressive disease that starts with fatty liver infiltration and then advances with progressive fibrosis that can lead to cirrhosis. One of the most common causes of cirrhosis. It can present with cirrhosis such as ascites and UGI bleeding from esophageal varices. Other presentations that are more common include fatigue, jaundice, edema, ascites, mental status changes of encephalopathy, and pruritis. History of alcohol use is the most common presentation.

Risk Factors: Men at risk at 14 drinks per week. Women are at risk at 7 drinks per week.

Pathophysiology: Induction of fibrosis of hepatocytes from alcohol and breakdown products of alcohol.

Examination: Patients with enlarged liver, bruising, skin excoriations from itching, edema of lower extremities, altered mental status, dilated veins of abdominal wall, Dupuytren's contractures, palmar erythema, testicular atrophy, painful gynecomastia and asterixis with advance disease.

Laboratory: AST/ALT elevations 2-3/1.

Rare AST and ALT over 300 IU.

Imaging: Ultrasound, CT scan, or MRI used for the diagnosis will show nodularity. Also uses for Hepatocellular carcinoma surveillance.

Associated symptoms/conditions: Can be complicated with acute alcoholic hepatitis with prolonged massive bilirubin elevation.

Diagnosis: Thorough history and physical exam with appropriate lab testing and imaging. Rule out other or concomitant liver disease.

Treatment: Avoid alcohol, sodium restriction, diuretics, and with advanced disease consider a liver transplant.

Management: Can be complicated with acute alcoholic hepatitis with prolonged massive bilirubin elevation.

Cholestatic Liver Disorders

Primary Sclerosing Cholangitis

Presentation: Cholestatic disorder with patchy inflammation of intra- and extrahepatic biliary tree. Associated with chronic ulcerative colitis and less frequent with Crohn's Disease.

Risk Factors: More common in men.

Pathophysiology: Cholestatic liver chemistries profile.

Examination/Laboratory: Cholestatic liver enzyme elevations (alkaline phosphatase).

Imaging: Imaging by MRCP.

Associated symptoms/conditions: Most common symptoms are abdominal pain, fatigue, and jaundice.

Cholestatic disorder with patchy inflammation of intra- and extrahepatic biliary tree.

Markedly increases the risk of colorectal carcinoma.

Diagnosis: ERCP can make a diagnosis but mostly for therapeutics.

Treatment: No specific treatment other than a liver transplant.

Management: Endoscopic treatment of biliary strictures. Monitor hepatic status and liver transplant with hepatic decompensation.

Primary Biliary Cholangitis

Presentation: Fatigue, pruritis including nocturnal and altered mental status.

Risk Factors: Most common in middle-aged women and most common cholestatic liver disease in adults in the USA.

Pathophysiology/Examination: Physical finding of skin excoriation and hyperpigmentation.

Laboratory: Anti-mitochondrial antibody positive lab is sensitive and specific.

Elevated liver enzymes in cholestatic pattern (serum alkaline phosphatase).

Imaging: MRCP.

Associated symptoms/conditions: Severe pruritis is a hallmark symptom and is associated with fatigue.

Diagnosis: Liver biopsy not necessary.

Treatment: Obeticholic Acid.

Management: Cool showers, moisturizing, cotton clothes.

Drug-Induced Liver Injury (DILI)

Presentation: Hepatocellular, cholestatic, or mixed abnormal liver enzymes possible.

Risk Factors: Supplements and herbals can cause DILI as can multiple prescriptions or over-the-counter medications.

Pathophysiology: Direct toxicity to hepatocytes or interference with normal metabolic activities of the liver.

Examination: Usually minimal physical findings but can present with jaundice, altered mental status, pruritis,

Laboratory: Elevated AST, ALT, serum bilirubin, alkaline phosphatase, or any combinations.

Associated symptoms/conditions: Can cause cholestatic, hepatocellular, or mixed pattern.

Diagnosis: High degree of suspicion and thorough review of current and recent medications. This should include intense questioning of over-the-counter medications and herbs and supplements. Always screen with a drug screen, especially for acetaminophen.

Treatment: Discontinue meds and monitor patient and liver enzymes. Acetaminophen has treatment.

Management: Multiple sites are available to find common and uncommon medications (e.g. www.livertox.nih.gov).

Other causes of chronic liver disease and abnormal liver enzymes include alpha 1 anti-trypsin deficiency, granulomatous parasitic disorders, multiple less common viruses, vascular disorders such as Budd-Chiari Syndrome, sarcoidosis, primary liver cancer, metastatic liver cancer, and cholangiocarcinoma.

Complications of Cirrhosis

Thrombocytopenia
Coagulopathy (INR prolonged)
Ascites
Edema
Sarcopenia
Encephalopathy
Varices (esophageal/gastric)
Hepatocellular carcinoma
Hypoalbuminemia
Hepatorenal syndrome
Spontaneous bacterial peritonitis
Hepatopulmonary syndrome
Painful gynecomastia
Loss of sex drive

Pharmacological Treatments of HBV

The goal of HBV therapies is to reduce morbidity and mortality via suppression of HBV replication. Sustained suppression translates to a reduction in hepatic aminotransferase levels (a marker of liver damage), histological improvement in the liver, loss of Hb e/s/c Ag (hepatitis B e/s/c antigen), and suppression of HBV DNA to undetectable levels. These endpoints translate to reduced necroinflammation, decreased risk of hepatocellular carcinoma and cirrhosis, and decreased need for liver transplantation. HBV eradication is not currently attainable.

Nucleoside and Nucleotide Analogues (NAs): Antiviral therapy with NAs is indicated for patients with fulminant HBV until HBsAg clearance is documented, or indefinitely in patients requiring liver transplantation. First-line oral NA therapy is tenofovir or entecavir. Second-line oral NtA therapy is adefovir. Patients with minimal disease and those who are unlikely to achieve SVR should not be treated with NAs to avoid resistance (the most potent NA should always be used). In NA-naive patients, lamivudine is associated with the highest rate of drug resistance, and tenofovir and entecavir with the lowest rate.

Adefovir

Adefovir, an adenine NtA that inhibits HBV replication. Adefovir (diphosphate) competes with deoxyadenosine 5'-triphosphate for incorporation into viral DNA. After incorporation, adefovir inhibits HBV polymerase and terminates the DNA chain.

Adverse effects: Well tolerated. Nephrotoxicity (at high doses only).

Black Box Warning: Severe acute exacerbations of HBV upon discontinuation.

Metabolic disorders: lactic acidosis and hepatomegaly (i.e., enlarged liver).

Lamivudine

Lamivudine is a cytosine NsA. Lamivudine competes with natural deoxycytidine triphosphate and causes DNA chain termination and inhibition of HBV replication. Chronic therapy is limited by lamivudine-resistant strains of HBV due to mutations (15–30% at 1 year; >70% at 5 years of therapy).

Adverse effects: Excellent safety profile.

Black Box Warning: Severe acute exacerbations of HBV upon discontinuation of treatment in HIV/HBV co-infected patients.

Metabolic disorders: lactic acidosis and hepatomegaly.

Telbivudine

Telbivudine is a thymidine NsA. Telbivudine competes with natural thymidine triphosphate and causes DNA chain termination resulting in the inhibition of HBV replication. Telbivudine was superior to lamivudine in a 2-year randomized study (N=1367). Switching from lamivudine to telbivudine resulted in a significantly greater reduction in HBV DNA load at 24 and 52 weeks in a randomized study (N=246).

Adverse effects: Mild. Fatigue, headache, cough, nausea, diarrhea, rash, fever, and myalgia.

Black Box Warning: Severe acute exacerbations of HBV upon discontinuation.

Metabolic disorders: lactic acidosis and hepatomegaly.

Entecavir

Entecavir is a guanosine NsA. Entecavir inhibits all three functions of HBV DNA polymerase: base priming, reverse transcription of negative strands, and synthesis of positive strands of DNA. Suppression of HBV DNA levels was greater with entecavir vs. lamivudine or adefovir in comparative trials. Entecavir should be taken on an empty stomach (+/-2 h from meals). The oral bioavailability of entecavir is ~100% (fasting) vs. ~45% (fed).

Adverse effects: Well tolerated.

Black Box Warning: Severe acute exacerbations of HBV upon discontinuation of treatment. Development of resistance to HIV nucleoside RT inhibitors in HIV/HBV co-infected patients. Metabolic disorders: lactic acidosis and hepatomegaly.

Tenofovir (an adenosine NsA)

Tenofovir competes with deoxyadenosine 5'-triphosphate for incorporation into viral DNA. After incorporation, tenofovir inhibits HBV polymerase. Tenofovir is similar in structure to adefovir but has a higher rate of SVR and histologic improvement. Tenofovir is effective against lamivudine- and entecavir-resistant HBV, but has reduced activity against adefovir-resistant strains.

Adverse effects: Nausea, abdominal pain, diarrhea, dizziness, fatigue, and rash.

Black Box Warning: Metabolic disorders: lactic acidosis and hepatomegaly.

Pharmacological Treatments of HCV

The goal of HCV therapies is viral eradication, i.e., sustained viral response (SVR) defined as the absence of HCV RNA 12/24 weeks after completion of therapy. SVR translates to improved liver histology, reduction in the risk of cirrhosis and hepatocellular carcinoma. Acute HCV infection shows a high risk (>80%) of progression to the chronic phase. HCV is a single-stranded RNA virus that is categorized into nine distinct genotypes. The HCV genotype (i.e., the viral strain) is an important variable. It is determined by a blood test. Genotypes of HCV are genetically distinct groups of the virus. Genotype 1 is the most common in the United States affecting >75% of all chronic HCV patients; 20-25% of patients have genotypes 2 or 3, with small numbers of patients infected with genotypes 4-6. Most HCV patients have only one principal genotype, rather than multiple genotypes. Genotype 4 is common in Africa; genotype 6 is common in Southeast Asia.

The concept of Directly Acting Antivirals (DAAs):

DAAs are molecules that target specific nonstructural (NS) proteins of the HCV and result in disruption of viral replication and infection. There are 4 classes of DAAs, which are defined by their mechanism of action and therapeutic target:

NS3/4A protease inhibitors (PIs),
NS5A inhibitors
NS5B nucleoside polymerase inhibitors (NIs)
NS5B non-nucleoside polymerase inhibitors (NNIs)

Note on SVR12 vs. SVR24: The FDA has reviewed results from clinical trials of HCV treatment in nearly 13,600 adult participants: 51.8% of participants had an undetectable viral load 12 weeks after cessation of therapy (i.e., SVR12). Overall, 50.6% of participants also had the same result at week 24 after cessation of therapy (i.e., SVR24). Thus, the vast majority (>98%) of participants had both an SVR12 and an SVR24. Thus, an SVR12 may be an important end-point in HCV clinical trials. Expect more pharmaceutical companies to focus on SVR12 in the future.

The FDA warning of the increased risk of HBV reactivation in co-infected patients treated with DAAs for HCV (supplementary reading). 24 cases with confirmed reactivation of HBV infection were identified between November 2013 and July 2016. All 24 patients received treatment with DAAs for the treatment of HCV. HBV reactivation occurred within 4-8 weeks of starting HCV treatment. Three of the patients decompensated: two died and one required hepatic transplantation. DAAs cause immunosuppression, but the mechanism of HBV reactivation is unknown. During the clinical trials for DAAs, HBV co-infection was one of the exclusion criteria. 12 of the 24 cases received antiviral treatment for HBV: tenofovir or entecavir. Information about other patients is unavailable. With HBV treatment, most patients had improvement in HBV DNA, elevated aminotransferase, and malaise or fatigue.

Daclatasvir

Daclatasvir, a DAA, inhibits HCV RNA replication and virion assembly by binding to NS5A preventing its interaction with host cell proteins required for replication. Daclatasvir is highly selective for HCV.

Monotherapy is not recommended. Instead, combination therapy with sofosbuvir is recommended.

Adverse effects: Nausea, headache, fatigue

Black Box Warning: HBV reactivation in HCV/HBV co-infected patients

Ombitasvir+paritaprevir+dasabuvir+ritonavir (HCV genotypes 1) (FDA: 12-2014)

A combination therapy of 4 drugs: ombitasvir, paritaprevir, dasabuvir, and ritonavir. Ombitasvir+paritaprevir+ritonavir are combined as a fixed-dose tablet and dasabuvir is a separate tablet.

Ombitasvir is an NS5A inhibitor with pan-genotypic (i.e., across all genotypes) activity. Paritaprevir is an inhibitor of the NS3/4A serine protease. Dasabuvir is a non-nucleoside NS5B polymerase inhibitor. Ritonavir inhibits CYP3A4 thereby increasing paritaprevir plasma levels with no effects on HCV. Ombitasvir, paritaprevir, dasabuvir target multiple steps of the HCV lifecycle and show non-overlapping resistance profiles.

Adverse reactions: Mild. Skin irritation, nausea, asthenia, insomnia, fatigue.

Black Box Warning: HBV reactivation in HBV/HCV co-infected patients.

Sofosbuvir+pegIFN+ribavirin (HCV genotypes 1-4) (FDA: 2013) – Not very effective

Sofosbuvir, a DAA, serves as a defective substrate for HCV NS5B protein and inhibits viral RNA replication. Monotherapy (sofosbuvir alone) is not recommended. Sofosbuvir is approved for combination therapy with pegIFN-a and ribavirin (SVR>70) for 12–24 weeks. Nucleotide inhibitors of the HCV RNA polymerase (e.g., sofosbuvir) exhibit a very low probability for resistance – an important advantage over HCV drugs that target other viral enzymes: e.g., the protease, for which resistance caused therapeutic failures.

Sofosbuvir+Ledipasvir (HCV genotypes 1,4,5,6) (FDA: 10-2014)

Sofosbuvir+ledipasvir, a DAA (similar to daclatasvir), inhibits HCV NS5A and is available as a combination treatment with sofosbuvir for chronic HCV genotype 1 with or without cirrhosis. Ledipasvir is fully active against sofosbuvir resistance and vice versa. Combination treatments: sofosbuvir ledipasvir for chronic HCV genotype 1,4-6 with or without cirrhosis. Sofosbuvir+ledipasvir results in SVR>93% after 12 weeks of treatment.

Adverse effects (S+L): Asthenia, headache, fatigue, insomnia.

Black Box Warning: HBV reactivation in HBV/HCV co-infected patients.

Sofosbuvir+Velpatasvir (HCV genotypes 1-6) (FDA: 06-2016)

Sofosbuvir+Velpatasvir (similar to ledipasvir) is a DAA, inhibits HCV NS5A, and is available as a combination treatment with sofosbuvir for chronic HCV genotype 1 with or without cirrhosis. Combination treatments: Sofosbuvir+Velpatasvir for chronic HCV genotype 1-6 with or without cirrhosis. Sofosbuvir+Velpatasvir result in SVR>95% after 12 weeks of treatment.

Contraindicated for patients taking antibiotic rifampin (potent CYP inducer).

Adverse effects (S+V): Nausea, headache, fatigue.

Black Box Warning: HBV reactivation in HBV/HCV co-infected patients.

Sofosbuvir+Velpatasvir+Voxilaprevir (HCV genotypes 1-6) (FDA: 07-2017)

Sofosbuvir+Voxilaprevir: a pan-genotypic HCV NS3/4A protease inhibitor. Combination treatments for chronic HCV genotype 1-6 with or without cirrhosis. Sofosbuvir+velpatsvir+voxilaprevir result in SVR12>96%.

Contraindicated for patients taking antibiotic rifampin (potent CYP inducer).

Adverse effects (S+V+V): Diarrhea, headache, fatigue.

Black Box Warning: HBV reactivation in HBV/HCV co-infected patients.

References

Bacon, B. R., P. C. Adams, K. V. Kowdley, L. W. Powell, A. S. Tavill, and D. American Association for the Study of Liver. 2011. Diagnosis and management of hemochromatosis: 2011 practice guideline by the American Association for the Study of Liver Diseases. *Hepatology* 54 (1):328-343.

Barton, J. C., and C. Q. Edwards. 1993. HFE Hemochromatosis. In *GeneReviews((R))*, edited by M. P. Adam, D. B. Everman, G. M. Mirzaa, R. A. Pagon, S. E. Wallace, L. J. H. Bean, K. W. Gripp, and A. Amemiya. Seattle (WA).

Cacoub, P., and D. Saadoun. 2021. Extrahepatic Manifestations of Chronic HCV Infection. *N Engl J Med* 384 (11):1038-1052.

Chalasani, N., Z. Younossi, J. E. Lavine, M. Charlton, K. Cusi, M. Rinella, S. A. Harrison, E. M. Brunt, and A. J. Sanyal. 2018. The diagnosis and management of nonalcoholic fatty liver disease: Practice guidance from the American Association for the Study of Liver Diseases. *Hepatology* 67 (1):328-357.

de Bruyn, G., and E. A. Graviss. 2001. A systematic review of the diagnostic accuracy of physical examination for the detection of cirrhosis. *BMC Med Inform Decis Mak* 1:6.

Dienstag, J. L. 2022. Acute viral hepatitis. In *Harrison's Principles of Internal Medicine*, edited by F. A. Loscalzo J, & Kasper D, & Hauser S, & Longo D, & Jameson J: McGraw .

Garcia-Tsao, G., J. G. Abraldes, A. Berzigotti, and J. Bosch. 2017. Portal hypertensive bleeding in cirrhosis: Risk stratification, diagnosis, and management: 2016 practice guidance by the American Association for the study of liver diseases. *Hepatology* 65 (1):310-335.

Gherlan, G. S. 2015. Liver ultrasound elastography: More than staging the disease. *World J Hepatol* 7 (12):1595-1600.

Heimbach, J. K., L. M. Kulik, R. S. Finn, C. B. Sirlin, M. M. Abecassis, L. R. Roberts, A. X. Zhu, M. H. Murad, and J. A. Marrero. 2018. MASLD guidelines for the treatment of hepatocellular carcinoma. *Hepatology* 67 (1):358-380.

Iloeje, U. H., H. I. Yang, J. Su, C. L. Jen, S. L. You, C. J. Chen, E. Risk Evaluation of Viral Load, and H. B. V. S. G. Associated Liver Disease/Cancer-In. 2006. Predicting cirrhosis risk based on the level of circulating hepatitis B viral load. *Gastroenterology* 130 (3):678-686.

Kappus, M. R., and R. K. Sterling. 2013. Extrahepatic manifestations of acute hepatitis B virus infection. *Gastroenterol Hepatol (N Y)* 9 (2):123-126.

Kudaravalli, P., and S. John. 2022. Nonalcoholic Fatty Liver. In *StatPearls*. Treasure Island (FL).

Lemon, S. M., J. J. Ott, P. Van Damme, and D. Shouval. 2017. Type A viral hepatitis: A summary and update on the molecular virology, epidemiology, pathogenesis and prevention. *J Hepatol*.

Martin, K., A. Hatab, V. S. Athwal, E. Jokl, and K. Piper Hanley. 2021. Genetic Contribution to Non-alcoholic Fatty Liver Disease and Prognostic Implications. *Curr Diab Rep* 21 (3):8.

Terrault, N. A., A. S. F. Lok, B. J. McMahon, K. M. Chang, J. P. Hwang, M. M. Jonas, R. S. Brown, Jr., N. H. Bzowej, and J. B. Wong. 2018. Update on Prevention, Diagnosis, and Treatment of Chronic Hepatitis B: MASLD 2018 Hepatitis B Guidance. *Clin Liver Dis (Hoboken)* 12 (1):33-34.

Varbobitis, I., and G. V. Papatheodoridis. 2016. The assessment of hepatocellular carcinoma risk in patients with chronic hepatitis B under antiviral therapy. *Clin Mol Hepatol* 22 (3):319-326.

Weiss, K. H. 1993. Wilson Disease. In *GeneReviews((R))*, edited by M. P. Adam, D. B. Everman, G. M. Mirzaa, R. A. Pagon, S. E. Wallace, L. J. H. Bean, K. W. Gripp and A. Amemiya. Seattle (WA).

Younossi, Z. M., M. Stepanova, J. Ong, G. Trimble, S. AlQahtani, I. Younossi, A. Ahmed, A. Racila, and L. Henry. 2021. Nonalcoholic Steatohepatitis Is the Most Rapidly Increasing Indication for Liver Transplantation in the United States. *Clin Gastroenterol Hepatol* 19 (3):580-589 e585.

Zoulim, F. 2011. Hepatitis B virus resistance to antiviral drugs: where are we going? *Liver Int* 31 Suppl 1:111-116.

Case Study Questions

Case Study

A 47-year-old recent immigrant from China is being evaluated for abnormal liver enzymes. The patient has diabetes, hypertension, hyperlipidemia, and is obese. The patient received a blood transfusion in 1993 after a moving vehicle accident that resulted in a splenectomy. The patient denies tobacco use but drinks one to two glasses of wine per day on weekends. Vital signs are stable but BMI is 42. The patient has no complaints of pruritus, dark urine, yellow eyes, or light-colored stool. A physical exam is normal except for an enlarged non-tender liver. Medications currently in use are metformin, aspirin, acetaminophen, hydrochlorothiazide, and atorvastatin. Laboratory findings are as follows:

AST	82 U/L (8-48)
ALT	111 U/L (7-55)
Total Bilirubin	1.7 mg/dl (.1-1.1)
INR	1.2 (.1-1.0)
Serum Albumin	3.7 grams (3.4-5.4)
Serum Alkaline Phosphatase	160 U/L (44-157)

1.1 What is the next test that should be done?
- A Ultrasound of the liver
- B Serology test for Hepatitis C virus
- C Serology test for Hepatitis B virus
- D Antinuclear antibody (ANA) serology
- E All of the above

1.2 Antibodies to Hepatitis C virus, Hepatitis B virus, Hepatitis B antigen, and ANA are all negative. The ultrasound of the liver is consistent with steatosis. What is the most likely cause of abnormal liver enzymes?
- A Alcoholic liver disease
- B Chronic Hepatitis C
- C Chronic Hepatitis B
- D Autoimmune hepatitis
- E Metabolic Dysfunction-Associated Steatotic Liver Disease

Quiz Questions

1. A 65-year-old female is complaining of severe pruritis. Following are her liver enzyme levels:
AST 97 IU (10-40)
ALT 96 IU (7-56)
Serum alkaline phosphatase 789 IU (30-120)
Total bilirubin 3.7 mg (.1-1.2)
Antimitochondrial antibodies positive
What is the diagnosis?
A Primary Biliary Cholangitis
B Primary Sclerosing Cholangitis
C Hepatocellular Carcinoma
D Wilson Disease
E Hemochromatosis

2. A 27-year-old man with a 15-year history of chronic ulcerative colitis has a significant increase in his serum alkaline phosphatase. His MRCP is abnormal with diffuse biliary tree strictures.
What is the diagnosis?
A Primary Biliary Cholangitis
B Primary Sclerosing Cholangitis
C Colorectal Cancer
D Drug-Induced Liver Injury
E Cholelithiasis

3. A 34-year Chinese native has immigrated to the USA. A test for which virus should be performed?
A Hepatitis A Virus
B Hepatitis B Virus
C Hepatitis C Virus
D Hepatitis D Virus
E Hepatitis E Virus

4. Drug Induced Liver Injury (DILI) can cause what pattern of abnormal liver enzymes?
A Hepatocellular
B Cholestatic
C Mixed
D All above
E None

5. What liver disease is common in obese patients with metabolic syndrome?
A Chronic Hepatitis C
B Chronic Hepatitis B
C Alcoholic liver disease
D Metabolic Dysfunction-Associated Steatotic Liver Disease
E Wilson Disease

6. A 44-year-old woman with chronic HBV was initially treated with lamivudine for 6 months and then with entecavir for the following 6 months. Both treatments were unsuccessful due to a developed resistance. Which treatment should be recommended next?
A Telbivudine
B Pegylated interferon
C Ribavirin
D Entecavir + pegylated interferon
E Tenofovir + entecavir

7. A 38-year-old female with chronic HBV was undergoing a drug treatment. Initially, the prescribed medication was taken once daily after dinner and it did not reduce the viral load after 24 weeks of treatment. For the following 24 weeks, the same medication was taken on an empty stomach and it significantly reduced the viral load. Which medication is likely discussed?
A Entecavir
B Tenofovir
C Lamivudine
D Adefovir
E Telbivudine

8. Viral resistance to HCV medications affects the effectiveness of drug therapy. Which class of HCV medications is characterized by the lowest resistance?

A DNA Polymerase Inhibitors
B NS3/4a Protease Inhibitors
C NS5B Nucleoside Polymerase Inhibitors
D NS5B Non-Nucleoside Polymerase Inhibitors
E NS5A Inhibitors

9. Which potent CYP3A4 inhibitor, with no direct effects on HCV, increases plasma levels of paritaprevir (which is metabolized by CYP3A4) and thus, boosts the effects of paritaprevir?

A Tenofovir
B Ritonavir
C Ledipasvir
D Sofosbuvir
E Velpatosvir

Case Study Answers

1.1 E. This patient has elevated liver enzymes with a broad list of possible causes. Ultrasound of the liver is needed to look for non-alcoholic liver disease due to her metabolic syndrome but also to exclude more advanced diseases no matter the cause. The patient has risk factors for both hepatitis C and B. Has had a previous blood transfusion and is from China which has high HBV rates. Young females with elevated liver chemistries should also be screened for autoimmune liver disease. The answer is E) i.e. all of the above.

1.2 E. With negative serology for Hepatitis B and C as well as negative ANA answers B, C, and D are not likely. The patient does not drink enough alcohol to have alcoholic liver disease. She has metabolic syndrome and therefore, is a candidate for nonalcoholic fatty liver disease.

Quiz Answers

1. A. Primary Biliary Cholangitis (PBC) is the most likely answer in this middle-aged woman complaining of pruritis. The abnormal liver chemistries are cholestatic patterns. The AMA test is positive making PBC the correct answer in this clinical setting with cholestasis.

2. B. Primary Sclerosing Cholangitis (PSC) is more common in men and is associated with ulcerative colitis. The pattern of elevated liver enzymes is cholestatic. The MRCP is abnormal.

3. B. Hepatitis B has a high carrier rate in China and recommendations are to test all natives from countries with high carrier rates.

4. D. DILI can cause abnormal liver enzymes in all three major patterns.

5. D. Metabolic Dysfunction-Associated Steatotic Liver Disease is one of the most common liver diseases and continues to increase in frequency. Metabolic syndrome is a major risk factor for it.

6. E. Tenofovir + entecavir is the preferred method of treating lamivudine-resistant HBV. Tenofovir is effective against entecavir-resistant and lamivudine-resistant HBV (but has reduced activity against adefovir-resistant strains). See also (Zoulim 2011).

7. A. Entecavir should be taken on an empty stomach (+/-2 h from meals). Note, oral bioavailability is ~100% (fasting) vs. ~45% (fed).

8. C. NS5B Nucleoside Polymerase Inhibitors have the lowest drug resistance in HCV by non-selectively destroying RNA replication i.e., casting a "wrench in gears", a mechanism difficult to resist.

9. B. While ritonavir (a potent CYP3A4 inhibitor) has no direct effects on HCV, it increases plasma levels of paritaprevir (which is metabolized by CYP3A4) and thus, boosts the effects of paritaprevir.

CHAPTER 8

NAUSEA AND VOMITING

MONTE TROUTMAN, DO[1], AND VICTOR V. UTESHEV, PHD[2]

[1] University of North Texas Health Science Center, Fort Worth, Texas, USA
[2] Epigen Biosciences Inc., San Diego, California, USA

Symptoms: Immuno-Infectious
Endo-Repro-Gastrointestinal

DRUG LIST FOR NAUSEA AND VOMITING

Central $5HT_3$ and D_2 receptors are located in the brainstem chemoreceptor trigger zone (CTZ) and the nucleus of the solitary tract (NTS).

$5\text{-}HT_3$ receptor antagonists: produce both central and peripheral effects and are used for chemotherapy/radiation-induced and postoperative nausea/vomiting as well as prophylaxis

- Ondansetron (+dexamethasone+aprepitant).
- Palonosetron.
- Has a very long half-life time, ~40 hrs.

D_2 receptor antagonists: direct central antiemetic and indirect peripheral pro-kinetic effects

- Metoclopramide.
- Like ondansetron, less effective.
- Dis-inhibits parasympathetic activity; increases esophageal sphincter tone; stimulates gastric emptying.
- FDA-approved for diabetic gastroparesis, GERD, postoperative and chemotherapy-induced NV (central anti-emetic effects).
- Antipsychotics.
- Chlorpromazine.
- Prochlorperazine.
- Droperidol.
- Use is limited; black box: QT prolongation & torsade de pointes.

H_1R Antagonists: motion sickness, postoperative nausea/vomiting, food poisoning.

- Promethazine.
- Meclizine (+ for vertigo).
- Diphenhydramine.

Cannabinoids.

- Dronabinol.
- Chemotherapy-induced nausea/vomiting.

Neurokinin 1 Receptor Antagonist (substance P is an endogenous NK1 receptor agonist):

- Aprepitant.
- Chemotherapy-induced and postoperative nausea/vomiting.

Anti-Muscarinics

- Not commonly used due to serious side effects (dry mouth, tachycardia, urinary retention).

Nausea and Vomiting

Nausea is the subjective sensation of impending vomiting. It is usually nonlocalized. It is usually associated with vomiting but can be isolated. It is often associated with salivation, perspiration, anorexia, flatus, and passage of stool.

Vomiting (emesis) is the act of forcefully expelling gastric and or intestinal contents via the mouth. It is usually associated with nausea. Regurgitation, in contrast to vomiting, is the spontaneous effortless reflux of gastric content into the mouth. Vomiting is coordinated by the vomiting center in the lateral reticular formation of the medulla of the brainstem. The vomiting center receives input from a number of different neural pathways that utilize various neurotransmitters, including dopamine, acetylcholine, histamine, and serotonin.

Establishing the causes of nausea and vomiting allows targeted therapy of the cause.

Pathophysiology: Vomiting requires synchronized contraction and relaxation of multiple muscles. Afferent neural signals from the brainstem control the motor elements of vomiting while neural signals in the medulla initiate vomiting. Neural signals from the gastrointestinal tract, heart, lungs, cerebral cortex, brainstem, and vestibular complex are also involved with vomiting. Another structure on the floor of the brain's fourth ventricle is the vomiting center (i.e. area postrema). This structure is stimulated by the chemotrigger zone which is outside the blood-brain barrier and therefore can be stimulated by compounds in the circulation. The perception of nausea involves neural circuits in the supratentorial regions of the brain. Afferent vagal signals mediate vomiting but nausea is mediated by this and alternate pathways. Clinically relevant receptors of the vomiting center are:

5-hydroxytryptamine receptors 3 (5HT3R).
dopamine receptors (D_2 primarily).
histamine receptors.
muscarinic receptors.
cannabinoid receptors.
neurokinin receptors.

Risk factors: Nausea and vomiting are more common in females and young patients who are more prone to motion sickness. Those who have a history of vomiting with pregnancy or from previous chemotherapy all have an increased risk of vomiting no matter the cause. Certain chemotherapeutic agents are more likely to cause nausea and vomiting and include the following:

cisplatin.
dacarbazine.
etoposide.
5-fluorouracil.
methotrexate.
nitrogen mustard.
tamoxifen.
vinblastine.

History and Examination

A thorough examination of the patient with nausea and vomiting is always indicated and should concentrate on medical and surgical history. A complete history of medications including over-the-counter medications, supplements, marijuana, or illicit drugs is necessary.

Physical examination includes vital signs, hydration status, oral, cardiovascular, pulmonary, and thorough abdominal exam. The abdominal examination should include observation, auscultation, palpation, and inspection for hernias. Nutritional assessment is also essential, especially in chronic vomiting syndromes.

Laboratory results: These should include a Complete Blood Count, a Comprehensive metabolic profile that includes serum electrolytes and kidney function and blood sugar and liver chemistries, lipase, and urine analysis. A pregnancy test should be performed in all women of reproductive age. Cultures of appropriate specimens when sepsis is suspected. A serum drug screen including illicit drugs should be collected early in the evaluation.

Imaging: This may be indicated depending on findings of history, physical, and lab. It includes standard X-rays, ultrasounds, CTs, and MRIs. Further investigation or treatment depends on the findings.

Endoscopy: Upper endoscopy is frequently performed in chronic nausea and vomiting cases when possible GI disorders are suspected.

Associated symptoms/conditions: Associated symptoms and conditions depend on the severity and longevity of nausea and vomiting. Severe nausea and vomiting occasionally cause acute upper gastrointestinal bleeding. This may present with hematemesis, coffee ground emesis, or melena (black tarry stool). GI bleeding can be caused by a condition known as Mallory-Weiss Syndrome, where forceful retching and vomiting lead to traumatic tears of the esophagus usually near the esophagogastric junction. When the esophagus completely ruptures, it's known as Boerhaave Syndrome.

Other conditions are dehydration, electrolyte imbalance, constipation, and depression.

Diagnosis: Diagnosis is made based on the history, physical, lab, and imaging. Endoscopy is occasionally required for the diagnosis.

Treatment: Appropriate treatment is based on the findings and cause. For severe vomiting, treatment includes intravenous fluids and pain relief.

Food and Poison Induced

CDC estimates that over 40 million Americans suffer from food poisoning each year. Most cases are secondary to food contaminated by bacteria or bacterial toxins (>50% of cases). Other etiologies include viruses (approximately 40%), parasites, and chemicals that may cause nausea, vomiting, and diarrhea.

History should include questions about raw food consumption especially raw seafood and vegetables. The foods most associated with food poisoning are beef, pork, eggs, fish, poultry, milk, cheese, shellfish, and vegetables.

A thorough history is essential for new-onset acute nausea and vomiting. Food poisoning should be suspected if multiple members of a party/family ingested the same food or have eaten at the same restaurant/event and became ill. Staying abreast of medical news on local, state, and national health department bulletins is crucial.

The following bacterial agents are listed in order of frequency as causes of nausea and vomiting:

- *Clostridium perfringens* presents with nausea, vomiting, and diarrhea caused by toxins from bacteria from poultry or beef cooked in bulk. It is preventable with proper food handling. Symptoms occur in 8-24 hours. Symptoms are nausea, vomiting, and diarrhea with crampy abdominal pain lasting 24 hours. Support therapy is the treatment.
- *Bacillus cereus* is a gram-positive rod that causes diarrhea and vomiting. The vomiting syndrome is caused by bacterial enterotoxin. Incubation is 2 hours. Nearly all victims admit to eating refried rice. Onset is usually within 2 hours and lasts 24 hours. Only supportive treatment is needed.
- *Vibrio species:* Over 10 species cause disease. V. cholera causes cholera. It is a gram-negative bacillus found naturally in water. The most common Vibrio species causing infection are parahaemolyticus, vulnificus, and alginolyticus. They occur from eating raw or undercooked seafood, especially oysters. Symptoms are nausea, vomiting, and diarrhea. Patients with chronic liver disease are most susceptible to more serious outcomes with overwhelming sepsis as the cause. Rapid diagnosis and treatment with clinical support and antibiotics are the treatment.

Other Causes

Cyclic Vomiting Syndrome (CVS):

- Recurrent episodes of acute clustered vomiting lasting less than a week with prolonged symptom-free periods in between. CVS is often associated with a personal or family history of migraine headaches. CVS is diagnosed when other causes are excluded by lab imaging, endoscopy, and cannabis use. Disorders that need to be excluded are gastroenteritis and peptic ulcer disease. (Li et al. 2008; Venkatesan et al. 2019) It is associated with other GI symptoms including abdominal pain, anorexia, fatigue, and headaches. Treatment during episodes is supportive with attention to dehydration, renal disorders, and electrolyte imbalance. Treatment is with lifestyle modifications and anti-emetics.

Cannabinoid Hyperemesis Syndrome

- This is a variant of CVS precipitated and worsened by chronic cannabis use. It is associated with abdominal pain. Onset and duration are similar to CVS. Patients frequently give the history that hot baths or showers relieve the symptoms. Treatment is discontinuation of cannabis and should be tried for at least 6 months. (Venkatesan et al. 2019)

Functional Vomiting

This is a diagnosis of exclusion. It is associated with eating disorders, rumination, self-induced vomiting, and major psychiatric disorders. Multiple etiologies are possible and no definitive cause is known. Comprehensive history and physical exam and endoscopic evaluation with GI imaging (ultrasound and/or CT scan). This is preceded by extensive lab evaluation. Treatment is psychiatric as well as anti-emetics.

Pregnancy
Pregnancy is a cause of nausea and vomiting and should be ruled out in females of reproductive age.

Neurologic Disorders
Migraine headaches and brain tumors can be causes of chronic nausea and vomiting. A thorough neurologic exam including an examination of the retina should be done. Middle ear infections should also be ruled out with an otoscopic exam.

GI Motility Disorders
The two most common motility disorders are gastroparesis and chronic intestinal pseudo-obstruction. Diabetes is the most common cause of gastroparesis and is often associated with peripheral polyneuropathy. Chronic or relapsing vomiting is caused by some of the same disorders that cause acute vomiting.

Motion sickness and vertigo are also causes of nausea and vomiting.

Acute Vomiting

Establish if extensive emergent evaluation and treatment are needed. This is done by assessing for shock, hypotension, volume depletion, and GI bleeding (hematemesis or coffee ground emesis). Pregnancy must be excluded. Labs besides pregnancy tests should include complete blood count, comprehensive metabolic profile, lipase, C-reactive protein, and urinalysis. Consideration should be given to thyroid function tests and toxicology tests. (Hang B. 2016)

Causes of acute vomiting include gastric outlet obstruction from peptic ulcer disease including pyloric stenosis from active or chronic disease. Other causes of acute vomiting can be an acute intestinal obstruction or acute pancreatitis from gallstones or alcohol. Other causes can be internal hernias, malignancies, and adhesions caused by previous surgery and pelvic organ disorders. Surgery plays a prominent role in the evaluation and treatment of these disorders.

Complications of Vomiting

electrolyte imbalance.
constipation.
kidney disorders such as acute kidney failure.
Mallory-Weiss esophageal tears.
Boerhaave's syndrome (esophageal rupture into mediastinum).
dental disease.
aspiration pneumonia.
dehydration.
depression.

Pharmacological Treatment of Nausea and Vomiting

A variety of drugs that block certain receptors expressed in the brainstem chemoreceptor trigger zone (CTZ; a nausea/vomiting center) have antiemetic properties. The prokinetic effects of some of these agents support their anti-emetic action because GI hypomotility supports nausea, vomiting, indigestion, and GERD. By contrast, fast GI kinetics reduce the chances of these symptoms. Note: direct antiemetic effects are primarily central, while direct prokinetic effects are primarily peripheral.

5-HT_3R Antagonists:
Ondansetron is an antagonist of serotonin 5-HT_3 receptors. These receptors mediate neurotransmission centrally and peripherally in afferent pathways controlling emesis including central (CTZ and the nucleus of the solitary tract) and peripheral (the stomach and small intestine) regions. Selective antagonists of these receptors (e.g., ondansetron) effectively inhibit emesis including that evoked by surgeries and chemo- or radiation therapy. These drugs have the plasma half-life of 3-4 h and are generally well tolerated.

D_2 Dopamine Receptor Antagonists:
Metoclopramide: A central and peripheral D_2 dopamine receptor antagonist; a 5-HT_4 receptor agonist; a 5-HT_3 receptor antagonist; and an acetylcholinesterase inhibitor. The central effect of metoclopramide within the brainstem CTZ and the nucleus of the solitary tract are directly antiemetic, while its peripheral effects on smooth muscles from the esophagus through the proximal small bowel are prokinetic and thus, indirectly antiemetic. Metoclopramide dis-inhibits parasympathetic activity, increases esophageal sphincter tone, and stimulates gastric emptying. Metoclopramide is FDA-approved for diabetic gastroparesis, GERD, and postoperative and chemotherapy-induced NV (via central anti-emetic effects). Metoclopramide should be taken before meals and at bedtime to control

nausea/vomiting in diabetic gastroparesis, esophageal reflux, and pregnancy. Metoclopramide is an effective antiemetic in cancer chemotherapy in combination with other drugs. Serious side effects include tardive dyskinesia and other extrapyramidal symptoms (Black Box warning; internet search keyword "Reglan diary"), nausea, headache, weakness/fatigue.

Prochlorperazine and chlorpromazine are common anti-nausea and anti-emetic agents. These drugs are not very effective in chemotherapy-induced emesis. However, they exhibit antihistaminic and anticholinergic activities and thus, can be used to treat motion sickness. The antiemetic effects of these drugs are dose-dependent. Side effects include hypotension, sedation, and extrapyramidal movement disorders that limit their chronic use.

Antihistamines (H1R blockers):

Promethazine (phenothiazine derivative).
Meclizine.
Diphenhydramine.

Histamine H_1-receptor antagonists with anticholinergic properties are effective in the treatment of motion sickness, vertigo, and postoperative emesis. Minor sedative effects are expected. However, these drugs are not very effective against chemotherapy-induced emesis. They can be used in combination therapies to reduce the extrapyramidal side effects of D_2 antagonists.

Cannabinoids:
Dronabinol is D^9-Tetrahydrocannabinol, an active ingredient of marijuana with antiemetic properties useful against post-chemotherapy emesis. It is orexigenic and can be useful in the treatment of AIDS and anorexia. Side effects are hallucinations, disorientation, and vertigo that limit their use.

Macrolide antibiotics: Erythromycin
Erythromycin binds to motilin receptors which are G protein-coupled receptors located throughout the enteric nervous system. Activation of motilin receptors increases the frequency and amplitude of antral contractions and initiates gastric phase III contractions.

Side effects of macrolide antibiotics include abdominal pain (~50%); nausea (37%); diarrhea (24%); and vomiting (7%). At higher intravenous doses, erythromycin may cause QT prolongation, cardiac depression, and possibly torsades de pointes. The chronic use of erythromycin may cause tachyphylaxis via desensitization of motilin receptors.

Indications for Use of Antiemetic Drugs:

motion sickness and vertigo.
postoperative recovery from anesthesia.
pregnancy.
cancer chemotherapy.
migraine.
gastric stasis.

Postoperative nausea and vomiting requiring treatment are uncommon (~5%). To prevent unnecessary side effects (e.g., hypotension, movement disorders) prophylactic treatments are discouraged. Patients at moderate to high risk for aspiration should receive prophylactic therapy. Serotonin antagonists (ondansetron) are most effective if given at the end of surgery. Metoclopramide may act as an effective postoperative treatment.

Nausea and vomiting associated with cancer chemotherapy can be quite severe and may negatively affect the patient's compliance with effective anticancer treatments. In practice, therapies utilizing combinations of antiemetic drugs exhibit the best efficacy for nausea and vomiting.

Ondansetron and other 5HT3 antagonists are the most effective agents available for preventing nausea and vomiting from chemotherapy. Combining ondansetron with dexamethasone improves efficacy.

Aprepitant, a neurokinin 1 (NK 1) receptor antagonist selectively blocks NK1 receptors in the brainstem's CTZ and area postrema. When used in combination therapy, aprepitant significantly enhances the anti-emetic efficacy of 5-HT3 receptor antagonists and corticosteroids. Side effects include fatigue, dizziness, and diarrhea.

GI motility is enhanced by cholinergic stimulation (parasympathetic inputs), adrenergic inhibition (sympathetic inputs), and dopaminergic/serotonergic modulation within the enteric nervous system. As a result, antagonists of D_2 and 5-HT_3 receptors support gastric motility. Motilin, a GI peptide is a potent prokinetic agent. Erythromycin and its analogs act as motilin receptor agonists in the antrum and duodenum. While muscarinic receptor agonists (e.g., bethanechol) are expected to produce anti-emetic effects, they often produce serious side effects and are avoided in practice.

Summary of adverse effects:
Promethazine:
Drowsiness.
Black Box: Fatal respiratory depression in children <2 years old.

Meclizine/diphenhydramine:
Xerostomia (anti-cholinergic efficacy).
Drowsiness.

Metoclopramide:
Nausea, headache, weakness/fatigue.
Black Box: Tardive dyskinesia and other extrapyramidal symptoms (use a search engine and keyword "Reglan Diary").

Erythromycin:
Abdominal pain, nausea/vomiting, diarrhea.
Arrhythmia, tachycardia, prolongation of the QT interval.

References

Hang B., B. S., Ditkoff J., Long B., and Koyfman A. 2016. Nausea and vomiting. In *Emergency Medicine: A Comprehensive Study Guide*, edited by S. J. Tintinalli J.E., Ma O., Yealy D.M., Meckler G.D., Cline D.M.: McGraw Hill.

Li, B. U., F. Lefevre, G. G. Chelimsky, R. G. Boles, S. P. Nelson, D. W. Lewis, S. L. Linder, R. M. Issenman, C. D. Rudolph, H. North American Society for Pediatric Gastroenterology, and Nutrition. 2008. North American Society for Pediatric Gastroenterology, Hepatology, and Nutrition consensus statement on the diagnosis and management of cyclic vomiting syndrome. *J Pediatr Gastroenterol Nutr* 47 (3):379-393.

Venkatesan, T., D. J. Levinthal, B. U. K. Li, S. E. Tarbell, K. A. Adams, R. M. Issenman, I. Sarosiek, S. S. Jaradeh, R. N. Sharaf, S. Sultan, C. D. Stave, A. A. Monte, and W. L. Hasler. 2019. Role of chronic cannabis use: Cyclic vomiting syndrome vs cannabinoid hyperemesis syndrome. *Neurogastroenterol Motil* 31 Suppl 2:e13606.

Case Study Questions

Case Study 1

1.1 A 52-year-old diabetic patient has increasing epigastric abdominal pain that is worse after meals. The patient has prolonged nausea with episodic vomiting after meals. A gastric emptying study showed delayed gastric emptying and the patient now returns to the clinic to discuss treatment plans. An upper endoscopy (EGD) performed one year ago for this complaint was normal including biopsies negative for H. pylori. A decrease in appetite, because of the recently increased severity of symptoms over the last two months, has resulted in a 10-pound weight loss. The patient eats three small meals a day that are low in fat and high in fiber as advised for the management of chronic constipation. Blood sugars are generally poorly controlled with a recent HgbA1C of 11.6% (normal 4-5.9%). A physical exam is normal except for epigastric tenderness. BMI = 24 kg/m^2 (normal 18.5-25). What is the next recommended step?

A CT angiography study
B CT scan of the abdomen
C Treat with promotility medication
D Repeat EGD
E Return to endocrinology for better control of blood sugars

Case Study 2

2.1 A 62-year-old female with breast cancer is undergoing a combination chemotherapy with doxorubicin. Which treatment should be used to reduce her chemotherapy-induced nausea and vomiting?

A Meclizine
B Ondansetron + dexamethasone
C Metoclopramide
D Meclizine + dexamethasone
E Aprepitant

2.2 Which medication can improve the efficacy of her anti-emetic treatment?

A Atropine
B Promethazine
C Bismuth subsalicylate
D Aprepitant
E Meclizine

Quiz Questions

1. A 32-year-old patient complains of recurring episodes of nausea and vomiting of non-bloody material. These episodes are periodic with periods that are symptom-free in between vomiting spells. Nausea and vomiting are often relieved with hot showers. The obtained drug screen is expected to be positive for which drugs?

A Cannabis
B Acetaminophen
C Methamphetamine
D Cocaine
E Alcohol

2. A patient with long-standing poorly controlled diabetes has frequent nausea and vomiting. His hemoglobin A1c is markedly elevated. His diabetes is complicated by peripheral neuropathy. What is causing his nausea and vomiting?

A Acute kidney disorder
B Gastric outlet obstruction
C Gastroparesis
D Drug-induced
E Esophageal cancer

3. Patient was started on chemotherapy for pancreatic cancer. Soon after, nausea and vomiting started. What structure in the brain is responsible for nausea and vomiting?

A Medulla
B Cerebellum
C Cerebral cortex
D Vomiting Center
E Chemical Trigger Zone

4. A 37-year-old patient with recurring episodes of nausea and vomiting that are separated by weeks with no symptoms. He is treated for migraine headaches and has a family history of migraine headaches. He denies illicit drug use. What is the diagnosis?

A Drug-induced vomiting
B Cyclic Vomiting Syndrome
C Cerebellar hypertension
D Intermittent alcohol binge drinking
E Colon cancer

5. Spontaneous occurrence of gastric contents in the hypopharynx with no retching is:

A Vomiting
B Rumination
C Regurgitation
D Hyperemesis
E Hypersalivation

6. A 32-year-old male complains of nausea and vomiting that continued for the second straight day after the patient ate some leftovers of Chinese take-out. No headache, diarrhea or fever were reported. Which treatment is the most appropriate for this patient?

A Metoclopramide
B Promethazine
C Ondansetron + dexamethasone
D Dronabinol
E Dicyclomine

Case Study Answers

1.1 E. Poor glucose control especially in diabetics can lead to gastroparesis. A repeat EGD would add little additional information. Treatment with a pro-motility medication should not precede an attempt to obtain better control of their diabetes and/or without a gastric emptying scan. CT angiogram would provide little additional information in someone that does not have suspected ischemia. Although a CT scan would probably be done, the best course of action is to obtain better control of this patient's diabetes.

2.1 B. 5-HT3R antagonists with both central and peripheral effects (e.g., ondansetron) are used in combination with dexamethasone for treatment and prophylaxis of chemotherapy/radiation-induced and postoperative nausea/vomiting. A combination therapy of ondansetron+dexamethasone is more efficacious than ondansetron or dexamethasone monotherapies. Metoclopramide is a dopamine D2 receptor antagonist with peripheral pro-kinetic effects (disinhibits parasympathetic activity increasing esophageal sphincter tone and gastric emptying) and central anti-emetic effects. However, metoclopramide has serious adverse effects (Black Box: Tardive Dyskinesia).

2.2 D. Aprepitant increases the anti-emetic efficacy of ondansetron+dexamethasone in chemotherapy/radiation-induced and postoperative nausea/vomiting. Other choices are not used in ondansetron+dexamethasone therapies.

Quiz Answers

1. A. This clinical scenario is classic for hyperemesis cannabinoid syndrome. The history of symptoms of periods of vomiting between symptom-free periods is typical. A key to the diagnosis is not only cannabis use but the relief of symptoms with a hot bath/shower. Symptom relief with hot showers is not present with acetaminophen, cocaine, alcohol, or meth amphetamine although they can cause vomiting.

2. C. The clinical scenario of poorly controlled diabetes with a high A1c level as well as peripheral neuropathy makes gastroparesis the most likely answer. Peripheral neuropathy implies intestinal tract neuropathic disorders and resultant gastroparesis. Esophageal cancer more likely would have dysphagia as a symptom. Gastric outlet obstruction would have symptoms of large-volume emesis and should have other symptoms such as abdominal distention. Drugs can always be a possible cause of nausea and vomiting but no drugs were listed for this patient.

3. E. The medulla, cerebellum, cerebral cortex, and vomiting center are all protected by the blood-brain barrier and toxins in the bloodstream cannot stimulate these areas. The chemical trigger zone is not protected by the blood-brain barrier and therefore, can be accessible to stimulants and thus, may trigger nausea and vomiting.

4. B. This clinical scenario of periods of nausea and vomiting separated by periods of no symptoms is therefore cyclic. It is often associated with migraine headaches or even a family history of migraines. There is no history of drug or alcohol use in his patient. These are not classic symptoms of colon cancer.

5. C. This question is the definition of regurgitation, it is spontaneous. Hypersalivation is also called water brash and indeed is the production of large amounts of saliva often leading to drooling. Vomiting is the forceful expulsion of gastric contents associated with retching. Hyperemesis is repeated bouts of vomiting. Rumination is associated with psychological disorders as the patient voluntarily forces regurgitation of gastric contents which are either spit out or re-swallowed.

6. B. Promethazine is a potent and safe antagonist of H1 Histamine receptors used to treat nausea and vomiting. Promethazine is the most suitable for this patient (food poisoning). Other anti-emetics listed are too strong for this case and can also be expensive. Dronabinol is a cannabinoid used for chemotherapy-induced nausea and vomiting. Ondansetron+dexamethasone are used for treatment and prophylaxis of chemotherapy/radiation-induced and postoperative nausea/vomiting. Metoclopramide is a dopamine D2 receptor antagonist with peripheral pro-kinetic effects (disinhibits parasympathetic activity increasing esophageal sphincter tone and gastric emptying) and central anti-emetic effects. However, metoclopramide has serious adverse effects (Black Box: Tardive Dyskinesia). Dicyclomine is a weak spasmolytic anti-muscarinic agent used in mixed IBS to reduce parasympathetic activity and thus, relax gastrointestinal smooth muscles and reduce gastrointestinal motility.

CHAPTER 9.1

JOINT PAIN AND DRUGS FOR GOUT

KNOX VAN DYKE, PHD[1] AND DAVID P. SIDEROVSKI, PHD[2]

[1] West Virginia University, Morgantown, WV
[2] University of North Texas Health Science Center, Fort Worth, TX

Symptoms: **Immuno-Infectious**
Musculoskeletal

DRUG LIST FOR GOUT

Colchicine	microtubule polymerization inhibitor
Uricosuric Drugs:	
Probenecid	renal uric acid reabsorption inhibitor
Sulfinpyrazone	renal uric acid reabsorption inhibitor
Xanthine Oxidase Inhibitors:	
Allopurinol	inhibitor of the uric acid synthesis
Oxypurinol	active metabolite of allopurinol
Febuxostat	inhibitor of the uric acid synthesis
Uricases:	
Pegloticase	recombinant uricase which oxidizes uric acid
Rasburicase	recombinant uricase which oxidizes uric acid
Lesinurad	urate transporter inhibitor

General Background

Each day, the human body excretes ~0.7 grams of uric acid into passed urine. Most of this uric acid is derived from the oxidation of the purines hypoxanthine and xanthine (Fig. 9.1.1) and exists as a urate salt at neutral pH. The glomerular filtrate of blood is usually acidified by the kidneys from a pH of ~7.4 to an acidic pH of about 6 in the urine. Uric acid has very limited solubility; therefore, as urate salts move through the renal tubular system, encountering a more acidic pH, the possibility of forming uric acid stones and thereby damaging the kidney increases. **Gout** (or "gouty arthritis") is caused by excessive uric acid deposition in peripheral joints and is frequently observed as an acute inflammation of a single joint within the large toe, forefoot, instep, heel, ankle, knee, or elbow. Uric acid, a product of the metabolic breakdown of purine nucleotides and a normal component of urine, is a sparingly soluble substance; unlike other mammals, humans lack the enzyme uricase to degrade uric acid to the more highly water-soluble allantoin (Fig. 9.1.1). Excessive uric acid levels (hyperuricemia) leading to gout occur either by biochemical overproduction or insufficient renal excretion, or a combination of both events. If hyperuricemia is untreated for years, monosodium urate (MSU) crystals may accumulate in joints, subcutaneous tissue, and renal parenchyma and pelvis; crystalline sodium urate deposits also frequently result in inflammatory bumps or bulges (tophi) that can be observed in the earlobes, elbows, hands, and base of the large toe. In addition, if hyperuricemia is left unchecked, uric acid stones may form in the urinary tract. Renal or urinary blockade can result in progressive renal failure in the later stages of untreated gout; this major complication of the disease can be avoided by early treatment.

The renal mechanisms engaged in moving uric acid into urine are complex and minimally involve filtration out of the bloodstream, reabsorption, secretion, and urinary excretion (Fig. 9.1.2). The proximal tubule of the nephron is the principal site of both carrier-mediated urate reabsorption back into the renal bloodstream and urate secretion back into the tubule. Urate concentration in the proximal tubule is thus ultimately determined by the balance between influx and efflux. *When urate transport from the peritubular fluid is high, there is net elimination of urate across the luminal membrane; in contrast, when urate transport from the luminal fluid is high, there is net reabsorption across the basolateral membrane.* Urate transport from the ultrafiltrate, via an active, anion-exchange mechanism in the luminal membrane, can be inhibited by drugs such as probenecid, sulfinpyrazone, and salicylate. Carrier-mediated secretion of urate can also be inhibited by a variety of drugs, including thiazide diuretics and loop diuretics. Urate excretion rate is subject to modification by various compounds, including uricosuric agents (those that stimulate urate excretion; see below), diuretics, radiographic contrast agents, and certain anti-cancer drugs. These drug effects on urate excretion may be biphasic, in that low doses may depress uric acid excretion whereas higher doses may elicit the opposing, uricosuric effect.

Figure 9.1.1

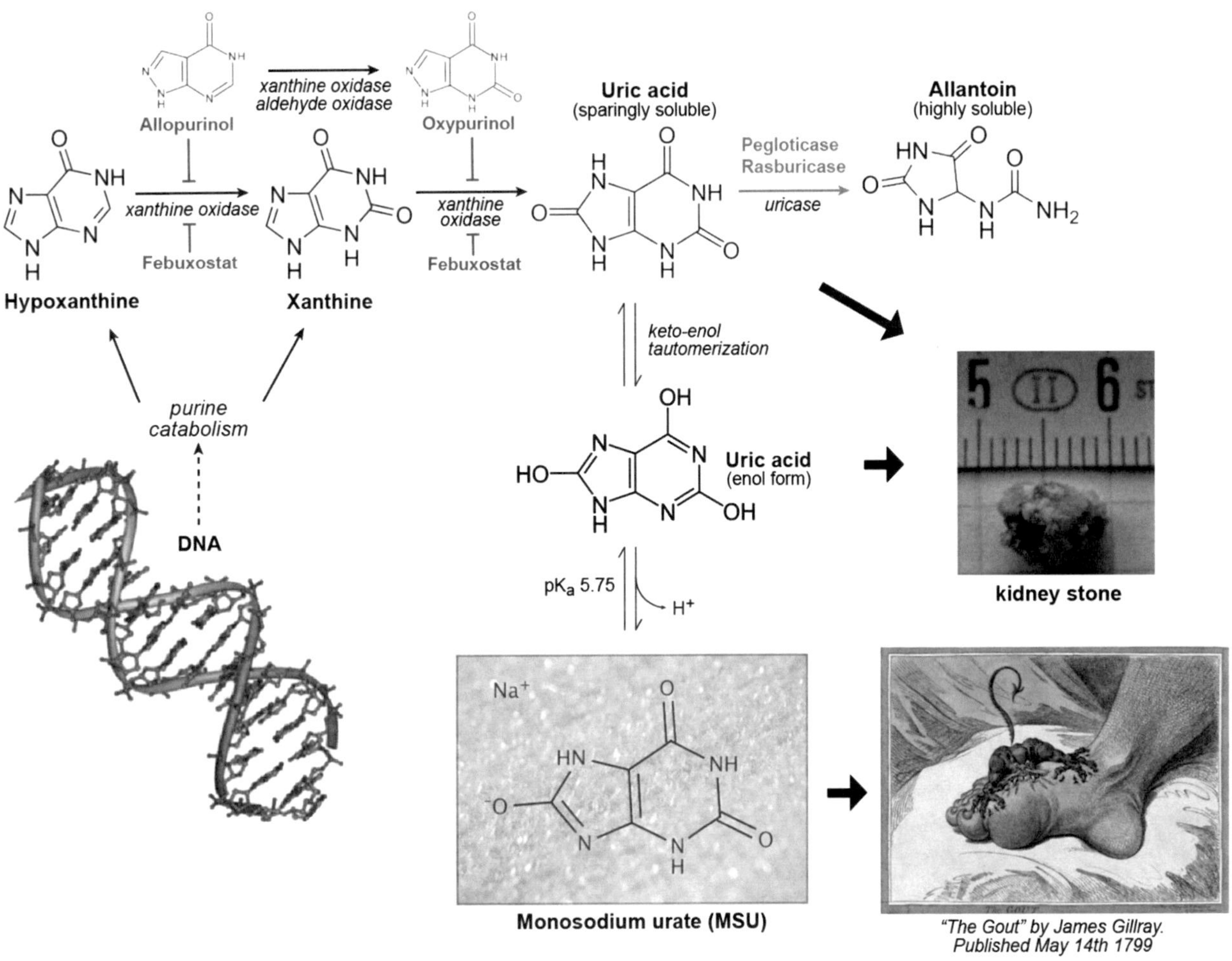

Source and disposition of uric acid. Uric acid is a direct product of hypoxanthine and xanthine oxidation and is a sparingly soluble substance; humans lack the enzyme uricase to degrade uric acid to highly water-soluble allantoin. Excessive uric acid levels lead to the formation of stones in the kidney or urinary tract. Monosodium urate (MSU) crystals can accumulate in joints, subcutaneous tissue, kidney, earlobes, elbows, hands, and large toes. The anti-gout drugs allopurinol and febuxostat (red) act as inhibitors of the xanthine oxidase that converts hypoxanthine and xanthine into uric acid; allopurinol is also metabolized in the body to oxypurinol (red), which also inhibits xanthine oxidase activity. The recombinant uricase proteins pegloticase and rasburicase convert uric acid into the highly soluble and easily excreted allantoin.

Presentation: Most commonly, the first metatarsophalangeal joint (the big toe) is involved (*podagra* or "gout of the foot"). Any (and potentially multiple) joint(s) may be involved in a gout attack, most frequently involving the feet, ankles, knees, and elbows. A typical gout flare in these joints is characterized by sudden severe pain, with redness, warmth, and swelling of the affected joint(s). Presentation of acute gouty arthritis is rather unique and rarely understated (*e.g.*, see lower right illustration of Fig. 9.1.1), and only needs to be distinguished from a bacterial infection.

Figure 9.1.2

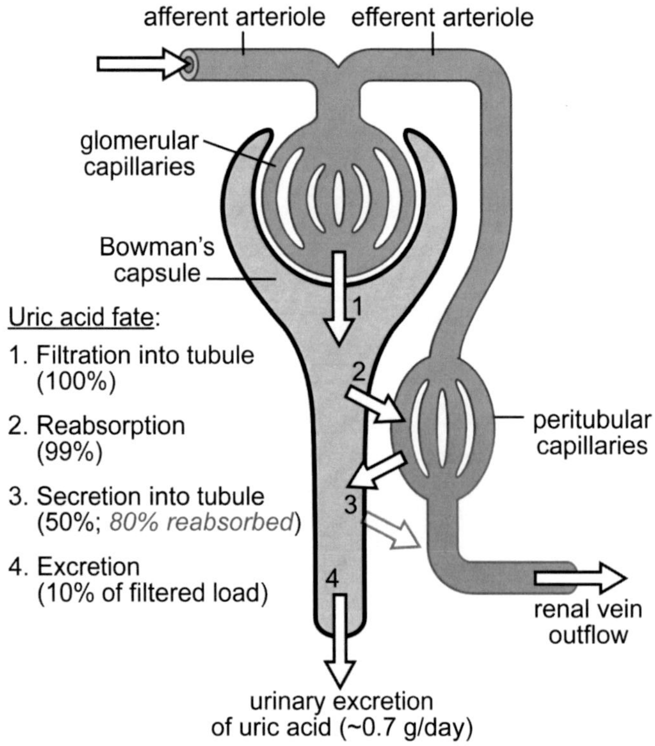

The fate of uric acid in the kidney. Uric acid is first filtered out of the glomerular blood flow into the Bowman's capsule. Nearly all of this uric acid is then actively reabsorbed into the renal blood flow. Half of this uric acid is secreted back into the tubule, but only 10% of the original filtered load of uric acid is ultimately excreted into the urine. Both passive and active transport mechanisms are involved in these uric acid handling processes.

Risk Factors: The risk of acquiring gout is primarily related to the duration and extent of hyperuricemia. There is little risk when blood uric acid level is below 7 mg/dL, which is the normal occurrence: adult men have mean serum urate levels of 6.8 mg/dL, and premenopausal women have mean serum urate values of 6 mg/dL. However, at serum urate concentrations of 10 to 11 mg/dL, the likelihood of gout is relatively high. The cause of hyperuricemia may be discerned by formal quantification of uric acid excretion. If a patient placed on a purine-restricted diet for one week is observed to excrete >0.6 g uric acid per day, the patient is likely an overproducer of urate. In contrast, if <0.35 g of uric acid is eliminated per day under a purine-restricted diet, impaired renal function is likely. The vast majority of gout patients exhibit such urate underexcretion; there are also gout patients who produce excessive uric acid and additionally exhibit underexcretion. Hyperuricemia can be either primary (*i.e.*, of genetic origin (Reginato et al. 2012)) or secondary to other diseases (often of hematological origin), rapid weight loss, or medicine/chemotherapy use. For example, cancer chemotherapy for lymphomas and leukemias, evoking sustained cellular death and the release and breakdown of nucleic acids, can lead to hyperuricemia and gout as part of a constellation of metabolic abnormalities labeled tumor lysis syndrome. Specific drugs can impair the renal elimination of uric acid and can produce hyperuricemia and gout; these include salicylates, pyrazinamide and ethambutol, nicotinic acid (niacin), cyclosporine, and certain diuretics (*e.g.*, thiazides, furosemide) (see Chapter 2 for pharmacovigilance). Similarly, a high dietary intake of ethanol or fructose, or a ketogenic (low-carbohydrate) diet generating high ketone levels can competitively inhibit uric acid transport.

Pathophysiology: Acute attacks of gouty arthritis (flares) are generally the result of urate phagocytosis by tissue-resident macrophages. Monosodium urate (MSU) crystals, once engulfed by the phagocytic cell, can directly activate the NLRP3 inflammasome (Martinon et al. 2006; Giguere et al. 2014), a multi-protein complex of the innate immune system consisting of the NOD-like receptor NLRP3 (*a.k.a.* NALP3 or cryopyrin), the adaptor protein ASC, and caspase-1 (formerly known as interleukin (IL)-1-converting enzyme). Once the NLRP3 inflammasome is activated, IL-1β is produced and secreted, leading to immune system cell infiltration (*e.g.*, neutrophil recruitment) and acute inflammatory processes. This newly-appreciated link between MSU deposition and IL-1β production has stimulated research into new inhibitor strategies with promise in blocking the inflammatory process underlying gout. Early clinical studies of anti-IL-1 agents rilonacept, canakinumab, and anakinra (Chapter 9.2), have suggested that these biologics may be effective against gout; (Sundy et al. 2014) however, their present cost may make them less competitive compared to present pharmacotherapy.

Examination: Involvement of single or multiple joints in inflammation (*synovitis*), warmth, tenderness, swelling, and erythema. Findings may also include features of systemic inflammation, such as fever (especially with a polyarticular flare), and tophi (subcutaneous MSU crystal deposition in fingers, toes, Achilles' tendons, knees, outer bump of the elbows, and/or auricle rim). MSU crystal deposition has also been seen in various parts of the eye (*e.g.*, cornea).

Laboratory: Serum uric acid levels fluctuate over short time-periods. Therefore, while the risk of gout does increase with the absolute level and duration of hyperuricemia, testing blood draws for serum urate levels from a patient presenting with an acute gouty flare (and thereby potentially diagnosing hyperuricemia) is not by itself diagnostic for gout. Indeed, serum urate at 9.0 mg/dL represents an incidence of acute gout of only ~5% per year. (Campion et al. 1987)

Imaging: Polarized-light microscopy of aspirated synovial fluid from an affected joint (or from a tophaceous deposit) can yield observation of yellow, needle-shaped, negatively-birefringent urate crystals; observing such crystal deposits resident within neutrophils from the aspirated fluid is common during an acute gouty attack.

Associated symptoms/conditions: Having gout increases the risk of developing diabetes and heart disease. Gout can cause kidney stones, which in turn can lead to symptoms such as severe flank or groin pain and (often) blood in the urine.

Diagnosis: A diagnosis of gout is confirmed by the identification of MSU crystals in the synovial fluid of the affected joint(s). (Martillo et al. 2014) As presenting features of a bacterial infection (a *septic* joint) *versus* an acute gouty attack can overlap, culturing the aspirated fluid from arthrocentesis is valuable to rule out bacterial infection. Joint infection and gout are not mutually exclusive conditions and can co-exist in the same joint.

Treatment: Gout produces a great deal of acute pain given its inherent inflammation. ***Treatments** for the hyperuricemia at the root of gout development with agents that lower blood uric acid levels (see below)* ***are generally contraindicated during an acute gouty attack, since such pharmacotherapy, at least in its initial stages, may exacerbate the condition***. Thus, the first step in gout treatment is often anti-inflammatory pain medication. Various non-steroidal anti-inflammatory drugs (NSAIDs; Chapter 9.2) can be individually prescribed, including ibuprofen, indomethacin, naproxen, and sulindac; these NSAIDs may also be given in combination with colchicine, a specific agent for acute gouty attacks. The first NSAID, phenylbutazone, was used for the treatment of gout starting in 1949; however, it is no longer approved for human use owing to severe adverse effects (e.g., aplastic anemia, bone marrow suppression). Data from clinical trials comparing oral glucocorticoids (Chapter 9.2) with NSAIDs suggest that glucocorticoids such as prednisone and prednisolone are at least as effective as NSAIDs for acute gout and may elicit fewer serious adverse effects. (Rainer et al. 2016) Intra-articular application of a glucocorticoid anti-inflammatory drug is also a common intervention in acute gout treatment.

Management: Once the acute attack is under control (see *Treatment* above), long-term management through the use of drug therapy, body weight management, and dietary control can be initiated to decrease uric acid production, increase its excretion, or both. As for dietary control, it would seem logical to consider restricting the intake of purine-rich foods such as red meat; however, as only ~10% of gout patients are urate overproducers, dietary control has only a minor effect on the gout population. Furthermore, only a small proportion of total blood uric acid is derived from dietary purine intake.

Pharmacological Treatment of Gout

Colchicine

As previously stated, gout is associated with local tissue accumulation of urate crystals by phagocytic cells and subsequent inflammasome activation, IL-1β production, and downstream inflammatory processes. Pro-inflammatory cytokines and chemokines that are locally produced by and for immune system cell infiltration are responsible for much of the inflammation and pain associated with acute gout attacks. The alkaloid colchicine, originally extracted from the autumn crocus (*Colchicum autumnale*), has long been used selectively for the treatment of acute gouty arthritis. Indeed, if the diagnosis of acute gout is uncertain, colchicine should be used since a response to this drug is generally taken as establishing the diagnosis of acute gouty arthritis. Colchicine has minimal effects on urate synthesis or excretion; instead, it decreases inflammation associated with this disorder.

Colchicine is not effective in reducing inflammation in other disorders; hence, its nearly exclusive use is as an anti-inflammatory agent in treating acute gouty arthritis. Colchicine reduces the frequency of subsequent acute gout attacks, particularly while starting drugs that lower urate levels. However, colchicine is not used in long-term prophylactic treatment (*e.g.*, over years), but rather should be viewed as a useful 'bridge' for progressing from an acute gout flare to longer-term, urate-lowering pharmacotherapy.

Oral colchicine dosing is usually initiated at the first sign of an acute attack and can be taken more than once a day without regard to meals. Colchicine is continued until either symptom subside (onset of pain relief ~18-24 hrs), adverse reactions appear, or a maximum daily dose has been reached. Oral colchicine is absorbed rapidly and concentrates in the gastrointestinal tract, spleen, kidney, and liver (with the latter organ the major site of its metabolism via CYP3A4-

mediated deacetylation). Leukocytes accumulate and store colchicine even after a single intravenous injection. Colchicine is mainly eliminated via fecal excretion since the alkaloid and its metabolites are readily secreted into bile. Only 15-30% is eliminated in the urine, except in those gout patients with liver disease for whom urinary excretion is more important.

At the molecular level, colchicine binds to intracellular tubulin and thereby inhibits microtubule polymerization; blockade of microtubule assembly dynamics can disrupt inflammasome activation, microtubule-based inflammatory cell chemotaxis, the generation of leukotrienes and cytokines, and the act of phagocytosis. In these ways, at the cellular level, colchicine is thought to inhibit neutrophil motility and activity, leading to a net anti-inflammatory effect at the site of acute gout flares.

Nausea, vomiting, abdominal cramping/pain, and diarrhea are major, limiting side effects that ultimately establish an individual's tolerated dosage of colchicine. These side effects occur in ~80% of patients and especially in those taking high dosages of colchicine. Its gastrointestinal toxicity stems from its anti-mitotic effect on cells that are rapidly turning over, such as those of the intestinal epithelium, compounded by its hepatobiliary recycling. These gastrointestinal side effects usually affect patient adherence with continued colchicine use before the onset of more serious toxicity, thereby providing a margin of safety to its administration. Large oral doses of colchicine are followed by throat-burning sensation, bloody diarrhea, bloody urine, reduced urine output, shock, and CNS depression. Colchicine is used with caution in gout patients with compromised heart, kidney, or gastrointestinal tract function, or with liver disease.

The Uricosuric Drugs

Uricosuric drugs compete with uric acid for urate transporters. In small doses, uricosuric drugs *decrease* total urate excretion by inhibiting its tubular secretion. This particular impact on urate secretion is relatively minor; however, at high dosages, uricosuric drugs *increase* total urate excretion by inhibiting its proximal tubular reabsorption (Fig. 9.1.2: phase 2 *versus* phase 3 of 'uric acid fate'). Uricosuric drugs, therefore, have a complex and dose-dependent effect on both serum and urinary uric acid levels: namely, *at low doses, these agents increase serum uric acid levels while decreasing the urinary levels; at high doses, they have the opposite effect at both locales.* Given this complexity, the initial phase of uricosuric agent pharmacotherapy is the most dangerous period for the patient. For the drug-naïve patient, until the body dose of the uricosuric agent builds up enough to fully inhibit uric acid reabsorption as well as secretion, there is a temporary increase in hyperuricemia, significantly increasing the risk of an acute gout attack. Therefore, anti-gout drug therapy is often initiated with small amounts of colchicine (*see above*) before adding a uricosuric agent. In addition, increasing urinary uric acid concentrations during uricosuric drug therapy elevates the risk of renal stone formation.

Probenecid

For controlling hyperuricemia and preventing tissue deposition of tophi, probenecid is effective and relatively safe; however, it is not useful in treating acute attacks of gouty arthritis. Its administration decreases the incidence of future acute gouty attacks as well as the complications usually associated with long-term hyperuricemia such as renal damage. Probenecid can also be given with colchicine and is formulated as a single tablet containing both drugs for the prevention of gout in patients with frequent, severe gout attacks; the colchicine dose in this combination is lower than that given during an acute gouty attack.

Probenecid is rapidly absorbed after oral administration, reaching its peak level in plasma within 2-4 hours; however, its half-life is somewhat variable (4-12 hours) given competing influences of its extensive plasma protein binding and its active clearance by proximal tubular secretion. Metabolism of probenecid involves oxidation of alkyl side chains and glucuronide conjugation. Upon elimination, the major metabolite of probenecid acyl glucuronide accounts for close to 50% of the original dose.

The uricosuric action of probenecid stems from the drug's ability to inhibit the active reabsorption of uric acid from the glomerular filtrate. When given in sufficient amounts, probenecid (an organic acid itself) blocks uric acid reabsorption by the organic anion transporter (OAT) in the proximal tubules (Fig. 9.1.2) and thus increases urinary uric acid elimination. However, at low doses, probenecid competes preferentially with plasma uric acid for the proximal tubule anionic transport system, thereby blocking uric acid its access to this active secretory system.

Adverse reactions to probenecid use include occasional rashes, allergic dermatitis, upper gastrointestinal tract irritation, and drowsiness. As probenecid use elevates urinary uric acid levels, and uric acid tends to crystallize out of acidic urine, liberal fluid intake should be recommended, as well as intake of sufficient sodium bicarbonate or potassium citrate to maintain an alkaline urine pH. Urine alkalization is recommended until hyperuricemia abates and existing tophi disappear; afterward, urine alkalization and restriction on purine-producing foods can be modestly relaxed. Probenecid elimination is increased with increasing urinary pH, given that tubular back-diffusion is decreased at alkaline urinary pH ranges. Probenecid is contraindicated in patients with a history of renal calculi.

Probenecid not only impairs the renal active secretion of uric acid, but also a variety of acidic drugs and compounds, including sulfinpyrazone, sulfonylureas, indomethacin, penicillin, sulfonamides, and 17-ketosteroids (Chapter 3). Additional important clinical interactions with probenecid use include those with captopril; cephalosporins; ketoprofen, naproxen, and ketorolac; lorazepam; methotrexate; quinolones; acyclovir and ganciclovir; and zidovudine/azidothymidine (AZT). The excretion of all these drugs is reduced by probenecid; therefore, if these agents are to be given concomitantly with probenecid, their dosage should be modified appropriately. The ability of probenecid to inhibit renal secretion of drugs has therapeutic utility in certain circumstances; it can be used in adjunctive pharmacotherapy to maintain high blood levels of penicillin, cephalosporin, acyclovir, and cyclosporine. Salicylates interfere with the clinical effects of probenecid and thus should be avoided in patients using this uricosuric agent.

Sulfinpyrazone

Sulfinpyrazone is chemically related to the first NSAID, phenylbutazone, and possesses antithrombotic and platelet-inhibiting effects; however, it lacks the anti-inflammatory, analgesic, and sodium-retaining properties of phenylbutazone. Sulfinpyrazone possesses several undesirable side effects that limit its therapeutic usefulness. The marketing of sulfinpyrazone under the brand-name Anturane has been discontinued in the US.

Sulfinpyrazone is rapidly absorbed after oral administration, reaching its peak level in plasma within 1-2 hours. It is highly bound to plasma protein (~99%), more so than probenecid (84-94%), and is a more potent uricosuric agent. Most of the drug is eliminated as the parent compound (90%) through active proximal tubular secretion. Sulfinpyrazone also undergoes CYP450-mediated hydroxylation to form an active uricosuric metabolite which contributes to the drug's prolonged activity (~10 hours) and increased potency relative to probenecid. In contrast to probenecid, the rate of sulfinpyrazone excretion is not increased by urine alkalinization; this lack of rate increase is because sulfinpyrazone is largely ionized at all urinary pH ranges and thus not a candidate for passive tubular back-diffusion.

The mechanism of sulfinpyrazone's uricosuric activity is similar to that of probenecid (*see above*). As with probenecid, during the initial period of sulfinpyrazone use, acute attacks of gout may increase in frequency and severity. Thus, it is recommended that colchicine or an NSAID be co-administered early on during sulfinpyrazone therapy. Abdominal pain, nausea/vomiting, and possible reactivation of peptic ulceration have all been reported under sulfinpyrazone use. It should be used cautiously in patients with compromised renal function; abundant fluid intake should accompany sulfinpyrazone administration to minimize the risk of renal stone formation.

The Xanthine Oxidase Inhibitors

Allopurinol and its metabolite Oxypurinol

Allopurinol is valued for treating chronic tophaceous gout and is especially beneficial for patients with renal insufficiency. Patients receiving allopurinol demonstrate pronounced decreases in serum and urinary uric acid levels. Given that allopurinol and its active metabolite, **oxypurinol**, do not rely on renal mechanisms for their efficacy in reducing uric acid levels, allopurinol is particularly useful for patients who have

- previously developed renal uric acid stones;
- excessively high urate excretion (*e.g.*, >1.2 g per day);
- one of many blood disorders (*e.g.*, polycythemia vera, leukemia);
- excessive deposition of tophi; or,
- failed in their responses to uricosuric agents.

Allopurinol also inhibits reperfusion injury that occurs when a transplanted or ischemic organ is reperfused with blood or an appropriate buffer. Reperfusion injury is caused primarily by the local formation of free radicals (reactive oxygen species, ROS), such as superoxide anion, hydroxyl free radicals, and peroxynitrite, which are strong oxidants and damaging to tissues. Various theories exist as to the effect(s) of allopurinol in this context: it may inhibit the irreversible breakdown of purine substrates, inhibit the formation of reactive oxygen species, and/or protect against mitochondrial membrane damage.

Allopurinol is highly absorbed after oral administration, reaching its peak level in plasma within 1 hour. Unlike the uricosuric agents, allopurinol is not appreciably bound to plasma proteins nor is it affected by renal secretory mechanisms. Allopurinol is rapidly and almost completely metabolized by xanthine oxidase (and, alternatively, by aldehyde oxidase) to form the active metabolite oxypurinol (Fig. 9.1.1). Oxypurinol accumulates during long-term allopurinol administration, contributing to the parent drug's long half-life (18–20 hours) and facilitating once-a-day dosing. Oxypurinol itself is not administered as an orally available drug, given that it is not well absorbed by this route of administration.

In contrast to the uricosuric agents, allopurinol reduces hyperuricemia via competitive inhibition of uric acid synthesis rather than by affecting renal urate reabsorption per se. Allopurinol inhibits xanthine oxidase, the enzyme involved in the metabolism of hypoxanthine and xanthine to uric acid (Fig. 9.1.1). Urinary and blood concentrations of uric acid are both greatly reduced upon xanthine oxidase inhibition, and there is a concomitant increase in excretion of the more soluble uric acid precursors hypoxanthine and xanthine.

Allopurinol can cause gout flares during the initiation of drug therapy and is not to be initiated during an acute gouty attack. As with uricosuric agents, allopurinol therapy should be accompanied by increased fluid intake to ensure water diuresis and by sodium bicarbonate or potassium citrate intake to maintain an alkaline urine pH. Concomitant use of colchicine can help prevent acute gouty attacks that may be elicited during the onset of allopurinol use.

Allopurinol administration is commonly associated with various skin rashes, fever, gastrointestinal distress, and hepatotoxicity – side effects that often require termination of use. Allopurinol can also cause the rare but life-threatening dermatological conditions of toxic epidermal necrolysis and Stevens-Johnson syndrome; the HLA-B*5801 allele is a genetic marker for these allopurinol-induced severe cutaneous adverse reactions. Patients with renal impairment may be particularly prone to a toxicity syndrome elicited two to four weeks after initiation of allopurinol termed DRESS (drug reaction with eosinophilia and systemic symptoms), characterized by rash, fever, internal organ inflammation, lymphadenopathy, and varied hematologic abnormalities such as eosinophilia, thrombocytopenia, and atypical lymphocytosis.

Allopurinol inhibits the oxidative inactivation of the chemotherapeutic/immunosuppressant prodrug azathioprine and its active metabolite 6-mercaptopurine; therefore, their individual administered doses must be decreased to as little as 25% of their original dose if either is given along with allopurinol. Allopurinol may also increase the activity and/or half-life of other immunosuppressive, cytotoxic, and anti-viral drugs (*e.g.*, cyclosporine, didanosine, vidarabine). Unlike with probenecid, the actions of allopurinol are not antagonized by salicylate co-administration.

Febuxostat

As with allopurinol, **febuxostat** is used to treat chronic gout and hyperuricemia. Febuxostat is generally only recommended for those patients who cannot tolerate allopurinol; it has been reported to be more effective than standard doses of allopurinol, but not more effective than higher doses of allopurinol. Following oral administration, febuxostat is over 99% bound to plasma proteins. It is conjugated by several of the uridine diphosphate glucuronosyltransferase (UGT) enzymes; it can also be oxidized by CYP1A2, CYP2C8, CYP2C9, and non-P450 enzymes to four active metabolites. Febuxostat metabolites are eliminated nearly equally in the urine and feces, primarily as metabolites and conjugates.

Febuxostat is not chemically related to purines, but it acts as a selective inhibitor of xanthine oxidase by non-competitively blocking the molybdenum pterin center within the enzyme's active site. Febuxostat inhibition of xanthine oxidase reduces the production of uric acid (Fig. 9.1.1). As with allopurinol, gout flares can occur during the initiation of febuxostat therapy, and similar precautions must be taken. Additional adverse effects associated with febuxostat therapy include rash, nausea, diarrhea, headache, and increased hepatic serum enzyme levels. Recent concerns from post-approval clinical safety studies have surfaced regarding the potential for more heart-related deaths with febuxostat usage as compared to allopurinol. Febuxostat should be used with caution in individuals with a history of cardiovascular disease. Similarly, febuxostat should be used cautiously in individuals with severe renal or hepatic disease; liver function tests should be performed in all individuals prior to initiation of this drug and at regular intervals thereafter.

As with allopurinol, febuxostat inhibits the xanthine oxidase-mediated metabolism of azathioprine and 6-mercaptopurine. The manufacturer of febuxostat recommends avoiding this combination.

The Uricases Pegloticase and Rasburicase

Intravenous infusion of **pegloticase** every two to four weeks is approved for the treatment of severe, treatment-refractory, chronic gout and represents an alternative for those intolerant of first-line therapies. In contrast, **rasburicase** is approved for the prevention and treatment of tumor lysis syndrome in patients receiving chemotherapy for hematologic cancers such as leukemias and lymphomas. Rasburicase has been used for hyperuricemia in gout and is being investigated for treating severely high blood levels of uric acid from other sources.

Pegloticase and rasburicase are injected intravenously. Pegloticase differs from rasburicase in that it is covalently modified with mono methoxyl-poly(ethylene glycol) to reduce its immunogenicity and greatly increase its elimination half-life (12 days *vs* 8 hours for the unmodified protein). The half-life of rasburicase is 16 – 22 hours.

Pegloticase and rasburicase are recombinant uricase enzymes that catalyze the oxidation of uric acid into hydrogen peroxide and 5-hydroxyisourate, the latter of which spontaneously decomposes into allantoin and carbon dioxide (Figure 9.1.1). Allantoin is highly soluble in plasma and easily excreted through the kidney. Rasburicase is produced in the yeast *S. cerevisiae* from a fungal clone of urate oxidase, whereas pegloticase is of porcine origin and produced in *E. coli*.

Pegloticase and rasburicase are contraindicated for individuals with glucose-6-phosphate dehydrogenase (G6PDH) deficiency, as the drugs may precipitate severe, life-threatening hemolysis with methemoglobinemia (stemming from enzymatic hydrogen peroxide generation). Pegloticase and rasburicase may also show immunogenicity. Pegloticase is associated with allergic reactions in approximately 25% of patients, even with antihistamine and glucocorticoid treatment prior to infusion.

Lesinurad

Lesinurad is used in combination with a xanthine oxidase inhibitor such as allopurinol for treating hyperuricemia associated with gout. The combination therapy is approved only for patients who cannot achieve target reductions in serum uric acid levels with a xanthine oxidase inhibitor alone. Following oral administration, lesinurad is absorbed and becomes highly bound to plasma proteins. It is eliminated by CYP2C9-mediated oxidation to inactive metabolites, and approximately 30% of a dose is eliminated as the parent compound in the urine. The half-life of lesinurad is approximately 5 hours.

Lesinurad inhibits the urate transporter and urate-anion exchanger **URAT1** (*a.k.a.* solute carrier family 22 [organic anion/cation transporter], member 12, or SLC22A12), an integral membrane protein responsible for reabsorption of uric acid in the kidneys. *This inhibition leads to increased urinary uric acid excretion and consequent lowering of hyperuricemia.* It also inhibits the transporter protein OAT4, which is associated with hyperuricemia caused by diuretics.

Dose-dependent side effects of elevated creatinine, nephrolithiasis, and renal failure have been observed and are more common if lesinurad is used alone; patients prescribed lesinurad are therefore advised to stay well hydrated and their renal function is closely monitored. Lesinurad is contraindicated in patients with Lesch–Nyhan syndrome (juvenile gout) or tumor lysis syndrome, as well as with severe renal impairment, including kidney transplant and hemodialysis. As lesinurad is a weak inducer of CYP3A4 levels in the liver, other drugs that are metabolized by this cytochrome P450 enzyme become less effective (*e.g.*, simvastatin, warfarin, hormonal contraceptives).

References For Chapter 9.1

Campion, E. W., R. J. Glynn, and L. O. DeLabry. 1987. Asymptomatic hyperuricemia. Risks and consequences in the Normative Aging Study. *American Journal of Medicine* 82 (3):421-426.

Giguere, P. M., B. J. Gall, E. A. Ezekwe, Jr., G. Laroche, B. K. Buckley, C. Kebaier, J. E. Wilson, J. P. Ting, D. P. Siderovski, and J. A. Duncan. 2014. G Protein signaling modulator-3 inhibits the inflammasome activity of NLRP3. *Journal of Biological Chemistry* 289 (48):33245-33257.

Martillo, M. A., L. Nazzal, and D. B. Crittenden. 2014. The crystallization of monosodium urate. *Curr Rheumatol Rep* 16 (2):400.

Martinon, F., V. Petrilli, A. Mayor, A. Tardivel, and J. Tschopp. 2006. Gout-associated uric acid crystals activate the NALP3 inflammasome. *Nature* 440 (7081):237-241.

Rainer, T. H., C. H. Cheng, H. J. Janssens, C. Y. Man, L. S. Tam, Y. F. Choi, W. H. Yau, K. H. Lee, and C. A. Graham. 2016. Oral Prednisolone in the Treatment of Acute Gout: A Pragmatic, Multicenter, Double-Blind, Randomized Trial. *Ann Intern Med* 164 (7):464-471.

Reginato, A. M., D. B. Mount, I. Yang, and H. K. Choi. 2012. The genetics of hyperuricaemia and gout. *Nat Rev Rheumatol* 8 (10):610-621.

Sundy, J. S., H. R. Schumacher, A. Kivitz, S. P. Weinstein, R. Wu, S. King-Davis, and R. R. Evans. 2014. Rilonacept for gout flare prevention in patients receiving uric acid-lowering therapy: results of RESURGE, a phase III, international safety study. *J Rheumatol* 41 (8):1703-1711.

CHAPTER 9.2

JOINT PAIN AND DRUGS FOR ARTHRITIS

ROBERT LUEDTKE, PHD[1], EDWARD SHADIACK, DO[2]
AND VICTOR V. UTESHEV, PHD[3]

[1] University of North Texas Health Science Center, Fort Worth, TX
[2] The Veterans Health Administration's War Related Illness and Injury Study Center, East Orange, NJ
[3] Epigen Biosciences Inc., San Diego, CA

Symptoms: **Immuno-Infectious**
Musculoskeletal

DRUG LIST FOR ARTHRITIS

Nonsteroidal anti-inflammatory drugs (NSAID):
Aspirin NSAID COX-1 & COX-2 inhibitor analgesic/antipyrogen
Ibuprofen NSAID COX-1 & COX-2 inhibitor
Naproxen NSAID COX-1 & COX-2 inhibitor

Neuropathic Pain Inhibitors:
Pregabalin neuropathic pain/ $\alpha_2\delta$-1 calcium channel inhibitor
Duloxetine neuropathic pain/ serotonin/norepinephrine reuptake inhibitor

Stronger NSAIDs (prescription required)
Diclofenac nonselective COX-1 & COX-2 inhibitor
Fenoprofen nonselective COX-1 & COX-2 inhibitor
Flurbiprofen nonselective COX-1 & COX-2 inhibitor
Ketorolac nonselective COX-1 & COX-2 inhibitor
Celecoxib preferential COX-2 inhibitor
Indomethacin preferential COX-2 inhibitor
Mefenamic acid preferential COX-2 inhibitor
Meloxicam preferential COX-2 inhibitor

Disease-Modifying Anti-Rheumatic Drugs (DMARDs)
Apremilast inhibits intracellular PDE4 which hydrolyses cyclic adenosine monophosphate (cAMP), increases levels of the anti-inflammatory cytokine IL10, and decreases TNF-α production.
Azathioprine blocks purine synthesis.
Baricitinib Janus Kinase pathway inhibitor
Hydroxychloroquine interferes with antigen processing by macrophages
Leflunomide dihydroorotate dehydrogenase inhibitor
Methotrexate reduces purines and pyrimidines in T-cells and increases adenosine
Sulfasalazine sulfa drug, mechanism of action unclear
Tofacitinib JAX enzyme inhibitor

Corticosteroids **b**ind intracellular glucocorticoid receptors (*e.g.*, prednisone, hydrocortisone, prednisolone, dexamethasone, methylprednisolone, triamcinolone, and betamethasone)

Biological Response Modifiers (BRM)
Tofacitinib JAX enzyme inhibitor
Baricitnib JAX enzyme inhibitor
Abatacept fusion protein, CD80/CD/86 checkpoint protein
Anakinra modified recombinant protein, IL-1 receptor blocker
Etanercept fusion protein, binds TNFα
Adalimumab humanized monoclonal antibody, binds TNFα
Infliximab chimeric monoclonal antibody, binds TNFα
Certolizumab pegol PEGylated Fab' humanized monoclonal antibody binds TNFα

Golimumab	human monoclonal antibody, binds TNFα
Rituximab	chimeric monoclonal antibody
Tocilizumab	humanized monoclonal antibody

General Background

Arthritic disorders are medical conditions that present with pain, stiffening, and/or swelling of the joints, leading to a decrease in motion. Arthritis can affect individuals of all ages including children. Some common conditions associated with arthritis include osteoarthritis, rheumatoid arthritis, systemic lupus erythematosus, psoriatic arthritis, and septic arthritis. Fibromyalgia is an extremely common condition that can present in the setting of an arthritic disorder but is a disorder of pain regulation (e.g., nociplastic pain), not an arthritic disorder. (Bailly et al. 2020; Kosek et al. 2016) Fibromyalgia can be primary (occurring in the absence of other conditions) or secondary (occurring in the presence of, and complicating other conditions that cause pain). (FitzGerald et al. 2020; Veale D.J. 2021)

Patients afflicted with arthritis experience severe pain and a limitation of normal motor skills. Repeated visits to the physician's office are common. Patients become physically inactive, which may lead to worsening debility and loss of income. In addition, patients who experience arthritic symptoms are at increased risk for sleep disturbances, depression, and heart disease.

Decreased mobility associated with arthritis contributes to an increased risk of obesity. Adipose cells play a role in arthritic conditions because they are a source of cytokines, chemokines, and adipokines. Adipokines, including adiponectin and leptin, are a family of hormones and cytokines secreted by adipose cells that can have either pro- or anti-inflammatory effects. Studies in obese mice and humans have found that high levels of serum tumor necrosis factor-alpha (TNF-α), interleukin-1 beta (IL-1β), and interleukin 6 (IL-6), are produced by macrophages derived from adipose tissue. These pro-inflammatory cytokines regulate the proliferation and apoptosis of adipocytes, promote lipolysis, inhibit lipid synthesis, and decrease blood lipids. Elevated levels of TNF-α, IL-1β, and IL-6 are also found in the synovial fluid, synovial membrane, subchondral bone, and cartilage of patients with osteoarthritis. Moreover, TNF-α, IL-1, and IL-6 can a) induce the production of other cytokines, matrix metalloproteinases, and prostaglandins, b) inhibit the synthesis of proteoglycans and type II collagen, and c) play a role in cartilage matrix degradation and bone resorption in osteoarthritis.

Diagnosis

While essentially all forms of arthritis include symptoms of joint pain, the location, timing, associated symptoms, and pattern of pain may differ depending on the type of arthritis. For example, the symptoms of rheumatoid arthritis generally present as a symmetric polyarthritis affecting the small joints (e.g., hands, toes, wrists), have joint stiffness that is generally most severe in the morning and lasting greater than 1 hour, and may have associated systemic features. Conversely, patients with osteoarthritis generally experience fewer and larger joints involved (e.g., spine, hip, knee) with morning stiffness lasting less than 30 minutes without any associated systemic symptoms.

Important features for an arthritis diagnosis include the: a) rapidity and age of symptom onset, b) pattern of joint pain (e.g., symmetry), c) presence of synovitis (i.e., objective swelling of the synovium), d) timing of symptoms, and e) therapies that lead to pain relief. Laboratory and imaging tests may help support the diagnosis of an arthritic disorder, for example: (1) Rheumatoid Factor (an autoreactive antibody that binds the Fc portion of human antibodies) may help support the diagnosis of Rheumatoid Arthritis; (2) Antinuclear antibodies are a group of autoreactive antibodies that bind to contents of the cell nucleus (extractable nuclear antigen antibodies are more specific antibodies to certain components of the cell nucleus); and (3) C-reactive protein (CRP) is a non-specific inflammatory marker that suggests the presence of systemic inflammation. None of these is 100% sensitive or specific, and patients without an arthritic disorder may still demonstrate low levels of various autoantibodies. In addition, X-rays can provide information on the extent of joint degeneration or possible effusion.

Common Types of Arthritic Conditions

Osteoarthritis:

Osteoarthritis is the most common arthritic condition in the world. It is a disease of the whole joint, involving structural alterations in the articular cartilage, subchondral bone, ligaments, capsule, synovial membrane, and periarticular muscles. (Hunter and Bierma-Zeinstra 2019) It is a degenerative joint disease in that the immune system is not invovled to the same degree as, say, Rheumatoid Arthritis.

Presentation: The knees are the most common site, followed by the hand and hip. Symptoms generally include joint pain (especially during or after movement), joint stiffness after periods of inactivity typically lasting <30 minutes ("gel phenomena"), joint tenderness and loss of range of motion, an abrasive sensation with popping/cracking ("crepitus") when using the affected joints, and joint swelling (e.g., Baker's cyst in the popliteal fossa). As compared to other arthritides, Osteoarthritis is generally slower to progress. Osteoarthritis of the fingers is more prevalent in the familial forms of the condition and affects the distal (DIP) and proximal (PIP) interphalangeal joints (whereas rheumatoid arthritis classically affects the wrist, metacarpophalangeal (MCP), and PIP joints). Osteoarthritis frequently involves the first carpometacarpal joint. The age of onset is generally >60 years old. Earlier onset may be secondary to a post-traumatic event or familial form.

Risk Factors: The prevalence of Osteoarthritis increases with age. Females are more likely to be affected than males. Genetics is felt to account for about 50% of the risk of developing Osteoarthritis. (Skousgaard et al. 2015) About 100 genetic variants have been identified, which account for about 20% of the heritability of osteoarthritis. (Aubourg et al. 2021) Abnormal biomechanics such as limb length discrepancy, abnormal limb alignment, and other conditions causing abnormal contact between joint surfaces plays a role in the development of osteoarthritis. (Glyn-Jones et al. 2015) There is some association between physically intensive jobs and the incidence of osteoarthritis. (Yucesoy et al. 2015) Obesity adds additional stress to weight-bearing joints which can lead to osteoarthritis. (Guilak 2011) A history of sports injuries or automobile accidents is thought to increase the risk of osteoarthritis. (Thomas et al. 2017) Metabolic diseases such as hemochromatosis (*a genetic disease leading to iron overload*) or metabolic syndrome/diabetes can also increase the risk of osteoarthritis. (Chadha 2016)

Pathophysiology: The pathophysiology of Osteoarthritis is complex and not completely understood. It is not just a disorder of "wear and tear," and involves dysfunction at a cellular level in conjunction with complicated metabolic processes and localized joint inflammation. (Martel-Pelletier et al. 2016) Pathways common to both osteoarthritis and cardiovascular disease have been identified, suggesting a role for fat metabolism and the innate immune system in the pathogenesis of Osteoarthritis. Ultimately, Osteoarthritis results when the cartilage that cushions the ends of a bone degenerates leading to joint space narrowing and bone damage. The pain, at least initially, is thought to be related to nociceptive sensation (pain sensed in relation to tissue damage itself). Over time, the pain may progress to include neuropathic (pain related to nerve damage or abnormal activity) and then centralize in a process where the central nervous system inappropriately modulates pain signaling leading to increased levels of (and possibly more widespread) pain ("nociplastic pain"). (Hunter and Bierma-Zeinstra 2019; Fitzcharles et al. 2021)

Examination: In the hands, patients with Osteoarthritis can have visually apparent bony bumps. When the PIP joints are affected, these are called Bouchard's nodes, and when the DIP joints are affected, these are called Heberden's nodes. In some cases of knee Osteoarthritis, a fluid-filled cyst (i.e., Baker's cyst) may be evident behind the knee in the popliteal fossa.

Laboratory: There are no specific laboratory findings for Osteoarthritis in the blood. Synovial fluid analysis can be used in the setting of significant effusion to rule out an underlying inflammatory etiology. Sometimes mildly elevated inflammatory markers can be seen, which are suspected to be secondary to inflammation arising from comorbid obesity and metabolic syndrome.

Imaging: Findings include loss of joint space (which is usually non-uniform), bone spur formation (i.e. osteophytes), subchondral sclerosis (thickening/hardening of bone beneath the affected cartilage), and cysts. (Braun and Gold 2012) A more specific finding in the hand is a central erosion at the distal or proximal interphalangeal joints known as a gull-wing (or seagull) erosion (whereas erosions in Rheumatoid Arthritis occur on more lateral aspects of the joint not covered by cartilage and known as "marginal erosions").

Associated symptoms/conditions: Osteoarthritis is associated with cardiovascular disease and its risk factors (e.g., diabetes, hyperlipidemia), and also with depression. (Hunter and Bierma-Zeinstra 2019)

Diagnosis: This is a clinical diagnosis based on symptoms from history, signs on physical exam, and supported by radiographic features, in the absence of signs or symptoms to suggest another etiology. Common features include joint pain, older age, clicking/popping with a restricted range of motion, and joint tenderness on exam. (Hunter and Bierma-Zeinstra 2019)

Treatment: Exercise and weight loss are the interventions best supported as a primary intervention to prevent further joint damage. Tylenol and NSAIDs are often the first line for the management of pain associated with Osteoarthritis. Joint injections with corticosteroids are often performed adjunctively. Although glucosamine and chondroitin have been used to promote healthy cartilage, research has largely been unrevealing of benefits. Duloxetine is a serotonin-norepinephrine reuptake inhibitor (SNRI) that can be used for the neuropathic and nociplastic aspects of pain associated with Osteoarthritis. (Hunter and Bierma-Zeinstra 2019)

Management: While osteoarthritic symptoms can be managed with medication, the joint damage is irreversible. Surgery is often explored for a variety of reasons, but these are beyond the scope of this text. Canes, walkers, or other mobility assistive devices may help keep a patient functional. Physical therapy may be very useful in addressing abnormal biomechanics and for strengthening synergistic muscles to provide some relief and allow for improved joint function.

Rheumatoid Arthritis:

Rheumatoid arthritis is an inflammatory disorder involving the joint capsule leading to the development of fibrous tissue in the synovium (i.e., *the soft tissue between the joint capsule and the joint cavity*) and ultimately to the destruction of articular cartilage (*i.e., tissue that covers the ends of bones that converge to form a joint*). (Smolen et al. 2016)

Presentation: A symmetric, small joint polyarthritis with tender, warm, and swollen joints secondary to inflammation of the synovium ("synovitis"), typically presenting in adults. Morning stiffness (and stiffness after prolonged inactivity in general) is more extensive than in osteoarthritis and classically lasts longer than 1 hour. Systemic symptoms (e.g., fever, fatigue, loss of appetite) are frequently reported during flares. Virtually any body system can be affected, with interstitial lung disease being a common association. (Smolen et al. 2016)

Risk Factors: Genetic factors are thought to represent about 40-50% of the risk of developing the condition. (Deane et al. 2017) A positive family history increases the risk of rheumatoid arthritis three to five times and concordance rates in twins are increased. Environmental contributors include smoking, periodontitis, obesity, hormonal factors; and occupational exposures to silica dust, organic solvents, and paints. (Klareskog et al. 2020; Kronzer and Davis 2021)

Pathophysiology: Autoreactive antibodies attack synovial tissue leading to synovial hypertrophy, inflammation, and bone erosions that result in joint deformity. (Rheumatoid arthritis 2018) The etiology of pain in Rheumatoid Arthritis is thought to be nociceptive secondary to inflammatory mediators, although there is a recognition that this can evolve to include neuropathic and nociplastic (i.e., centralized) processes. (Zhang and Lee 2018)

Examination: As the pathological state progresses, the accompanying inflammation erodes the joint surface leading to impairment of movement and deformation of the involved joint. Classically reported findings in severe disease of the hands and feet include swan-neck deformity (*hyperextension of the proximal interphalangeal joint and flexion of the distal interphalangeal joint*), boutonniere deformity (*flexion of the proximal interphalangeal joint and hyperextension of the proximal interphalangeal joint*), and "hammer toe" deformity (*a deformation of the muscles and ligaments of the second, third, fourth, or fifth toe causing the toes of the foot to bend*). (Harb et al. 2013)

Laboratory: During a flare, inflammatory markers (e.g., erythrocyte sedimentation rate, C-reactive protein) may be elevated. Rheumatoid Factor, an antibody against the Fc portion of a human antibody (predominantly, though not exclusively, IgM) may be elevated though is non-specific. Anti-citrullinated protein/peptide antibodies, such as anti-cyclic citrullinated peptide (anti-CCP), are more specific indicators of the condition. Elevations of anti-CCP may predict the later development of rheumatoid arthritis in patients not currently meeting criteria for the condition.

Imaging: Joint space narrowing with juxta-articular osteopenia, marginal erosions (i.e. along the outer border of a joint not covered by cartilage), and soft tissue swelling help differentiate this from osteoarthritis. (Chang et al. 2016)

Associated symptoms/conditions: Patients with severe rheumatoid arthritis can also experience symptoms beyond the joints including the skin, sclera of the eye, pericardium of the heart, kidneys, nervous tissue, blood vessels, as well as hematologic abnormalities. (Cojocaru et al. 2010) Commonly present are peripheral neuropathies (*damage to the peripheral nervous system*), carpel tunnel syndrome (*compression of the median nerve causing hand numbness, tingling, or weakness*), and/or poor coordination that can increase the risk of accidents or serious injury. Interstitial lung disease and lung nodules are seen in RA. (Conforti et al. 2021) Patients are more prone to atherosclerosis and to early mortality from cardiovascular disease. (Provan et al. 2020)

Diagnosis: Rheumatoid arthritis is a clinical diagnosis based on signs and symptoms and supported by laboratory and radiographic findings. American College of Rheumatology (ACR) criteria (used for research) require active synovitis (inflammation of the synovial membrane) in at least one joint. Points are then assigned for the number and type of joints (small joints get more points than large ones), supportive laboratory findings (i.e., ESR, CRP, Rheumatoid Factor, and anti-CCP), and symptom duration. Six out of 10 points clinches the diagnosis (Aletaha et al. 2010)

Treatment: Methotrexate is the first-line pharmaceutical for the treatment of Rheumatoid Arthritis. There are many other diseases modifying anti-rheumatic drugs that may be used, including hydroxychloroquine, sulfasalazine, leflunomide, TNF-inhibitors (e.g., etanercept), abatacept, IL-6 inhibitors (tocilizumab), the B-cell depleting agent rituximab, and JAK inhibitors (e.g. tofacitinib). Glucocorticoids are additive and typically used in low doses given their significant side effect profile. (Smolen et al. 2016; Fraenkel et al. 2021)

Management: As this disorder progresses a hammer toe joint can become rigid and immobile, and surgery may be required to reinstate some degree of flexibility. Physical Therapy and Occupational Therapy are helpful to maintain function.

Psoriatic Arthritis:

Psoriatic arthritis is inflammatory condition that develops in as many as 25% of patients who suffer from psoriasis. (Alinaghi et al. 2019) Psoriasis is a noninfectious skin disorder that causes skin cells to multiply faster than normal, leading to a characteristic rash.

Presentation: Psoriatic arthritis presents most often in adults between the ages of 30 and 50 years old. There are five common patterns of joint involvement associated with Psoriatic Arthritis: (1) primarily distal interphalangeal joints of the hands (and/or feet), (2) symmetric small joint polyarthritis (similar to Rheumatoid Arthritis), (3) oligoarticular (≤4 joints), (4) spine and sacroiliac joint arthritis, and (5) arthritis mutilans. (Moll and Wright 1973) Arthritis mutilans, the most severe joint manifestation of psoriatic arthritis, is a condition of actual bone destruction leading to shortened and deformed joints, primarily affecting the small joints in the fingers. The axial/sacroiliac type presents with inflammatory back pain features such as insidious onset, night pain that improves with getting up, pain >3 months, younger age of onset (typically <40), improvement with exercise, and no improvement despite rest; it may also be exquisitely responsive to NSAIDs. (Rudwaleit et al. 2009)

Risk Factors: Some patients who develop psoriatic arthritis have a family history of either psoriasis or psoriatic arthritis. The HLA B27 allele has been associated with axial/spine involvement in individuals with Psoriatic arthritis. (Chandran et al. 2009) HLA B27 is associated with a class of conditions known as the spondyloarthritides (pleural of Spondyloarthritis) that, in addition to psoriatic arthritis, include *ankylosing spondylitis, reactive arthritis, and enteropathic, or inflammatory bowel disease associated, Spondyloarthritis*. HLA B27 is a class I cell surface antigen encoded by the B locus in the major histocompatibility complex (MHC). This genetic locus codes for proteins involved in presenting antigenic peptides to T cells. In addition to genetic risk factors, physical trauma, infections, obesity, and smoking are thought to increase the risk of psoriatic arthritis in people with this genetic predisposition. (Veale and Fearon 2018)

Pathophysiology: The pathogenesis of psoriasis (and psoriatic arthritis) is incompletely understood. Psoriatic arthritis appears to be primarily a T-cell mediated process, with key contributions of multiple different types of T-cells (Th1, Th17, Treg, Th22). Unlike Rheumatoid Arthritis, Psoriatic Arthritis does not have an associated pathogenic antibody (which is produced by B-lymphocytes). There is a multitude of inflammatory mediators thought to play a role in the development of psoriasis, including interleukins: IL-17, IL-22, IL-23, IL-1β, and TNFα, among others. (Cai et al. 2012) These lead to synovial inflammation and thickening (pannus formation) with subsequent bone and cartilage destruction. (Veale and Fearon 2018) As with all other inflammatory conditions, pain may nociceptive (i.e., from joint inflammation and local damage), but may progress to involve neuropathic and nociplastic (i.e., centralized pain) pathways.

Examination: The swelling of an entire finger or toe is known as *dactylitis* or more colloquially called a "sausage digit." Pain and inflammation where tendons (especially the Achilles tendon) and ligaments attach to bone are known as *Enthesitis*. Psoriatic skin lesions are red patches covered with a fine white scale classically over extensor surfaces (e.g., elbows, knees), scalp, and low back, and pitting of the nails. The Koebner phenomenon refers to the appearance of skin lesions subsequent to trauma to the skin.

Laboratory: Inflammatory markers (e.g., erythrocyte sedimentation rate, C-reactive protein) may be elevated during flares, though are non-specific. HLA-B27 is present in about 25% of cases, though is non-specific. There should be absence of Rheumatoid Factor and Anti-CCP antibodies.

Imaging: X-ray may note irregular erosions with new bone growth. This bony growth can occur at the sites of Enthesitis and results in enthesophytes (i.e., bone spurs). Bones may appear to fuse together, referred to radiographically as "ankylosis." Thickening of the periosteum may also be visible (*periostitis*). (Poggenborg et al. 2015) Bone erosions at the joint (classically in the hands and feet) can get so bad that there is a distal narrowing of the bone to the point that it may look like a pencil (the bone) sitting in a cup (the joint) and is referred to as "Pencil-in-cup" changes. (Ory et al. 2005)

Associated symptoms/conditions: Psoriatic skin lesions, although not necessary to make a diagnosis, are extremely prevalent in the condition. Psoriatic arthritis is accompanied by changes in the appearance of fingernails and toenails, ranging from small pits to a complete crumbling of the nails (i.e., onycholysis). Inflammation of the uvea of the eye (*uveitis)* may also be seen. There is an association with cardiovascular disease and its risk factors (e.g., diabetes, dyslipidemia), and also with inflammatory bowel disease, gout, and depression. (Perez-Chada and Merola)

Diagnosis: The diagnosis of psoriatic arthritis is a clinical one, though classification criteria do exist to support a diagnosis. These criteria include: (1) evidence of psoriasis, (2) onycholysis, pitting, or hyperkeratosis of the nails, (3) absence of Rheumatoid Factor on lab work, (4) dactylitis, and (5) ossification of joint margins. (Taylor et al. 2006)

Treatment: Both the American College of Rheumatology (ACR) and the European Union League against Rheumatism (EULAR) have competing recent guidelines for the pharmaceutical treatment of psoriatic arthritis. ACR recommends that TNF inhibitors be the first-line treatment, whereas EULAR recommends methotrexate for polyarthritis (>4 joints). Regardless, both find a role in the early treatment of patients with Psoriatic Arthritis. Other agents include sulfasalazine, leflunomide, and inhibitors of the IL-17 and IL-12/23 pathways. NSAIDs and corticosteroids are adjunctive. (Singh et al. 2019; Gossec et al. 2020)

Management: Since there is no cure for psoriatic arthritis, the clinical focus is to control the symptoms and prevent further damage to inflamed joints, without which, the condition can evolve into a disabling disorder. Low-impact exercise, physical and occupational therapies, and other complementary therapies (e.g., acupuncture, massage) are recommended to help improve physical functioning and pain. (Gossec et al. 2020)

Systemic Lupus Erythematosus (SLE):

Systemic lupus erythematosus (SLE, *also colloquially referred to as Lupus*) is a chronic inflammatory systemic autoimmune disorder characterized by the production of autoantibodies that bind human DNA.

Presentation: The symptoms of SLE are very numerous and diverse. It can be problematic to diagnose SLE because its symptoms can mimic symptoms associated with other arthritic disorders. (Aringer et al. 2019) Some of the most common symptoms at presentation include fatigue, muscle pain (myalgia), joint pain (arthralgia), cutaneous photosensitivity, hair loss, and rashes (most specifically a malar rash). (Metry et al. 2019). This symptom can either arise suddenly or develop slowly. Most patients with lupus have a disease characterized by episodic flares where symptoms worsen and then improve. Approximately 90% of SLE patients are females, who are generally afflicted during childbearing age. Photosensitivity is commonly observed in patients with SLE, where skin rash, itching, and/or burning skin worsen after exposure to sunlight or artificial ultraviolet light.

Risk Factors: While SLE and other autoimmune disorders appear to have a genetic component, the inheritance pattern is complex. Patients may inherit a genetic variation that increases the risk of SLE but, in most cases, one gene does not directly cause the disorder. Certain ethnic groups (i.e., Africans, Asians, Hispanics/Latinos, Native Americans, Native Hawaiians, or Pacific Islanders) have a greater risk of developing SLE. Environmental factors have been proposed to possibly trigger the disorder in genetically predisposed individuals. The strongest epidemiologic evidence exists for exposure to crystalline silica, current cigarette smoking, use of oral contraceptives, and postmenopausal hormone replacement therapy, while there is an inverse association with alcohol use. (Parks et al. 2017) Symptoms are also reported after infections, drug administration, or even exposure to sunlight. Drug-induced lupus is a variety of its own, with its own antibody (*anti-histone antibodies*), and classically associated with hydralazine, procainamide, and TNF-inhibitors. (Almoallim et al. 2012)

Pathophysiology: It is known that both the innate and adaptive aspects of the immune system play an important role in the development of disease. This process is incompletely understood, though patients ultimately develop autoreactive B-cells which produce auto-antibodies that bind to components of human DNA. These auto-antibodies and inflammatory cytokines lead to tissue damage. (Choi et al. 2012) Immune complexes are deposited in a variety of tissues (e.g., kidney) and lead to further tissue damage. (Bao et al. 2015) How auto-reactivity initially develops is still the topic of debate, though some suggest that a defect in the ability to clear cellular nuclear proteins leads to these autoantigens being present in blood and exposing them directly to immune cells which go on to become sensitized to these antigens. (Arneth 2019)

Examination: A malar (aka "butterfly") rash is present in about 30% of patients with SLE. This is an erythematous rash of both cheeks and nasal bridge which spares the nasolabial fold. There are a number of other skin findings known to occur with SLE (e.g., discoid lupus). Hair loss in patches or diffusely thinned (nonscarring alopecia) is also common. Examination of the mouth may identify (aphthous) ulcers on the buccal mucosa, tongue, or palate. Other less specific signs may be present based on the involved organ system. (Kiriakidou and Ching 2020)

Laboratory: Non-specific laboratory findings include cytopenias (e.g., low white blood cells, red blood cells, or platelets), evidence of renal damage (e.g., hematuria, proteinuria, elevated creatinine), low complement levels (C3, C4), or evidence of inflammation (i.e., elevated ESR, CRP). Anti-nuclear antibodies are typically present in a high titer (>1:80). (Bossuyt et al. 2020) More specific antibodies (e.g., anti-Smith, anti-double-stranded DNA) may also be seen and may be predictive of certain manifestations of the disease (e.g., anti-dsDNA and renal manifestations).

Imaging: As SLE can affect essentially any organ, radiographic findings vary widely. There are only a very few imaging findings that can be considered more specific. On echocardiogram, there may be non-infectious vegetation on multiple cardiac surfaces, most commonly the mitral valve, known as Libman-Sack endocarditis. (Lalani et al. 2004) Imaging may also show a non-erosive deformation of the joints of the hands (typically) known as Jaccoud arthropathy. (Santiago et al. 2015)

Associated symptoms/conditions: About 50% of SLE patients experience severe complications, which can include nephritis, central nervous system vasculitis, pulmonary hypertension, interstitial lung disease, and/or stroke. Lupus nephritis can occur when autoantibodies are deposited in the renal glomeruli, causing chronic complement-dependent inflammation, blood in the urine, high blood pressure, renal insufficiency, or kidney failure. About 25% of patients with SLE also have the anti-phospholipid syndrome, which is a disorder of hypercoagulability (e.g., more frequent deep venous thromboses) and recurrent pregnancy morbidity (e.g., miscarriages) in the presence of anti-phospholipid and/or anti-cardiolipin antibodies. (McMahon et al. 2006) Patients with SLE are at increased risk for the development of cardiovascular disease. (McMahon et al. 2011)

Diagnosis: SLE is a clinical diagnosis, supported by laboratory and radiographic data. There do exist classification criteria (2019 ACR/EULAR criteria) to help in establishing a diagnosis, but these are considered more specific criteria meant for research studies. (Aringer et al. 2019) General features of diagnosis include identifying appropriate symptoms with more specific organ involvement on laboratory assessment in the setting of a high titer anti-nuclear antibody.

Treatment: Hydroxychloroquine is the first-line treatment for essentially all lupus patients. (Schrezenmeier and Dorner 2020) Glucocorticoids are especially used during acute flares of the condition, but may be used chronically in low doses (preferably <7.5 mg/day of prednisone) due to the risks of long-term administration. Calcineurin inhibitors are often recommended in lupus nephritis. Cyclophosphamide and rituximab are used for more severe disease. Other immunosuppressive drugs that find utility in treating SLE include methotrexate, azathioprine, and mycophenolate mofetil. (Fanouriakis et al.)

Management: The use of sunscreen is advisable due to the prevalence of photosensitivity in individuals with SLE. Smoking cessation should be strongly advised, especially as tobacco is thought to play a role in the pathogenesis of the disease. (Fanouriakis et al. 2019) Exercise and interventions like cognitive behavioral therapy have been shown to improve symptoms. (Fangtham et al. 2019)

Juvenile Idiopathic Arthritis:

Juvenile idiopathic arthritis (JIA) is not one disease but a diverse group of arthritides with varied characteristics, grouped together based on their chronicity, younger age of onset, and unknown etiologies. In 2001, the International League of Associations for Rheumatology developed what are now the most commonly recognized different categories of JIA. (Petty et al. 2004) JIA, as a group, is the most common type of arthritis observed in children. (Cimaz 2016) Further classification into one of the seven defined categories of JIA helps in selecting treatments and in monitoring for complications.

Presentation: Symptoms of JIA vary from category to category, though commonalities includes joint pain, swelling, and stiffness, in a child (<16 years old), lasting >6 weeks. One specific condition, systemic JIA, also includes ≥2 weeks of fever occurring in close proximity to the onset of arthritis and is associated with (at least one of) an evanescent rash, lymphadenopathy, hepatosplenomegaly, and serositis (e.g., pleuritis, pericarditis, peritonitis). Oligoarthritic JIA is defined by its affecting ≤4 joints in the first 6 months (though can have more involved joints later), whereas Polyarthritis JIA affects ≥5 joints during the first 6 months (and is divided into Rheumatoid Factor Positive and Negative varieties). Psoriatic JIA has arthritis with psoriasis (or with dactylitis, nail pitting/onycholysis, or psoriasis in a first-degree relative). Enthesitis Related JIA has arthritis and enthesitis, or either with at least two of sacroiliac/lumbosacral pain, HLA B27, acute anterior uveitis, onset in a male >6 years old, or history of other conditions under the Spondyloarthritis umbrella. Those who meet the criteria for JIA and none of the above OR more than one of the above would be classified as Undifferentiated JIA. (Petty et al. 2004)

Risk Factors: Given the heterogeneity of conditions, risk factors vary from condition to condition. Some monogenetic etiologies have been identified in the years since the most recent classification criteria were put forth. Additionally, there are an increasing number of genetic risk factors being identified including HLA (e.g., HLA B27) and non-HLA alleles. (Nigrovic et al. 2019) As a class, there is some evidence to support an association with intrauterine and maternal exposure to inhaled pollutants such as cigarette smoke, ozone, fine dust, and volatile vapors; however, these studies may be the subject of recall bias. (Franca et al. 2018)

Pathophysiology: Systemic JIA is purported to be secondary to dysfunction localized primarily to the innate immune system, with the elaboration of several proinflammatory cytokines (e.g., IL-1β, IL-6, IL-18). (Frosch and Roth 2008) Genetic studies do provide support for the hypothesis that some of the JIAs may be a juvenile onset of their adult counterparts, (Nigrovic et al. 2019) with similar pathophysiology (e.g., enthesitis-related JIA and Spondyloarthritis).

Examination: Joints can be swollen, tender to palpation, with both pain and reduced range of motion. Oligoarthritic JIA (≤ 4 joints) and Polyarthritic JIA (≥ 5 joints) are differentiated based on the number of affected joints in the first 6 months after presentation. Patients with Psoriatic JIA may have red patches with a fine white scale on the extensor surfaces (this is often misdiagnosed as eczema given the rarity of psoriasis in children), nail pitting/onycholysis, or dactylitis (e.g., swelling of an entire digit). Enthesitis (e.g., pain and inflammation at the insertion of tendons, ligaments, or joint capsules) and sacroiliac joint tenderness may be present in Enthesitis related JIA. Systemic symptoms (e.g., fever, chills) and diffuse lymphadenopathy, hepatosplenomegaly, and an evanescent rash may be present in Systemic JIA. (Petty et al. 2004)

Laboratory: A positive Rheumatoid Factor may be present in Polyarthritic JIA. HLA B27 is often found in Enthesitis JIA variety. Inflammatory markers (erythrocyte sedimentation rate, C-reactive protein) are variably, and non-specifically, elevated. Anemia in chronic disease or leukocytosis (i.e., elevated white blood cell count) is sometimes observed but, again, is non-specific. (Kim and Kim 2010)

Imaging: Imaging is useful in evaluating the joint and in helping to rule out other etiologies of joint pain (e.g., malignancy, fracture). MRI is finding more frequent use in the evaluation of JIA. (Kim and Kim 2010)

Associated symptoms/conditions: JIA can result in serious complications, such as interference with a child's growth and bone development (which can also be secondary to the use of corticosteroids). Some JIA is associated with eye inflammation (*uveitis*), cataracts, glaucoma, or blindness. Children with juvenile idiopathic arthritis are also at increased risk for a life-threatening condition called Macrophage Activation Syndrome.

Diagnosis: This is a clinical diagnosis and is often considered if a child (<16 years old) has more than 6 weeks of arthritis with a negative evaluation for infection or malignancy.

Treatment: Medications used to treat juvenile idiopathic arthritis include nonsteroidal anti-inflammatory drugs, disease-modifying anti-rheumatic drugs, biological agents, and corticosteroids. Corticosteroids can also inhibit growth and should be used for the shortest possible duration.

Management: Pharmaceuticals (e.g., NSAIDs) and other modalities (such as physical therapy) are used for controlling pain and improving function. Some patients with JIA (particularly those positive for HLA B27) need to be monitored for the development of uveitis. Attention to growth and development is essential. Standard vaccinations are recommended for children with JIA though live virus vaccines may be contraindicated when on a biologic immunosuppressant. (Moore 2018)

Septic Arthritis:

Septic arthritis refers to infectious causes of arthritis, but does not imply the presence of actual sepsis. Etiologic agents include bacterial, viral, and fungal organisms. What follows is a discussion of bacterial septic arthritis, with viral and fungal being beyond the scope of this chapter. Bacterial septic arthritis represents a medical emergency and may lead to permanent joint damage or progress to a life-threatening systemic infection. It should be suspected in a patient with the acute onset of arthritis in a single joint, regardless of the existence of pre-existing joint disease (e.g., Rheumatoid Arthritis).

Presentation: Bacterial septic arthritis typically presents as an acutely swollen, stiff, and painful joint, often in the setting of fever. (Weston et al. 1999) Native joints most commonly reported to be involved include the knees and hips. (Kaandorp et al.)

Risk Factors: Antecedent joint disease (e.g., Rheumatoid Arthritis) or prior joint arthroplasty (i.e., replacement) significantly increase risk for septic arthritis. New joint pain in patients with a compromised immune system (e.g., primary immunodeficiency, diabetes, cancer, or taking immunosuppressive medications) should also raise red flags. (Ross 2017) Septic arthritis can complicate a joint injection due to introducing an infectious agent into the joint. (Mohamed et al. 2019) A skin or soft tissue infection near a joint may spread locally to include the joint. More distant infections may spread hematogenously (i.e., through the blood) to settle in the joint, so IV drug users are at an elevated risk for septic arthritis.

Pathophysiology: Septic arthritis is caused by the introduction of an infectious agent directly into a joint, which can be either derived from another part of the body (hematogenous spread or local invasion) or from penetration directly into the joint (trauma, injection). The most common bacterial cause of septic arthritis in adults is *Staphylococcus aureus*. *Neisseria gonorrhea* is the most common cause of atraumatic septic arthritis among sexually active adults. (Momodu and Savaliya 2021) Joint damage occurs both due to the bacteria itself and due to the resultant inflammation. (Colavite and Sartori 2014)

Examination: Patients almost universally exhibit a painful and limited range of motion of the joint, though this is non-specific. Joint effusion is also extremely common, and its acute onset should raise suspicion for septic arthritis. The joint may appear red or be warm to the touch; however, these are variably reported and their absence does not rule out the condition. The patient may also be febrile. (Carpenter et al. 2011)

Laboratory: Commonly obtained blood studies often identify an elevated white blood cell count and inflammatory markers, though these are nonspecific. Procalcitonin may be a more specific for test bacterial infections, though is more useful in systemic infections such that a low procalcitonin does not rule out septic arthritis. (Carpenter et al. 2011) Blood cultures may reveal the etiologic organism. (Coakley et al. 2006) Synovial fluid analysis is essential for confirming the diagnosis of septic arthritis and for identifying the organism. Synovial fluid white blood cells >50 x 10^9/L are very suggestive, though septic arthritis can be present with lower counts. (Carpenter et al. 2011)

Imaging: X-rays may demonstrate swelling and can help to provide evidence of pre-existing joint disease. (Horowitz et al. 2011) CT and MRI may help to identify any co-occurring osteomyelitis. (Coakley et al. 2006; Ross 2017)

Associated symptoms/conditions: Patients with septic arthritis may present with signs of a systemic infection or sepsis (e.g., fever, elevated heart rate, elevated respiratory rate). When joint infection is secondary to seeding from another site, that infectious process may be readily apparent (e.g., cellulitis) or obscure (e.g., bacterial endocarditis).

Diagnosis: Septic arthritis may be strongly suggested based on history and physical exam, and supported by laboratory findings in blood. When suspected, the joint fluid must be obtained, though failure to identify the organism on Gram stain or culture still does not rule out the condition. (Coakley et al. 2006)

Treatment: The treatment for septic arthritis generally includes promptly and repeatedly draining any accumulated joint fluid and the administration of empirically selected broad-spectrum antibiotics (e.g., vancomycin). (Coakley et al. 2006) If treatment is delayed, septic arthritis can lead to joint degeneration and permanent joint damage.

Management: In addition to treating acute septic arthritis, it is important to manage any risk factors which may have predisposed the patient to develop the condition (e.g., diabetes, corticosteroid use, etc.). Physical therapy and assistive devices may be helpful in the aftermath of joint damage secondary to septic arthritis.

Fibromyalgia:

Fibromyalgia is a disorder of pain processing at the level of the central nervous system. It is not an arthritic condition but can co-occur with one.

Presentation: Fibromyalgia is characterized by chronic (i.e., >6 months), widespread (i.e., left and right side, upper and lower body extremities, and axial) pain, in association with chronic fatigue, unrefreshing sleep and cognitive symptoms (i.e., "brain fog"). Patients will often report symptoms in a wide variety of systems (e.g., headaches, irritable bowel syndrome, depression, chemical sensitivities).

Risk Factors: Fibromyalgia may be co-occur with another painful condition (e.g., inflammatory arthritis), and is known to be associated with prior physical and emotional trauma. It has been proposed that 10-20% of patients with Rheumatoid Arthritis also have Fibromyalgia. (Zhao et al. 2019) Genetics are thought to account for about 50% of the risk of developing fibromyalgia. (D'Agnelli et al. 2019) Fibromyalgia is reported to occur much more commonly in females, possibly secondary to hormonal differences.

Pathophysiology: Putative mechanisms include abnormality of ascending pain pathways, integration of pain signals at the level of the brain, and descending inhibitory pain signaling, all leading to amplification of pain-sensing. This has been referred as central sensitization. (Sluka and Clauw 2016)

Examination: There are no specific physical examination features, other than widespread pain and subjectively increased tenderness to painful stimuli. The 1990 American College of Rheumatology diagnostic criteria for fibromyalgia included the identification of 11 out of 18 specific tender points. (Wolfe et al. 1990) The tender point exam was subsequently removed in the updated 2010 diagnostic criteria (modified again in 2016), because (1) these points were found not to be specific to the condition, (2) most clinicians did not use them, and (3) when clinicians did use them, most used them improperly. (Wolfe et al. 2016)

Laboratory: Laboratory studies (e.g., inflammatory markers, auto-antibodies) may be used to exclude other conditions that mimic fibromyalgia.

Imaging: Functional magnetic resonance imaging has demonstrated differences in brain activity between groups of patients with fibromyalgia and healthy controls in research studies, but the applicability to individual clinical patients has not been establsiehd and these are not clinically available. (Lopez-Sola et al. 2017; Gracely et al. 2002)

Associated symptoms/conditions: Fibromyalgia is associated with multiple other pain and non-pain conditions such as: tension and migraine headaches, temporomandibular joint disorder, irritable bowel syndrome, anxiety, and depression, as all may be related to central sensitization. (Yunus 2007) Fibromyalgia is often comorbid with rheumatic disorders.

(Lichtenstein et al. 2018) Patients with fibromyalgia have demonstrably worse sleep than those without the condition, and some speculate that impaired sleep is a primary contributor to the development of the condition. (Choy 2015) Insomnia, obstructive sleep apnea, and restless legs syndrome all occur at higher rates in patients with fibromyalgia. (Roizenblatt et al. 2011)

Diagnosis: The diagnosis of fibromyalgia is a clinical one. The 2016 modification to the 2010 American College of Rheumatology diagnostic criteria bases a diagnosis of fibromyalgia on a point system that includes the presence of chronic, generalized, widespread pain, in association with fatigue, unrefreshing sleep, cognitive symptoms, headache, pain/cramping in the lower abdomen, and depression. (Wolfe et al. 2016)

Treatment: Medications for fibromyalgia include serotonin-norepinephrine reuptake inhibitors (e.g., duloxetine, venlafaxine, and milnacipran), tricyclic antidepressants (e.g., nortriptyline, amitriptyline) and agents that bind the alpha-2-delta site on voltage-gated calcium channels (e.g., gabapentin, pregabalin). (Bair and Krebs 2020). Despite there being some data to show improvement with these agents, and several being FDA approved for this indication, both clinical experience and recent studies suggest that the effectiveness of these agents in chronic pain may not be clinically meaningful for many suffering from this condition. (Mascarenhas et al. 2021)

Management: Fibromyalgia is best managed with a multimodal approach in addition to pharmaceutical agents. The addition of cognitive behavioral therapy for pain, physical therapy, and manipulative physical modalities can help patients in a setting where medications may not be as effective. Interventions to improve sleep should be pursued, as there is some indication that poor sleep may be contribute to central sensitization. Addressing stress is vital, and mind-body interventions have demonstrated some utility. Physical activity, especially aerobic exercise, is strongly advised. (Bair and Krebs 2020)

General Treatment Strategies for Arthritic Conditions

There are three fundamental goals for the treatment of all arthritic conditions. The first goal is to alleviate patient pain. The second goal is to minimize joint inflammation. The third goal is to arrest the progression of an arthritic disorder. A physical exam, imaging tests, and laboratory tests are used in concert to help elucidate the type of arthritis that is being presented so that an appropriate therapeutic strategy can be developed. Treatment of an arthritic condition can include both non-pharmacological and pharmacological strategies.

Non-pharmacological treatment strategies can include physical, occupational, and nutritional therapies. For instance, weight loss (exercise + diet) is the most important treatment for osteoarthritis affecting the weight-bearing joints. The efficacy of nutritional therapies is controversial (Thomas et al. 2018; Philippou et al. 2021; Aparicio-Soto et al. 2017) and may include the intake of anti-inflammatory foods, including foods rich in omega-3 fatty acids and vitamin D.

Conditions are broadly divided into systemic inflammation (e.g., rheumatoid arthritis, SLE) and local arthritis (e.g., osteoarthritis). Pharmaceuticals help to reduce pain and inflammation (e.g., NSAIDs, steroids), attenuate the immune system (i.e., disease-modifying anti-rheumatic drugs), or modulate contributing metabolites (e.g., urate-lowering therapy). Although there are general guidelines for the prescription of various pharmaceuticals in each condition, every patient is an individual and the choice of medication should be tailored to their symptoms, tolerances, and preferences.

Pharmacological Treatment of Arthritic Disorders

Osteoarthritis is the most prevalent arthritic disorder worldwide and is characterized by chronic pain and impaired physical function. Although there is no cure for osteoarthritis, medications can be used to alleviate joint pain and swelling. Common pain medications generally include over-the-counter analgesic medications such as aspirin and acetaminophen. Nonsteroidal anti-inflammatory drugs (NSAIDs; see also Chapter 14) are often the first line of pharmacotherapy used to relieve pain and reduce inflammation. The major advantage of NSAIDs is that they are readily available and that over-the-counter NSAIDs are inexpensive.

Acetaminophen is in a drug category of its own. Acetaminophen is not classified as an *NSAID* because it does not possess anti-inflammatory activity. *However,* it is an analgesic that can alleviate mild arthritic pain. The American College of Rheumatology recommends acetaminophen as one of several treatment options for patients with hip, hand, or knee arthritis pain that does not improve with exercise and weight loss. It should be noted that while the analgesics aspirin and acetaminophen can be administered safely, both drugs can be toxic if they are used chronically or if administered at high doses.

If an arthritic disorder increases in severity, more potent NSAIDs, requiring a physician's prescription, can be used, including the nonselective COX-1/COX-2 inhibitors Diclofenac (Voltaren), Fenoprofen (Nalfon), Flurbiprofen (Ocufen) and Ketorolac (Toradol), as well as the COX-2 preferential inhibitors Celecoxib (Celebrex), Indomethacin (Indocin), Mefenamic acid (Ponstel) and Meloxicam (Mobic).

If arthritic disorder continues to progressively develop, corticosteroids, which are anti-inflammatory drugs that can be administered by mouth, injected, or applied as topical creams, can be included in the treatment regimen. Corticosteroids, such as prednisone, are only available by a physician's prescription. One reason for that is that injectable steroids provide temporary relief but can hasten the worsening of the condition and thus, the treatment has to be closely monitored by an expert. Additional drugs that are approved by the Federal Drug Administration (FDA) for the treatment of osteoarthritic pain include the anti-depressant duloxetine and the anti-seizure drug pregabalin.

Aspirin (Figure 9.2.1)

Figure 9.2.1

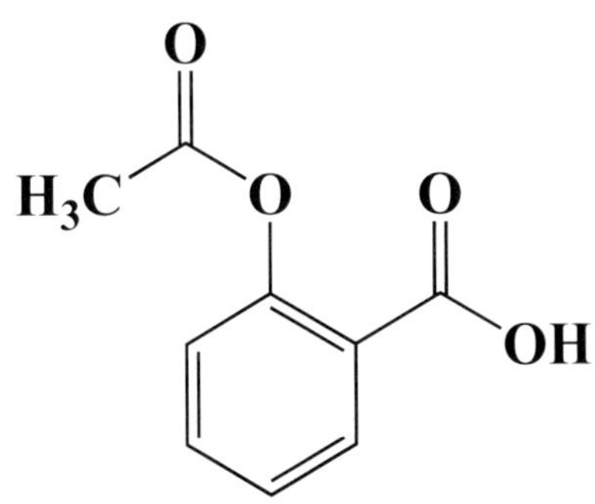

Acetylsalicylic acid

Aspirin (acetylsalicylic acid), is a common NSAID that can reduce the symptoms of inflammation and exhibits a broad range of pharmacologic activities, including analgesic and antipyretic properties. Aspirin and other NSAIDs do not generally change the course of arthritic disorders. They are primarily used for symptomatic relief. The inhibition of cyclooxygenase enzymes is the central mechanism of action of both aspirin and other NSAIDs. Mammalian cells contain two isozymes of cyclooxygenase: prostaglandin-endoperoxide H2 synthase-1 and -2 (COX-1 and COX-2, respectively). Prostaglandin H_2 (PGH_2) is a type of prostaglandin that is synthesized from arachidonic acid by COX-1 and COX-2. The enzymatic conversion of arachidonic acid to PGH_2 occurs by these two enzymes. Both enzymes are inhibited by aspirin and NSAIDs.

Aspirin was at one time the most common cause of accidental poisoning in children. Additionally, the administration of aspirin to children or teenagers recovering from the flu or chicken pox can cause swelling of the liver (*hepatomegaly*) and the brain (*Reye's syndrome*). The earliest symptoms of acute aspirin poisoning can include ringing in the ears (*tinnitus*) or impaired hearing. Additionally, symptoms of aspirin overdose can include rapid breathing (*hyperventilation*), vomiting, dehydration, fever, arrhythmias, alterations in mental status, hepatic injury, and double vision. Aspirin should not be used if the patient has a history of bleeding disorders such as hemophilia or a recent history of stomach or intestinal bleeding.

Acetaminophen (Figure 9.2.2)

Figure 9.2.2

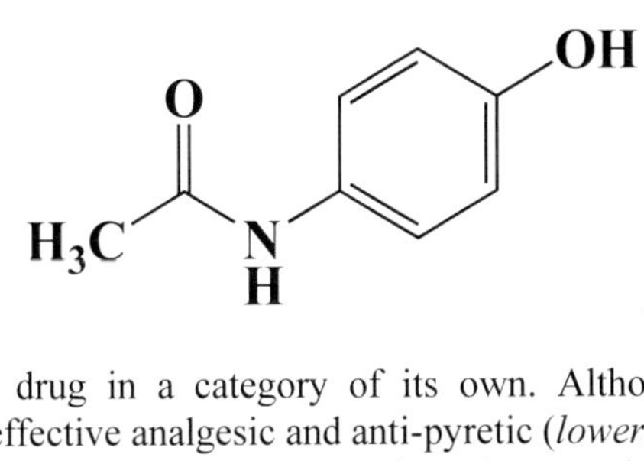

Acetaminophen (a.k.a. paracetamol)

Acetaminophen is a drug in a category of its own. Although it is not used to treat inflammatory symptoms, acetaminophen is an effective analgesic and anti-pyretic (*lowers fever*) agent as long as the recommended dosage is not exceeded. Acetaminophen overdose can cause hepatic necrosis, especially if administered with alcohol. If a high dose of acetaminophen (up to 4000 mg/day) is initiated, a patient should avoid taking any other medications that might contain acetaminophen, including over-the-counter cold remedies.

Current clinical guidelines recommend the use of acetaminophen for the treatment of mild-to-moderate symptoms of osteoarthritis. The precise analgesic *mechanism of action* of acetaminophen has not been fully elucidated. Comparisons of the treatment of osteoarthritis with acetaminophen with a variety of NSAIDs have been performed and generally, acetaminophen has greater efficacy than NSAIDs. Many of these short-term studies have reported little or no difference in safety between acetaminophen and NSAIDs.

Acetaminophen is found in numerous medicinal products and since it is an over-the-counter drug, patients can underestimate its potential for toxicity. Patients may accidentally develop clinically significant hepatic toxicity following repeated ingestions of supratherapeutic doses of acetaminophen in an attempt to relieve pain or to reduce fever. Repeated administration of acetaminophen at even slightly excessive doses can cause hepatic toxicity, especially in patients who abuse alcohol. This category of patients is most likely to present for medical care when the toxic effects of acetaminophen are already established. Acetaminophen overdose is a common cause of acute liver failure leading to approximately 20 percent of liver transplant cases in the USA.

Duloxetine (Figure 9.2.3) is a second-line agent for the treatment of osteoarthritis that does not respond to acetaminophen or NSAIDs. Duloxetine can also be used as an add-on medication for patients who have had a partial response to acetaminophen or NSAIDs. Duloxetine does not improve osteoarthritis but it does reduce pain.

Figure 9.2.3

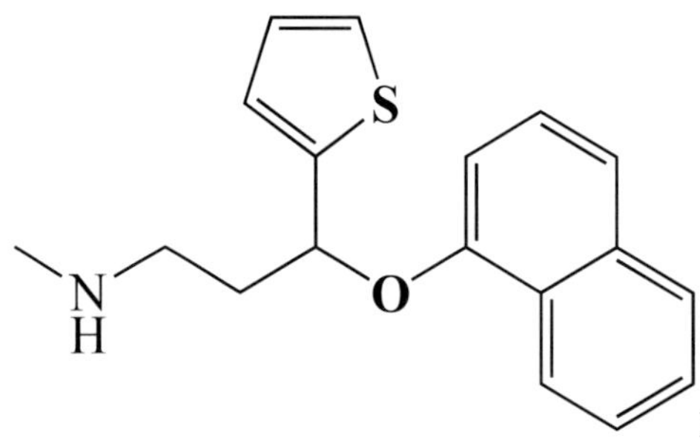

Duloxetine

In the initial stages of osteoarthritis, some patients report that pain worsens with joint use and improves with rest. In the later stages of the disease, patients may experience pain after minimal motion and pain at rest. Patients with high levels of pain may be experiencing centrally mediated pain processing. Changes in the central nervous system can lead to either an increase or a decrease in pain sensation. Neurological pathways involved with pain perception are thought to involve ascending nociceptive pathways that transmit a pain signal from the periphery to the brain. A pain signal is transmitted to central nerves in the spinal dorsal horn where peripheral nociceptors form synapses with neurons in the dorsal horn. Various neurotransmitters and neuromodulators, including substance P and glutamate, are involved in the amplification of the gating process for pain. Conversely, gamma aminobutyric acid (GABA), glycine, endocannabinoids, endorphins, monoamines, and neurosteroids are associated with the inhibition of pain signaling. Through ascending pathways, the pain signal is conducted until it reaches the brain.

If the patient does not have a satisfactory clinical response to the maximum dose of acetaminophen, oral or topical NSAIDs, intra-articular corticosteroid injections can be initiated. If these measures prove to be ineffective, duloxetine administration can be initiated in an attempt to diminish pain. Duloxetine is a serotonin/norepinephrine reuptake inhibitor that is thought to potentiate serotonin and norepinephrine activity in the CNS, resulting in an inhibition of the sensation of pain.

Common adverse side effects of duloxetine can include:

a) difficulty sleeping,
b) headaches,
c) vertigo (dizziness),
d) blurred vision,
e) constipation or diarrhea,
f) nausea or vomiting,
g) dry mouth and/or
h) sweating.

Pregabalin (Figure 9.2.4)

Figure 9.2.4

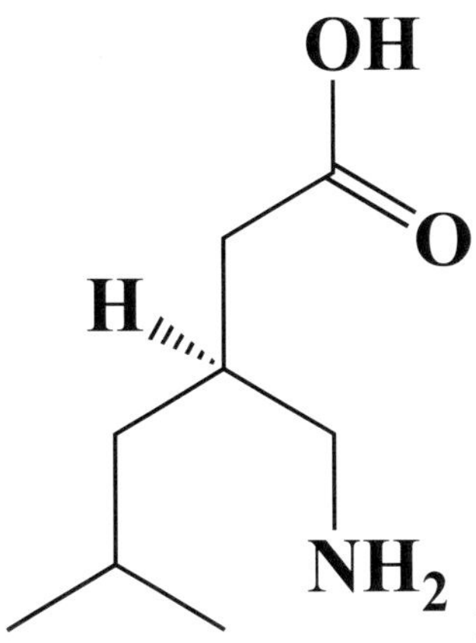

Pregabalin

Like duloxetine, pregabalin (Lyrica) is also used to treat severe hand pain associated with osteoarthritis. Pregabalin is also used to treat epilepsy, neuropathic pain (pain caused by stimuli that are normally not painful), and fibromyalgia. The calcium channel alpha$_2$-delta type-1 (α_2 δ -1) protein subunit in the neocortex, hippocampus, amygdala, and spinal cord appears to be the major therapeutic target for pregabalin. Pregabalin is thought to reduce abnormal pain-associated neuronal excitability by reducing the release of a variety of neurotransmitters, including substance P, noradrenalin, acetylcholine, glutamate, and/or glycine. Pregabalin is also thought to reduce the antiallodynic effects (*where the pain is caused by a stimulus that does not normally elicit pain*) by reducing membrane expression of the $\alpha_2\delta$-1 protein. Pregabalin impairs the normal trafficking of $\alpha_2\delta$-1 protein, resulting in a decrease in $\alpha_2\delta$-1 protein expression in presynaptic terminals. Consequently, reduced expression of $\alpha_2\delta$-1 protein results in reduced neurotransmitter release leading to a reduction of pain sensation.

Common side effects of pregabalin include:

a) headache or dizziness,
b) sleepiness,
c) confusion,
d) trouble with memory,
e) poor coordination,
f) dry mouth,
g) vision problems,
h) weight gain.

Nonsteroidal Anti-inflammatory Drugs (NSAIDs)

Although over-the-counter NSAIDs such as ibuprofen and naproxen sodium can be initially used to alleviate pain and reduce inflammation, if required, stronger NSAIDs (obtained only by prescription) can be used. These NSAIDs, including Celecoxib (Celebrex), Diclofenac (Voltaren), Fenoprofen (Nalfon), Flurbiprofen (Ocufen), Indomethacin (Indocin), Ketorolac (Toradol), Mefenamic acid (Ponstel) or Meloxicam (Mobic), can be prescribed if the arthritic symptoms worsen. However, these drugs can have adverse side effects including, stomach irritation, heart problems, and/or kidney damage. In general, NSAIDs are contraindicated if the patient a) consumes more than three alcoholic drinks per day, b) takes anticoagulants, c) has ulcers, d) has a liver disorder, d) has kidney disease, or e) has coronary illnesses.

Ibuprofen (Figure 9.2.5)

Ibuprofen (Addaprin, Advil, Dyspel, Genpril, I-Prin, KS Ibuprofen, Motrin, TH Ibuprofen) is an NSAID that is widely used in the management of inflammatory, musculoskeletal, and rheumatic disorders because it is highly effective and has minimal toxicities. Ibuprofen's mechanism of action is the nonselective inhibition of cyclooxygenase enzymes COX-1 and COX-2. Ibuprofen is administered as a racemic mixture; however, the S-enantiomer is believed to be the pharmacologically active enantiomer. Following oral administration, the peak serum concentration of ibuprofen is achieved within 1–2 hours. The majority of ibuprofen is metabolized and eliminated within 24 hours.

Figure 9.2.5

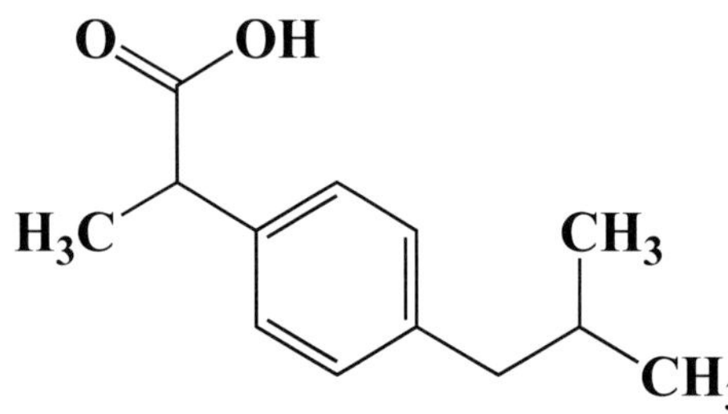

Ibuprofen

Ibuprofen can be administered orally or by intravenous injection. Ibuprofen is suitable for self-medication because of its wide spectrum of indications and good safety profile. Ibuprofen should not be taken with low-dose aspirin because it could interfere with aspirin's ability to prevent heart attacks. Drinking alcohol with ibuprofen may increase the risk of gastrointestinal bleeding.

Adverse side effects of ibuprofen can include:

a) abdominal cramps,
b) diarrhea,
c) dizziness,
e) drowsiness,
f) gastrointestinal bleeding,
g) headache,
h) heartburn,
i) high blood pressure,
j) nausea or vomiting,
k) peptic ulcer,
l) swelling of feet,
m) skin rash and/or
n) tinnitus (ringing in the ears).

Naproxen (Figure 9.2.6)

Figure 9.2.6

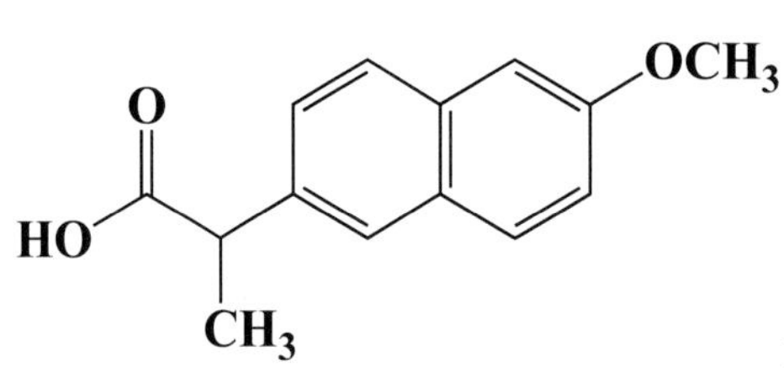

Naproxen

Naproxen (Aleve) is another NSAID that can be used to reduce joint pain and inflammation in patients with rheumatoid arthritis and osteoarthritis. As with ibuprofen, **Naproxen** inhibits the COX-1 and COX-2 enzymes, leading to the inhibition of prostaglandin synthesis. As with ibuprofen, using naproxen with low-dose aspirin may interfere with aspirin's ability to prevent heart attacks. Naproxen is often administered orally as an extended-release tablet formulation which is a slow-acting form of the drug for treating chronic arthritic conditions. Naproxen can also cause stomach or intestinal bleeding, especially in older adults.

Since ibuprofen is a short-acting NSAID with a rapid onset, it is better suited than naproxen for treating acute pain. Ibuprofen is administered every four or six hours, while naproxen is a long-acting NSAID with a slower therapeutic onset but it is better suited for the treatment of chronic arthritic conditions.

Common adverse side effects of naproxen may include:

a) indigestion,
b) heartburn,
c) stomach pain,
d) nausea,
e) headache,
f) dizziness,
g) drowsiness,
h) bruising,
i) itching or rash,
j) swelling and/or
k) tinnitus.

Corticosteroids

Corticosteroid treatment includes the use of prednisone, hydrocortisone (Figure 9.2.7), prednisolone (Figure 9.2.8), dexamethasone (Figure 9.2.9), methylprednisolone, triamcinolone or betamethasone. Prednisone is a commonly used steroid for the treatment of rheumatoid arthritis. The actions of glucocorticoids are predominantly mediated through the intracellular glucocorticoid receptor, which is a member of the nuclear receptor family of ligand-activated transcription factors.

Figure 9.2.7

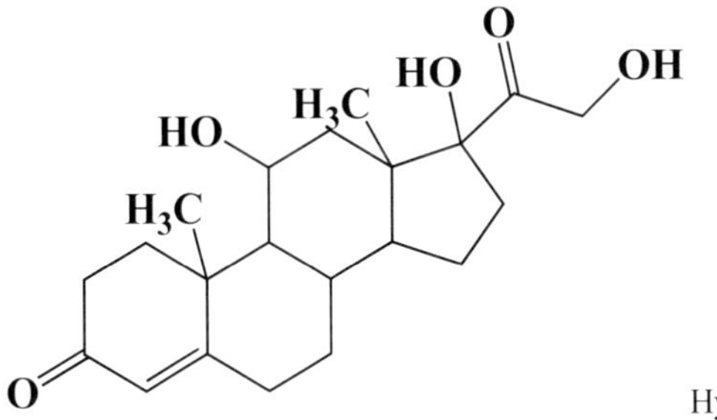

Hydrocortisone

Figure 9.2.8

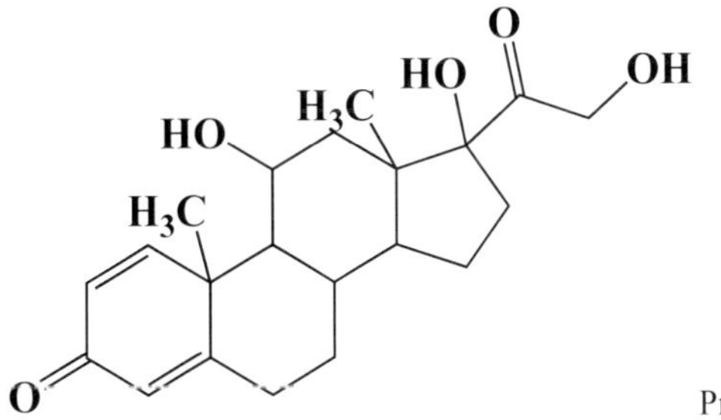

Prednisolone

Figure 9.2.9

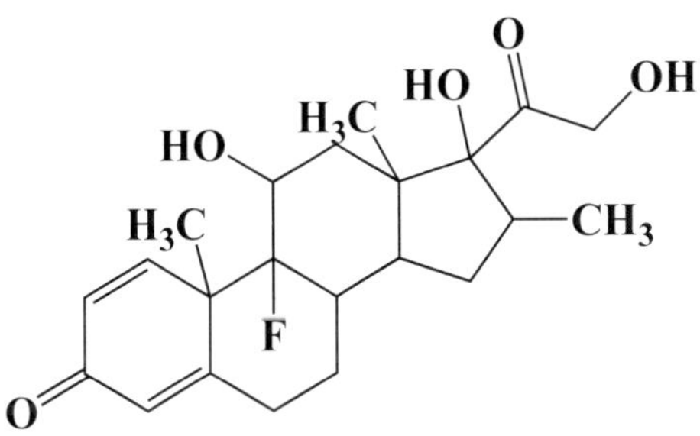

Dexamethasone

Corticosteroids are used in arthritis for two reasons. First, these drugs are anti-inflammatory drugs that can mitigate the damage caused by the inflammation in rheumatoid arthritis and systemic lupus erythematosus when the patient does not respond to NSAIDs or if an NSAID produces adverse side effects. Second, corticosteroids are immunosuppressive and decrease the adverse effects of autoimmunity.

However, the adverse side effects associated with corticosteroid administration can be problematic. These adverse side effects can include thinning of bones, weight gain, and the development of diabetes. Corticosteroids are often prescribed initially to relieve acute symptoms to gradually reduce the dose and eventually terminate the medication. This strategy is often called a "burst-and-taper" therapeutic strategy. Patients can often tolerate a high dose of corticosteroid for less than 5 days and then either stop the drug or return to a low dose of the steroid without a dose taper. Although corticosteroid treatment can be of benefit to patients with rheumatoid arthritis, it can also lead to long-term side effects, such as skin thinning, easy skin bruising, weight gain, progression to diabetes, and/or bone loss that can lead to osteoporosis. Therefore, the risks of using corticosteroids must be balanced with the benefits when prescribing or continuing corticosteroid administration for treating rheumatoid arthritis.

The adverse side effect associated with corticosteroid administration for more than a few weeks include:

a) mild arm or leg muscle weakness,
b) blurred vision,
c) thinning or excessive hair growth
d) increased bruising,
e) slow healing of cuts and wounds,
f) elevated levels of WBC/neutrophils,
g) acne,
h) round face (corticosteroid-induced lipodystrophy/moon face),
i) slowed growth in children and adolescents and
j) osteoporosis (loss of bone calcium) especially in women.

Disease-Modifying Anti-Rheumatic Drugs (DMARDs).

Clinical studies indicate that the remission of symptoms of rheumatoid arthritis may occur if a patient is treated early in the course of their disease with disease-modifying anti-rheumatic drugs (DMARDs). DMARDs are immunosuppressive agents. The American College of Rheumatology divides DMARDs into conventional (e.g., hydroxychloroquine, sulfasalazine, leflunomide, methotrexate) and biological that target specific immune pathways (e.g., adalimumab, infliximab, etanercept, rituximab, abatacept, tocilizumab, tofacitinib). Biologic DMARDs are prescribed if treatments with conventional DMARDs have failed. DMARDs can slow the progression of rheumatoid arthritis and prevent permanent damage to the joints and other tissues. In general, these drugs attenuate components of the immune response to slow the progression of inflammatory arthritic disorders.

Hydroxychloroquine (Schrezenmeier and Dorner 2020) **(Figure 9.2.10) and sulfasalazine** (Kerschbaumer et al. 2023) **(Figure 9.2.11)** are used for milder cases of rheumatoid arthritis, psoriatic arthritis or juvenile idiopathic arthritis. These two drugs are generally well tolerated. Hydroxychloroquine is used to treat moderate inflammation, swelling, stiffness and to relieve joint pain. It has been proposed that the anti-rheumatic properties of hydroxychloroquine result from the ability to interfere with antigen processing by macrophages. Patients taking hydroxychloroquine should be examined yearly by an ophthalmologist to avoid potential ocular problems. While short-term hydroxychloroquine treatment does not appear to increase the risk of major adverse side effects in patients with rheumatoid arthritis, long-term use of hydroxychloroquine may be associated with increased cardiovascular mortality. Both the European League Against Rheumatism and the American College of Rheumatology identify hydroxychloroquine as the first line medical treatment for SLE.[19]

Sulfasalazine is used for the treatment of rheumatoid arthritis, juvenile arthritis, psoriatic arthritis, ankylosing spondylitis, and ulcerative colitis. (Kerschbaumer et al. 2023) Sulfasalazine is most effective for treating mild to moderate arthritic symptoms. Sulfasalazine helps reduce joint pain, swelling, and stiffness associated with arthritis. Sulfasalazine also may prevent joint damage and decrease the risk of reduced joint function.

Figure 9.2.10

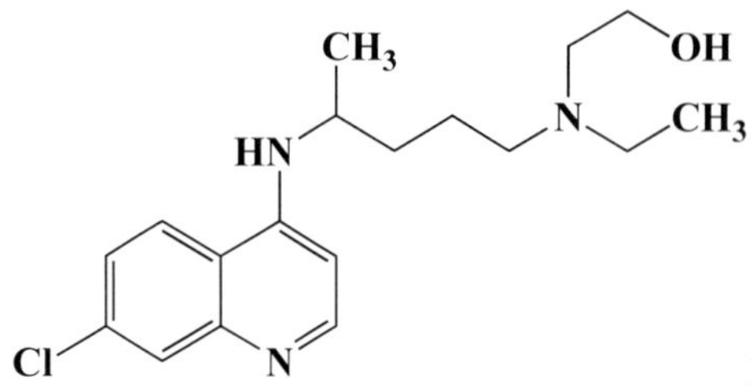

Hydroxychloroquine

Figure 9.2.11

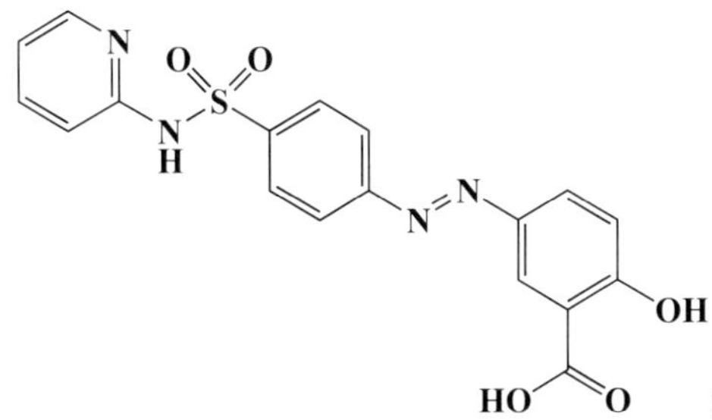

Sulfasalazine

Sulfasalazine is most effective for treating mild to moderate symptoms. (Kerschbaumer et al. 2023) Typically, patients who respond to sulfasalazine notice improvement within 12 weeks. Sulfasalazine is a sulfa drug that tends to have a slow onset of action when compared to corticosteroids. The exact mechanism of action of sulfasalazine has not been fully elucidated. Furthermore, it is not known whether sulfasalazine or its metabolites, sulfapyridine and 5-aminosalicylic acid, are responsible for anti-inflammatory effects. The most common side effect associated with sulfasalazine is headaches. Additional side effects can include indigestion, nausea, diarrhea, rash, itchiness, and fever. It may also cause a metallic taste in the mouth.

Leflunomide (Figure 9.2.12) is an immunosuppressive anti-rheumatic drug approved to treat adult moderate to severe rheumatoid arthritis and psoriatic arthritis. Leflunomide is an immunomodulatory drug that selectively inhibits the mitochondrial enzyme dihydroorotate dehydrogenase, which plays a key role in the synthesis of the pyrimidine ribonucleotide uridine monophosphate, which is essential for rapidly proliferating cells such as those associated with the immune response. Suppression of the immune system leads to a reduction of inflammation, joint swelling, and joint damage associated with rheumatoid arthritis. Importantly, leflunomide is teratogenic (*causes fetal malformations*) and is not used if a patient is pregnant or is anticipating a pregnancy.

Figure 9.2.12

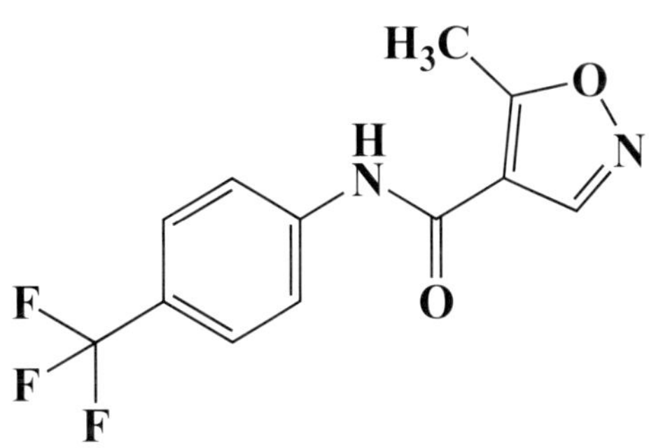

Leflunomide

Leflunomide and methotrexate are both efficacious for the treatment of rheumatoid arthritis and may be additively efficacious if administered in combination.

The side effects associated with leflunomide include:

a) diarrhea, abdominal pain, and indigestion,
b) cough and respiratory tract infections,
c) hair loss,
d) high blood pressure,
e) rash,
f) nausea,
g) bronchitis, chest pain,
h) headache,
i) back pain,
j) indigestion,
k) vertigo,
l) loss of appetite and weight loss,
m) vomiting,
n) weakness,
o) chest pain,
p) dry skin, eczema,
q) paresthesia (*abnormal skin sensation*),
r) rhinitis (inflammation and swelling of the mucous membrane of the nose,
s) cholelithiasis (*gallstone formation*) and/or
t) shortness of breath.

Methotrexate (Figure 9.2.13) is a cancer chemotherapeutic and immunosuppressive drug that is used for the treatment of inflammatory forms of arthritis. It not only reduces pain and swelling, but it may also slow joint damage and disease progression. Methotrexate can be used as a first-line therapy for patients with rheumatoid arthritis, psoriatic arthritis, or juvenile idiopathic arthritis. Methotrexate can also be used in combination with other DMARDs, including leflunomide, sulfasalazine, or hydroxychloroquine. A common drug combination is the use of methotrexate with tumor necrosis factor (TNF) inhibitors such as etanercept, adalimumab, infliximab, or certolizumab pegol. Methotrexate combines effectively with other biologics, such as abatacept, rituximab, or tocilizumab.

Figure 9.2.13

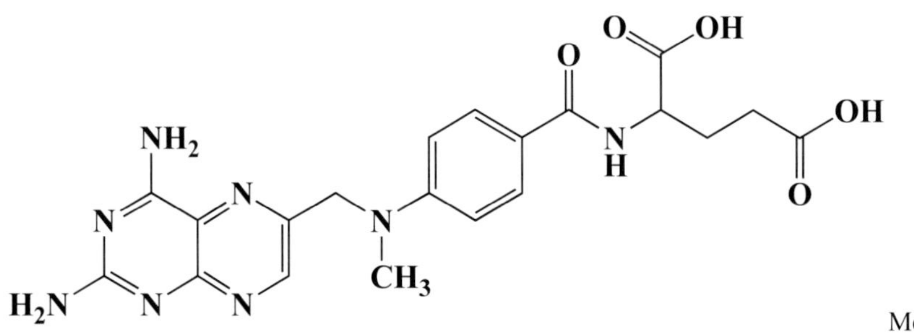

Methotrexate

Methotrexate was originally designed as an antagonist of the folate synthetic pathway for treating patients with leukemia by inhibiting the enzyme dihydrofolate reductase. However, much lower doses (15–25 mg/week) of methotrexate are used to treat patients with rheumatoid arthritis. This low-dose clinical efficacy of methotrexate is unaffected by the administration of folic acid, indicating that the mechanism of action of methotrexate is different for patients being treated for cancer compared to arthritis. At the dose used to treat arthritis methotrexate reduces the level of both purines and pyrimidines in primary human T-cells and increases adenosine levels. These effects inhibit T cell function, suppress adhesion molecules expressed by T cells and inhibit the binding of IL-1β to its receptors. At these doses, there is also an overexpression of adenosine receptors in the immune cells of patients with rheumatoid arthritis. The clinical effects of methotrexate treatment in patients with rheumatoid arthritis may be due to enhanced signaling through the A2A adenosine G-protein coupled receptor, which binds adenosine with high affinity, leading to immune suppression. A major advantage of using methotrexate for the treatment of arthritic conditions is that it is safe when taken for long periods and can be used in children.

The side effects associated with the doses of methotrexate to treat arthritic disorders include:

a) GI problems including nausea and vomiting,
b) mouth ulcers or sores,
c) headaches,
d) fatigue,
e) a general sense of malaise,
f) rashes,
g) dyspepsia (*stomach upset*),
h) hepatic dysfunction and/or
i) myelosuppression.

Apremilast (Figure 9.2.14)

Figure 9.2.14

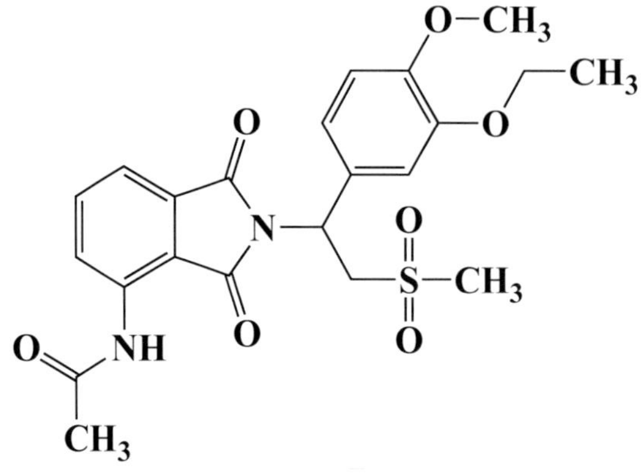

Apremilast

Apremilast is used to treat psoriatic arthritis and severe plaque psoriasis. Apremilast is a small molecular weight drug that specifically inhibits intracellular phosphodiesterase-4 (PDE4), which is a member of the class of phosphodiesterases that hydrolyze the intracellular second messenger, cyclic adenosine monophosphate (cAMP). Apremilast has been shown to alter the activity of inflammatory mediators involved in psoriasis arthritis and is thought to increase levels of the anti-inflammatory cytokine IL10 and decrease TNF-α production by human synovial cells *in vitro*. Apremilast has been found to have a favorable safety profile and efficacy.

Common side effects associated with apremilast can include:

a) nausea, vomiting, and diarrhea,
b) upper respiratory tract infection,
c) abdominal pain,
d) fatigue,
e) indigestion, heartburn,
f) decreased appetite and weight loss,
g) insomnia,
h) back pain,
i) depression,
j) inflammation of the airways in the lungs (*bronchitis*) and
k) sinus headache.

Azathioprine (Figure 9.2.15)

Figure 9.2.15

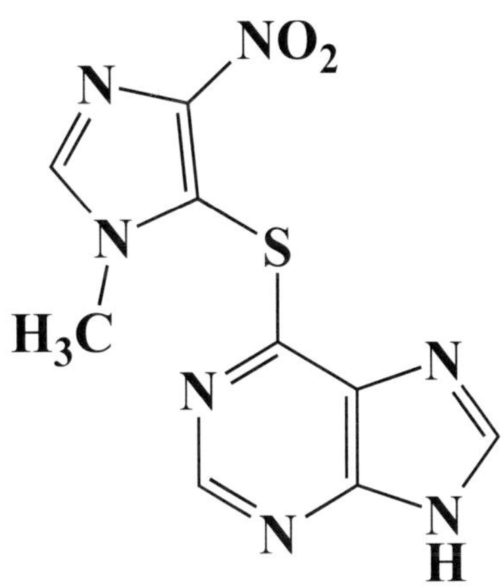

Azathioprine

Azathioprine is metabolized to 6-mercaptopurine and then enzymatically converted to 6-thiouric acid, 6-methyl-MP, and 6-thioguanine. Ultimately, these metabolites block the pathway for purine synthesis. Azathioprine is thought to specificity inhibit DNA and RNA formation in lymphocytes because these cells lack a salvage pathway. By inhibiting purine synthesis, the rate of replication of immune cells is decreased, thus leading to immunosuppression. It has also been proposed that the 6-thioguanine metabolite may inhibit CD28-mediated signaling in T-cells.

Azathioprine is used for the treatment of both systemic lupus erythematosus and rheumatoid arthritis. Azathioprine should not be administered if the patient is pregnant.

Adverse side effects of azathioprine include:

a) stomach irritation/abdominal pain,
b) nausea or vomiting,
c) changes in hair color/texture, hair loss,
d) loss of appetite,
e) blood in the urine or stool,
f) bruising,
g) fatigue or
h) mouth sores and ulcers.

Biological Response Modifiers

Biologic Response Modifiers (BRM) are disease-modifying anti-rheumatic drugs that include monoclonal antibodies and recombinant proteins. They also include the synthetic compounds baricitinib and tofacitinib that inhibit the Janus Kinase-Signal Transducer and Activator of Transcription Pathway (JAK-STAT pathway). In general, BRMs target portions of the immune system that causes inflammation and joint damage. As with other anti-arthritic drugs they are not capable of curing the arthritic disorder, but they are used to slow the progression of the disease and/or help put it into remission.

Tofacitinib (Figure 9.2.16)

Tofacitinib is a small molecular weight BRM that selectively inhibits two JAK enzymes of the Janus Kinase-Signal Transducer and Activator of Transcription Pathway (JAK-STAT pathway), which is a principal signaling cascade for the production of cytokines and growth factors. The two JAK kinases that are primarily affected by the binding of tofacitinib are JAK1 and JAK3.

Figure 9.2.16

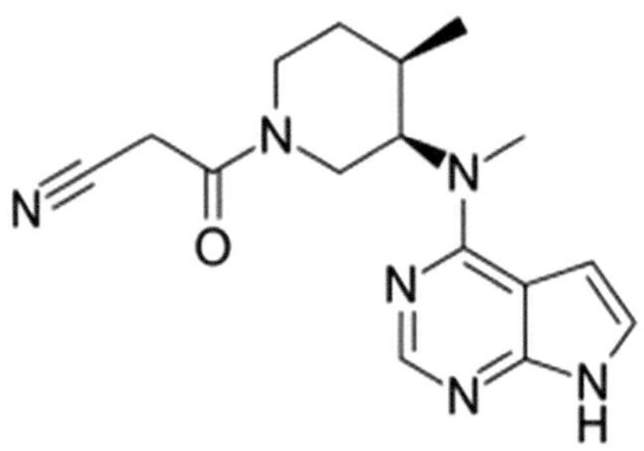

Tofacitinib

The JAK-STAT system consists of three components; (1) the cell membrane-associated type I and II cytokine receptors, (2) the Janus kinases which phosphorylate the receptors; and (3) the Signal Transducer and Activator of Transcription (STAT) complex which enters the cell nucleus and regulates the transcription of target genes. After the cytokine binds to the gamma-interferon gamma receptor (IFNγR) and the interleukin-10 receptor (IL-10R), the JAK enzymes phosphorylate the receptor. These phosphorylated STAT proteins then form a dimer that translocates into the cell nucleus. This protein dimer binds to DNA and initiates gene transcription.

JAK activation stimulates cell proliferation, cell differentiation, and cell migration (which are critical to the development of an immune response). JAK activation is also involved in the development of the mammary gland, adipogenesis (formation of fat cells), and sexual dimorphism (where the two sexes of the same species exhibit different characteristics beyond the differences in their sexual organs). The Janus kinase (JAK)-signal transducers and activators of transcription (STAT) also play an important role in the coordination of cytokine receptor signaling. The JAK-STAT signaling pathway has been implicated in the pathogenesis of inflammatory and autoimmune diseases, including rheumatoid arthritis, psoriasis, and inflammatory bowel disease. Mutations in JAK and STAT genes have been found to cause immunodeficiency syndromes and autoimmunity.

The dysregulation of the JAK-STAT pathway in T helper cells is thought to be responsible for various types of autoimmune disorders. While tofacitinib administration increases B-cell count, it does not change the serum levels of IgG, IgM, or IgA immunoglobulins. In addition, although tofacitinib does not change the total T-cell count, long-term use of tofacitinib decreases the number of CD4- and CD8-positive T-cells.

Tofacitinib has been approved for use in the treatment of patients with moderate to severe active rheumatoid arthritis. Tofacitinib is also approved for the treatment of patients with rheumatoid arthritis who do not respond to other DMARD(s). Tofacitinib is recommended for use either alone or in combination with methotrexate.

The most common adverse reactions associated with tofacitinib during the first three months of treatment include:

a) headache,
b) nausea,
c) diarrhea,
d) upper respiratory tract infections and/or
e) nasopharyngitis (cold symptoms associated with the swelling of the nasal passages and the back of the throat).

Baricitinib (Figure 9.2.17)

Baricitinib is a synthetic BRM that is used for the treatment of adults with moderate to severe rheumatoid arthritis. In an analogous manner to tofacitinib, the mechanism of action of baricitinib is to inhibit enzymes associated with the Janus Kinase pathway. This drug can be administered alone or in combination with methotrexate in patients who responded inadequately to or are intolerant of other DMARDs. A once-daily administration of baricitinib, with/without methotrexate, can improve the symptoms of rheumatoid arthritis patients who are DMARD-naive or who have had an inadequate response to methotrexate or other DMARDs. Baricitinib plus methotrexate is more effective than the adalimumab plus methotrexate drug combination in patients with an inadequate response to methotrexate alone. The onset of these beneficial effects is rapid and once-daily treatment with baricitinib alone or in combination with methotrexate is generally well tolerated.

Figure 9.2.17

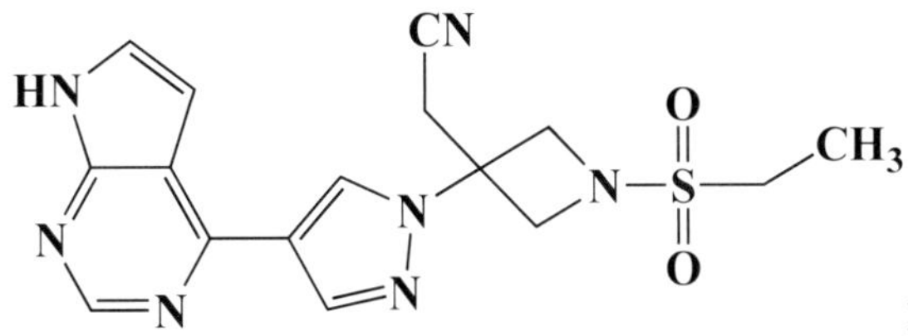

Baricitinib

The most commonly reported adverse drug reactions include:

a) upper respiratory tract infections,
b) increased LDL cholesterol,
c) nausea and/or
d) thrombocytosis (excessive number of platelets in the blood).

Abatacept

Abatacept is used for the treatment of moderate to severe rheumatoid arthritis after previous DMARD treatments have failed to alleviate symptoms. Abatacept can also be used as a first-line therapy for the treatment of psoriatic arthritis and juvenile idiopathic arthritis. Abatacept may be used alone or in combination with other DMARDs.

Abatacept is a fusion protein composed of the Fc region of an IgG1 immunoglobulin protein juxtaposed to the extracellular domain of the cytotoxic T-lymphocyte-associated protein 4 (CTLA-4). CTLA-4 functions as an immune checkpoint protein that can downregulate an immune response. Checkpoint protein-associated pathways play an important role in the development and maintenance of self-tolerance. For a T-cell response to be activated an antigen-presenting cell must initiate two signals to a T-cell. One signal involves the interaction of the major histocompatibility complex (MHC) with an antigen and the second signal involves the activation of CD80/CD86 proteins expressed on B-cells, which operate in tandem to prime CD4+ T-cell to respond to an antigen. After treatment of rheumatoid arthritis patients with abatacept, there is an internalization of the CD80/CD86 proteins. Abatacept is thought to bind to the CD80/CD86 proteins and prevent the second signal that is required for CD4+ T cell activation. Patients with rheumatoid arthritis who are treated with abatacept have a progressive decrease in immature B-cells that can internalize an antigen and present it to T-cells. Thus, abatacept acts by binding to CD80/CD86 proteins expressed by B-cells, resulting in a reduction of the expression of CD80/CD86 protein, which impairs CD4+ T-cell activation.

Abatacept is administered as a 30-minute intravenous infusion. Following the initial administration abatacept is administered 2 and 4 weeks after the first infusion. Alternatively, abatacept can be administered weekly by subcutaneous injection without the need for an intravenous (IV) loading dose. Concurrent therapy with abatacept and a tumor necrosis factor antagonist is not recommended.

Adverse side effects of Abatacept can include:

a) lung infections in patients with chronic obstructive pulmonary disease (COPD),
b) acceleration of the growth and metastasis of slow-growing cancers,
c) increase the risk of lower respiratory tract, urinary, or herpes infections,
d) high blood pressure,
e) nausea, upset stomach, diarrhea, vomiting,
f) fatigue,
g) increased risk of pneumonia or flu,
h) cough,
i) mouth sores and/or
j) elevated transaminases indicating possible liver damage.

Anakinra

Interleukin-1α (IL-1α) and interleukin-1β (IL-1β) are proinflammatory cytokines that are thought to play a role in the pathophysiology of rheumatoid arthritis. IL-1-mediated inflammation has been found in numerous inflammatory disorders including rheumatoid arthritis, type 2 diabetes, atherosclerosis, and acute myocardial infarction. In addition, there is a naturally occurring interleukin-1 receptor antagonist (IL-1αR) protein that can competitively block the binding of cytokines IL-1α and IL-1β to interleukin receptors. IL-1αR has been shown to inhibit the effects of IL-1 to reduce the severity of inflammatory disorders.

Anakinra is a modified recombinant protein that blocks the binding of IL-1α and IL-1β to the interleukin receptors without eliciting a receptor-mediated response. Therefore, it acts as an interleukin receptor antagonist. The amino acid sequence of anakinra differs from the sequence of the human IL-1αR protein antagonist by the addition of one methionine located at the N-terminus. It also differs from the human protein in that it is not glycosylated, because it is produced in *E. coli* bacterial cells and recombinant proteins made in bacterial cells are not glycosylated. Since anakinra is capable of blocking the binding and the function of IL-1α and IL-1β receptors, anakinra has been used to attenuate a variety of interleukin-1-related autoimmune inflammatory disorders.

Anakinra is administered by subcutaneous injection and can be used alone or in combination with other medications. Subcutaneous injection of 100 mg of anakinra can provide clinical benefits within days and anakinra has been used daily in patients for over 12 years, demonstrating a record of safety. Anakinra is used primarily to reduce the pain and swelling associated with rheumatoid arthritis. Although immunosuppression can lead to the reactivation of opportunistic infections, the reactivation of *Mycobacterium tuberculosis* infections is rare in patient populations at risk.

Adverse side effects of anakinra can include:

a) worsening of rheumatoid arthritis symptoms,
b) nausea, vomiting, diarrhea, stomach pain,
c) headaches,
d) joint pain,
e) flu-like symptoms such as stuffy nose, sneezing, sore throat, and/or
f) redness, bruising, pain, or swelling at the injection site.

Tumor Necrosis Factor (TNF) Inhibitors

Tumor necrosis factor (**TNF**) is a cytokine that is produced by activated macrophages, helper T-cells cells, natural killer cells, neutrophils, mast cells, eosinophils, and neurons. TNF binds to two receptors, TNFR1 and TNFR2. Dysregulation of TNF production has been implicated in the development of Alzheimer's disease, cancer, psoriasis, and inflammatory bowel disease. Although anti-TNF therapy has only modest effects as a cancer chemotherapeutic agent, TNF inhibitors are used for the treatment of arthritic disorders.

The most significant side effect is an increased risk for all types of infections, including tuberculosis (TB) and fungal infections. Some of these infections can be severe. Patients should be tested for TB before starting therapy because TB infections can worsen during treatment. Other side effects associated with TNF inhibitors include the occurrence of rare white blood cell cancers, an increased risk of bacterial, fungal, viral, and mycobacterial parasitic opportunistic infections, as well as the initiation or exacerbation of multiple sclerosis-like disorders. Long-term use of TNF inhibitors may increase the risk of lymphomas and skin cancer. People with significant heart failure should not use a TNF inhibitor, because their heart disease could worsen.

Etanercept

Etanercept is a 159 kDa fusion protein used to treat autoimmune disorders. Etanercept binds TNF-α and inhibits its binding to the TNF-α receptor. Etanercept contains amino acid sequences for both the TNF-α receptor and the constant region of an IgG1 antibody. TNF-α is a cytokine produced primarily by macrophages. TNF-α acts by attracting white blood cells to the sites of inflammation; therefore the competitive inhibition of TNF-α by etanercept reduces an autoinflammatory response.

Etanercept is used in adults to prevent joint damage caused by rheumatoid arthritis, psoriatic arthritis, or ankylosing spondylitis (*also known as Bechterew's disease*), which is a rare long-term arthritic condition that results in pain and stiffness of the spine. Etanercept is also used to treat plaque psoriasis in adults.

Some of the common side effects associated with the administration of etanercept include:

a) runny nose and/or sore throat,
b) nausea and/or vomiting,
c) a mild fever,

d) headaches,
e) dizziness,
f) rash and/or
g) stomach pain.

Humanized Monoclonal Antibodies

The term antibody (*Antikörper in German*) was first used in the late 1800s to describe substances found in the serum that could neutralize a pathogen or toxin. The study of how antibodies are formed, how they bind antigens, their amino acid, their three-dimensional structure, and the genetic mechanisms that give rise to antibody formation has been a central focus for the field of immunology. Antibodies are glycoproteins belonging to the immunoglobulin superfamily. The terms antibody and immunoglobulin are commonly used interchangeably.

The mammalian antibody protein response is elicited in response to immunization and is composed of five fundamental antibody classes IgA, IgD, IgE, IgG, and IgM. In addition, the antibody response is described as being heterogeneous. That is, the antibody response is comprised of a variety of antibody proteins with a different amino acid sequence, where each antibody can bind a single antigen with a different affinity. This phenomenon is referred to as antibody diversity. One of the long-term goals of molecular immunology research has been to use antibodies to treat human immunological abnormalities, arthritic disorders, cancer, or pathological infections.

The term monoclonal antibody (mAb) refers to a single unique antibody obtained by the cloning of a single plasma B cell which secrets multiple antibody molecules that all have the same amino acid sequence and bind to the antigenic determinant with the same affinity. The ability to produce monoclonal antibodies has become an important research tool in biochemistry and an important technique for developing therapeutics.

A humanized monoclonal antibody is originally obtained from non-human species (generally a mouse or rat) but whose amino acid sequence has been modified to increase its similarity to a human antibody. This humanization process is performed because it minimizes the potential immunogenicity of a monoclonal antibody if it is to be administered to a human patient. The names of therapeutic antibodies generally end in the suffices *zumab* (as in the humanized antibody certolizumab), *imab* (as in the chimeric antibody infliximab), or *umab* (as in the human monoclonal adalimumab), which are used clinically for the treatment of rheumatoid arthritis and psoriatic arthritis. Humanized antibodies are distinct from chimeric antibodies, where the protein sequence of a chimeric antibody retains stretches of amino acids not found in humans. Antibody-based therapies are routinely administered by injection.

Common adverse side effects of humanized monoclonal antibodies can include:

a) pain, swelling, soreness, redness, itchiness, and/or rash at the injection site,
b) flu-like symptoms such as chills, fatigue, fever, muscle aches and pains, vomiting, and/or diarrhea, and
c) cytokine release or "cytokine storm" syndrome can sometimes occur following monoclonal antibody administration. Symptoms of cytokine storm can include intense flu-like symptoms such as nausea, headache, rapid heartbeat, low blood pressure, or trouble breathing.

Adalimumab

Adalimumab is a human monoclonal antibody used to treat rheumatoid arthritis, psoriatic arthritis, psoriasis, or juvenile idiopathic arthritis. Adalimumab acts by binding to the TNF-α protein, which is primarily produced by activated macrophages, but also by T helper cells, natural killer cells, neutrophils, mast cells, eosinophils, mast cells, and neurons. TNF-α is an endogenous pyrogen. In addition to arthritic conditions, dysregulation of TNF-α production has been implicated in Alzheimer's disease, asthma, tumor growth, graft versus host reactions, and inflammatory bowel disorders.

Adalimumab has been used alone or in concert with other DMARDs for the treatment of arthritic disorders and it is also used for patients who have not responded to other treatments.

Adalimumab is used for the treatment of rheumatoid arthritis, either alone, or with methotrexate. Adalimumab is administered by subcutaneous injection. Using adalimumab injection may increase the risk that the patient may experience a severe fungal, bacterial, or viral infection.

Common side effects of adalimumab can include:

1) upper respiratory tract infections,
2) pain at the injection site,
3) rash or
4) headache.

Infliximab

Infliximab is a chimeric monoclonal antibody used for the treatment of rheumatoid arthritis, psoriasis, and psoriatic arthritis. Infliximab was originally developed as a mouse monoclonal antibody, where several of the mouse immunoglobulin domains were substituted with human antibody domains. Infliximab binds and neutralizes TNF-α.

Adverse side effects of infliximab can include:

a) infections,
b) reactivation of hepatitis B or tuberculosis,
c) drug-induced lupus,
d) vertigo and
e) allergic reactions including swelling of the lips, difficulty breathing and low blood pressure.

Certolizumab pegol

Certolizumab pegol is a PEGylated Fab fragment of a humanized monoclonal antibody that binds TNF-α. PEGylation is the attachment of polyethylene glycol polymers to a drug or therapeutic protein to diminish immunogenicity and reduce renal clearance. PEGylation can also increase water solubility. Certolizumab pegol can bind TNF in both its soluble form and when it is bound to the cell membrane. Consequently, incubation of monocytes with certolizumab pegol results in the inhibition of LPS-induced TNFα and IL-1ß production in human monocytes.

Golimumab

Golimumab is a human monoclonal antibody that binds protein TNFα, resulting in a reduction in the expression of C-reactive protein (CRP) levels, IL-6, intercellular adhesion molecules (ICAM)-1, matrix metalloproteinase (MMP-3) and vascular endothelial growth factor (VEGF). Golimumab is capable of binding both the soluble and transmembrane forms of TNFα.

Golimumab has been approved for the treatment of rheumatoid arthritis, psoriatic arthritis, and ulcerative colitis. Golimumab can be self-administered once monthly by subcutaneous injection or intravenous injection. Treatment with golimumab is not recommended for patients with rheumatoid arthritis who have failed to find symptom relief with prior treatment BRMs that target TNF.

Rituximab

Rituximab is a chimeric monoclonal antibody that binds protein CD20 expressed on the plasma membrane of B cells. Rituximab has been used in combination with methotrexate to treat moderate to severe rheumatoid arthritis when an inadequate response to one or more TNF antagonist therapies has been obtained.

In addition to rheumatoid arthritis, rituximab has also been used to treat non-Hodgkin lymphoma and chronic lymphocytic leukemia.

In 2020 a three-dimensional cryogenic electron microscopy (cryo-EM) characterization of CD20 complexed with rituximab showed that CD20 was a compact double-barrel-shaped protein dimer that interacted with two rituximab molecules. Cross-linking of the CD20 protein with rituximab results in a circular assembly that was postulated to lead to complement recruitment. This interaction was thought to lead to the preferential downregulation of CD20-positive B-cells via a mechanism of antibody-dependent cellular cytotoxicity (ADCC) and/or complement-dependent cytotoxicity (CDC).

Tocilizumab

Tocilizumab (also known as Atlizumab) is a humanized monoclonal antibody used for the treatment of moderate to severe rheumatoid arthritis and juvenile idiopathic arthritis. Tocilizumab is an effective treatment for rheumatoid arthritis with a rapid and sustained improvement of arthritic disorders, including a reduction of joint damage and improved motor function. Tocilizumab is often used therapeutically if DMARD drugs or TNF-α blockers are found to be ineffective or not tolerated.

Tocilizumab binds both the membranous and soluble forms of interleukin-6 receptor (IL-6R) and competitively inhibits the binding of IL-6 to the IL-6R. Tocilizumab binds with high affinity at the IL-6R and acts like a competitive antagonist at the IL-6R. Although IL-6 had initially been classified as a proinflammatory cytokine, the IL-6R appears to be involved in both pro-inflammatory and anti-inflammatory functions.

IL-6 is found in the synovial fluid and serum of patients with rheumatoid arthritis. The levels of IL-6 in the synovial fluid correlate with disease status and the extent of joint destruction. IL-6 appears to promote synovitis and joint destruction by stimulating neutrophil migration, osteoclast (multinucleated cell involved in the dissolution and absorption of bone) maturation, and vascular endothelial growth factor-stimulated pannus (growth in joints that can cause bone pain, swelling, and damage) proliferation.

IL-6 may also mediate the induction of C-reactive protein anemia via the hypothalamic-pituitary-adrenal axis. C-reactive protein is found in the plasma when there is increased system inflammation. The physiological role of C-reactive protein is thought to activate complement after binding lysophosphatidylcholine expressed on the surface of dead or dying cells. Therefore, IL-6 may be involved in the development of chronic inflammatory diseases associated with CRP elevation.

IL-6 may contribute to the induction and maintenance of autoimmunity by acting through the maturation of B-cells and the activation of T helper 17 cells (T_h17). T_h17 cells are pro-inflammatory T helper cells that produce IL-17. These cells are a subclass of T cells that signal T regulatory cells to differentiate and enable the T_h17 cells to maintain mucosal barriers, which contributes to pathogen clearance. Autoreactive T_h17 cells are associated with autoimmune diseases including multiple sclerosis, rheumatoid arthritis, and psoriasis. The overactivation of T_h17 cells can lead to complement-mediated hypersensitivity. In addition, IL-6 is classified as a myokine (a cytokine produced by muscle cells) that is secreted into the blood in response to the *muscle contractions associated with physical exertion such as exercise. Thus,* IL-6 *is thought to* act as both a pro-inflammatory *cytokine* and an anti-inflammatory myokine.

Surgery

If pharmacotherapy inadequately alleviates pain or is unable to prevent or slow joint damage, surgery to repair damaged joints may be considered. Surgery can help to reduce pain and improve function. Rheumatoid arthritis surgery may involve one or more of the following procedures:

a) removal of the inflamed lining of the joint, knees, elbows, wrists, fingers, and hips joints (Synovectomy),
b) repair the tendons surrounding a joint,
c) surgical fusing of a joint to realign and stabilize a joint when replacement of the joint isn't an option (joint fusion) or
d) removal of the damaged parts of a joint and the insertion of a prosthesis (total joint replacement).

References For Chapter 9.2

Aletaha, D., T. Neogi, A. J. Silman, J. Funovits, D. T. Felson, C. O. Bingham, 3rd, N. S. Birnbaum, G. R. Burmester, V. P. Bykerk, M. D. Cohen, B. Combe, K. H. Costenbader, M. Dougados, P. Emery, G. Ferraccioli, J. M. Hazes, K. Hobbs, T. W. Huizinga, A. Kavanaugh, J. Kay, T. K. Kvien, T. Laing, P. Mease, H. A. Menard, L. W. Moreland, R. L. Naden, T. Pincus, J. S. Smolen, E. Stanislawska-Biernat, D. Symmons, P. P. Tak, K. S. Upchurch, J. Vencovsky, F. Wolfe, and G. Hawker. 2010. 2010 Rheumatoid arthritis classification criteria: an American College of Rheumatology/European League Against Rheumatism collaborative initiative. *Arthritis & Rheumatism* 62 (9):2569-2581.

Alinaghi, F., M. Calov, L. E. Kristensen, D. D. Gladman, L. C. Coates, D. Jullien, A. B. Gottlieb, P. Gisondi, J. J. Wu, J. P. Thyssen, and A. Egeberg. 2019. Prevalence of psoriatic arthritis in patients with psoriasis: A systematic review and meta-analysis of observational and clinical studies. *J Am Acad Dermatol* 80 (1):251-265 e219.

Almoallim, H., Y. Al-Ghamdi, H. Almaghrabi, and O. Alyasi. 2012. Anti-Tumor Necrosis Factor-alpha Induced Systemic Lupus Erythematosus(). *Open Rheumatol J* 6:315-319.

Aparicio-Soto, M., M. Sanchez-Hidalgo, and C. Alarcon-de-la-Lastra. 2017. An update on diet and nutritional factors in systemic lupus erythematosus management. *Nutr Res Rev* 30 (1):118-137.

Aringer, M., K. Costenbader, D. Daikh, R. Brinks, M. Mosca, R. Ramsey-Goldman, J. S. Smolen, D. Wofsy, D. T. Boumpas, D. L. Kamen, D. Jayne, R. Cervera, N. Costedoat-Chalumeau, B. Diamond, D. D. Gladman, B. Hahn, F. Hiepe, S. Jacobsen, D. Khanna, K. Lerstrom, E. Massarotti, J. McCune, G. Ruiz-Irastorza, J. Sanchez-Guerrero, M. Schneider, M. Urowitz, G. Bertsias, B. F. Hoyer, N. Leuchten, C. Tani, S. K. Tedeschi, Z. Touma, G. Schmajuk, B. Anic, F. Assan, T. M. Chan, A. E. Clarke, M. K. Crow, L. Czirjak, A. Doria, W. Graninger, B. Halda-Kiss, S. Hasni, P. M. Izmirly, M. Jung, G. Kumanovics, X. Mariette, I. Padjen, J. M. Pego-Reigosa, J. Romero-Diaz, I. Rua-Figueroa Fernandez, R. Seror, G. H. Stummvoll, Y. Tanaka, M. G. Tektonidou, C. Vasconcelos, E. M. Vital, D. J. Wallace, S. Yavuz, P. L. Meroni, M. J. Fritzler, R. Naden, T. Dorner, and S. R. Johnson. 2019. 2019 European League Against Rheumatism/American College of Rheumatology Classification Criteria for Systemic Lupus Erythematosus. *Arthritis Rheumatol* 71 (9):1400-1412.

Arneth, B. 2019. Systemic Lupus Erythematosus and DNA Degradation and Elimination Defects. *Front Immunol* 10:1697.

Aubourg, G., S. J. Rice, P. Bruce-Wootton, and J. Loughlin. 2021. Genetics of osteoarthritis. *Osteoarthritis Cartilage*.

Bailly, F., A. Cantagrel, P. Bertin, S. Perrot, T. Thomas, T. Lansaman, L. Grange, D. Wendling, C. Dovico, and A. P. Trouvin. 2020. Part of pain labelled neuropathic in rheumatic disease might be rather nociplastic. *RMD Open* 6 (2).

Bair, M. J., and E. E. Krebs. 2020. Fibromyalgia. *Ann Intern Med* 172 (5):ITC33-ITC48.

Bao, L., P. N. Cunningham, and R. J. Quigg. 2015. Complement in Lupus Nephritis: New Perspectives. *Kidney Dis (Basel)* 1 (2):91-99.

Bossuyt, X., E. De Langhe, M. O. Borghi, and P. L. Meroni. 2020. Understanding and interpreting antinuclear antibody tests in systemic rheumatic diseases. *Nat Rev Rheumatol* 16 (12):715-726.

Braun, H. J., and G. E. Gold. 2012. Diagnosis of osteoarthritis: imaging. *Bone* 51 (2):278-288.

Cai, Y., C. Fleming, and J. Yan. 2012. New insights of T cells in the pathogenesis of psoriasis. *Cell Mol Immunol* 9 (4):302-309.

Campion, E. W., R. J. Glynn, and L. O. DeLabry. 1987. Asymptomatic hyperuricemia. Risks and consequences in the Normative Aging Study. *American Journal of Medicine* 82 (3):421-426.

Carpenter, C. R., J. D. Schuur, W. W. Everett, and J. M. Pines. 2011. Evidence-based diagnostics: adult septic arthritis. *Acad Emerg Med* 18 (8):781-796.

Chadha, R. 2016. Revealed aspect of metabolic osteoarthritis. *J Orthop* 13 (4):347-351.

Chandran, V., C. T. Schentag, J. E. Brockbank, F. J. Pellett, S. Shanmugarajah, S. M. Toloza, P. Rahman, and D. D. Gladman. 2009. Familial aggregation of psoriatic arthritis. *Annals of the Rheumatic Diseases* 68 (5):664-667.

Chang, E. Y., K. C. Chen, B. K. Huang, and A. Kavanaugh. 2016. Adult Inflammatory Arthritides: What the Radiologist Should Know. *Radiographics* 36 (6):1849-1870.

Choi, J., S. T. Kim, and J. Craft. 2012. The pathogenesis of systemic lupus erythematosus-an update. *Current Opinion in Immunology* 24 (6):651-657.

Choy, E. H. 2015. The role of sleep in pain and fibromyalgia. *Nat Rev Rheumatol* 11 (9):513-520.

Cimaz, R. 2016. Systemic-onset juvenile idiopathic arthritis. *Autoimmunity Reviews* 15 (9):931-934.

Coakley, G., C. Mathews, M. Field, A. Jones, G. Kingsley, D. Walker, M. Phillips, C. Bradish, A. McLachlan, R. Mohammed, V. Weston, Guidelines British Society for Rheumatology Standards, and Group Audit Working. 2006. BSR & BHPR, BOA, RCGP and BSAC guidelines for management of the hot swollen joint in adults. *Rheumatology (Oxford)* 45 (8):1039-1041.

Cojocaru, M., I. M. Cojocaru, I. Silosi, C. D. Vrabie, and R. Tanasescu. 2010. Extra-articular Manifestations in Rheumatoid Arthritis. *Maedica (Bucur)* 5 (4):286-291.

Colavite, P. M., and A. Sartori. 2014. Septic arthritis: immunopathogenesis, experimental models and therapy. *J Venom Anim Toxins Incl Trop Dis* 20:19.

Conforti, A., I. Di Cola, V. Pavlych, P. Ruscitti, O. Berardicurti, F. Ursini, R. Giacomelli, and P. Cipriani. 2021. Beyond the joints, the extra-articular manifestations in rheumatoid arthritis. *Autoimmunity Reviews* 20 (2):102735.

D'Agnelli, S., L. Arendt-Nielsen, M. C. Gerra, K. Zatorri, L. Boggiani, M. Baciarello, and E. Bignami. 2019. Fibromyalgia: Genetics and epigenetics insights may provide the basis for the development of diagnostic biomarkers. *Mol Pain* 15:1744806918819944.

Deane, K. D., M. K. Demoruelle, L. B. Kelmenson, K. A. Kuhn, J. M. Norris, and V. M. Holers. 2017. Genetic and environmental risk factors for rheumatoid arthritis. *Best Pract Res Clin Rheumatol* 31 (1):3-18.

Fangtham, M., S. Kasturi, R. R. Bannuru, J. L. Nash, and C. Wang. 2019. Non-pharmacologic therapies for systemic lupus erythematosus. *Lupus* 28 (6):703-712.

Fanouriakis, A., M. Kostopoulou, A. Alunno, M. Aringer, I. Bajema, J. N. Boletis, R. Cervera, A. Doria, C. Gordon, M. Govoni, F. Houssiau, D. Jayne, M. Kouloumas, A. Kuhn, J. L. Larsen, K. Lerstrom, G. Moroni, M. Mosca, M. Schneider, J. S. Smolen, E. Svenungsson, V. Tesar, A. Tincani, A. Troldborg, R. van Vollenhoven, J. Wenzel, G. Bertsias, and D. T. Boumpas. 2019. 2019 update of the EULAR recommendations for the management of systemic lupus erythematosus. *Annals of the Rheumatic Diseases* 78 (6):736-745.

Fitzcharles, M. A., S. P. Cohen, D. J. Clauw, G. Littlejohn, C. Usui, and W. Hauser. 2021. Nociplastic pain: towards an understanding of prevalent pain conditions. *Lancet* 397 (10289):2098-2110.

FitzGerald, J. D., N. Dalbeth, T. Mikuls, R. Brignardello-Petersen, G. Guyatt, A. M. Abeles, A. C. Gelber, L. R. Harrold, D. Khanna, C. King, G. Levy, C. Libbey, D. Mount, M. H. Pillinger, A. Rosenthal, J. A. Singh, J. E. Sims, B. J. Smith, N. S. Wenger, S. S. Bae, A. Danve, P. P. Khanna, S. C. Kim, A. Lenert, S. Poon, A. Qasim, S. T. Sehra, T. S. K. Sharma, M. Toprover, M. Turgunbaev, L. Zeng, M. A. Zhang, A. S. Turner, and T. Neogi. 2020. 2020 American College of Rheumatology Guideline for the Management of Gout. *Arthritis Care Res (Hoboken)* 72 (6):744-760.

Fraenkel, L., J. M. Bathon, B. R. England, E. W. St Clair, T. Arayssi, K. Carandang, K. D. Deane, M. Genovese, K. K. Huston, G. Kerr, J. Kremer, M. C. Nakamura, L. A. Russell, J. A. Singh, B. J. Smith, J. A. Sparks, S. Venkatachalam, M. E. Weinblatt, M. Al-Gibbawi, J. F. Baker, K. E. Barbour, J. L. Barton, L. Cappelli, F. Chamseddine, M. George, S. R. Johnson, L. Kahale, B. S. Karam, A. M. Khamis, I. Navarro-Millan, R. Mirza, P. Schwab, N. Singh, M. Turgunbaev, A. S. Turner, S. Yaacoub, and E. A. Akl. 2021. 2021 American College of Rheumatology Guideline for the Treatment of Rheumatoid Arthritis. *Arthritis Care Res (Hoboken)* 73 (7):924-939.

Franca, C. M. P., A. M. E. Sallum, A. L. F. Braga, F. L. Strufaldi, C. A. A. Silva, and S. C. L. Farhat. 2018. Risk Factors Associated with Juvenile Idiopathic Arthritis: Exposure to Cigarette Smoke and Air Pollution from Pregnancy to Disease Diagnosis. *J Rheumatol* 45 (2):248-256.

Frosch, M., and J. Roth. 2008. New insights in systemic juvenile idiopathic arthritis--from pathophysiology to treatment. *Rheumatology (Oxford)* 47 (2):121-125.

Giguere, P. M., B. J. Gall, E. A. Ezekwe, Jr., G. Laroche, B. K. Buckley, C. Kebaier, J. E. Wilson, J. P. Ting, D. P. Siderovski, and J. A. Duncan. 2014. G Protein signaling modulator-3 inhibits the inflammasome activity of NLRP3. *Journal of Biological Chemistry* 289 (48):33245-33257.

Glyn-Jones, S., A. J. Palmer, R. Agricola, A. J. Price, T. L. Vincent, H. Weinans, and A. J. Carr. 2015. Osteoarthritis. *Lancet* 386 (9991):376-387.

Gossec, L., X. Baraliakos, A. Kerschbaumer, M. de Wit, I. McInnes, M. Dougados, J. Primdahl, D. G. McGonagle, D. Aletaha, A. Balanescu, P. V. Balint, H. Bertheussen, W. H. Boehncke, G. R. Burmester, J. D. Canete, N. S. Damjanov, T. W. Kragstrup, T. K. Kvien, R. B. M. Landewe, R. J. U. Lories, H. Marzo-Ortega, D. Poddubnyy, S. A. Rodrigues Manica, G. Schett, D. J. Veale, F. E. Van den Bosch, D. van der Heijde, and J. S. Smolen. 2020. EULAR recommendations for the management of psoriatic arthritis with pharmacological therapies: 2019 update. *Annals of the Rheumatic Diseases* 79 (6):700-712.

Gracely, R. H., F. Petzke, J. M. Wolf, and D. J. Clauw. 2002. Functional magnetic resonance imaging evidence of augmented pain processing in fibromyalgia. *Arthritis & Rheumatism* 46 (5):1333-1343.

Guilak, F. 2011. Biomechanical factors in osteoarthritis. *Best Pract Res Clin Rheumatol* 25 (6):815-823.

Harb, A., K. Shawwa, A. H. Alraiyes, and M. C. Alraies. 2013. Severe rheumatoid arthritis hand deformity. *BMJ Case Rep* 2013.

Horowitz, D. L., E. Katzap, S. Horowitz, and M. L. Barilla-LaBarca. 2011. Approach to septic arthritis. *American Family Physician* 84 (6):653-660.

Hunter, D. J., and S. Bierma-Zeinstra. 2019. Osteoarthritis. *Lancet* 393 (10182):1745-1759.

Kaandorp, C. J., H. J. Dinant, M. A. van de Laar, H. J. Moens, A. P. Prins, and B. A. Dijkmans. 1997. Incidence and sources of native and prosthetic joint infection: a community based prospective survey. *Annals of the Rheumatic Diseases* 56 (8):470-475.

Kerschbaumer, A., A. Sepriano, S. A. Bergstra, J. S. Smolen, D. van der Heijde, R. Caporali, C. J. Edwards, P. Verschueren, S. de Souza, J. E. Pope, T. Takeuchi, K. L. Hyrich, K. L. Winthrop, D. Aletaha, T. A. Stamm, J. W. Schoones, and R. B. M. Landewe. 2023. Efficacy of synthetic and biological DMARDs: a systematic literature review informing the 2022 update of the EULAR recommendations for the management of rheumatoid arthritis. *Annals of the Rheumatic Diseases* 82 (1):95-106.

Kim, K. H., and D. S. Kim. 2010. Juvenile idiopathic arthritis: Diagnosis and differential diagnosis. *Korean J Pediatr* 53 (11):931-935.

Kiriakidou, M., and C. L. Ching. 2020. Systemic Lupus Erythematosus. *Ann Intern Med* 172 (11):ITC81-ITC96.

Klareskog, L., J. Ronnelid, S. Saevarsdottir, L. Padyukov, and L. Alfredsson. 2020. The importance of differences; On environment and its interactions with genes and immunity in the causation of rheumatoid arthritis. *J Intern Med* 287 (5):514-533.

Kosek, E., M. Cohen, R. Baron, G. F. Gebhart, J. A. Mico, A. S. C. Rice, W. Rief, and A. K. Sluka. 2016. Do we need a third mechanistic descriptor for chronic pain states? *Pain* 157 (7):1382-1386.

Kronzer, V. L., and J. M. Davis, 3rd. 2021. Etiologies of Rheumatoid Arthritis: Update on Mucosal, Genetic, and Cellular Pathogenesis. *Curr Rheumatol Rep* 23 (4):21.

Lalani, T. A., J. P. Kanne, G. A. Hatfield, and P. Chen. 2004. Imaging findings in systemic lupus erythematosus. *Radiographics* 24 (4):1069-1086.

Lichtenstein, A., S. Tiosano, and H. Amital. 2018. The complexities of fibromyalgia and its comorbidities. *Current Opinion in Rheumatology* 30 (1):94-100.

Lopez-Sola, M., C. W. Woo, J. Pujol, J. Deus, B. J. Harrison, J. Monfort, and T. D. Wager. 2017. Towards a neurophysiological signature for fibromyalgia. *Pain* 158 (1):34-47.

Martel-Pelletier, J., A. J. Barr, F. M. Cicuttini, P. G. Conaghan, C. Cooper, M. B. Goldring, S. R. Goldring, G. Jones, A. J. Teichtahl, and J. P. Pelletier. 2016. Osteoarthritis. *Nat Rev Dis Primers* 2:16072.

Martillo, M. A., L. Nazzal, and D. B. Crittenden. 2014. The crystallization of monosodium urate. *Curr Rheumatol Rep* 16 (2):400.

Martinon, F., V. Petrilli, A. Mayor, A. Tardivel, and J. Tschopp. 2006. Gout-associated uric acid crystals activate the NALP3 inflammasome. *Nature* 440 (7081):237-241.

Mascarenhas, R. O., M. B. Souza, M. X. Oliveira, A. C. Lacerda, V. A. Mendonca, N. Henschke, and V. C. Oliveira. 2021. Association of Therapies With Reduced Pain and Improved Quality of Life in Patients With Fibromyalgia: A Systematic Review and Meta-analysis. *JAMA Intern Med* 181 (1):104-112.

McMahon, M. A., M. Keogan, P. O'Connell, and G. Kearns. 2006. The prevalence of antiphospholipid antibody syndrome among systemic lupus erythematosus patients. *Ir Med J* 99 (10):296-298.

McMahon, M., B. H. Hahn, and B. J. Skaggs. 2011. Systemic lupus erythematosus and cardiovascular disease: prediction and potential for therapeutic intervention. *Expert Rev Clin Immunol* 7 (2):227-241.

Metry, A. M., I. Al Salmi, F. Al Balushi, M. A. Yousef, F. Al Ismaili, A. Hola, and S. Hannawi. 2019. Systemic Lupus Erythematosus: Symptoms and Signs at Initial Presentations. *Antiinflamm Antiallergy Agents Med Chem* 18 (2):142-150.

Mohamed, M., S. Patel, K. Plavnik, E. Liu, K. Casey, and M. A. Hossain. 2019. Retrospective Analysis of Septic Arthritis Caused by Intra-Articular Viscosupplementation and Steroid Injections in a Single Outpatient Center. *J Clin Med Res* 11 (7):480-483.

Moll, J. M., and V. Wright. 1973. Psoriatic arthritis. *Semin Arthritis Rheum* 3 (1):55-78.

Momodu, II, and V. Savaliya. 2021. Septic Arthritis. In *StatPearls*. Treasure Island (FL).

Moore, D. L. 2018. Immunization of the immunocompromised child: Key principles. *Paediatr Child Health* 23 (3):203-205.

Nigrovic, P. A., M. Martinez-Bonet, and S. D. Thompson. 2019. Implications of juvenile idiopathic arthritis genetic risk variants for disease pathogenesis and classification. *Current Opinion in Rheumatology* 31 (5):401-410.

Ory, P. A., D. D. Gladman, and P. J. Mease. 2005. Psoriatic arthritis and imaging. *Annals of the Rheumatic Diseases* 64 Suppl 2:ii55-57.

Parks, C. G., A. de Souza Espindola Santos, M. Barbhaiya, and K. H. Costenbader. 2017. Understanding the role of environmental factors in the development of systemic lupus erythematosus. *Best Pract Res Clin Rheumatol* 31 (3):306-320.

Perez-Chada, L. M., and J. F. Merola. 2020. Comorbidities associated with psoriatic arthritis: Review and update. *Clinical Immunology* 214:108397.

Petty, R. E., T. R. Southwood, P. Manners, J. Baum, D. N. Glass, J. Goldenberg, X. He, J. Maldonado-Cocco, J. Orozco-Alcala, A. M. Prieur, M. E. Suarez-Almazor, P. Woo, and Rheumatology International League of Associations for. 2004. International League of Associations for Rheumatology classification of juvenile idiopathic arthritis: second revision, Edmonton, 2001. *J Rheumatol* 31 (2):390-392.

Philippou, E., S. D. Petersson, C. Rodomar, and E. Nikiphorou. 2021. Rheumatoid arthritis and dietary interventions: systematic review of clinical trials. *Nutrition Reviews* 79 (4):410-428.

Poggenborg, R. P., M. Ostergaard, and L. Terslev. 2015. Imaging in Psoriatic Arthritis. *Rheum Dis Clin North Am* 41 (4):593-613.

Provan, S. A., S. Lillegraven, J. Sexton, K. Angel, C. Austad, E. A. Haavardsholm, T. K. Kvien, and T. Uhlig. 2020. Trends in all-cause and cardiovascular mortality in patients with incident rheumatoid arthritis: a 20-year follow-up matched case-cohort study. *Rheumatology (Oxford)* 59 (3):505-512.

Rainer, T. H., C. H. Cheng, H. J. Janssens, C. Y. Man, L. S. Tam, Y. F. Choi, W. H. Yau, K. H. Lee, and C. A. Graham. 2016. Oral Prednisolone in the Treatment of Acute Gout: A Pragmatic, Multicenter, Double-Blind, Randomized Trial. *Ann Intern Med* 164 (7):464-471.

Reginato, A. M., D. B. Mount, I. Yang, and H. K. Choi. 2012. The genetics of hyperuricaemia and gout. *Nat Rev Rheumatol* 8 (10):610-621.

Roizenblatt, S., N. S. Neto, and S. Tufik. 2011. Sleep disorders and fibromyalgia. *Curr Pain Headache Rep* 15 (5):347-357.

Ross, J. J. 2017. Septic Arthritis of Native Joints. *Infect Dis Clin North Am* 31 (2):203-218.

Rudwaleit, M., R. Landewe, D. van der Heijde, J. Listing, J. Brandt, J. Braun, R. Burgos-Vargas, E. Collantes-Estevez, J. Davis, B. Dijkmans, M. Dougados, P. Emery, I. E. van der Horst-Bruinsma, R. Inman, M. A. Khan, M. Leirisalo-

Repo, S. van der Linden, W. P. Maksymowych, H. Mielants, I. Olivieri, R. Sturrock, K. de Vlam, and J. Sieper. 2009. The development of Assessment of SpondyloArthritis international Society classification criteria for axial spondyloarthritis (part I): classification of paper patients by expert opinion including uncertainty appraisal. *Annals of the Rheumatic Diseases* 68 (6):770-776.

Santiago, M. B., V. Galvao, D. S. Ribeiro, W. D. Santos, P. R. da Hora, A. P. Mota, E. Pimenta, I. Oliveira, A. M. Atta, M. G. Reis, E. A. Reis, and C. Lins. 2015. Severe Jaccoud's arthropathy in systemic lupus erythematosus. *Rheumatol Int* 35 (10):1773-1777.

Schrezenmeier, E., and T. Dorner. 2020. Mechanisms of action of hydroxychloroquine and chloroquine: implications for rheumatology. *Nat Rev Rheumatol* 16 (3):155-166.

Singh, J. A., G. Guyatt, A. Ogdie, D. D. Gladman, C. Deal, A. Deodhar, M. Dubreuil, J. Dunham, M. E. Husni, S. Kenny, J. Kwan-Morley, J. Lin, P. Marchetta, P. J. Mease, J. F. Merola, J. Miner, C. T. Ritchlin, B. Siaton, B. J. Smith, A. S. Van Voorhees, A. H. Jonsson, A. A. Shah, N. Sullivan, M. Turgunbaev, L. C. Coates, A. Gottlieb, M. Magrey, W. B. Nowell, A. M. Orbai, S. M. Reddy, J. U. Scher, E. Siegel, M. Siegel, J. A. Walsh, A. S. Turner, and J. Reston. 2019. Special Article: 2018 American College of Rheumatology/National Psoriasis Foundation Guideline for the Treatment of Psoriatic Arthritis. *Arthritis Rheumatol* 71 (1):5-32.

Skousgaard, S. G., J. Hjelmborg, A. Skytthe, L. P. Brandt, S. Moller, and S. Overgaard. 2015. Probability and heritability estimates on primary osteoarthritis of the hip leading to total hip arthroplasty: a nationwide population based follow-up study in Danish twins. *Arthritis Res Ther* 17:336.

Sluka, K. A., and D. J. Clauw. 2016. Neurobiology of fibromyalgia and chronic widespread pain. *Neuroscience* 338:114-129.

Smolen, J. S., D. Aletaha, and I. B. McInnes. 2016. Rheumatoid arthritis. *Lancet* 388 (10055):2023-2038.

Sundy, J. S., H. R. Schumacher, A. Kivitz, S. P. Weinstein, R. Wu, S. King-Davis, and R. R. Evans. 2014. Rilonacept for gout flare prevention in patients receiving uric acid-lowering therapy: results of RESURGE, a phase III, international safety study. *J Rheumatol* 41 (8):1703-1711.

Taylor, W., D. Gladman, P. Helliwell, A. Marchesoni, P. Mease, H. Mielants, and Caspar Study Group. 2006. Classification criteria for psoriatic arthritis: development of new criteria from a large international study. *Arthritis & Rheumatism* 54 (8):2665-2673.

Thomas, A. C., T. Hubbard-Turner, E. A. Wikstrom, and R. M. Palmieri-Smith. 2017. Epidemiology of Posttraumatic Osteoarthritis. *J Athl Train* 52 (6):491-496.

Thomas, S., H. Browne, A. Mobasheri, and M. P. Rayman. 2018. What is the evidence for a role for diet and nutrition in osteoarthritis? *Rheumatology (Oxford)* 57 (suppl_4):iv61-iv74.

Veale, D. J., and U. Fearon. 2018. The pathogenesis of psoriatic arthritis. *Lancet* 391 (10136):2273-2284.

Veale D.J., Fearon U., Low C., and Miller L.D. 2021. *Rheumatoid arthritis.* edited by S. J. H. (Ed.). 4 ed: McGraw Hill.

Weston, V. C., A. C. Jones, N. Bradbury, F. Fawthrop, and M. Doherty. 1999. Clinical features and outcome of septic arthritis in a single UK Health District 1982-1991. *Annals of the Rheumatic Diseases* 58 (4):214-219.

Wolfe, F., D. J. Clauw, M. A. Fitzcharles, D. L. Goldenberg, W. Hauser, R. L. Katz, P. J. Mease, A. S. Russell, I. J. Russell, and B. Walitt. 2016. 2016 Revisions to the 2010/2011 fibromyalgia diagnostic criteria. *Semin Arthritis Rheum* 46 (3):319-329.

Wolfe, F., H. A. Smythe, M. B. Yunus, R. M. Bennett, C. Bombardier, D. L. Goldenberg, P. Tugwell, S. M. Campbell, M. Abeles, P. Clark, and et al. 1990. The American College of Rheumatology 1990 Criteria for the Classification of Fibromyalgia. Report of the Multicenter Criteria Committee. *Arthritis & Rheumatism* 33 (2):160-172.

Yucesoy, B., L. E. Charles, B. Baker, and C. M. Burchfiel. 2015. Occupational and genetic risk factors for osteoarthritis: a review. *Work* 50 (2):261-273.

Yunus, M. B. 2007. Fibromyalgia and overlapping disorders: the unifying concept of central sensitivity syndromes. *Semin Arthritis Rheum* 36 (6):339-356.

Zhang, A., and Y. C. Lee. 2018. Mechanisms for Joint Pain in Rheumatoid Arthritis (RA): from Cytokines to Central Sensitization. *Curr Osteoporos Rep* 16 (5):603-610.

Zhao, S. S., S. J. Duffield, and N. J. Goodson. 2019. The prevalence and impact of comorbid fibromyalgia in inflammatory arthritis. *Best Pract Res Clin Rheumatol* 33 (3):101423.

Case Study Questions For Chapters 9.1-9.2

Case Study

A 60-year-old man who is 50 lbs overweight arrives at the physician's office complaining of acute pain in the left ankle spreading from the toes of his left foot. He woke up at 2:25 AM last night feeling that this large toe "*had been doused with kerosene and set on fire*". Examination of the extremities reveals redness and tenderness over the ankle and toes of his left foot; the man complains of severe pain when slight pressure is applied to the ankle. He reports consuming red meat at least 6 times a week and always has dinner with three or more glasses of red wine. What should his physician do?

Quiz Questions For Chapters 9.1-9.2

1. A 62-year-old man is recovering from an injury to his right arm received in a recent motorcycle accident and tells his doctor that he plans to take over-the-counter (OTC) aspirin "to deal with the pain". The doctor reviews his medical history and recommends replacing aspirin with acetaminophen/paracetamol. What underlying health condition does the patient likely have to drive this doctor's recommendation?

A Rheumatoid arthritis
B Chronic migraine
C A prior ischemic stroke
D Lupus erythematosus
E Gout syndrome

2. A 46-year-old man is prescribed a first-line drug for prophylaxis of acute gouty attacks. Which is the most likely medication prescribed to the man?

A Allopurinol
B Lesinurad
C Colchicine
D Febuxostat
E Pegloticase

3. A 54-year-old man has gout attacks every 1 - 2 months. He has a moderate degree of renal impairment (estimated glomerular filtration rate = 52 mL/min) due to many previous episodes of nephrolithiasis. Which drug would be the safest for him to use for the long-term management of his gout?

A Allopurinol
B Lesinurad
C Colchicine
D Febuxostat
E Aspirin

4. For what reason(s) should febuxostat and pegloticase not be used as first-line drugs for prophylaxis of acute gouty attacks?

A Less effective than allopurinol
B Heightened risk of myocardial infarction and allergy development, respectively
C Heightened risk of hepatic toxicity and renal toxicity, respectively
D Each will likely become first-line therapy as physicians gain more experience with their use
E Heightened risk of developing DRESS (drug reaction with eosinophilia and system symptoms)

5. A 52-year-old female patient with gout is prescribed a drug that inhibits the active reabsorption of uric acid from the glomerular filtrate, blocks uric acid reabsorption by the organic anion transporter in the proximal tubules and thus, increases urinary uric acid elimination. The same drug can be given in combination with colchicine. Which drug is prescribed?

A Allopurinol
B Lesinurad
C Aspirin
D Febuxostat
E Probenecid

6. A pharmaceutical company develops a new treatment for acute and chronic gout. The novel agent is an inhibitor targeting the product(s) of NLRP3 inflammasome activation by monosodium urate crystals (MSU). Which is the best protein target?

A Matrix Metalloproteinase 19
B Interleukin 1β
C Interleukin 6
D Interleukin 10
E Transforming Growth Factor β (TGF-β)

7. A 38-year-old female makes an appointment with her doctor and complains of a facial rash around her nose in a shape of a butterfly. This rash is likely a symptom of which condition?

A Sjögren syndrome
B Psoriasis
C Rheumatoid arthritis
D Systemic lupus erythematosus
E Gout

8. A 52-year-old female is prescribed hydroxychloroquine to treat systemic lupus erythematosus. Which is the mechanism of action of hydroxychloroquine?

A It decreases the production of red blood cells.
B It interferes with antigen processing by macrophages and inhibits macrophage phagocytosis and superoxide production by neutrophils.
C It has reduces fever by inhibiting synthesis of cyclooxygenase-1.
D It inhibits metabolism of both cyclooxygenase-1 and cyclooxygenase-2.
E It inhibits the synthesis of uric acid.

9. A 62-year-old man is prescribed leflunomide which is a prodrug for rheumatoid arthritis. Which is the mechanism of action of leflunomide?

A It inhibits liver metabolism of pyrimidine.
B It increases synthesis of P-glycoproteins.
C It is anti-inflammatory by inhibiting synthesis of pyrimidine.
D It increases the turnover of tumor necrosis factor receptors.
E It decreases the production of red blood cells.

10. A 48-year-old male with severe long-standing rheumatoid arthritis has been taking high doses of an anti-inflammatory medicine daily for 4 years. A few months ago, he developed epigastric distress, and his medication was replaced with a disease-modifying anti-rheumatic drug (DMARD). While the new DMARD prescription was effective, it was soon replaced with a non-DMARD drug because the patient complained of headache, nausea, and diarrhea. Which new drug is a likely new replacement?

A Aspirin
B Duloxetine
C Acetaminophen
D Tocilizumab
E Methotrexate

11. Which statement best describes the mechanism of action of adalimumab?

A It inhibits both cyclooxygenase-1 and cyclooxygenase-2.
B It is a humanized monoclonal antibody that inactivates tumor necrosis factor α.
C It is a glucocorticoid that inhibits gastric motility and B-cell production.
D It inhibits $\alpha 4$ integrins and may cause leukoencephalopathy.
E It inhibits $\alpha 4\beta 7$ integrins in white blood cells.

Case Study Answers For Chapters 9.1-9.2

Take a blood sample to determine his serum uric acid level to validate a preliminary diagnosis of acute gout. Pending the results of the serum urate determination, the physician should prescribe an NSAID such as ibuprofen 800 mg three to four times daily or indomethacin 25 to 50 mg four times daily. Upon finding a serum uric acid level of 11 mg/dL and continuing pain, colchicine should be added to his pharmacotherapy. The patient should be instructed to strongly consider dietary restrictions, particularly avoiding meat products and decreasing alcohol intake. If his attacks return despite lifestyle changes, other drug measures, such as allopurinol, will be likely in his future.

Quiz Answers For Chapters 9.1-9.2

1. E. Aspirin is suggested to increase serum uric acid by decreasing uric acid excretion. It has been reported to be associated with more frequent gout flares. Although aspirin may be contraindicated after hemorrhagic stroke, given its anti-platelet effects, it is not contraindicated after ischemic stroke. Aspirin is not contraindicated in other disorders.

2. A. The American College of Rheumatology, in its 2020 guidelines for the management of gout, suggests allopurinol as the preferred first-line agent for the prophylaxis of gout.

3. D. Febuxostat is the correct answer. Allopurinol is relatively contraindicated in this man because he has renal impairment, and people with renal impairment are at elevated risk of experiencing DRESS as an adverse effect of allopurinol. Similarly, lesinurad should be avoided because it can cause renal toxicity, and it should only be used with allopurinol, which is relatively contraindicated. Colchicine is absolutely contraindicated for individuals with renal impairment. Therefore, febuxostat is the safest choice; note, however, that its use is cautioned in those with severe renal impairment

4. B. Although febuxostat and pegloticase are very efficacious agents, they are not first-line drugs for gout attack prophylaxis. Febuxostat is associated with a greater number of cardiac-related deaths than allopurinol, and pegloticase is a foreign protein that causes allergic reactions in about 25% of individuals. While febuxostat can increase liver enzyme levels and precipitate hepatic damage, pegloticase is not associated with nephrotoxicity, so this answer choice (C) is incorrect.

5. E. Probenecid is a potent inhibitor of renal uric acid reabsorption. Allopurinol and febuxostat inhibit uric acid synthesis. Lesinurad inhibits urate transporters. Aspirin is an NSAID.

6. B. MSU crystals, once engulfed by the phagocytic cell, can directly activate the NLRP3 inflammasome. Once the NLRP3 inflammasome is activated, IL-1β is produced and secreted, leading to immune system cell infiltration (*e.g.*, neutrophil recruitment) and acute inflammatory processes. This link between MSU deposition and IL-1β production defines the best target for blocking the inflammatory process underlying gout. Other listed options are not directly linked to MSU.

7. D. There are several rheumatologic conditions with characteristic rashes. The malar, or butterfly, rash is specific for lupus and is erythema of the cheeks sparing the nasolabial folds. Psoriasis typically occurs with psoriatic patches and can also have nail pitting. Other options do not show characteristic rashes.

8. B. Hydroxychloroquine, a conventional disease-modifying anti-rheumatic drug (DMARD), is the first-line treatment for SLE. Immunosuppressive effects including those listed are its main mechanism of action as a DMARD. (Schrezenmeier and Dorner 2020)

9. C. Leflunomide selectively inhibits the mitochondrial enzyme dihydroorotate dehydrogenase, which plays a key role in the synthesis of the pyrimidine ribonucleotide uridine monophosphate, which is essential for the rapidly proliferating cells such as those associated with the immune response. Other options are incorrect.

10. D. Tocilizumab (also known as Atlizumab) is a humanized monoclonal antibody used for the treatment of moderate to severe rheumatoid arthritis. Tocilizumab is often used therapeutically if DMARD drugs or TNF-α blockers are found to be ineffective or not tolerated. Other listed options are incorrect.

11. B. Adalimumab a human monoclonal antibody used to treat rheumatoid arthritis, psoriatic arthritis, psoriasis, or juvenile idiopathic arthritis. Adalimumab acts by binding to the TNF-α protein, which is primarily produced by activated macrophages, but also by T helper cells, natural killer cells, neutrophils, mast cells, eosinophils, mast cells, and neurons. Biological activities attributed to TNFα in disease pathogenesis include inducing proinflammatory cytokines (e.g., IL-1 and IL-6), enhancing leukocyte migration into tissues (by increasing blood vessel permeability), and increasing adhesion molecule release.

SYMPTOMS 2 –

CARDIO-RENAL-RESPIRATORY SYMPTOMS TO TREATMENT

CHAPTER 10

CARDIAC ARRHYTHMIAS AND TREATMENT

RACHEL PITTMAN, PHARMD AND ROBERT ALLEN, DO, FACEP

University of the Incarnate Word School of Osteopathic Medicine, San Antonio, Texas, USA

Symptoms: **Cardio-Renal-Respiratory**

DRUG LIST FOR ARRHYTHMIAS

Class I Antiarrhythmics:

Disopyramide	Class 1a Antiarrhythmic	Blockade of sodium channels
Procainamide	Class 1a Antiarrhythmic	Blockade of sodium channels
Quinidine	Class 1a Antiarrhythmic	Blockade of sodium channels
Lidocaine	Class 1b Antiarrhythmic	Blockade of sodium channels
Mexiletine	Class 1b Antiarrhythmic	Blockade of sodium channels
Flecainide	Class 1c Antiarrhythmic	Blockade of sodium channels
Propafenone	Class 1c Antiarrhythmic	Blockade of sodium channels

Class 2 Antiarrhythmics:

Esmolol	Class 2 Antiarrhythmic	Blockade of β_1 receptors
Propranolol	Class 2 Antiarrhythmic	Blockade of β_1 receptors
Nadolol	Class 2 Antiarrhythmic	Blockade of β_1 receptors
Sotalol	Class 2 (3) Antiarrhythmic	Blockade of β_1 receptors, prolongation of action potential

Class 3 Antiarrhythmics:

Amiodarone
Class 3 Antiarrhythmic Prolongation of action potential
Dofetilide
Class 3 Antiarrhythmic Prolongation of action potential
Dronedarone
Class 3 Antiarrhythmic Prolongation of action potential
Ibutilide
Class 3 Antiarrhythmic Prolongation of action potential

Class 4 Antiarrhythmics:

Diltiazem	Class 4 Antiarrhythmic	Blockade of calcium channels
Verapamil	Class 4 Antiarrhythmic	Blockade of calcium channels

Miscellaneous Antiarrhythmics:

Adenosine	Misc. Antiarrhythmic	Inhibition of AV current
Atropine	Anticholinergic agent	Inhibition of muscarinic ACh receptors

Cardiac Arrhythmias

General Background

Cardiac arrhythmias are generally due to disturbances in the normal cardiac electrical conduction system. A quick review of this system shows that under normal conditions, the electrical impulse that stimulates the cardiac muscle to contract originates in the upper right atrium, in an area called the sinoatrial (SA) node. This impulse is then conducted through both the left and right atria until it arrives at the atrioventricular (AV) node. At the AV node, the impulse is delayed slightly to allow the proper sequence of contraction. Contraction of the atria and the generation of atrial pressure pushes blood through the atrioventricular valves and into the ventricles, allowing the passive filling of the ventricles. From the AV node, the impulse is then conducted into the ventricles via the Bundle of His into the ventricles proper, where the conduction system divides into left and right bundle branches, and from there into the ventricular myocardium via Purkinje fibers, ultimately aiding in ventricular contraction.

Disturbances to the cardiac conduction system can occur in both the atria and ventricles. Disturbances that originate in the atria are usually referred to as supraventricular arrhythmias, and those arising in the ventricles are called ventricular arrhythmias. Disturbances in the conduction system can be congenital or can be the result of many different types of conditions such as myocardial hypertrophy, ischemia/infarct, toxins, electrolyte disturbances, and physical disturbances such as impact or electrical shock.

Cardiac arrhythmias can present in a variety of ways, from relatively benign presentations to sudden cardiac death. In some cases, an irregular cardiac rhythm is not noticed by the patient, but the effects of that arrhythmia may be noticed, such as hypotension, chest pain, and shortness of breath. In other cases, the patient may notice an irregular heartbeat with no other symptoms being noticed. For example, it is possible for some individuals to have atrial fibrillation and notice no effects at all. Other individuals can feel a sudden onset of weakness and near-syncope, while still, others may notice a decrease in exercise tolerance and mild shortness of breath. In cases of ventricular fibrillation, sudden loss of consciousness and no pulse is the rule.

There are many risk factors for cardiac arrhythmias including cardiac ischemia due to atherosclerotic cardiovascular disease, cardiac hypertrophy, hypertension, diabetes, congenital abnormalities in the conduction system, malformation of or damage to the cardiac valves, and electrolyte disturbances, to name a few.

Diagnosis

Diagnosis of cardiac arrhythmias is best done by performing a 12-lead ECG while the arrhythmia is present. In most cases, this will provide sufficient information to determine the etiology and treatment needed. However, a standard 12-lead ECG may only capture a few seconds of cardiac activity which may not be enough time to capture an intermittent or transient arrhythmia. In cases of intermittent arrhythmias, ambulatory ECG monitoring via Holter monitors or by event recording is frequently necessary. In some cases, invasive cardiac electrophysiological studies are required to determine the etiology of cardiac arrhythmias. This is usually done with the intention of performing catheter ablation of irritable foci or accessory cardiac conduction pathways at the same time.

The first consideration in the evaluation and treatment of cardiac arrhythmias is determining if the patient is stable or unstable. Some cardiac arrhythmias are by definition unstable, most notably ventricular fibrillation (VF or V-Fib), while the remaining majority can be stable or unstable depending on the condition of the patient. A cardiac arrhythmia is considered unstable if as a result of the arrhythmia the patient has:

-Hypotension (systolic BP below 90 mm Hg)
-Hypoperfusion manifested by
  -Altered mentation
  -Chest pain due to cardiac ischemia
  -Shortness of breath
-A very rapid heart rate (usually defined as 220 beats per minute or higher in an adult)

In unstable patients, rapid action is required to return the patient to a stable rhythm. This is usually done by electrical means such as transcutaneous (external) cardiac pacing, synchronized cardioversion, or defibrillation. Pharmacologic therapy in unstable patients is usually done after electrical therapy to prevent the recurrence of unstable arrhythmia. Stable patients can be treated electrically or with medications depending on the type of arrhythmia and its etiology.

Arrhythmias can be classified into two general categories: bradydysrhythmias and tachydysrhythmias.

Bradydysrhythmias are defined as arrhythmias having ventricular rates below 60 beats per minute (in adults). Common bradydysrhythmias include sinus bradycardia, junctional rhythm, idioventricular rhythm, 3rd-degree heart block, and less frequently, 2nd-degree heart block.

Presentation: Presentation of bradydysrhythmias can range from completely asymptomatic to unstable. For example, it is not unusual for well-conditioned athletes to have sinus bradycardia with resting heart rates in the middle-to-low 50s: This is not considered pathological and is a result of good aerobic fitness. Symptomatic bradydysrhythmias can present with dizziness, lightheadedness, nausea, vomiting, near-syncope, syncope, chest pain, and shortness of breath.

Pathophysiology: The majority of bradydysrhythmias result from factors outside the cardiac electrical system, including cardiac ischemia, drug effects or overdose, hypoxia, and acute coronary syndrome. Bradycardia can also result from structural disease of the infranodal conduction system.

Examination: As noted above, symptoms of bradycardia can range from asymptomatic to significant instability. In all cases, the ventricular rate and the pulse must be below 60.

Laboratory/imaging: Lab and imaging are not usually required in the diagnosis of bradycardia. Lab studies and imaging may be useful to determine underlying pathology causing bradycardia such as ischemia or valve pathology.
Associated symptoms/conditions: Symptomatic bradycardia can present with chest pain, shortness of breath, hypotension, altered mentation, and loss of consciousness. Conditions that can cause bradycardia include myocardial infarction, especially inferior wall myocardial infarction. Bradycardia can be associated with myocarditis, hypothyroidism, hypothermia, and both congenital and acquired heart disease.

Diagnosis: Diagnosis of bradycardia is generally by 12-lead ECG. Diagnosis of the underlying cause may be complicated and require extensive workup, but in general symptomatic bradycardia is self-evident.

Treatment: Symptomatic or unstable bradycardia is best treated by transcutaneous (external) cardiac pacing, which is fast, effective, and safe. It is usually well tolerated, although sedation is frequently required, as it is uncomfortable if the patient is awake. Once the symptomatic bradycardia is treated then the underlying cause can be addressed and corrected.

Symptomatic but stable bradycardia is best treated by determining and correcting the underlying cause. Bradycardia may be treated with atropine to increase the SA node rate; however, the side effects of atropine limit its use.

Sinus bradycardia:
Sinus bradycardia is the most common bradycardia. In many cases, sinus bradycardia is a normal finding, particularly associated with athletic conditioning and sleep. It can be an early manifestation of sinus node dysfunction. It can also occur due to medication or drug use (opiates in particular), obstructive sleep apnea, increased intracranial pressure, some infectious diseases, hypothermia, hypothyroidism, and severe hypoxia. In the setting of acute myocardial infarction, bradycardia is associated with obstruction of the right coronary artery (RCA), most likely due to increased vagal activity.

In most cases, sinus bradycardia should be treated (if at all) by treating the underlying cause. In cases where treatment is required, it usually responds well to the administration of atropine, however, the side effects of atropine limit its use to cases where transcutaneous pacing is not immediately available.

Atrioventricular blocks:
Atrioventricular blocks are delayed, intermittent or complete blockages of electrical impulses from the AV node to the ventricles. Clinically, these can range from a benign finding to a medical emergency. First-degree heart blocks and second-degree Mobitz Type I are usually asymptomatic, whereas second-degree Mobitz Type II and third-degree heart block frequently present with hemodynamic instability.

In a first-degree AV block, an electrical impulse from the atria to the ventricles is conducted, however, there is a longer than normal delay, resulting in a prolonged PR interval (by definition, over 200 milliseconds). It is occasionally found in completely normal hearts; however, it can appear due to increased vagal tone, myocardial infarction, myocarditis, and medication toxicity. First-degree heart block does not require treatment, however underlying causes should be sought, and progression to higher-degree heart blocks can occur.

In a second-degree heart block, Mobitz Type I, there is a gradually increasing delay of impulse conduction across the AV node until there is a complete block of AV conduction resulting in a 'dropped' QRS complex. After the dropped QRS the AV conduction returns to normal, then gradually increases again, starting the cycle over again. Second-degree heart block type I can be the result of myocarditis, myocardial ischemia, medication toxicity, and cardiac surgery. Specific treatment is not necessary unless there is significant bradycardia. Atropine or transcutaneous pacing can be used in the event of symptomatic bradycardia.

In second-degree heart block Mobitz type II, the PR interval remains normal with a QRS following each P-wave, until there is a 'dropped' QRS, where the P-wave is not conducted across the AV node and no QRS follows. QRS complexes are usually widened. If more than one P-wave is not conducted consecutively this is referred to as a 'high-grade' second-degree type II block. These blocks usually occur in the infranodal conducting system and can rapidly progress to a complete heart block. Second-degree Type II blocks are frequently associated with myocardial ischemia. Patients found to have a second-degree heart block type II should have external pacing pads applied in anticipation of a sudden deterioration to significant bradycardia, or progression to third-degree heart block. Even if there is no progression to third-degree heart block, permanent transvenous pacing is usually required.

In third-degree AV block (also known as AV dissociation or complete heart block), no P-waves are conducted to the ventricles at all. The atria beat at their intrinsic rate, and the ventricles contract at the idioventricular rate, with no relationship between P-waves and QRS complexes seen on ECG. The most common cause of third-degree heart block is myocardial ischemia, specifically in the left ventricle. Nodal third-degree heart block occurs when the blockage is at the level of the AV node: in these cases, the junctional pacemaker takes over and the QRS complex can be narrow. If the blockage is below the level of the node (infranodal) the QRS complex is wide and frequently very slow. This usually results in severe bradycardia with hemodynamic compromise and must be treated immediately. In any event, a patient with a third-degree heart block should have transcutaneous pacing pads put in place with anticipation of starting immediate pacing if signs/symptoms of hemodynamic instability appear.

Junctional bradycardia:
Junctional bradycardia, junctional rhythm, or junctional escape beats can occur if the discharge from the SA node is slowed or blocked from reaching the AV node and the intrinsic rate of the AV node (usually 40-60 beats/minute) takes over ventricular activation. No p-wave is seen, but the QRS complex is usually of normal duration. Junctional escape beats can occur with sinus bradycardia if the pause between beats is long enough, or after premature atrial beats. It can also be caused by digitalis toxicity, hypokalemia, heart failure, and myocarditis. Accelerated junctional beats or junctional tachycardia can occur from medication toxicity, inferior wall myocardial ischemia, and acute rheumatic fever. Digitalis toxicity can also produce junctional tachycardia as well as junctional bradycardia. Junctional escape beats do not usually require treatment, however, if necessary, atropine can be used to increase the rate by decreasing vagal tone. Transcutaneous pacing is also effective. Junctional tachycardia is best treated by identifying and treating the underlying cause.

Idioventricular rhythms:
Idioventricular rhythms originate from the ventricles and are seen on ECG as a wide QRS complex without evidence of atrial activity. The intrinsic rate of the ventricles is generally between 30 and 50 beats per minute, so idioventricular rhythms are normally bradycardic. Accelerated idioventricular rhythms can occur with rates of 50-120 beats per minute. Idioventricular rhythms are most frequently seen in the setting of acute myocardial infarction. Symptoms include weakness, dizziness, hypoperfusion, and chest pain. Accelerated idioventricular rhythms are seen in drug toxicity (digitalis, cocaine), myocarditis, and hyperkalemia. Accelerated idioventricular rhythms are frequently asymptomatic unless the patient requires an intact atrial function to maintain perfusion.

Treatment of symptomatic idioventricular rhythms generally relies on correcting the underlying cause. Symptomatic idioventricular bradycardias are unlikely to respond to atropine and are usually treated by transcutaneous pacing, with eventual conversion to transvenous pacing if needed. Importantly, accelerated idioventricular rhythms should not be treated with antiarrhythmic medications, as in the absence of any other pacemaker activity, this could lead to asystole.

Tachydysrhythmias:
Presentation: Tachycardia is defined as a ventricular heart rate greater than 100 beats per minute. In most cases, Tachydysrhythmias usually present with a pulse rate of greater than 100 beats per minute although in some cases (for example pulseless ventricular tachycardia and ventricular fibrillation) it may present with no pulse at all. Patients experiencing tachycardia may have no symptoms at all or may present with chest pain, shortness of breath, hypotension, altered mental status, or a subjective sensation of 'fluttering' in the chest.

Pathophysiology: Tachydysrhythmias are usually divided into supraventricular and ventricular. Supraventricular tachycardias (SVT) originate at or above the AV node, usually present with a narrow QRS complex (duration less than 100 milliseconds), and are called narrow-complex tachycardias.

Not all SVTs will present with a narrow complex tachycardia: in some cases, such as SVT with aberrant conduction, bundle–branch block, ventricular preexcitation syndrome (such as Wolff-Parkinson-White syndrome) SVT can present as a wide-complex tachycardia.

Ventricular tachycardias originate below the AV node in the ventricular myocardium, usually present with a wide QRS complex (duration over 100 milliseconds), and are referred to as wide-complex tachycardias.

Examination: Patients with tachycardia will generally have a pulse rate of greater than 100 beats per minute. ECG monitoring will usually show a heart rate of over 100 beats per minute and may be regular or irregular. Blood pressure can be normal but hypertension and hypotension can occur. Patients with pulseless ventricular tachycardia or ventricular fibrillation will be pulseless, apneic, have no detectable blood pressure, and be unresponsive.

Laboratory/Imaging: As with bradydysrhythmias, laboratory, and imaging are not usually required in the diagnosis of tachycardia. Lab studies and imaging may be useful to determine underlying pathology causing tachycardia such as ischemia or valve pathology.

Associated Symptoms/Conditions: Tachydysrhythmias can present with a variety of symptoms, or with none at all. Some patients will present with a subjective sensation of 'fluttering' or pounding sensation in the chest. Unstable tachycardias can present with chest pain, shortness of breath, hypotension, or altered mental status. Conditions associated with tachycardia include physiologic responses to exercise, anxiety, and fear: These tend to be self-limiting. Other conditions include pain, hyperpyrexia, hyperthyroidism, myocardial ischemia, hypoxia, pulmonary embolism, use of stimulants (especially cocaine or methamphetamine), and alcohol use/withdrawal.

Diagnosis: As with bradydysrhythmias, diagnosis of tachydysrhythmia is usually done by ECG, either 12-lead or rhythm strip. However, in cases of intermittent or paroxysmal tachydysrhythmias, it may be difficult to capture the dysrhythmia on ECG. Ambulatory ECG monitoring or cardiac event monitoring may be required in these cases. In some cases, formal cardiac electrophysiological studies may be required to elicit the type of dysrhythmia and its etiology.

Treatment: In cases of physiologic tachycardia, such as exercise-induced tachycardia, treatment is usually unnecessary. In cases where tachycardia is due to underlying pathologies, such as hyperthyroidism or alcohol withdrawal, treatment of the underlying pathology is required. If necessary, tachycardia in these cases can be controlled with beta-blockers or calcium channel blockers while the underlying problem is addressed.

Stable tachydysrhythmias are usually treated by treating the anatomical or physiological cause of the tachydysrhythmia. For supraventricular tachydysrhythmias, rate control with beta-blockers or calcium channel blockers may be needed. For ventricular tachycardias treatment with agents such as amiodarone may be required.
Treatment of tachycardia associated with anatomical variants such as accessory cardiac conduction pathways can be treated by determining the location of the pathway (usually by electrophysiologic studies) and if possible, treated by catheter-based ablation of the accessory pathway.

In cases of unstable tachydysrhythmias (where unstable is defined as being associated with chest pain, shortness of breath, or hypotension), immediate treatment with DC cardioversion is usually recommended.

In cases of pulseless ventricular tachycardia or ventricular fibrillation, treatment is immediate defibrillation, or if no defibrillator is on-hand, immediate initiation of high-quality CPR until a defibrillator is available.

Some of the common types of tachydysrhythmias and their treatment are noted below:

Stable narrow-complex tachycardia:
Stable narrow-complex tachycardia can be further divided into regular and irregular rhythms.

Regular narrow-complex tachycardia is initially treated by vagal maneuvers, which attempt to decrease the heart rate by increasing vagal tone. If vagal maneuvers are unsuccessful or unfeasible, then it can be treated by giving 6 mg adenosine IV push followed by 12 mg IV push if the rhythm does not convert.

If the rhythm converts to normal sinus rhythm with either vagal maneuvers or adenosine, it is likely that the underlying cause is an AV nodal reentrant tachycardia or an AV reentrant tachycardia. Rate control should then be possible by the use of AV nodal blocking agents such as beta-blockers or diltiazem. After control is achieved, then consideration of EP studies with accessory pathway ablation should be considered.

If two 12 mg doses of adenosine are unsuccessful in converting SVT, then heart rate control using beta-blockers or diltiazem may be needed.

In cases of irregular narrow complex tachycardia, the most likely rhythms are atrial fibrillation/atrial flutter with rapid ventricular response or multifocal atrial tachycardia. In these cases, rate control with beta-blockers or diltiazem is needed while addressing any underlying causes.

Sinus tachycardia:
In the majority of cases, sinus tachycardia is a physiologic response to increased demand for cardiac output. Sinus tachycardia is diagnosed by an ECG showing a normal sinus rhythm with a rate of over 100 beats per minute. Probably the most common cause of sinus tachycardia is exercise. Other, less benign causes include pain, fear,

anxiety, hyperthyroidism, shock, fever, drug abuse, hypoxia, anemia, and myocardial infarction. In most cases, the treatment of sinus tachycardia is to treat the underlying cause.

Paroxysmal Supraventricular Tachycardia:
Paroxysmal Supraventricular Tachycardia (PSVT) is a condition where there is a sudden onset and just as sudden cessation of atrial tachycardia. It is most common in young women but can occur in either sex at any age. Symptoms of PSVT are a sudden onset of palpitations and rapid heartbeat, frequently associated with lightheadedness, dizziness, and occasionally chest pain. Symptoms usually stop as abruptly as they began but can last from minutes to hours. Heart rates of over 170 beats per minute are not uncommon. ECG usually shows a rapid narrow-complex ventricular rate with no apparent sinus-type P waves or PR interval. The cause of the majority of PSVT is due to an atrioventricular nodal reentrant pathway (referred to as an 'atrioventricular nodal reentrant tachycardia', or AVNRT), where there is an accessory pathway to the AV node so that a cyclical reentry excitation can occur. Other causes include an ectopic atrial focus.

PSVT can frequently be terminated by vagal maneuvers, such as a Valsalva maneuver, carotid sinus massage, or cold-water facial immersion, particularly if these are done early in the episode. In cases where vagal maneuvers have been unsuccessful, adenosine is usually effective. In refractory cases, synchronized cardioversion may be necessary.

Multi-focal atrial tachycardia:
Multi-focal atrial tachycardia (MFAT) is defined as a tachycardia where there are three or more separate atrial foci competing to pace the ventricle. This usually presents as an irregular tachycardia that may be difficult to distinguish from atrial flutter or atrial fibrillation. ECG shows multiple different P-wave morphologies, with no consistent P to P or PR to PR intervals. There must be at least three different P-wave morphologies in a single ECG lead to diagnose MFAT. QRS complexes are usually normal, and the rhythm is usually irregularly irregular. MFAT is usually the result of severe chronic lung disease and can frequently signal decompensation. Treatment is to treat the underlying pathology; antiarrhythmic treatment is not usually effective unless underlying hypoxia and/or electrolyte abnormalities are corrected first. After these have been corrected, beta-blockers or calcium channel blockers can be considered.

Atrial fibrillation/flutter:
Atrial fibrillation is one of the most common supraventricular arrhythmias. It is classically associated with myocardial ischemia or valvular heart disease; however, it can also be caused by many other entities such as myocarditis, cardiomyopathy, binge alcohol drinking (so-called 'holiday heart syndrome'), chest trauma, and hyperthyroidism. Patients with left atrial enlargement are highly susceptible to chronic atrial fibrillation.

In atrial fibrillation, there are multiple areas of atrial myocardium with chaotic electrical discharges and contraction, leading to quivering atrial walls. There is no smooth, rhythmic contraction of the atria, which leads to ineffective ventricular filling and decreased cardiac output.

The symptom primarily associated with atrial fibrillation is an irregularly irregular heartbeat. Some patients are relatively asymptomatic; however, others who are reliant on atrial contraction to maintain cardiac output can have hypotension and symptoms of hypoperfusion. Ventricular response to atrial fibrillation is usually rapid, resulting in elevated heart rates. Clinical examination can show an irregularly irregular heartbeat auscultated with a pulse deficit noted at the wrist or carotid.

On ECG there is an irregularly irregular rate noted with no discernable P-waves, usually with a chaotic baseline. The ventricular rate is usually elevated and can be upwards of 120-170 beats per minute ('atrial fibrillation with a rapid ventricular response').

Atrial flutter is a condition where there is a rapid atrial rate, frequently 300 beats per minute. There is variable AV conduction, so the ventricular response could be 150 if there is a 2:1 conduction, or 100 if there is a 3:1 conduction. P-waves are present, but they are abnormal, and frequently found in a 'sawtooth' baseline. Atrial flutter usually has a regular ventricular rhythm.
In both atrial fibrillation and atrial flutter there is a loss of effective atrial contraction. In many cases, loss of effective left atrial contraction leads to decreased left ventricular filling, thus less cardiac output: this can precipitate hypotension, hypoperfusion, and heart failure in some patients. Patients with atrial fibrillation are highly susceptible to both arterial and venous thromboembolism, which can result in strokes and pulmonary emboli.

The treatment of atrial fibrillation is complicated and dependent on many individual factors: no two patients are alike. In general, there are three issues that must be addressed: rate control, rhythm control/conversion, and anticoagulation.

In unstable patients with acute onset of atrial fibrillation with a rapid ventricular response, treatment is urgent and involves synchronized cardioversion, preferably after anticoagulation.

Unstable patients with long-duration atrial fibrillation may not respond to cardioversion so resuscitation with rate control, anticoagulation (if not already anticoagulated) and life support measures should be done.

In stable patients with acute onset of atrial fibrillation, treatment can be via rate control or via rhythm conversion. If rate control is chosen, the ventricular rate is controlled by diltiazem or by beta-blockers, anticoagulation is initiated, and the patient is re-evaluated in several weeks for elective cardioversion. If rhythm control is chosen, synchronized cardioversion can be done with adequate sedation, or pharmacologic conversion with ibutilide, procainamide, or flecainide can be attempted.

Atrial fibrillation can lead to the formation of atrial thrombi in the right or left atria. If an atrial thrombus has formed, conversion from atrial fibrillation to sinus rhythm can propel the thrombus into the pulmonary or systemic circulation. The risk of thrombus formation increases with the duration of the dysrhythmia. In general, atrial fibrillation of longer than 48 hours duration should not be converted to normal sinus rhythm until the patient has been anticoagulated for 3-4 weeks.

Wide-complex tachycardia:
Wide complex tachycardias present with a QRS complex greater than 100 milliseconds and a ventricular rate of greater than 100. Wide complex tachycardias include ventricular tachycardia, ventricular fibrillation, and supraventricular tachycardia with aberrant conduction. Wide-complex tachycardias are considered more dangerous than narrow-complex tachycardias and are usually treated more aggressively.

Ventricular fibrillation/pulseless ventricular tachycardia:
Ventricular fibrillation is chaotic electrical activity in the ventricular myocardium leading to disorganized, asynchronous contraction of the ventricular myocardium. Instead of a smooth, rhythmic contraction, there are rapid, ineffective fasciculations of the ventricular myocardium with no effective cardiac contraction. A patient with ventricular fibrillation has zero cardiac output, no blood pressure, and no pulse. Patients with ventricular fibrillation are unconscious and unresponsive. Ventricular tachycardia without a pulse (see below) is considered to be ventricular fibrillation and is treated the same.

The etiology of ventricular fibrillation is generally due to cardiac ischemia, particularly as a result of blockage of the left anterior descending coronary artery. It is the most common cause of sudden cardiac death in coronary artery disease. Other causes are electrical shock (especially with alternating current), and blunt trauma to the chest (commotio cordis).

Treatment of ventricular fibrillation is by immediate cardiopulmonary resuscitation followed by rapid defibrillation. Time for defibrillation is the most important variable in survival from ventricular fibrillation, which has resulted in the widespread placement of automatic external defibrillators (AEDs). Once advanced life support is available, the primary treatment of ventricular fibrillation is still defibrillation. If that is unsuccessful, medications such as amiodarone, lidocaine, or procainamide can be administered. If defibrillation is successful, amiodarone, lidocaine, or procainamide can be used to raise the ventricular fibrillation threshold and prevent a recurrence. However, the key to successful resuscitation from ventricular fibrillation remains immediate CPR followed by defibrillation as soon as possible.

Unstable wide-complex tachycardia:
Unstable wide-complex tachycardia is treated according to the degree of instability present. For example, a patient with ventricular tachycardia without a pulse is treated as if they have ventricular fibrillation, with immediate CPR followed by defibrillation as rapidly as possible. However, if there is a pulse present, but the patient with ventricular tachycardia is unstable, they are treated by synchronized cardioversion. In fact, for any unstable tachycardia (other than pulseless ventricular tachycardia), the treatment of choice is immediate synchronized cardioversion.

Ventricular tachycardia:
Ventricular tachycardia is defined as a sequence of three or more consecutive depolarizations from an ectopic ventricular source at a rate of 100 beats per minute or greater. It is most commonly due to cardiac ischemia or infarction, although valvular heart disease, cardiomyopathy hypoxia, and hyperkalemia are other causes. As it is arising from ectopic ventricular foci, it is seen as a wide-complex QRS on ECG. There are other conditions such as SVT with aberrant conduction that can mimic ventricular tachycardia, and diagnosis based on ECG can be challenging.

Ventricular tachycardia can present as pulseless, unstable, and stable. As noted above, the treatment for pulseless ventricular tachycardia is the same as for ventricular fibrillation, i.e. immediate CPR with defibrillation as soon as possible. The treatment of unstable ventricular tachycardia is synchronized cardioversion (with or without sedation depending on the condition of the patient). Stable ventricular tachycardia can be treated with amiodarone, lidocaine, or procainamide. A variant of ventricular tachycardia, torsades de pointes, can be treated with magnesium IV.

Stable ventricular tachycardia:
As noted above, ventricular tachycardia can be found in a hemodynamically stable patient. In such cases, treatment is with amiodarone, lidocaine, or procainamide.

SVT with aberrant conduction:
Not all wide-complex tachycardias are due to ventricular beats. In some cases, supraventricular tachycardia with aberrant conduction can present as a wide complex tachycardia. The most common presentation of this is Wolff-Parkinson-White syndrome (WPW syndrome).

WPW syndrome is a ventricular preexcitation syndrome caused by an accessory conduction pathway that bypasses the AV node, creating a direct connection between the atria and ventricles. It is normally found on an ECG while the patient is in sinus rhythm. The WPW ECG is characterized by a short PR interval (less than 120 milliseconds), a 'slurring' of the initial QRS called a delta wave, and a slightly widened QRS complex.

WPW can cause atrial fibrillation, but its most common presentation is with atrioventricular reciprocating tachycardia (AVRT). This presents most commonly as a narrow-complex tachycardia, but in some cases can be present as a wide-complex tachycardia.

Narrow-complex AVRT in WPW syndrome is treated as with any narrow-complex tachycardia, with vagal maneuvers, adenosine, and AV nodal blocking agents such as beta-blockers or calcium channel blockers.

Wide-complex tachycardia in WPW syndrome is known as antidromic AV reciprocating tachycardia. There is anterograde conduction down the accessory pathways and retrograde conduction of the impulse up to the atria via the AV node. This results in a very rapid wide-complex tachycardia that can be difficult to differentiate from ventricular tachycardia. The clinical significance of wide-complex tachycardia in WPW syndrome is that the use of agents that can block conduction in the AV node or enhance conduction in the accessory tract is contraindicated: this includes adenosine, amiodarone, calcium channel blockers, and beta-blockers. The treatment of choice in wide-complex tachycardia or atrial fibrillation secondary to WPW syndrome is synchronized cardioversion or procainamide.

General Treatment Strategies for Arrhythmias:
The widely used Singh-Vaughan Williams classification system groups antiarrhythmic medications into four classes based on their mechanism of action:

Class 1 antiarrhythmics block sodium channels. They are further subdivided into 1a, 1b, and 1c groups based on their effects on the action potential duration and their robustness of sodium channel blockade. Class 1a medications increase the duration of the action potential and exhibit moderate blockade of sodium channels; class 1b reduces the duration of the action potential and are weak sodium channel blockers, and class 1c has no effect on the action potential duration and is strong sodium channel blockers.

Class 2 antiarrhythmics antagonize beta-adrenergic (β_1) receptors in the heart, which slows conduction velocity through the AV node and decreases automaticity.

Class 3 antiarrhythmics prolong the duration of the action potential, generally through blockade of the rapid component of the delayed rectifier potassium current, I_{Kr} (although ibutilide blocks sodium channels).

Class 4 antiarrhythmics block calcium channels, which slows conduction in the SA and AV nodes.

Importantly, many antiarrhythmics exhibit activity of more than one class, such as amiodarone, which possesses class 1, 2, 3, and 4 activities. Thus, medications are classified according to their predominant mechanism of action. Additionally, some antiarrhythmics, like adenosine, do not fall into any of the Singh-Vaughan Williams classes.

Pharmacological Treatment of Arrhythmias:

Disopyramide
Disopyramide is a class 1a antiarrhythmic which decreases the rate of diastolic depolarization, decreases the upstroke velocity, and increases the action potential duration of cardiac cells. It lengthens the effective refractory period of the atria while having little effect on the refractory period of the AV node. Disopyramide has significant antimuscarinic activity in the heart and negative inotropic effects. In the U.S., disopyramide is only available in an oral formulation, which is rapidly and almost completely absorbed from the GI tract. Approximately 50% of a given dose is excreted unchanged in the urine, while the other 50% is metabolized to inactive metabolites by the liver, which is then also renally excreted. Renal impairment increases the elimination half-life of the drug, and heart failure increases both its peak serum concentration (C_{max}) and the time required to reach peak serum concentration (T_{max}). Because of its negative inotropic properties, disopyramide may precipitate heart failure or exacerbate pre-existing heart failure, and

its use should generally be avoided in patients with heart failure. Since disopyramide lengthens the QT interval, it is contraindicated in patients with congenital QT prolongation. Other adverse effects are mainly due to either negative inotropy or anticholinergic effects and include hypotension, dry mouth, urinary retention, constipation, and worsening of glaucoma. Although it is effective in the treatment of a variety of supraventricular arrhythmias, disopyramide is only approved for the treatment of life-threatening ventricular arrhythmias (e.g., sustained ventricular tachycardia). It is sometimes used off-label for the maintenance of sinus rhythm in patients with atrial fibrillation, usually in combination with ventricular rate-controlling medications.

Procainamide

Procainamide is a class 1a antiarrhythmic, though its metabolite, *N*-acetylprocainamide (NAPA), also has class 3 activity. It increases the effective refractory period of the atria and ventricles, thereby slowing conduction velocity. It also increases the threshold for myocardial excitation, which decreases myocardial excitability. Procainamide is available in both parenteral formulations and an oral formulation that is 75-95% bioavailable. It is hepatically metabolized to NAPA, and the amount of an administered dose that is converted to NAPA ranges from 16 to 21 percent in "slow acetylators" to 24 to 33 percent in "fast-acetylators". Both procainamide and NAPA are primarily eliminated by the kidneys, so the procainamide dose must be reduced in patients with renal impairment. Procainamide has a boxed warning for causing positive anti-nuclear antibody tests with prolonged administration, and in around 20% of patients per year, this is accompanied by a lupus erythematosus-like syndrome consisting of arthralgia, pleural or abdominal pain, and sometimes arthritis, pleural effusion, and pericarditis. Other adverse effects associated with procainamide include hypotension, rash, nausea, diarrhea, and rarely, agranulocytosis. Procainamide is contraindicated in patients with complete heart block, torsade des pointes, and an established diagnosis of systemic lupus erythematosus. Although procainamide is effective against most atrial and ventricular arrhythmias, its proarrhythmic properties and high incidence of lupus-like syndrome with prolonged administration limit its uses. The intravenous formulation of procainamide is used in the treatment of sustained ventricular arrhythmias associated with acute myocardial infarction, although other agents, such as lidocaine and amiodarone are preferred. Oral procainamide is rarely used.

Quinidine

Quinidine is an antimalarial and a class 1a antiarrhythmic with mechanisms of action similar to procainamide. It slows conduction and prolongs the action potential duration by blockade of sodium, potassium, and calcium channels. Like disopyramide, quinidine has antimuscarinic actions in the heart, although they are less pronounced. IV quinidine is no longer available in the USA. Oral quinidine is readily absorbed from the GI tract and is extensively hepatically metabolized to inactive metabolites which are excreted in the urine. Quinidine has marked proarrhythmic effects and can cause QT prolongation, which may progress to torsade de pointes. Quinidine carries a boxed warning for increased mortality based on the results of two meta-analyses, one of which showed a risk of death approximately three times higher in the quinidine group than in the placebo group. Other adverse effects associated with quinidine use include cinchonism (usually with chronic use of high doses), fever, diarrhea, and rarely, hepatitis, dermatitis, and visual disturbances. Due to its proarrhythmic effects, quinidine has been largely replaced by safer antiarrhythmics and nonpharmacological treatments. It is indicated for patients with Brugada syndrome who are not good ICD candidates or who are experiencing symptomatic ventricular arrhythmias in spite of ICD placement.

Lidocaine

Lidocaine is a class 1b antiarrhythmic that exerts its action by blocking activated and inactivated sodium channels, thereby decreasing the action potential duration and effective refractory period of Purkinje fibers and ventricular cardiac myocytes. It also raises the ventricular fibrillation threshold. Lidocaine is rapidly and extensively metabolized by the liver, which necessitates parenteral administration. Lidocaine has a duration of action of 10-20 minutes and an elimination half-life of 1.5-2 hours following an IV bolus administration. Liver disease may increase the half-life of lidocaine by twofold or more, and conditions that alter blood flow to the liver, such as heart failure or shock may similarly increase the half-life. Most of the lidocaine's adverse effects are neurologic in nature and include light-headedness, apprehension, dizziness, tremors, and convulsions. Proarrhythmic effects are less common with lidocaine than with other antiarrhythmics, but cardiovascular effects like hypotension and bradycardia can occur with high doses. Lidocaine is used in the acute management of ventricular arrhythmias such as pulseless ventricular tachycardia or cardiac arrest due to ventricular fibrillation. Although once used prophylactically to reduce ventricular fibrillation during acute myocardial infarction, lidocaine was found to increase mortality in this setting and is no longer used for this indication.

Mexiletine

Mexiletine is a class 1b antiarrhythmic that is structurally and functionally similar to lidocaine but orally active. Mexiletine is ~90% absorbed from the GI tract, but, unlike lidocaine, its first-pass metabolism is low. It has a half-life of 10-12 hours, which is approximately doubled in the setting of moderate to severe hepatic impairment. The most commonly reported adverse effect associated with the use of mexiletine is nausea, followed by dizziness, tremor, and nervousness. It can rarely cause hepatotoxicity and blood dyscrasias. Mexiletine is used in the treatment of ventricular arrhythmias such as long QT syndrome type 3.

Flecainide

Flecainide is a class 1c antiarrhythmic that slows conduction in cardiac tissue by blocking sodium and potassium channels. It decreases conduction in all parts of the heart but exhibits the greatest effect on the His-Purkinje system. Flecainide does not prolong the action potential or the QT interval, and it has no antimuscarinic effects. The absorption of flecainide following oral administration is nearly 100%, although milk may decrease its absorption. The half-life of flecainide is ~20 hours but is quite variable (ranging from 12-27 hours in adults). Approximately 30% of a given dose is excreted unchanged in the urine, the remainder having been converted to weakly active or inactive metabolites by the liver prior to renal excretion. Flecainide has a boxed warning for increased mortality because of the results of the Cardiac Arrhythmia Suppression Trial (CAST), which was terminated prematurely due to a more than twofold increase in mortality in patients treated with flecainide compared with placebo. Flecainide use is contraindicated in patients with heart block or chronic atrial fibrillation, and according to the American College of Cardiology/American Heart Association/European Society of Cardiology, its use is also contraindicated in patients with ischemia, prior MI, and structural heart disease. Adverse effects associated with flecainide use include dizziness, dyspnea, and visual disturbances. Flecainide is indicated to prevent paroxysmal atrial fibrillation/flutter and paroxysmal supraventricular tachycardias associated with disabling symptoms; it is also approved to prevent life-threatening ventricular tachycardias.

Propafenone

Propafenone is a class 1c antiarrhythmic with local anesthetic effects that reduce the upstroke velocity of the action potential, blocks the fast inward sodium current, and prolongs the effective refractory period. It also exhibits weak β-blocking activity due to structural similarities to propranolol. Orally administered propafenone is almost completely absorbed but exhibits dose-dependent bioavailability; i.e., larger doses have higher absolute bioavailability than do smaller doses. There are also two genetic variations in propafenone metabolism. In over 90% of patients, it is metabolized into two active metabolites by the CYP450 enzymes, with an elimination half-life of 2-10 hours. In less than 10% of patients, the ability to form one of the two metabolites is diminished or absent, resulting in an extended half-life. Severe liver dysfunction markedly increases the bioavailability of propafenone, and close monitoring of patients with hepatic impairment is recommended. The most commonly reported adverse effects of propafenone are an unusual taste, nausea/vomiting, and constipation. It can also cause exacerbation of heart failure and new or worsened arrhythmias. Propafenone is indicated to prolong the time to recurrence of paroxysmal atrial fibrillation/flutter (PAF) or paroxysmal supraventricular tachycardia (PSVT) in patients with disabling symptoms without structural heart disease. It can also be used in the treatment of life-threatening ventricular arrhythmias.

Esmolol

Esmolol is a short-acting class 2 antiarrhythmic (β-blocker) that is given IV and used to gain rapid control of ventricular rate in patients with atrial fibrillation or atrial flutter in perioperative, postoperative, or other emergent circumstances. It is also indicated for the short-term treatment of tachycardia and hypertension that occur during surgery or anesthesia.

Propranolol

Propranolol is a non-cardioselective β-blocker that has a wide variety of labeled and off-label indications, including migraine prophylaxis, essential tremor, and performance anxiety. It is used to control supraventricular and ventricular tachycardias. Following oral administration, propranolol is completely absorbed and extensively metabolized by the liver into active and inactive metabolites. The metabolites are excreted by the kidneys with an elimination half-life of 3-6 hours for the immediate release formulation. Propranolol should be used with caution in patients with hepatic or renal impairment. Adverse effects are similar to other β-blockers and include bronchospasm, new or worsening heart failure, and bradycardia/heart block.

Nadolol

Nadolol is a non-cardioselective β-blocker with mechanisms of action similar to those of propranolol and sotalol. Unlike propranolol and sotalol, nadolol is only about 30% absorbed following oral administration. It is not metabolized by the liver but is excreted unchanged by the kidneys. It has a longer elimination half-life than any other available beta antagonist (20-24 hours), which allows for once-daily dosing. Dosage adjustments are necessary for patients with renal impairment. Like other β-blockers, nadolol can cause bronchospasm, heart failure, and bradycardia/heart block. Although nadolol does not have a labeled indication for arrhythmias, it is used off-label in the treatment of both supraventricular and ventricular tachycardias.

Sotalol

Sotalol is formulated as a racemic mixture that has both class 2 (in the L-isomer) and class 3 (in both the D- and L-isomers) activity. The results of its class 2 (beta-blockade) activity are slowed heart rate, decreased AV nodal conduction, and increased AV nodal refractoriness. The class 3 electrophysiological effects include prolongation of the action potential and effective refractory period in both atria and ventricles. Following oral administration, it is almost 100% absorbed and is not metabolized by the liver. It is excreted unchanged by the kidneys with an elimination half-life of 12 hours. Dosage adjustments must be made in the setting of renal impairment, and sotalol is contraindicated in patients with CrCl < 40 mL/min. The most serious adverse effect of sotalol use is an increased risk of ventricular arrhythmias, including Torsades de Pointes, due to sotalol's prolongation of the QT interval. Other adverse effects related to sotalol's beta-blocking activity are new or worsened heart failure, bradycardia, and heart block. Because the beta-blocking of activity is not cardioselective, this medication should be avoided in patients with bronchospastic diseases to prevent inhibition of bronchodilation mediated by β_2 receptors. Sotalol is indicated for the maintenance of normal sinus rhythm in patients with symptomatic atrial fibrillation or flutter and in the treatment of life-threatening ventricular arrhythmias.

Amiodarone

As a class 3 antiarrhythmic, amiodarone mainly exerts its effects on the heart by blocking I_{Kr}, although it also blocks sodium channels significantly and adrenergic and calcium channels weakly. The net effect of amiodarone is to prolong the cardiac refractory period. Amiodarone is available in both oral and IV formulations. Orally dosed amiodarone is absorbed slowly from the gastrointestinal tract, with a bioavailability of ~50%. The rate and extent of absorption are increased by food. The onset of action is approximately 2-3 weeks, and the mean half-life associated with consistent oral therapy is 40-55 days. Amiodarone is metabolized by the liver to an active metabolite, N-desethylamiodarone, and this metabolite is excreted into the bile and eliminated primarily in the feces. Amiodarone is a substrate of CYP3A4 and an inhibitor of several P450 enzymes, which results in many significant drug interactions. Although no specific guidelines exist, it is likely that dosage adjustments should be made in the setting of hepatic impairment. Amiodarone has a boxed warning for several potentially fatal toxicities, the most common of which is pulmonary toxicity. The incidence of hypersensitivity pneumonitis or interstitial/alveolar pneumonitis has been as high as 10-17% in some studies and is fatal about 10% of the time. In addition to pulmonary toxicity, amiodarone also carries a boxed warning for liver injury (which normally manifests as elevated liver enzymes but can rarely result in overt liver disease) and symptomatic bradycardia and heart block (particularly in patients with preexisting sinus or AV node disease). Amiodarone accumulates in the skin, which can cause photosensitivity and a blue-gray discoloration of the skin in areas exposed to the sun. Micro-deposits of amiodarone occur in the corneas of most patients, and although visual acuity is not typically affected, some patients develop optic neuritis that can progress to blindness. Amiodarone contains iodine and also blocks the peripheral conversion of thyroxine (T_4) to triiodothyronine (T_3); for these reasons, it can cause either hyperthyroidism or hypothyroidism. Because of its significant toxicities, some of which can be life-threatening, amiodarone is only indicated for the treatment of recurrent ventricular fibrillation and recurrent hemodynamically unstable ventricular tachycardia in patients refractory to or intolerant of other antiarrhythmics. Despite the limited spectrum of labeled indications, amiodarone is used off-label to maintain normal sinus rhythm in patients with atrial fibrillation and as an adjunct treatment in patients with ventricular tachycardia and implanted cardioverter-defibrillators (ICDs) to decrease the frequency of painful shocks delivered by the ICD. Amiodarone is contraindicated in patients who have cardiogenic shock, severe sinus-node dysfunction, second- or third-degree AV block, or hypersensitivity to iodine. Several monitoring parameters are required at the initiation of amiodarone and periodically during treatment, including pulmonary function tests, liver function tests, thyroid function tests, chest X-rays, and ophthalmic exams.

Dronedarone

Dronedarone is a structural analog of amiodarone which lacks iodine atoms and has a methanesulfonyl group. These changes were intended to prevent effects on thyroxine metabolism and reduce the half-life of the drug. Dronedarone is available only as an oral tablet, and bioavailability is increased threefold when the tablet is taken with a high-fat meal. The half-life of dronedarone is much shorter than that of amiodarone (13-19 hours). The drug is metabolized extensively by the liver and is primarily eliminated in the feces. Since dronedarone is a substrate and an inhibitor of CYP3A4, it interacts with other medications that are substrates of or affect the activity of this enzyme. Although dronedarone has not been associated with thyroid dysfunction and appears to be less likely to cause pulmonary toxicity, it does have many adverse effects, some of which are serious. The ANDROMEDA trial found that dronedarone doubled the risk of death in patients hospitalized with symptomatic heart failure and severe left ventricular systolic dysfunction. The PALLAS trial showed that dronedarone doubles the risk of death, stroke, and hospitalization for heart failure in patients with high-risk permanent AF. As a result of these trials, dronedarone carries a boxed warning for increased risk of death in patients with decompensated heart failure and increased risk of death, stroke, and heart failure in patients with permanent atrial fibrillation, and use is contraindicated in these patients. Other significant adverse effects associated with the use of dronedarone are liver injury (including acute liver failure requiring transplant), increases in serum creatinine, and QT interval prolongation. Dronedarone is pregnancy category X based on observed teratogenicity in rats. Dronedarone is only indicated to reduce the risk of hospitalization for atrial fibrillation in patients in sinus rhythm with a history of paroxysmal or persistent atrial fibrillation.

Dofetilide

Dofetilide is a class 3 antiarrhythmic that exerts its effects by blockade of the rapid component of the delayed rectifier potassium current (I_{Kr}). Dofetilide is 100% bioavailable after oral administration, and 80% is excreted unchanged by the kidneys. The elimination half-life is approximately 10 hours, but this can be increased in the setting of renal impairment or in the presence of inhibitors of the renal cation transport system like cimetidine. Because the proarrhythmic qualities of dofetilide, such as Torsade de Pointes, are directly related to plasma concentration, the dosage must be based on creatinine clearance. Administration of dofetilide should be initiated in a facility that can measure baseline QT interval for three days, and creatine clearance must be calculated before initiation. Severe renal impairment (CrCl < 20mL/min) is a contraindication to dofetilide use, as are hypokalemia and baseline QTc >440 msec (500 msec in patients with ventricular conduction abnormalities). Dofetilide is indicated for the maintenance of normal sinus rhythm in patients with symptomatic atrial fibrillation or atrial flutter and can also be used to restore normal sinus rhythm in patients with atrial fibrillation/flutter.

Ibutilide

Ibutilide is a class 3 antiarrhythmic that delays repolarization by activation of a slow, inward sodium current. This mechanism differs from that of most class 3 drugs, which exert their antiarrhythmic effects by blocking outward potassium currents. Although ibutilide also inhibits the rapid component of I_{Kr}, the relative contribution of this mechanism to the antiarrhythmic activity of ibutilide is not known. Ibutilide is administered IV and rapidly metabolized by the liver to mostly inactive metabolites. These metabolites are primarily excreted in the urine, with an average elimination half-life of six hours that varies widely between individual patients (ranging from 2-12 hours). Ibutilide is indicated for the conversion of new-onset atrial fibrillation or atrial flutter to normal sinus rhythm. Since ibutilide can cause potentially fatal arrhythmias like sustained polymorphic ventricular tachycardia, patients must be observed with continuous ECG monitoring for at least 4 hours following infusion or until QTc has returned to baseline.

Diltiazem

Diltiazem is a class 4 antiarrhythmic that blocks L-type calcium channels on cardiac and smooth muscle cells, thereby inhibiting the influx of calcium ions that occurs during membrane depolarization. This results in the prolongation of AV nodal conduction time and effective refractory period, as well as dilation of coronary arteries (giving diltiazem antianginal effects). It is available as both an IV and an oral formulation, which have different labeled indications. Diltiazem tablets are indicated for the management of chronic stable angina and vasospastic angina but are used off-label for chronic rate control in patients with atrial fibrillation/atrial flutter. IV diltiazem is indicated for temporary control of rapid ventricular rate in patients with atrial fibrillation/atrial flutter and rapid conversion of paroxysmal supraventricular tachycardias to normal sinus rhythm. Oral diltiazem is well absorbed from the gastrointestinal tract and is subject to extensive first-pass metabolism, which gives it an absolute oral bioavailability of about 40%. The elimination half-life of IV or immediate-release oral diltiazem is 3-5 hours. Metabolites are excreted in the urine and feces. Although no specific dosage recommendations are given in the prescribing information, caution is advised when administering diltiazem to patients with renal or hepatic impairment. Diltiazem can cause bradycardia, heart block, cutaneous hypersensitivity reactions, and rarely, acute hepatic injury.

Verapamil

Verapamil is a class 4 antiarrhythmic with a mechanism of action identical to that of diltiazem. Like diltiazem, it is available as both an oral and an IV formulation, and the indications differ depending on the formulation. The IV formulation is indicated for rapid conversion to sinus rhythm of paroxysmal supraventricular tachycardias, although it seems to be less effective than diltiazem in this setting. The IV formulation can also be used to gain temporary control of rapid ventricular rate in atrial flutter and/or atrial fibrillation, except when these conditions are associated with accessory pathways, as in Wolff-Parkinson-White syndrome. The oral formulation is indicated for angina, control of ventricular rate in atrial fibrillation/flutter, hypertension, and prophylaxis of supraventricular tachycardia. Like diltiazem, orally administered verapamil is well-absorbed but subject to extensive first-pass metabolism. Norverapamil, a metabolite of verapamil, is weakly active. Metabolites are excreted in the urine and feces with an elimination half-life of 2.8-7.4 hours. The half-life may be increased by repetitive dosing and hepatic impairment and is also increased in the elderly. The dose of verapamil given to patients with severe hepatic impairment should be approximately 30% of the dose given to patients with normal liver function. Due to its negative inotropic and vasodilatory properties, verapamil can precipitate acute decompensation in patients with left ventricular dysfunction and should be avoided in patients with an ejection fraction of less than 30%. Other adverse effects include hypotension, bradycardia, heart block, and elevated liver enzymes.

Adenosine

Adenosine is a nucleoside that occurs in all cells of the body. Exogenous adenosine has antiarrhythmic properties that do not fall into any of the Singh-Vaughan Williams classes. Its mechanism of action involves the activation of an inward rectifier K^+ current and inhibition of calcium current, thereby slowing conduction through the AV node and prolonging the AV nodal refractory period. Adenosine is given as an IV bolus which is rapidly cleared from the circulation by cellular uptake, with a half-life of fewer than ten seconds. Because it is not metabolized by the liver nor excreted by the kidneys, hepatic and renal dysfunction does not affect dosing. Flushing, chest pain, and dyspnea occur commonly with adenosine administration and may persist for up to 24 hours after the infusion is complete. Adenosine is highly effective in the acute treatment of paroxysmal supraventricular tachycardia and is currently the drug of choice for this indication.

Atropine

Atropine is an anticholinergic medication rather than an antiarrhythmic but is included in this chapter because it is used in the treatment of bradyasystolic cardiac arrest. Atropine exerts its antiarrhythmic effects by antagonizing muscarinic acetylcholine receptors on cardiac myocytes, thereby abolishing parasympathetic slowing of the heart rate. Atropine is given as an IV bolus which is rapidly distributed throughout the body and metabolized by the liver via enzymatic hydrolysis to inactive metabolites. Between 13 and 50% of the administered dose is excreted unchanged in the urine along with the metabolites. Atropine can cause a variety of arrhythmias, as well as agitation, delirium, hot/flushed skin, dry mouth, and mydriasis.

References

Al-Khatib, S. M., Stevenson, W. G., Ackerman, M. J., Bryant, W. J., Callans, D. J., Curtis, A. B., Deal, B. J., Dickfeld, T., Field, M. E., Fonarow, G. C., Gillis, A. M., Granger, C. B., Hammill, S. C., Hlatky, M. A., Joglar, J. A., Kay, G. N., Matlock, D. D., Myerburg, R. J., & Page, R. L. (2018). 2017 AHA/ACC/HRS Guideline for Management of Patients with Ventricular Arrhythmias and the Prevention of Sudden Cardiac Death. *Circulation, 138*(13). https://doi.org/10.1161/cir.0000000000000549.

Arnaud, L., Mertz, P., Gavand, P. E., Martin, T., Chasset, F., Tebacher-Alt, M., Lambert, A., Muller, C., Sibilia, J., Lebrun-Vignes, B., & Salem, J. E. (2019). Drug-induced systemic lupus: revisiting the ever-changing spectrum of the disease using the WHO pharmacovigilance database. *Annals of the Rheumatic Diseases*, *78*(4), 504–508. https://doi.org/10.1136/annrheumdis-2018-214598.

Boehringer-Ingelheim. Flecainide [package insert]. U.S. Food and Drug Administration website. https://www.accessdata.fda.gov/drugsatfda_docs/label/2013/019151s012lbl.pdf. Accessed April 30, 2022.

Boehringer-Ingelheim. Mexitil (mexiletine) [package insert]. Boerhinger-Ingelheim website. https://docs.boehringer-ingelheim.com/Prescribing%20Information/ PIs/Mexitil%20Caps/Mexitil.pdf. Accessed April 30, 2022.

Brady WJ, Glass III GF. Cardiac Rhythm Disturbances. In: Tintinalli JE, Ma O, Yealy DM, Meckler GD, Stapczynski J, Cline DM, Thomas SH. eds. *Tintinalli's Emergency Medicine: A Comprehensive Study Guide, 9e*. McGraw Hill; 2020. https://accessmedicine.mhmedical.com/content.aspx?bookid=2353&sectionid=218687685.

Connolly, S. J., Camm, A. J., Halperin, J. L., Joyner, C., Alings, M., Amerena, J., Atar, D., Avezum, L., Blomström, P., Borggrefe, M., Budaj, A., Chen, S. A., Ching, C. K., Commerford, P., Dans, A., Davy, J. M., Delacrétaz, E., di Pasquale, G., Diaz, R., . . . Hohnloser, S. H. (2011). Dronedarone in High-Risk Permanent Atrial Fibrillation. *New England Journal of Medicine*, *365*(24), 2268–2276. https://doi.org/10.1056/nejmoa1109867.

Coplen, S. E., Antman, E. M., Berlin, J. A., Hewitt, P., & Chalmers, T. C. (1990). Efficacy and safety of quinidine therapy for maintenance of sinus rhythm after cardioversion. A meta-analysis of randomized control trials. *Circulation*, *82*(4), 1106–1116. https://doi.org/10.1161/01.cir.82.4.1106.

Echt, D. S., Liebson, P. R., Mitchell, L. B., Peters, R. W., Obias-Manno, D., Barker, A. H., Arensberg, D., Baker, A., Friedman, L., Greene, H. L., Huther, M. L., & Richardson, D. W. (1991). Mortality and Morbidity in Patients Receiving Encainide, Flecainide, or Placebo. *New England Journal of Medicine*, *324*(12), 781–788. https://doi.org/10.1056/nejm199103213241201.

Giardina, E. G. V. (1984). Procainamide: Clinical Pharmacology and Efficacy against Ventricular Arrhythmias. *Annals of the New York Academy of Sciences*, *432*(1 Clinical Phar), 177–188. https://doi.org/10.1111/j.1749-6632.1984.tb14519.x.

GlaxoSmithKline. Rythmol (propafenone) [package insert]. U.S. Food and Drug Administration website. https://www.accessdata.fda.gov/drugsatfda_docs/label/2013/019151s012lbl.pdf. Accessed May 2, 2022.

Grandi, E., & Ripplinger, C. M. (2019). Antiarrhythmic mechanisms of beta blocker therapy. *Pharmacological Research*, *146*, 104274. https://doi.org/10.1016/j.phrs.2019.104274.

Kirchhof, P., Camm, A. J., Goette, A., Brandes, A., Eckardt, L., Elvan, A., Fetsch, T., van Gelder, I. C., Haase, D., Haegeli, L. M., Hamann, F., Heidbüchel, H., Hindricks, G., Kautzner, J., Kuck, K. H., Mont, L., Ng, G. A., Rekosz, J., Schoen, N., . . . Breithardt, G. (2020). Early Rhythm-Control Therapy in Patients with Atrial Fibrillation. *New England Journal of Medicine*, *383*(14), 1305–1316. https://doi.org/10.1056/nejmoa2019422.

Køber, L., Torp-Pedersen, C., McMurray, J. J., Gøtzsche, O., Lévy, S., Crijns, H., Amlie, J., & Carlsen, J. (2008). Increased Mortality after Dronedarone Therapy for Severe Heart Failure. *New England Journal of Medicine*, *358*(25), 2678–2687. https://doi.org/10.1056/nejmoa0800456.

Lei, M., Wu, L., Terrar, D. A., & Huang, C. L. H. (2018). Modernized Classification of Cardiac Antiarrhythmic Drugs. *Circulation*, *138*(17), 1879–1896. https://doi.org/10.1161/circulationaha.118.035455.

Meridian Medical Technologies, Inc. Atropine [package insert]. U.S. Food and Drug Administration website. https://www.accessdata.fda.gov/drugsatfda_docs/label/2015/021146s015lbl.pdf. Accessed May 19, 2022.

Pfizer Inc. Adenosine [package insert]. U.S. Food and Drug Administration website. https://www.accessdata.fda.gov/drugsatfda_docs/label/2011/019937s026lbl.pdf. Accessed May 12, 2022.

Pfizer Inc. Calan SR (verapamil) [package insert]. U.S. Food and Drug Administration website. https://www.accessdata.fda.gov/drugsatfda_docs/label/2017/019152s041lbl.pdf. Accessed May 14, 2022.

Pfizer Inc. Corvert (ibutilide) [package insert]. Pfizer medical information website. https://labeling.pfizer.com/showlabeling.aspx?id=673. Accessed April 17, 2022.

Pfizer Inc. Lidocaine [package insert]. Pfizer medical information website.

https://labeling.pfizer.com/ShowLabeling.aspx?id=4497. Accessed April 27, 2022.

Pfizer Inc. Norpace (disopyramide) [package insert]. Pfizer medical information website. https://labeling.pfizer.com/ShowLabeling.aspx?format=PDF&id=634. Accessed April 20, 2022.

Pfizer Inc. Procainamide [package insert]. Pfizer medical information website. https://labeling.pfizer.com/ShowLabeling.aspx?id=4587. Accessed April 22, 2022.

Pfizer Inc. Tikosyn (dofetilide) [package insert]. U.S. Food and Drug Administration website. https://labeling.pfizer.com/showlabeling.aspx?id=639. Accessed April 29, 2022.

Podrid, P. J., Schoeneberger, A., & Lown, B. (1980). Congestive Heart Failure Caused by Oral Disopyramide. *New England Journal of Medicine*, *302*(11), 614–617. https://doi.org/10.1056/nejm198003133021106.

Sadowski, Z. P., Alexander, J. H., Skrabucha, B., Dyduszynski, A., Kuch, J., Nartowicz, E., Swiatecka, G., Kong, D. F., & Granger, C. B. (1999). Multicenter randomized trial and a systematic overview of lidocaine in acute myocardial infarction. *American Heart Journal*, *137*(5), 792–798. https://doi.org/10.1016/s0002-8703(99)70401-1.

Sauer WH, Koplan BA, Zei PC. Principles of Clinical Cardiac Electrophysiology. In: Loscalzo J, Fauci A, Kasper D, Hauser S, Longo D, Jameson J. eds. *Harrison's Principles of Internal Medicine, 21e*. McGraw Hill; 2022. https://accessmedicine.mhmedical.com/content.aspx?bookid=3095&sectionid=265437361.

Wyeth-Ayerst Laboratories. Cordarone (amiodarone) [package insert]. U.S. Food and Drug Administration website. https://www.accessdata.fda.gov/drugsatfda_docs/label/2018/018972s054lbl.pdf. Accessed May 3, 2022.

Valeant Pharmaceuticals. Cardizem (diltiazem) [package insert]. U.S. Food and Drug Administration website. https://www.accessdata.fda.gov/drugsatfda_docs/label/2010/020062s040lbl.pdf. Accessed May 25, 2022.

Covis Pharma. Betapace (sotalol) [package insert]. U.S. Food and Drug Administration website. https://www.accessdata.fda.gov/drugsatfda_docs/label/2011/021151s010lbl.pdf. Accessed May 5, 2022.

Pfizer Inc. Corgard (nadolol) [package insert]. U.S. Food and Drug Administration website. https://www.accessdata.fda.gov/drugsatfda_docs/label/2008/018063s060lbl.pdf. Accessed May 21, 2022.

Baxter International, Inc. Brevibloc (esmolol) [package insert]. U.S. Food and Drug Administration website. https://www.accessdata.fda.gov/drugsatfda_docs/label/2007/019386s039lbl.pdf. Accessed May 21, 2022.

ANI Pharmaceuticals, Inc. Inderal (propranolol) [package insert]. U.S. Food and Drug Administration website. https://www.accessdata.fda.gov/drugsatfda_docs/label/2011/016418s080,016762s017,017683s008lbl.pdf. Accessed May 21, 2022.

Case Study Questions

Case Study

A 72-year-old female presents to her primary care provider with a concern of increasing fatigue over the prior three months. Her history is notable for longstanding hypertension which is controlled with lisinopril. A physical examination demonstrates a blood pressure of 120/70 mm Hg and an irregular pulse of approximately 120 bpm at rest. The remainder of her examination is normal with no clinical evidence of right- or left-sided congestive heart failure. An electrocardiogram confirms the diagnosis of atrial fibrillation with a ventricular response of 120 bpm. What pharmacological treatments should be considered as the next steps for this patient?

Quiz Questions

1. A 65-year male patient is started on amiodarone for rhythm control of atrial flutter. Which test should be ordered before starting amiodarone and periodically during treatment?
   A. Creatinine clearance
   B. Pulmonary function tests
   C. Complete blood count
   D. Hemoglobin A1c
   E. Lipid panel

2. Which medication is used first-line in the acute treatment of paroxysmal supraventricular tachycardia?
   A. Adenosine
   B. Atropine
   C. Esmolol
   D. Lidocaine
   E. Verapamil

3. To which Singh-Vaughan Williams drug class does propafenone belong?
   A. Class 1a
   B. Class 1b
   C. Class 1c
   D. Class 2
   E. Class 3

4. Which mechanism of action most accurately describes the mechanism of action of class 4 antiarrhythmics?
   A. Blockade of β-adrenergic receptors
   B. Blockade of calcium channels
   C. Inhibition of AV current
   D. Blockade of sodium channels
   E. Prolongation of the action potential

5. A 72-year-old female patient presents to her primary care provider for management of chronic atrial flutter that remains symptomatic despite ventricular rate control with verapamil. Her medical history is significant for an MI four years ago. Which treatment would be contraindicated in this patient?
   A. Catheter ablation
   B. Amiodarone
   C. Apixaban
   D. Dofetilide
   E. Flecainide

6. A 53-year-old man is brought to the emergency department with bradycardia that progresses to bradyasystolic cardiac arrest. Which medication is considered the first-line for his treatment?
   A. Adenosine
   B. Atropine
   C. Dronedarone
   D. Mexiletine
   E. Propranolol

7. Which medication causes a lupus erythematosus-like syndrome in approximately 20% of treated patients?
   A. Amiodarone
   B. Lidocaine
   C. Procainamide
   D. Nadolol
   E. Verapamil

8. Which medication can be used to restore normal sinus rhythm in a patient with atrial fibrillation/flutter?
   A. Adenosine
   B. Atropine
   C. Esmolol
   D. Ibutilide
   E. Oral verapamil

9. Which medication should generally be avoided in a patient with asthma?
   A. Dofetilide
   B. Dronedarone
   C. Flecainide
   D. Propranolol
   E. Verapamil

10. A 70-year-old female patient who is being treated for atrial fibrillation presents to her primary care provider with increased fatigue, weight gain, and increased sensitivity to cold. Lab tests confirm a diagnosis of hypothyroidism. Which medication could be contributing to this condition?
    A. Amiodarone
    B. Diltiazem
    C. Procainamide
    D. Propranolol
    E. Quinidine

Case Study Answers

Initial reduction of ventricular rate with a beta blocker or a nondihydropyridine calcium channel blocker will likely improve the patient's fatigue. Depending on this patient's risk for cardiovascular complications and her preference, the provider will then decide on either rate or rhythm control for the long-term management of her atrial fibrillation. Rate control is preferred for most patients, with a goal of reducing the resting heart rate to <100 bpm (though some guidelines favor a stricter rate control of 60-80 bpm). Either a beta blocker or a nondihydropyridine calcium channel blocker can be used for chronic control of ventricular rate. For patients at high risk of cardiovascular complications due to atrial fibrillation (as this patient is due to her age and female sex), there may be slightly improved survival with rhythm control. If rhythm control is chosen, electrical cardioversion may be necessary to restore sinus rhythm. An antiarrhythmic such as amiodarone, flecainide, or propafenone should be started prior to electrical cardioversion and continued to maintain sinus rhythm. Additionally, this patient's $CHADS_2$ or CHA_2DS_2-VASc score should be calculated, and if it is ≥ 2, anticoagulation with either warfarin or one of several recommended direct oral anticoagulants should be initiated to prevent thromboembolism. Anticoagulation should be initiated 3-6 weeks before electrical cardioversion if the rhythm control treatment strategy is chosen, but anticoagulation is indicated for all patients with a $CHADS_2$/CHA_2DS_2-VASc score ≥ 2 whether rate or rhythm control is chosen.

Quiz Answers

1.. B. Since amiodarone can cause lung toxicities such as pulmonary fibrosis, monitoring pulmonary function tests is an important aspect of long-term amiodarone therapy.

2. A. Adenosine, when given as an IV bolus, is highly effective in the acute treatment of paroxysmal supraventricular tachycardia.

3. C. Propafenone is a Class 1c antiarrhythmic, which works by blocking sodium channels.

4. B. Class 4 antiarrhythmics, such as diltiazem and verapamil, exert their activity through the blockade of calcium channels.

5. E. Flecainide is contraindicated in patients with ischemia, prior MI, and/or structural heart disease.

6. B. Atropine is an anticholinergic that is used in the management of bradyasystolic cardiac arrest.

7. C. In approximately 20% of patients, procainamide causes a lupus-like syndrome consisting of arthralgia, pleural or abdominal pain, and sometimes arthritis, pleural effusion, and pericarditis.

8. D. While esmolol and verapamil can be used to control heart rate in a patient with atrial fibrillation/flutter, only ibutilide can be used to restore normal sinus rhythm. Adenosine and atropine are not used in the management of these conditions.

9. D. Non-selective beta blockers like propranolol are contraindicated in asthma because they can cause exacerbations.

10. A. Amiodarone blocks the peripheral conversion of thyroxine (T_4) to triiodothyronine (T_3) and can cause either hyperthyroidism or hypothyroidism.

CHAPTER 11

CARDIOVASCULAR CHEST PAIN AND TREATMENT

ROBERT ALLEN, DO, FACEP AND RACHEL PITTMAN, PHARMD

University of the Incarnate Word School of Osteopathic Medicine, San Antonio, Texas, USA

Symptoms: **Cardio-Renal-Respiratory**

DRUG LIST FOR CARDIOVASCULAR CHEST PAIN:

Nitrates:	
Isosorbide Dinitrate	Increased release of NO
Isosorbide Mononitrate	Increased release of NO
Nitroglycerin	Increased release of NO
Calcium Channel Blockers:	
Diltiazem	Blockade of calcium channels
Verapamil	Blockade of calcium channels
Amlodipine	Blockade of calcium channels
Felodipine	Blockade of calcium channels
Nifedipine	Blockade of calcium channels
Beta Blockers:	
Metoprolol	Blockade of β_1 receptors
Atenolol	Blockade of β_1 receptors
Drugs for Unstable Angina and Acute Coronary Syndrome:	
Morphine	Agonist of mu opioid receptors
Nitrates	Increased release of NO
Aspirin	Inhibition of COX-1 and COX-2
Clopidogrel	Blockade of $P2Y_{12}$ receptor

Cardiovascular Chest Pain

General Background:

Chest pain of cardiac origin is generally the result of ischemia or infarction of myocardial tissue. Like any other muscle, the myocardium requires a steady supply of oxygen and nutrients to maintain proper function. Increased activity of the muscle requires additional oxygen/nutrients, meaning there must be increased perfusion of myocardial tissue. Cardiac ischemia occurs when the myocardial demand for oxygen and nutrients exceeds the available supply. If the demand continues without being met, myocardial infarction or death of myocardial tissue can result. Therefore, the approach to relieving chest pain of cardiac origin can be to decrease myocardial activity, thus decreasing oxygen and nutrient demand, and/or increasing myocardial perfusion, thus increasing oxygen/nutrient delivery.

Myocardial perfusion can be limited by the narrowing of the coronary arteries, generally due to the build-up of atherosclerotic plaques in the walls of the coronary arteries (atherosclerotic cardiovascular disease; i.e. ASCV). This limits myocardial perfusion and can eventually cause ischemia when the blood supply from the narrowed arteries is insufficient to meet the metabolic demands of increased cardiac activity. This can result in exertional angina, or chest pain associated with exercise. If the exertion is decreased or the blood flow in the coronary artery is increased, the ischemia resolves and angina subsides. If the ischemia persists, eventually there will be ischemic death of cardiac muscle; a myocardial infarction, or a heart attack.

Cardiac ischemia/infarct can also occur in the absence of increased myocardial activity if the perfusion of the myocardial tissue is interrupted or blocked in any way. Classically this occurs with blockage of a coronary artery by a blood clot, usually caused by a ruptured or disrupted atherosclerotic plaque in the wall of the vessel.

Diagnosis

Presentation: The classic presentation of ischemic heart disease (IHD) is exertional angina: as the patient increases myocardial activity, the blood supply of the myocardium is insufficient to maintain the metabolic demands, resulting in myocardial ischemia. This can cause chest pain, usually noticed as a sensation of pressure around the chest, sometimes with radiation of the pain to the jaw and left arm. Chest pain can be accompanied by nausea/vomiting, diaphoresis, feelings of dread, and shortness of breath. There are many variants of chest pain, some of which can seem unrelated to the heart; for example, myocardial ischemia of the inferior wall of the heart can give symptoms very similar to acid reflux or heartburn. In middle-aged women, chest pain of cardiac origin can present as sudden onset of extreme fatigue, vague feelings of chest pressure, or nausea. A high index of suspicion is needed when evaluating chest pain or its equivalent in adults. Angina is usually relieved by rest or by the use of medications such as nitroglycerine. More severe angina that is not relieved by rest/medications, or lasts longer than usual is called unstable angina and is an indication for immediate work-up.

Chest pain associated with acute myocardial infarction (AMI) is similar to anginal chest pain, however, it is usually more severe, can occur at rest or be associated with exertion, and is not usually relieved by rest or anti-anginal medications. Chest pain associated with myocardial infarction is frequently the first recognized presentation of ischemic heart disease.

Risk Factors: There are multiple risk factors for cardiac chest pain. The primary risk factor for cardiac chest pain is a history of myocardial infarction or myocardial ischemia: this risk factor dwarfs all others, so a patient with a history of prior cardiac ischemia/infarct is automatically considered to be the highest risk for recurrence. Other risk factors are commonly grouped into two categories: modifiable risk factors and non-modifiable risk factors. Non-modifiable risk factors include family history (people with first-degree relatives who had/have IHD) and gender (males tend to have an earlier onset of IHD than females). Modifiable risk factors are those where some kind of therapeutic intervention can decrease the risk of IHD. These include a history of hypertension, diabetes, tobacco use, and hypercholesterolemia/dyslipidemia.

Pathophysiology: In most cases of IHD, the coronary arteries are slowly narrowed by the buildup of atherosclerotic plaques in the walls of the coronary arteries. This gradually decreases the flow of blood through the arteries so that eventually the metabolic demand of the myocardium exceeds the ability of the arteries to supply it. At first, this usually occurs during exertion when the myocardial metabolic demands are increased (exertional angina) and are relieved when the metabolic demand returns to normal. As the narrowing increases, less and less exertion is needed to exceed the capacity of the narrowed vessel.

In an AMI, a coronary artery becomes partially or completely blocked, usually as a result of an ASCV plaque 'rupturing' and causing a blood clot within the lumen of the artery, thereby restricting blood flow. The myocardium supplied by that vessel then becomes ischemic and will quickly die (infarct) if blood flow is not rapidly restored.

Examination: Physical examination of cardiovascular chest pain is limited, as in many cases there are minimal signs and a multitude of symptoms. A new-onset arrhythmia may present with chest pain if cardiac output is compromised by the rhythm, as is the case with some individuals with new-onset atrial fibrillation. Atrial fibrillation can sometimes be diagnosed by finding an irregular pulse with a pulse deficit. In most cases, the evaluation of cardiovascular chest pain is by history, EKG, and lab evaluation.

EKG: The 12-lead electrocardiogram (EKG or ECG) is one of the most important tools available for the evaluation of cardiovascular chest pain. A 12-lead EKG is done while the patient is experiencing chest pain that shows characteristic changes associated with cardiac ischemia (ST segment depression) that return to normal baseline when the chest pain resolves are considered diagnostic for chest pain of cardiovascular origin. Similarly, an EKG that shows signs of myocardial infarction (ST-segment elevation of at least 1 mm in two contiguous leads) is considered diagnostic for myocardial infarction. These are called ST-elevation myocardial infarctions, or STEMI. However, the EKG is not foolproof: there are many cases of myocardial infarction proven by cardiac enzyme elevation or cardiac catheterization that show no acute changes in the EKG. These are called non-ST-elevation myocardial infarctions or NSTEMI. So, while an abnormal EKG can rule in a myocardial infarction/ischemia, a normal EKG does not rule out myocardial ischemia/infarction.

Exercise stress testing, which involves EKG monitoring while undergoing exercise, is commonly used to diagnose cardiovascular chest pain. The patient is attached to an EKG monitor and undergoes a specific amount of exercise, usually while on a treadmill. EKG changes showing myocardial ischemia associated with exercise are considered diagnostic for ASCV. However, there are many false positives and false negatives associated with exercise stress testing. Nuclear medicine testing associated with exercise stress testing (see below) is more accurate and specific for ischemic heart disease.

Laboratory: Cardiac enzyme determination is one of the most important methods of evaluating cardiovascular chest pain. In cases of ischemia, cardiac enzymes generally do not become elevated, however, with infarction, cardiac enzymes will be elevated. Of cardiac enzyme measurements, currently the most useful is cardiac troponin (cTn), which if elevated is a good indicator of myocardial injury. It takes some time post-infarct for the enzymes to become elevated, meaning that it is usually necessary to draw several sets of enzymes several hours apart and determine if the enzymes are increasing. Of late, high-sensitivity troponin testing (also known as 5th Generation troponin testing) has become available which has increased the sensitivity of cTn testing. Other cardiac problems such as cardiac contusion, congestive heart failure, aortic valve disease, inflammatory cardiac disease, pulmonary embolism, and extreme exertion can elevate cTn, so history is still an important part of the evaluation of chest pain.

Imaging: The 'gold standard' for diagnosing IHD is imaging of the coronary arteries via cardiac catheterization. In the case of AMI, immediate cardiac catheterization and localization of atherosclerotic lesions can in some cases be followed by percutaneous transluminal coronary angioplasty (PTCA) with or without stent placement to clear blockages and restore coronary artery blood flow. As noted above, exercise stress testing can be combined with nuclear medicine imaging to determine myocardial perfusion. More recently, CT imaging looking for calcium build-up in coronary artery atherosclerotic plaques has been used as a non-invasive way of estimating coronary atherosclerosis. Ultrasound can be used in the setting of AMI and congestive failure to look for heart wall motion abnormalities and/or cardiac valve pathology.

Associated symptoms/conditions: As noted above, IHD is frequently associated with diabetes, hypertension, hypercholesterolemia, and tobacco use.

Diagnosis: Diagnosis of IHD can be difficult, as there is no one test (other than coronary angiography) that is highly sensitive and highly specific for IHD. In most cases, IHD is first suspected by history. Follow-up testing can include resting EKG, exercise EKG, exercise EKG combined with nuclear medicine imaging, cardiac ultrasound, CT calcium scoring, and cardiac catheterization. Acute myocardial infarction can be diagnosed by history and supported by ST elevation in two contiguous EKG leads in the case of STEMI and by elevation of cardiac enzymes in the case of NSTEMI.

Treatment: Treatment of IHD is by two general approaches: increasing coronary artery blood flow and decreasing myocardial oxygen demand. In terms of increasing coronary artery blood flow, coronary artery angiography can show the location of coronary artery stenosis, which can then be treated by PTCA, or if not reachable by catheter, by coronary artery bypass grafting (CABG). Pharmacological management of decreased coronary blood flow mainly uses nitrates, such as nitroglycerine or isosorbide dinitrate. In acute myocardial infarction, nitroglycerin can be used to increase coronary artery blood flow while awaiting PTCA, CABG, or thrombolytic therapy. Medications that can decrease myocardial oxygen demand include beta blockers and calcium channel blockers. Antiplatelet medications such as low-dose aspirin and clopidogrel can be used to help prevent blood clots in the coronary arteries and in stents placed during PTCA.

Management: Management of IHD is usually multifaceted. It is not unusual for patients with IDH to be treated with anti-platelet medications and beta-blockers, and also have nitroglycerin tablets prescribed for acute anginal attacks. Treatment of underlying conditions such as diabetes, hypercholesterolemia, and hypertension is necessary to reduce the risk of IHD, while CABG or PTCA may be necessary to reduce the frequency and severity of anginal symptoms. Lifestyle modifications including diet, exercise, weight loss, smoking cessation, and stress reduction should also be considered as part of a comprehensive management plan.
Management of acute myocardial infarction focuses on maintaining adequate cardiac output by control of lethal arrhythmias and rapid restoration of coronary artery blood flow.

General Treatment Strategies for Cardiovascular Chest Pain:
The initial treatment of cardiovascular chest pain is to establish life support measures: the patient is connected to a cardiac monitor and pulse oximeter, oxygen is given if indicated, IV access is obtained, EKG is performed, and a chest X-ray is ordered. Once life support measures are in place, treatment may include nitroglycerin, morphine, antiplatelet therapy, thrombolytic therapy, or immediate transport to the cardiac catheterization suite. If the chest pain appears to be secondary to a cardiac arrhythmia, treatment will likely include interventions to return the patient to a stable cardiac rhythm: this may include synchronized cardioversion or pharmacologic intervention.

Pharmacological Treatment of Cardiovascular Chest Pain:

Nitroglycerin
Nitroglycerin, the prototypical nitrate, was first used to treat angina in 1876. Because the liver contains a highly efficient nitrate reductase that rapidly inactivates nitroglycerin, it must be given via a route of administration that avoids first-pass metabolism. Currently, available dosage forms include transdermal patches and sublingual tablets, and sprays. Of these, sublingual tablets are used most commonly. Even with sublingual dosing, the mean half-life of

nitroglycerin tablets is only 2-3 minutes, which is likely due to extrahepatic metabolism by red blood cells and the smooth muscle cells of the vascular walls. Upon administration, nitroglycerin is bioactivated via the reduction of the nitrate group by mitochondrial aldehyde dehydrogenase and glutathione *S*-transferase, with subsequent release of nitric oxide (NO). Once released, NO activates soluble guanylyl cyclase, leading to increased levels of cGMP and smooth muscle relaxation. The vasodilation that results from smooth muscle relaxation of the blood vessels is most pronounced in the veins, although it also occurs in the arteries. Nitroglycerin, therefore, reduces preload, afterload, blood pressure, and myocardial oxygen demand, which explains its use in the treatment of angina pectoris. Sublingual nitroglycerin is administered under the tongue or in the buccal pouch at the first sign of an acute anginal attack. An additional tablet may be administered every five minutes until relief is obtained up to a maximum of three tablets. If angina persists after a total of three tablets within 15 minutes, the patient should seek prompt medical attention. Sublingual nitroglycerin can also be used prophylactically 5-10 minutes prior to engaging in activities that might prompt an acute anginal attack. The use of nitroglycerin is associated with the development of tolerance; although the mechanisms underlying the development of tolerance are not completely understood, both decreased bioactivation and systemic compensation have been implicated. Common adverse effects associated with the use of nitroglycerin are due to vasodilation and include headache, hypotension, and tachycardia. Nitroglycerin use is contraindicated in patients that are taking PDE-5 inhibitors such as sildenafil and tadalafil because concomitant use can cause severe hypotension and myocardial ischemia. Administration of large doses of nitroglycerin can cause the production of nitrite, which can cause the oxidation of hemoglobin to methemoglobin and could exacerbate anemia. For this reason, nitroglycerin use is also contraindicated in patients with severe anemia. Nitroglycerin sublingual tablets must be stored in the original glass container in which they are dispensed, and the container should be tightly capped to prevent loss of potency.

Isosorbide Dinitrate

Isosorbide dinitrate, like nitroglycerin, is an organic nitrate. The mechanism of action of this medication is almost identical to that of nitroglycerin, although different enzymes may be involved in the initial bioactivation of isosorbide dinitrate. Absorption of isosorbide dinitrate following oral administration is nearly 100%, but the drug is extensively metabolized to the 2-mononitrate and the 5-mononitrate form. Both metabolites have biological activity, but the 5-mononitrate form is highly active, and is itself commercially available as an oral dosage form (see below). These active metabolites are themselves metabolized, and the inactive metabolites are renally excreted with a half-life of 2-5 hours. Because the onset of action of isosorbide dinitrate is significantly slower than that of sublingual nitroglycerin (~1 hour), isosorbide dinitrate is not indicated for the treatment of acute anginal episodes but can be used to prevent angina pectoris. The adverse effect profile and contraindications are the same as those of nitroglycerin, and tolerance can also develop with chronic use.

Isosorbide Mononitrate

As mentioned above, isosorbide mononitrate is an active metabolite of isosorbide dinitrate. Unlike isosorbide dinitrate, it is not subject to first-pass metabolism when administered orally, so it has an absolute bioavailability of 100%. The indications, adverse effect profile, and contraindications are the same as those of isosorbide dinitrate. Clinically, isosorbide mononitrate is more commonly used for the prevention of angina than isosorbide dinitrate.

Diltiazem

Diltiazem is a non-dihydropyridine calcium channel blocker; it blocks L-type calcium channels on cardiac and smooth muscle cells, thereby inhibiting the influx of calcium ions that occurs during membrane depolarization. This results in the dilation of peripheral and coronary arteries, which increases coronary blood flow, decreases blood pressure and improves symptoms of angina and exercise tolerance. Diltiazem also has class 4 antiarrhythmic activity. It is available as both an IV and an oral formulation, which have different labeled indications. Diltiazem tablets are indicated for the management of chronic stable angina and vasospastic angina. IV diltiazem is indicated for the treatment of arrhythmias, which is discussed in detail in Chapter 10. Oral diltiazem is well absorbed from the gastrointestinal tract and is subject to extensive first-pass metabolism, which gives it an absolute oral bioavailability of about 40%. The elimination half-life of immediate-release oral diltiazem is 3-5 hours. Metabolites are excreted in the urine and feces. Although no specific dosage recommendations are given in the prescribing information, caution is advised when administering diltiazem to patients with renal or hepatic impairment. Diltiazem can cause bradycardia, heart block, cutaneous hypersensitivity reactions, and rarely, acute hepatic injury.

Verapamil

Verapamil is another non-dihydropyridine calcium channel blocker with a mechanism of action identical to that of diltiazem. Like diltiazem, it is available as both an oral and an IV formulation, and the indications differ depending on the formulation. The IV formulation is indicated for the treatment of arrhythmias, as verapamil also has class 4 antiarrhythmic activity. The oral formulation is indicated for angina, control of ventricular rate in atrial fibrillation/flutter, hypertension, and prophylaxis of supraventricular tachycardia. Like diltiazem, orally administered verapamil is well-absorbed but subject to extensive first-pass metabolism. Norverapamil, a metabolite of verapamil, is weakly active. Metabolites are excreted in the urine and feces with an elimination half-life of 2.8-7.4 hours. The half-life may be increased by repetitive dosing and hepatic impairment and is also increased in the elderly. The dose of verapamil given to patients with severe hepatic impairment should be approximately 30% of the dose given to patients with normal liver function. Due to its negative inotropic and vasodilatory properties, verapamil can precipitate acute decompensation in patients with left ventricular dysfunction and should be avoided in patients with an ejection fraction of less than 30%. Other adverse effects include hypotension, bradycardia, heart block, and elevated liver enzymes.

Amlodipine

Amlodipine is a dihydropyridine calcium channel blocker that is indicated for the treatment of hypertension, vasospastic or chronic stable angina, and coronary artery disease in the absence of heart failure. Like other dihydropyridine calcium channel blockers, amlodipine binds to a different site on the calcium channel than the non-dihydropyridine calcium channel blockers, and it binds more selectively to calcium channels in the vasculature rather than those in the heart. As a result, it does not have the antiarrhythmic activity that diltiazem and verapamil have but is able to treat angina by causing vasodilation of the coronary arteries and peripheral vasculature, thereby improving blood flow to the heart and reducing afterload, respectively. After oral administration, amlodipine is rapidly absorbed, with an absolute bioavailability of 64-90%. It is extensively metabolized by the liver and the inactive metabolites are excreted in the urine. The initial dose should be reduced in the setting of hepatic impairment, but dose adjustment in patients with renal dysfunction is not required. The most common adverse effect associated with amlodipine use is peripheral edema, although dizziness, hypotension, and flushing may also occur. Amlodipine is the only calcium channel blocker that can be used safely in patients with heart failure with reduced ejection fraction (HFrEF), although its use has no effect on functional status or mortality.

Felodipine

Felodipine is a dihydropyridine calcium channel blocker with a mechanism of action very similar to that of amlodipine. Although it does not have an FDA indication for angina, it is used off-label for the treatment of chronic stable angina. Following oral administration, felodipine is almost completely absorbed and extensively metabolized by the liver, giving it a bioavailability of approximately 20%. The half-life of felodipine is shorter than that of amlodipine (11-16 hours for felodipine versus 30-50 hours for amlodipine) but an extended-release formulation of felodipine exists that is expected to provide antianginal and antihypertensive effects for 24 hours. As with amlodipine, dosage adjustment of felodipine is required for hepatic dysfunction but not for renal impairment. The most common adverse effects of felodipine are headache and peripheral edema, and unlike amlodipine, felodipine should not be used in patients with HFrEF.

Metoprolol

Metoprolol is a cardioselective β-blocker, meaning that it binds selectively to β_1 receptors, found in the heart. Two oral formulations exist which differ in pharmacokinetics and indications: metoprolol succinate and metoprolol tartrate. The half-life of metoprolol succinate is longer than that of the tartrate formulation, which allows for once-daily dosing. Both dosage forms are rapidly absorbed after oral administration and about 50% metabolized by the liver. Polymorphisms in CYP2D6, the cytochrome that predominantly metabolizes metoprolol, can affect the bioavailability of the drug, as can inducers or inhibitors of CYP2D6. Both formulations are used in the treatment of angina pectoris, though their use is contraindicated in patients with vasospastic angina because they leave alpha-mediated vasoconstriction intact, which may aggravate a coronary artery spasm. Due to its negative inotropic effect, metoprolol is also contraindicated in patients with sinus bradycardia, sick sinus syndrome, and second or third-degree heart block. Patients taking beta-blockers like metoprolol should not abruptly discontinue their use as this can lead to exacerbation of angina and in some cases to myocardial infarction. Common adverse effects associated with metoprolol use include bradycardia, fatigue, and hypotension. Because metoprolol is cardioselective, it can be used with extreme caution in patients with bronchospastic disease.

Atenolol

Atenolol is a cardioselective β-blocker with a mechanism of action identical to that of metoprolol. After oral administration, atenolol is approximately 50% absorbed from the gastrointestinal tract, with the remaining 50% of the dose excreted unchanged in the feces. Unlike metoprolol, atenolol undergoes little hepatic metabolism, and the absorbed portion is excreted unchanged by the kidneys with an elimination half-life of 6-7 hours. The dose must be reduced for patients with renal impairment. The adverse effects and contraindications of atenolol are similar to those for metoprolol, although atenolol is more clearly contraindicated during pregnancy than metoprolol. Like metoprolol tartrate, atenolol is indicated for hypertension, angina pectoris (but not vasospastic angina), and acute myocardial infarction (the indications for metoprolol succinate differ slightly since it is indicated for heart failure but not acute myocardial infarction).

Surgery

In most cases of acute myocardial infarction, treatment with thrombolytics or cardiac catheterization with PTCA are the first interventions considered. In cases where the patient is in cardiogenic shock or otherwise needs urgent reperfusion therapy and thrombolysis and/or PTCA is not feasible or unsuccessful, then urgent coronary artery bypass graft surgery might be considered.

References

Abshagen UW. (1992, November 27). Pharmacokinetics of isosorbide mononitrate. *Am J Cardiol.*, 70(17):61G-66G. doi: 10.1016/0002-9149(92)90028-w. PMID: 1449102.

Hollander JE, Chase, M: Evaluation of the Adult with Chest Pain in the Emergency Department. Up To Date, Wolters Kluwer Health 2022 https://www.uptodate.com/contents/evaluation-of-the-adult-with-chest-pain-in-the-emergency department.

Ignarro, L. J. (2002, June 11). After 130 years, the molecular mechanism of action of nitroglycerin is revealed. *Proceedings of the National Academy of Sciences*, *99*(12), 7816–7817 https://doi.org/10.1073/pnas.132271799.

Kook, H. (2020, September 11). *Comparison of nebivolol versus diltiazem in improving coronary artery spasm and quality of life in patients with hypertension and vasospastic angina: A prospective, randomized, double-blind pilot study*. PLOS ONE. Retrieved October 20, 2022, from https://journals.plos.org/plosone/article?id=10.1371/journal.pone.0239039.

Marsh, N., and Marsh, A. (2000, April 1) A Short History of Nitroglycerine and Nitric Oxide in Pharmacology and Physiology - PubMed. *PubMed* pubmed.ncbi.nlm.nih.gov/10779131.

Opie LH. (1997, January) Pharmacological differences between calcium antagonists. Eur Heart J.;18 Suppl A:A71-9. doi: 10.1093/eurheartj/18.suppl_a.71. PMID: 9049541.

Pfizer. Norvasc (amlodipine) [package insert]. U.S. Food and Drug Administration website. https://www.accessdata.fda.gov/drugsatfda_docs/label/2011/019787s047lbl.pdf. Accessed May 31, 2022.

Smith, LM, Mahler SA: Chest Pain. Chapter 48 in Tintinalli's Emergency Medicine: A Comprehensive Study Guide, 9th ED McGraw Hill Education 2020.

Valeant Pharmaceuticals. Cardizem (diltiazem) [package insert]. U.S. Food and Drug Administration website. https://www.accessdata.fda.gov/drugsatfda_docs/label/2010/020062s040lbl.pdf. Accessed May 25, 2022.

AstraZeneca Pharmaceuticals. Plendil (felodipine) [package insert]. U.S. Food and Drug Administration website. https://www.accessdata.fda.gov/drugsatfda_docs/label/2012/019834s025lbl.pdf. Accessed May 29, 2022.

Pfizer Inc. Calan SR (verapamil) [package insert]. U.S. Food and Drug Administration website. https://www.accessdata.fda.gov/drugsatfda_docs/label/2017/019152s041lbl.pdf. Accessed May 29, 2022.

Novartis Pharmaceuticals. Lopressor (metoprolol tartrate) [package insert]. U.S. Food and Drug Administration website. https://www.accessdata.fda.gov/drugsatfda_docs/label/2008/017963s062,018704s021lbl.pdf. Accessed May 26, 2022.

Almatica Pharma. Tenormin (atenolol) [package insert]. U.S. Food and Drug Administration website. https://www.accessdata.fda.gov/drugsatfda_docs/label/2011/018240s031lbl.pdf. Accessed May 30, 2022.

Midas Pharma. Isosorbide dinitrate [package insert]. U.S. Food and Drug Administration website. https://www.accessdata.fda.gov/drugsatfda_docs/label/2019/020727s010lbl.pdf. Accessed June 2, 2022.

Pfizer Inc. Nitrostat (nitroglycerin sublingual tablets) [package insert]. U.S. Food and Drug Administration website. https://www.accessdata.fda.gov/drugsatfda_docs/label/2011/021134s005lbl.pdf. Accessed May 24, 2022.

Case Study Questions

Case Study

A 67-year-old male smoker with hypertension presents to his primary care provider with a concern of exertional chest pain for the last three months. Physical examination is unremarkable except for elevated blood pressure of 152/90 mm Hg. The resting ECG and lab results are normal. The physician administers a stress test, during which the patient exercises for 8 minutes, experiences chest pain and dyspnea, and is found to have a 2-mm ST-segment depression in the inferolateral leads at the end of the exercise. What pharmacological treatments should be considered as the next steps for this patient?

Quiz Questions

1. Which medication should not be used for a patient with asthma, COPD or chronic stable angina?
   A. Atenolol
   B. Isosorbide dinitrate
   C. Isosorbide mononitrate
   D. Propranolol
   E. Verapamil

2. Which medication can be used in the setting of acute unstable angina?
   A. Felodipine
   B. Diltiazem
   C. Isosorbide dinitrate
   D. Sublingual nitroglycerin
   E. Transdermal nitroglycerin

3. A 62-year-old male patient who is being treated for exertional angina asks his primary care provider about using tadalafil for erectile dysfunction. The physician should not prescribe this medication to the patient if he is taking which class of medication?
   A. Beta-blockers
   B. Calcium channel blockers
   C. Nitrates
   D. Statins
   E. Low-dose aspirin

4. Which medication class is contraindicated for vasospastic angina?
   A. Beta-blockers
   B. Calcium channel blockers
   C. Nitrates
   D. Statins
   E. Low-dose aspirin

5. A patient who is being treated with metoprolol succinate after a recent myocardial infarction develops significant bradycardia despite normal liver and kidney function. This patient is most likely to have a polymorphism that affects which enzyme?
   A. 1A2
   B. 2C9
   C. 2C19
   D. 2D6
   E. 3A4

Case Study Answers

The goals of therapy for chronic stable angina are reduction of symptoms, improved angina-free exertion capability, and prevention of subsequent cardiovascular events. Beta-blockers are the standard of care for most patients with chronic stable angina. Beta-blockers, by antagonizing β_1 adrenergic receptors in the heart, decrease heart rate and contractility, and therefore myocardial oxygen demand. A cardioselective β-blocker like atenolol or metoprolol can be used as monotherapy to reduce anginal episodes, improve exercise tolerance, and reduce the risk of myocardial infarction. In patients who cannot tolerate a β-blocker, a calcium channel blocker or long-acting nitrate is a reasonable alternative. Additional treatment considerations include smoking cessation and initiation of low-dose aspirin, an ACE inhibitor or ARB, and a statin if the patient is not already taking these medications.

Quiz Answers

1. D. Non-selective β-blockers are contraindicated in patients with asthma, COPD or chronic stable angina because they can exacerbate those conditions.

2. D. Sublingual nitroglycerin is the only one of the possible answers with an onset of action sufficiently rapid to allow it to be used acutely to treat unstable angina.

3. C. Co-administration of nitrates and tadalafil is contraindicated because of the risk of severe hypotension and myocardial ischemia.

4. A. Beta blockers are contraindicated for vasospastic angina because they may aggravate a coronary artery spasm.

5. D. The enzyme 2D6 extensively metabolizes metoprolol, so polymorphisms in the gene that encodes this enzyme can result in significant differences between patients in the activity of metoprolol.

CHAPTER 12

DRUGS FOR HYPERLIPIDEMIA

DAVID P. SIDEROVSKI, PHD[1] AND KENDRA UNGER, MD[2]

[1] University of North Texas Health Science Center, Fort Worth, Texas, USA
[2] West Virginia University, Morgantown, West Virginia, USA

Symptoms: **Cardio-Renal-Respiratory**
Endo-Repro-Gastrointestinal

DRUG LIST FOR HYPERLIPIDEMIA

Statins:
Atorvastatin 3-hydroxy-3-methyl glutaryl coenzyme-A (HMG CoA) reductase inhibitor
Fluvastatin HMG CoA reductase inhibitor
Lovastatin HMG CoA reductase inhibitor
Pitavastatin HMG CoA reductase inhibitor
Pravastatin HMG CoA reductase inhibitor
Rosuvastatin HMG CoA reductase inhibitor
Simvastatin HMG CoA reductase inhibitor

Bempedoic acid adenosine triphosphate-citrate lyase (ACL) inhibitor

Bile Acid Binding Resins:
Colestipol bile acid sequestrant
Cholestyramine bile acid sequestrant
Colesevelam bile acid sequestrant

Ezetimibe NPC1L1 protein inhibitor, which prevents intestinal cholesterol absorption

Nicotinic Acid (Niacin) NIACR1/2 activator, which inhibits free fatty acid mobilization

Fibric Acid Derivatives (Fibrates):
Clofibrate activator of peroxisome proliferator-activated receptor alpha (PPARα)
Gemfibrozil PPARα activator
Fenofibrate PPARα activator

PCSK9 Inhibitors:
Alirocumab antibody against proprotein convertase subtilisin/kexin type 9 (PCSK9)
Evolocumab antibody against PCSK9
Inclisiran small interfering-RNA (siRNA) inhibitor of PCSK9 translation

Nutraceuticals:
Fish oils rich in omega-3 fatty acids, which reduce triglyceride storage
Omega-3-acid ethyl esters ethyl eicosapentaenoic acid and ethyl docosahexaenoic acid

General Background

Given limited solubility in aqueous solutions such as blood, much of the cholesterol, triglycerides, and phospholipids transit within plasma as large, noncovalent agglomerations in association with lipid-binding proteins ("apolipoproteins"); these protein/lipid aggregates are collectively called **lipoprotein** particles. The lipids these particles ferry through the blood are vital in establishing membrane structure and serve as precursors for the biochemical synthesis of other critical molecules, including arachidonic acid, bile salts, prostaglandins, and steroid hormones. Most lipids can be synthesized *de novo* in the body, but several essential fatty acids must be obtained from dietary sources. While levels of lipoprotein particles can fluctuate widely due to nutritional and lifestyle factors, persistent changes in the levels of individual lipids and/or lipoprotein particles are collectively known as the **dyslipidemias.** These conditions can arise from genetic variations in biosynthetic enzymes and apolipoprotein-encoding genes (Table 12.1). **Hypercholesterolemia,** or elevation of plasma cholesterol, is the most clinically relevant of these dyslipidemias, given its association with the development of atherosclerosis ("artery hardening/blockage") and risk of heart disease. **Hypertriglyceridemia,** or elevation of plasma triglycerides, is also considered detrimental to long-term health.

Table 12.1

	Inherited hyperlipidemia	Cause & Outcome
Type Ia	Familial hyperchylomicronemia (Buerger-Gruetz syndrome)	Deficiency of the enzyme lipoprotein lipase; Increased chylomicrons
Type Ib	Familial apolipoprotein C2 deficiency	Altered ApoC2; Increased chylomicrons
Type IIa	Familial hypercholesterolemia	LDL receptor deficiency (1:500, autosomal dominant); Increased plasma LDL
Type IIb	Familial combined (mixed) hyperlipidemia	Decreased LDL receptor and increased ApoB; Increased plasma LDL & triglycerides, often with decreased HDL
Type III	Familial dysbetalipoproteinemia	Defect in ApoE2 metabolism; Increased LDL, triglyceride, and cholesterol levels, and decreased HDL
Type IV	Familial hypertriglyceridemia	~1:100 autosomal dominant disorder; Increased triglycerides but not cholesterol
Type V	Familial mixed hypertriglyceridemia	Genetically heterogeneous; Increased triglycerides, slightly increased cholesterol

A principal cause of death and disability in the Western world is coronary artery disease (CAD) which is the direct result of atherosclerosis. (Hansson 2005) Hypercholesterolemia is a proven risk factor for cardiovascular diseases (CVD), as plasma cholesterol plays a vital role in the development and progression of atherosclerosis. Lowering plasma levels of cholesterol, especially cholesterol borne by **low-density lipoprotein** particles ("LDL-C"), has well-established benefits in promoting the survival of patients without clinical evidence of CVD (primary prevention) and in patients with established CVD (secondary prevention).

Diagnosis of Hyperlipidemia

Presentation: Most people with hyperlipidemia cannot tell that they have it. Their first clinical presentation may be secondary to diagnosis with atherosclerosis after a cardiovascular or cerebrovascular incident such as a stroke, a heart attack caused by coronary artery disease (CAD), or peripheral arterial disease (PAD).

Risk Factors: While several genetic variations responsible for familial dyslipidemias have been characterized to date (Table 12.1), the vast majority of patients with hyperlipidemia have hypercholesterolemia or hypertriglyceridemia that has arisen from a multifactorial basis in the individual. These factors include a diet high in lipids, obesity, lack of exercise, and other comorbid conditions. The 2015-2020 version of "Dietary Guidelines for Americans" (published by the US Office of Disease Prevention and Health Promotion (2015)) saw the abandonment of its long-standing, strict limit on the intake of dietary cholesterol, stepping back from one of the most prominent public health messages since the 1960s on the perceived risk of dietary cholesterol intake. Their original recommendation to limit cholesterol consumption to only 300 mg per day was in response to clear epidemiological evidence that high levels of cholesterol in the bloodstream increased a person's risk of developing atherosclerosis and, thereby, one of several cardiovascular diseases including coronary artery disease (CAD), stroke, or peripheral arterial disease (PAD). Discontinuation of this original recommendation is an acknowledgement that most lipids, like cholesterol, are derived not only from dietary sources but also by *de novo* biochemical synthesis in body organs such as the liver. The recent removal of this dietary restriction recommendation regarding cholesterol also coincides with a recent sizeable increase in an already large armamentarium of cholesterol- and triglyceride-lowering drugs that can ameliorate hyperlipidemia conditions.

Pathophysiology: Atherosclerosis is characterized by plaque formation along the inner surface of arteries that develops asymptomatically over many years and can ultimately occlude blood flow or become unstable and serve as the nidus of acute thrombus formation; therefore, CVD prevention by eliminating the causative factors of plaque formation is the primary focus of anti-hyperlipidemia pharmacotherapy. While high LDL-C levels and low levels of **high-density lipoprotein-borne cholesterol** (HDL-C) are each considered independent risk factors for atherosclerosis and resultant CAD, neither LDL-C nor HDL-C are directly responsible for disease progression. Instead, cholesterol-enriched macrophages, called "foam cells", contribute much of the cholesterol associated with atherosclerotic plaques. These foam cells acquire their cholesterol after LDL particles are modified by oxidation. This modification promotes binding to receptors on the plasma membrane of foam cells, such as the **scavenger receptor class BI (SR-BI)** and **CD36**. As cholesterol accumulates, these scavenger receptors do not down-regulate in abundance at the plasma membrane. The resultant excessive cholesterol accumulation in foam cells causes mitochondrial dysfunction and, ultimately, cellular death. As a result, proteases and pro-inflammatory cytokines are released along with free cholesterol accumulating in the lipid core of the growing atherosclerotic plaque. Given this presumed functional linkage between the cholesterol borne within LDL particles and atherosclerotic plaque formation, LDL-C is characterized as the "bad cholesterol", and multiple different drug classes are now employed to lower LDL-C levels in plasma.

HDL particles are a significant part of the mechanics of reverse cholesterol transport by transporting excess cholesterol from macrophages and other body tissues to the liver for elimination in the bile and feces. In contrast to LDL particles being the repository of "bad cholesterol", HDL particles represent the so-called "good cholesterol" as these lipoprotein particles are believed to protect against atherosclerosis; in blood lipid profiling, ≥60 mg/dL of HDL has been considered a negative risk factor for CVD. HDL particles are also thought to lessen atherosclerosis by multiple other mechanisms, such as inhibiting oxidation of LDL particles, decreasing inflammation of the arterial inner-surface lining (endothelium), preventing platelet aggregation, and promoting prostacyclin availability and nitric oxide release.

Examination: In adults older than 19 years, a blood lipoprotein profile test should be performed (once every five years) upon phlebotomy/blood draw, right after the individual has concluded a recent 8+ hour fasting phase. If a fasting lipid panel can not be done, only the total cholesterol and HDL levels should be considered from the resultant laboratory report (see below).

Laboratory: Fasting blood levels of total cholesterol, low-density lipoprotein cholesterol (LDL-C), high-density lipoprotein cholesterol (HDL-C), and triglycerides (TG) should be obtained.

Imaging: Doppler ultrasound or conventional, CT-, or MR-guided angiography can be used to evaluate the extent of atherosclerosis (*e.g.*, as reviewed in (Galanakis et al. 2022)).

Associated symptoms/conditions: Carotid bruits ("*whooshing sounds*") may be heard via stethoscope over an atherosclerotic carotid artery upon auscultation during systole, reflecting turbulent blood flow caused by the partial obstruction; similar bruits may be heard in other regions upon auscultation (*e.g.*, renal artery stenosis caused by atherosclerosis). As carotid auscultation is reported to have limited sensitivity in detecting significant carotid stenosis, additional imaging modalities, including digital subtraction angiography, Doppler ultrasound, computed tomography angiography, and magnetic resonance angiography, are being increasingly utilized (*e.g.*, as reviewed in (Raman et al. 2012)).

Diagnosis: Based on the Third Report of the National Cholesterol Education Program (NCEP) Expert Panel, the following assessments regarding hypercholesterolemia can be made from a fasting blood lipid profile lab report.

LDL-C: <100 mg/dL is optimal; <130 mg/dL is near/above optimal; ≥130 mg/dL is high.

Total Cholesterol: <200 mg/dL is desirable; ≥240 mg/dL is high.

HDL-C: <40 mg/dL is low (*undesirable*); ≥60 mg/dL is high (*desirable*).

Guidelines for treating hypertriglyceridemia are less well-defined than those for hypercholesterolemia. Very high triglyceride levels **(> 1000 mg/dL)** should be treated immediately to avoid acute pancreatitis; however, the benefit of treating mild to moderate triglyceride elevations **(200-500 mg/dL)** is not yet clear.

Treatment: Especially for non-familial dyslipidemia diagnoses, statins are generally the first-line therapeutic agent to consider for hypercholesterolemia and mixed hyperlipidemia, whereas fibrates are usually the first-line therapeutic agent for hypertriglyceridemia. Suppose single-agent pharmacotherapy does not produce the desired changes in blood lipid profile after months of trial and evaluation. In that case, combination pharmacotherapy can also be considered across the drug classes listed below. For example, combining statin use with a cholesterol absorption inhibitor or a bile acid sequestrant generally leads to additive effects on lowering LDL-C levels without necessarily increasing adverse effects.

Management: Besides prescribing lipid-lowering drugs, physicians advise patients with hyperlipidemia to incorporate lifestyle changes that include aerobic exercise, stress management, weight loss, and dietary modifications to decrease total fat, cholesterol, saturated fatty acids, and trans-fatty acids. Therefore, advocating for lifestyle and diet changes should accompany prescriptions for lipid-lowering drugs. For example, the PREDIMED trial examined the influence of diet on CVD. (Estruch et al. 2018) This trial observed that, by recommending a traditional Mediterranean diet high in olive oil, nuts, fruits, vegetables, and grains, and low in animal fats, a relative risk reduction of ~30% was found among high-risk persons initially free of CVD.

General Treatment Strategies for Hyperlipidemia

Guidelines presented here for treating hypercholesterolemia to prevent CVD (see Table 12.2) follow a joint report from the American College of Cardiology and the American Heart Association which is based on a systematic evidence review conducted by the Cholesterol Expert Panel of the National Heart, Lung, and Blood Institute (NHLBI). (Stone et al. 2014) Along with elevated LDL-C levels, major risk factors for CVD include tobacco use, hypertension, low HDL-C levels, familial history of premature CVD, and age. Epidemiologic data also suggests that obesity, sedentary lifestyle, impaired fasting glucose, inflammation, abnormal homocysteine levels, clotting abnormalities, and impaired endothelium function may contribute to CVD risk. Elevated serum triglyceride is also considered a risk factor for CVD, especially in the presence of low HDL levels. As triglyceride levels are highly responsive to lifestyle interventions such as diet and exercise, recommending therapeutic lifestyle changes should precede and accompany all plans for pharmacotherapy.

Table 12.2. Summary of Recommendations from ACC/AHA for Treating Blood Cholesterol Levels to Reduce Atherosclerosis-associated Cardiovascular Disease (ASCVD) Risk in Adults

A.	Healthy lifestyle habits should be encouraged for all individuals
B.	Appropriate intensity (lo/mid/hi) of statin therapy should be initiated or continued:
1.	***Presence of atherosclerosis-associated cardiovascular disease (ASCVD)?***
a.	High-intensity statin therapy if age ≤ 75 & no drug safety concerns
b.	Moderate-intensity statin therapy if age > 75 or drug safety concerns
2.	***If LDL-C is ≥190 mg/dL and no ASCVD?***
a.	Investigate and resolve potential secondary cause of elevated LDL-C*
b.	High-intensity statin therapy if age > 21
c.	Use pharmacotherapy to achieve at least 50% reduction in LDL-C levels
d.	Non-statin, LDL-C lowering therapy could be considered to further reduce levels
3.	***If LDL-C is 70-190 mg/dL and person is a diabetic 40-75 years old?***
a.	Moderate-intensity statin therapy
b.	High-intensity statin therapy if calculated ASCVD risk^ ≥7.5% over ten years
4.	***If LDL-C is 70-190 mg/dL and person is NOT a diabetic, but 40-75 years old?***
a.	Re-emphasize healthy lifestyle habits and address other risk factors
b.	Calculate ASCVD risk^
i.	≥7.5% 10-year ASCVD risk? Moderate- or high-intensity statin
ii.	5.0 to 7.5% 10-year ASCVD risk? Consider moderate-intensity statin
iii.	Consider other factors that might lead to statin use (e.g., LDL-C >160 mg/dL, family history of premature ASCVD)
5.	***If LDL-C is <190 mg/dL and person is <40 or >75 years old or <5.0 10-year ASCVD risk?***
a.	Statin therapy may be considered for select persons (e.g., LDL-C >160 mg/dL, family history of premature ASCVD)

* Secondary causes of elevated LDL-C include unhealthy diet (e.g., too much saturated or *trans* fats, anorexia nervosa), drug use (e.g., amiodarone, cyclosporine, diuretics, glucocorticoids), diseases or disorders (e.g., biliary obstruction, hypothyroidism, obesity);

^ https://tools.acc.org/ASCVD-Risk-Estimator/

Pharmacological Treatment of Hyperlipidemia

Statins

There is now a vast body of evidence that statins lower LDL-C levels and significantly reduce CVD risk in many different groups, including those with or without cardiovascular disease, those with diabetes or kidney transplants, the elderly, and even patients with moderate CVD risk without significantly elevated LDL-C levels. (Sadowitz et al. 2010) While statins have also been reported to exert non-LDL-directed effects thought to be beneficial, only their extent of lowering LDL-C via inhibition of synthesis of the precursor to cholesterol predicts their ability to reduce CVD risk. Given their proven efficacy and relative safety record, statins are considered first-line pharmacotherapy for treating hypercholesterolemia (e.g., Table 12.2) and mixed dyslipidemias; they are also routinely prescribed following acute coronary syndrome syndromes like CAD regardless of lipid level status.

All statins act as competitive inhibitors of the enzyme 3-hydroxy-3-methylglutaryl coenzyme A reductase (**HMG CoA reductase**), which is the enzyme that catalyzes the rate-limiting step in endogenous cholesterol biosynthesis (Figure 12.1). Several statins are currently approved in the United States: **atorvastatin, fluvastatin, lovastatin, pitavastatin, pravastatin, rosuvastatin,** and **simvastatin**. Salient differences between these statins are summarized in Table 12.3. Statins target the liver – the organ that produces and utilizes cholesterol in creating bile acids critical to intestinal absorptive processes; most statins have first-pass hepatic metabolism in the range of 40 – 80%, except atorvastatin which ranges from 20 – 30%. Decreased hepatic cholesterol synthesis in the presence of a constant need to create bile acids from cholesterol ultimately leads the liver to increase its removal of LDL particles from the circulation via increased expression of LDL receptors (Figure 12.2). With its constant inhibition by daily statin use, the hepatic enzyme HMG CoA reductase becomes upregulated (via increased expression); however, this upregulation does not lead to a significant increase in cholesterol synthesis so long as the statin is used daily. Statin use can decrease LDL-C levels by 25 – 55%, raise HDL-C by 5 – 15%, and achieve a 10 – 35% reduction in triglyceride levels; the latter effect is thought to result from decreased hepatic production of very low-density lipoprotein (VLDL) particles and/or increased clearance of VLDL particles via increased LDL receptor levels.

Figure 12.1 Mechanism of action of the statins. All seven of the statins approved for use in the United States work by the same mechanism, namely hepatic inhibition of the rate-limiting enzyme to cholesterol synthesis: HMG-CoA reductase.

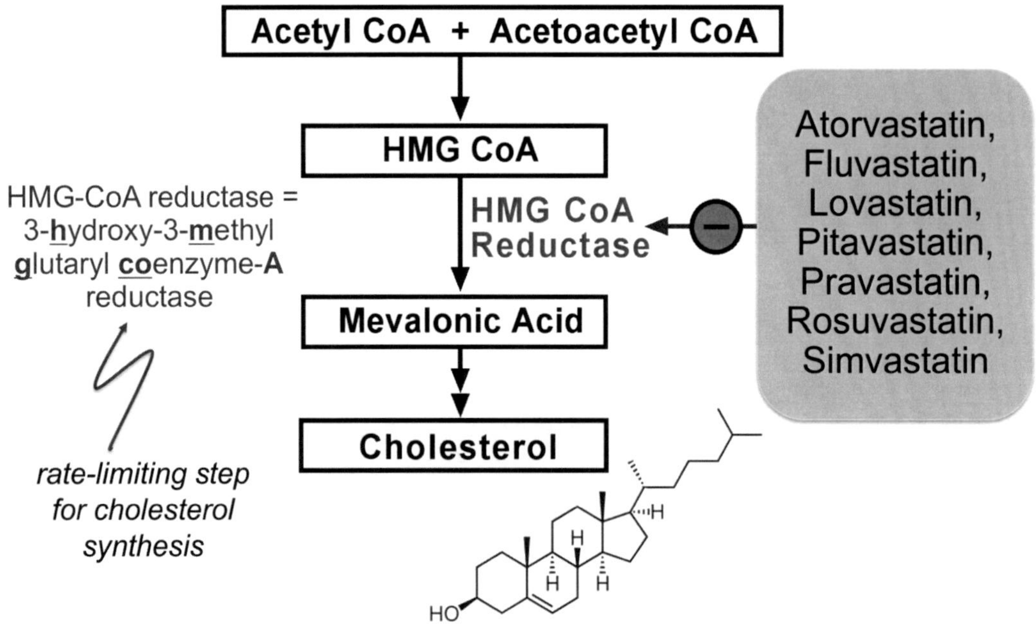

Figure 12.2 Changes to hepatic function caused by statin inhibition of HMG-CoA reductase. (A) Typically, the liver uses two sources of cholesterol to produce bile acids: cholesterol retrieved from plasma LDL-C uptake and cholesterol synthesized *de novo* within hepatocytes. (B) When cholesterol synthesis is reduced by statin-mediated inhibition of HMG-CoA reductase, the liver responds with an upregulation of LDL receptors to increase plasma LDL-C uptake.

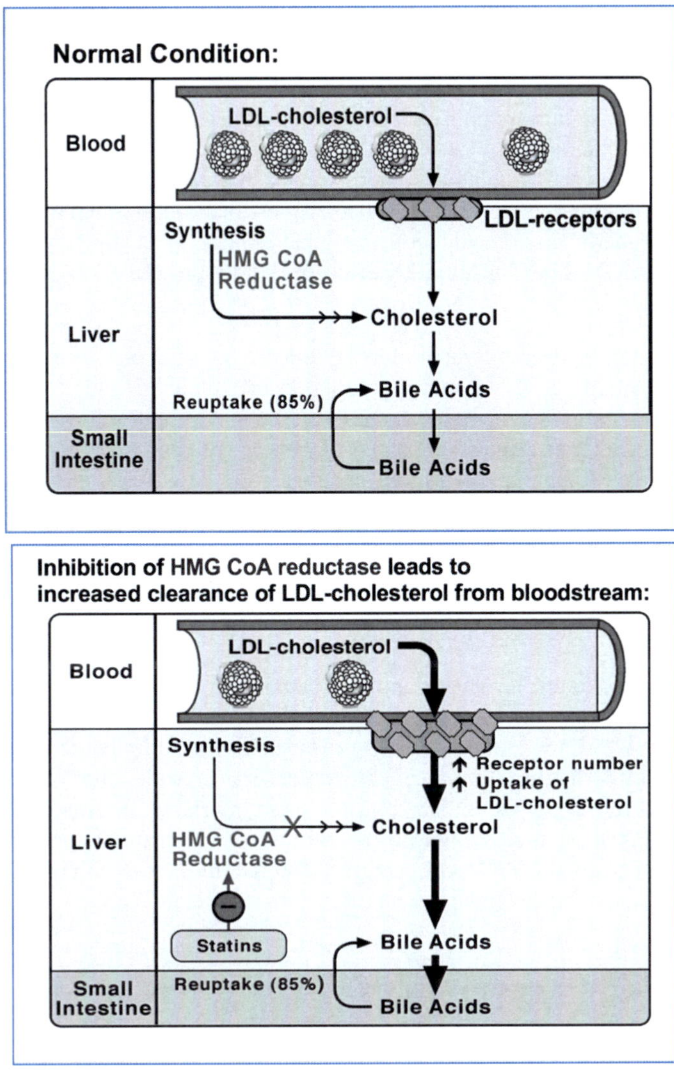

(A)

(B)

While some apparent differences exist among the various FDA-approved statins (*e.g.*, Table 12.3), they are all effective in treating the most common types of hypercholesterolemia and dyslipidemia. Suppose statin monotherapy is not observed to produce the desired degree of lipid-lowering. In that case, statins may be combined with some (but not all) lipid-lowering drugs of differing mechanisms of action. The combination of a statin with niacin, a drug that reduces VLDL and LDL production by the liver (*see below*), was initially considered valuable for patients with both elevated LDL-C and low HDL-C levels. The AIM-HIGH clinical trial showed that using extended-release niacin added to simvastatin (to raise low HDL-C levels) did not cause a superior benefit to simvastatin alone.(Investigators et al. 2011)

Table 12.3

Statin	Low intensity therapy*	Moderate intensity therapy*	High intensity therapy*
Lovastatin	20 mg	40 mg	
Simvastatin	*10 mg*	20 – 40 mg	
Pravastatin	10 – 20 mg	40 – 80 mg	
Fluvastatin	*20 – 40 mg*	80 mg	
Pitavastatin	*1 mg*	*2 – 4 mg*	
Atorvastatin		10 – 20 mg	40 – 80 mg
Rosuvastatin		5 – 10 mg	20 – 40 mg

* As reviewed by Stone et al. (2014) in consideration of specific statins and their doses previously evaluated in randomized controlled trials (RCTs); doses in *italics* have been FDA approved but were not tested in RCTs reviewed within Stone et al. (2014).

Statins should not be given with the fibrates (triglyceride-lowering drugs), especially gemfibrozil, since this particular combination may significantly increase statin-related toxicity (which is discussed later in this chapter). Several statins have also been shown to lower plasma triglycerides and are approved for this use (e.g., **atorvastatin**, **pravastatin,** **rosuvastatin** and **simvastatin**). Their effect on lowering plasma triglycerides is thought to be related to decreasing liver cholesterol levels to such a degree that the liver's formation of VLDL becomes impaired. Atorvastatin, rosuvastatin and simvastatin are also approved for patients with homozygous familial hypercholesterolemia, a genetic condition often fatal in childhood or early adulthood.

Beyond their lipid-lowering effects, statins are considered to have other effects contributing to lowered cardiovascular disease risk. These effects include attenuating vascular inflammation, improving endothelial cell function, stabilizing atherosclerotic plaques, reducing the risk of plaque rupture, decreasing vascular smooth muscle cell migration and proliferation, and inhibiting platelet aggregation. Studies also suggest that long-term statin use may decrease the risk of stroke, dementia, and Alzheimer's disease and improve bone density in postmenopausal women. Such broad protective actions may be related to either the lipid-lowering or pleiotropic effects of statins or some combination thereof.

The statins are presently considered the best tolerated of all lipid-lowering drug classes and have the lowest incidence of adverse effects. Minor adverse side effects commonly reported include abdominal pain, constipation or diarrhea, headache and nausea. The most significant adverse effect is myopathy and/or myositis. This adverse effect is characterized by skeletal muscle inflammation accompanied by muscle pain and weakness that may affect upwards of 1% of patients prescribed statins. Rhabdomyolysis can occur in rare cases (0.44 cases per 10,000 person-years). Rhabdomyolysis is a life-threatening condition involving rapid muscle disintegration with urinary excretion of myoglobin, which results in kidney damage. (Cziraky et al. 2013) Higher doses of statins or the more potent statins (Table 12.3) are more likely to cause rhabdomyolysis; statins that have a higher likelihood of causing rhabdomyolysis include simvastatin and atorvastatin. (Mendes et al. 2014) The risk of muscle damage increases upon the simultaneous use of triglyceride-lowering fibrates and statins.

As mentioned in **Table 12.4**, atorvastatin, lovastatin and simvastatin are each metabolized by the cytochrome P450 enzyme CYP3A4 to more soluble metabolites that are excreted in both the bile and urine; rosuvastatin also undergoes some metabolism by this pathway. Many commonly-used drugs such as amlodipine (and other dihydropyridine-type calcium channel blockers), cyclosporine, erythromycin, fluoxetine, itraconazole, and sertraline inhibit the CYP3A4 enzyme. This inhibition can dramatically potentiate plasma statin levels to increase the risk of myopathy and rhabdomyolysis. In addition, grapefruit juice should not be consumed within two hours of statin administration, as grapefruit juice can also inhibit intestinal CYP3A4. In contrast, **fluvastatin** is metabolized by CYP2C9, which is also responsible for warfarin metabolism. The only statin without significant metabolism by cytochrome P450 pathways is **pravastatin**.

Table 12.4. The seven statins currently approved for use in the United States

Statin	Distinguishing characteristic(s)
atorvastatin	Metabolized by cytochrome P450 enzyme CYP3A4, but less than lovastatin and simvastatin; many drugs significantly inhibit its metabolism through CYP3A4 inhibition, including amlodipine, erythromycin, clarithromycin, telithromycin, itraconazole, verapamil, nefazodone, protease inhibitors, cyclosporine, and grapefruit juice
fluvastatin	Metabolized primarily by CYP2C9; few significant interactions with CYP2C9 inhibitors
lovastatin	Naturally occurring compound found in food items such as oyster mushrooms, red yeast rice, and dark, fermented Chinese tea
pitavastatin	Sizeable effect in elevating HDL and possible benefits on glucose control; likely appropriate for patients with metabolic syndrome plus high LDL, low HDL and diabetes mellitus
pravastatin	Metabolism not 'bottlenecked' by a single, liver cytochrome P450 enzyme (*i.e.*, both enzymatic and nonenzymatic/chemical degradation pathways in play); therefore, less likely to be involved in drug-drug interactions
rosuvastatin	Rosuvastatin levels in hemodialysis patients are ~50% higher than levels in patients with normal renal function
simvastatin	Simvastatin is derived from a chemical modification of lovastatin and thus does not differ much in structure from lovastatin

Bempedoic Acid

A much newer drug than the statins, **bempedoic acid**, shares the statins' ability to lower LDL-C levels but does so by serving as an inhibitor of hepatic adenosine triphosphate-citrate lyase (ACL), another critical enzyme in the synthetic pathway of endogenous cholesterol. Clinical trials establishing bempedoic acid's benefits were performed in the context of patients already on a low-cholesterol diet and the highest dose of a statin tolerable to the patient. (Ray et al. 2019)

Bile Acid Binding Resins

The bile acid–sequestering drugs **colestipol** and **cholestyramine** originally served as primary pharmacotherapy for lowering plasma cholesterol before the clinical introduction of the statins for this indication. The most potent member of this class, **colesevelam**, was introduced after colestipol and cholestyramine to address the unpleasant gastrointestinal side effects of these latter two bile acid-binding resins. As a drug class, these bile acid–sequestering agents are second-line drugs that can safely be added to statin monotherapy to enhance the overall degree of cholesterol-lowering. Bile acid sequestrants can also be used alone as an alternative treatment for those patients unable to tolerate statins or for patients who are concerned with the potential for myopathy or rhabdomyolysis while on statin monotherapy. On their own, the bile acid binding resins can achieve LDL-C reductions of 20 to 25%; when combined with a statin, reductions of 50% or more in LDL-C levels are achievable.

As their name suggests, these cholesterol-lowering drugs are positively charged anion exchange resins that bind intestinal bile acids in the gut but are not significantly absorbed from the gut into the bloodstream. Thus, these drugs bind bile acids and significantly increase bile acid excretion into feces. The result of lowering bile acid levels that return to the liver by the enterohepatic circulation for 'reuse' causes the derepression of 7-α-hydroxylase, the rate-limiting enzyme for the conversion of cholesterol into bile acids. As a result, hepatic cholesterol use is increased to replace the bile acids lost to fecal excretion. This process causes an overall lowering of hepatic cholesterol levels. Hence, in parallel to the statins, the ultimate action of the bile acid–sequestering drugs is increased LDL receptor expression leading to increased liver clearance of LDL particles (**Figure 12.3**). These same regulatory mechanisms also lead to increased biosynthesis of hepatic cholesterol and triglycerides, which stimulates VLDL production and may increase plasma triglyceride levels.

The bile acid sequestering resins are used to treat mild to moderate LDL-C elevations. However, given that the resins can increase plasma VLDL and triglyceride levels in some patients, they are not recommended for those with high LDL-C and VLDL/triglyceride levels or in other conditions of hypertriglyceridemia. Several clinical studies have illustrated that **colesevelam** causes concomitant improvements in glycemic control along with its cholesterol-lowering effect. Although the mechanism of action of colesevelam is poorly understood, it is often used in patients with both diabetes and hyperlipidemia. (Handelsman 2011)

As bile acid sequestrants are designed to stay within the gastrointestinal tract, these drugs generally do not have systemic side effects. Therefore, they are relatively safe and may be the drug of choice for treating hypercholesterolemia in children and pregnant women. However, significant constipation, bloating and dyspepsia often limit patient compliance with taking these resins; complaints also extend to the poor taste of these drugs. The resins are given as the chloride salt. The chloride ion is exchanged for the negatively charged bile salt upon binding. Due to this exchange, bile acid sequestrant use can lead to hyperchloremic acidosis in vulnerable users such as children and patients with renal failure.

Given the mechanism of action of the bile acid sequestrants as anion exchange resins, their use raises the possibility of impaired absorption of other orally-administered drugs being used concurrently. Oral medications such as digitalis, phenobarbital, warfarin, aspirin, tetracycline, and phenylbutazone are examples of this limited absorption. Drugs that possess a negative charge in the acidic environment of the gut will bind to the resins and thereby have their absorption delayed, decreased or wholly abrogated. Other drugs should be taken at least 1 hour before or 4 to 6 hours after the bile acid sequestrant is taken. The resins can also decrease the absorption of fat-soluble vitamins A, D, E and K, and may restrict blood clotting secondary to vitamin K deficiency.

Figure 12.3 Mechanism of action of the bile acid binding resins. (A) Typically, 85% of the bile acids secreted by the liver into the small intestine are returned and reused, obviating de novo synthesis from cholesterol. (B) By sequestering bile acids and forcing their fecal elimination rather than reuse, the bile acid binding resins cause the liver to respond with an upregulation of LDL receptors to increase plasma LDL-C uptake, as well as some increase in endogenous cholesterol biosynthesis.

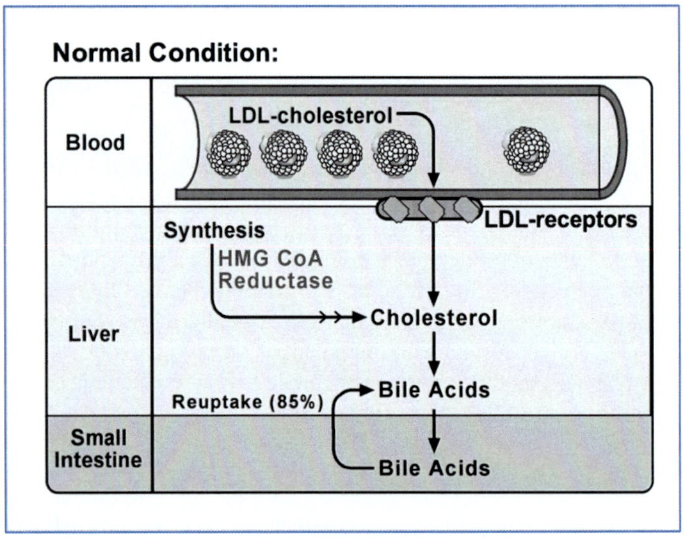

(A)

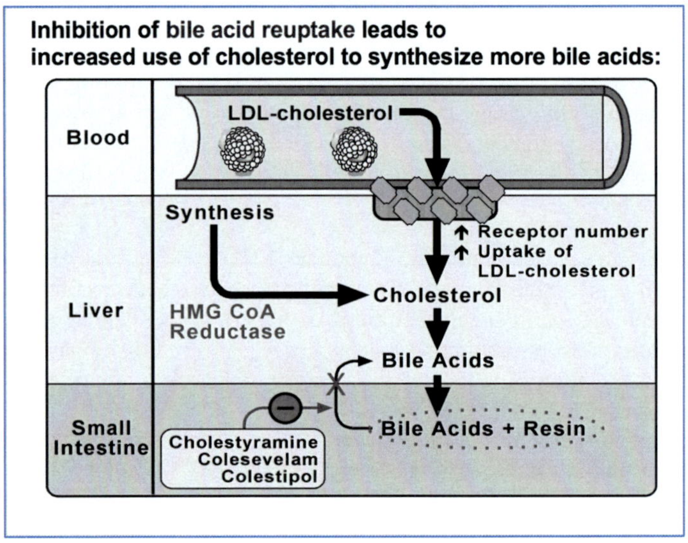

(B)

Cholesterol Absorption Inhibitors

While considered a drug 'class' of cholesterol absorption inhibitors, ezetimibe is presently the only member of this drug class. Several plant sterols and stanols, present naturally in fruits and vegetables, are also known to inhibit cholesterol absorption by the gut. Unfortunately, these natural products must be consumed in vast quantities to have any significant effect on plasma LDL-C levels. **Ezetimibe** is currently approved as either monotherapy or combined with statins or fenofibrate for treating hypercholesterolemia; moreover, a single pill combining ezetimibe with simvastatin is now available. The IMPROVE-IT clinical trial established that, when added to statin therapy, ezetimibe results in an incremental lowering of LDL-C levels and CVD risk. (Cannon et al. 2015)

Ezetimibe selectively reduces the absorption of dietary cholesterol and the reabsorption of biliary cholesterol by inhibiting cholesterol transport across the intestinal wall. The drug specifically binds to and inhibits the activity of the **Niemann-Pick C1-Like 1** (**NPC1L1**) protein located on the brush border of the small intestine. The NPC1L1 protein is a sterol transporter responsible for the uptake of cholesterol-bearing micelles into enterocytes. This action of ezetimibe ultimately reduces plasma LDL-C levels by decreasing the amount of cholesterol available to hepatocytes. This reduced availability leads the hepatocytes to absorb more cholesterol from the circulation, thus lowering circulating cholesterol levels. Ezetimibe does not affect the absorption of fatty acids or fat-soluble vitamins nor intestinal cholesterol ester hydrolysis.

As monotherapy, ezetimibe yields only a mild reduction in total and LDL-borne cholesterol. This muted response is due to the liver's compensatory increase in endogenous cholesterol synthesis. However, in combination with a statin, such a compensatory increase in cholesterol synthesis is avoided, and the resultant lowering of LDL-C levels may reach 55 – 60%. A similar synergistic response is observed upon the combined administration of ezetimibe and fenofibrate.

Ezetimibe is a well-tolerated drug, although a low incidence of reversible impairment of liver function has been observed. Liver impairment is more likely when ezetimibe is combined with a statin; this combination is also considered to elevate the risk of rhabdomyolysis. No dosage adjustments are necessary for the elderly or patients with renal or mild liver impairment. Ezetimibe is not prescribed to pregnant women, although there is a dearth of clinical evidence suggesting risk to the mother or fetus.

Nicotinic Acid (Niacin)

Nicotinic acid, also known as niacin or vitamin B3, is one of the essential human dietary nutrients necessary to avoid the disease of pellagra. The utility of nicotinic acid in lowering lipid levels is unrelated to its well-established role as a water-soluble vitamin. Its beneficial effect in lowering plasma lipids requires 1 – 3 grams per day, an amount far greater than the dietary requirement as an essential nutrient. The recommended daily allowance of niacin is 2–12 mg/day for children and 14–16 mg/day for adults. Furthermore, only the acid form of niacin, nicotinic acid, is active in lipid lowering.

Nicotinic acid inhibits the normal mobilization of free fatty acids from peripheral adipose tissue, thereby decreasing VLDL particle formation by the liver. The therapeutic effect of nicotinic acid is derived chiefly through its activation of the G protein-coupled receptors niacin receptor 1 (NIACR1) and niacin receptor 2 (NIACR2). These receptors are highly expressed in adipose tissue. The activated receptors inhibit cyclic adenosine monophosphate (cAMP) production, thus inhibiting fat breakdown in adipose tissue. This process reduces the amount of free fatty acids available for producing triglycerides and very low-density lipoproteins (VLDL). Since plasma VLDL is ultimately the source of LDL particles, lowering VLDL levels in turn lowers plasma LDL levels. Nicotinic acid is also seen to favorably increase plasma HDL levels by as much as 35%, an effect significantly higher than any other lipid-altering drug class. The action of nicotinic acid in raising HDL levels is less well understood but may involve a constellation of other effects, including increasing apolipoprotein A-I levels and inhibiting HDL hepatic uptake.

Because of its ability to raise HDL substantially (15 – 35%), nicotinic acid benefits patients with elevated cholesterol and/or triglycerides with low HDL levels. Nicotinic acid used as monotherapy can decrease plasma LDL-C levels by up to 25% and augment the overall reduction of very high LDL levels when combined with a statin or bile acid–sequestering resin. Because nicotinic acid can also lower plasma triglycerides by up to 50%, it is instrumental in treating mixed dyslipidemias, where both cholesterol and triglycerides may be elevated.

While nicotinic acid is a widely available lipid-lowering drug, given its over-the-counter availability, it requires very close physician management. A significant limitation of nicotinic acid use is poor patient compliance due to the production of intense cutaneous flushing in most users. For this reason, various extended-release formulations of niacin have been created to minimize this adverse flushing reaction. Taking nicotinic acid with aspirin and on a full stomach is also recommended to reduce the severity of the flushing reaction. As the prostaglandin D_2 receptor appears to be associated with this significant flushing side effect, a combination of niacin with a specific prostaglandin D_2 receptor inhibitor (MK-0524) was examined in a pharmaceutical company clinical trial (HPS2-THRIVE). Still, no additional benefit was found compared to statin treatment. The trial also showed an alarming increase in adverse effects, including diabetes complications, new-onset diabetes, and higher risks of infection, bleeding and hemorrhagic stroke. (Villines et al. 2012) Nicotinic acid use is also seen to cause gastrointestinal distress and liver dysfunction at high doses, as well as decreased glucose tolerance, hyperglycemia, and hyperuricemia. For these reasons, nicotinic acid use for lipid lowering is contraindicated in patients with hepatic dysfunction, peptic ulcer, hyperuricemia, or diabetes mellitus.

Fibric Acid Derivatives (Fibrates)

Clofibrate is the prototype of this family of lipid-lowering drugs. Clofibrate became the most widely prescribed lipid-lowering agent upon its approval for use in the United States. However, its association with gastrointestinal cancer led to its discontinuation. Other fibrate derivatives, such as **gemfibrozil** and **fenofibrate,** remain important lipid-lowering therapeutics.

Fibrates are the most effective drug class for lowering plasma triglycerides by as much as 50%. These drugs also beneficially raise HDL levels by 10 – 20% and cause a modest decline (~10%) in LDL levels. Fibrates work at the molecular level by activating the peroxisome proliferator-activated receptor α (PPARα). The PPAR proteins are members of the nuclear hormone receptor superfamily of transcription factors and are expressed widely in the liver, skeletal muscle, macrophages and heart. PPARα regulates many genes involved in lipid and lipoprotein metabolism: (i) increased lipoprotein lipase expression leads to decreased plasma triglyceride levels; (ii) modulation of various apolipoprotein levels leads to an increased clearance of triglyceride-rich particles; and (iii) modulation of various biosynthetic enzymes leads to decreased synthesis of triglycerides. These (and other) levels of metabolic regulation by activated PPARα all contribute to the fibrates' overall beneficial effects on plasma lipid levels. For example, increased lipoprotein lipase expression in muscle, combined with decreased expression of apolipoprotein CIII (a protein that inhibits the uptake of triglyceride-rich lipoproteins), contributes to the decline in plasma triglyceride and reduction of hepatic VLDL production.

Fibrates are helpful in treating hypertriglyceridemia, hypertriglyceridemia with low HDL, and dysbetalipoproteinemia (see **Table 12.1**) – the latter being a rare condition in which cholesterol-enriched VLDL remnants accumulate in the plasma and accelerate atherosclerotic plaque formation. However, fibrates are less effective for treating the mixed hyperlipidemias in which both LDL and triglyceride levels may need to be reduced. Combining statins and fibrates can be done carefully to obtain an enhanced reduction in LDL and triglyceride levels and a desired increase in HDL levels. In such cases, the risk of myopathy and rhabdomyolysis is enhanced over the risk of statin alone. Still, this heightened risk is less so for fenofibrate plus a statin than for gemfibrozil plus a statin.

PCSK9 Inhibitors

In 2015, two monoclonal antibodies, **alirocumab** and **evolocumab**, each binding and inhibiting proprotein convertase subtilisin/kexin type 9 (PCSK9), received FDA approval. (Abifadel et al. 2014) Both of these antibody therapeutics are considered second-line treatments that have the promise to lower LDL-C levels in adults with severe forms of hereditary high cholesterol, as well as in people with atherosclerosis when lifestyle modifications and statin use have not worked. Given that both are antibodies, alirocumab and evolocumab require delivery by subcutaneous injection twice a month. In 2021, the FDA approved a new approach to PCSK9 inhibition: **inclisiran**, a small interfering RNA that inhibits translation of the *PCSK9* mRNA and therefore leads to reduced PCSK9 protein expression.

PCSK9 degrades the LDL receptor and, therefore, normally opposes the stable expression of hepatic LDL receptors; thus, the binding of PCSK9 by alirocumab or evolocumab inhibits LDL receptor degradation and enhances LDL receptor stability and, hence, hepatic LDL-C uptake (**Figure 12.4**). The novel idea of targeting PCSK9 in this fashion came from observing mutations within the PCSK9 gene in people with very low cholesterol.

Figure 12.4 Mechanism of action of the PCSK9-binding inhibitory monoclonal antibodies alirocumab and evolocumab. (A) Typically, liver-localized PCSK9 (proprotein convertase subtilisin/kexin type 9) degrades the active form of the LDL receptor, leading to low steady-state levels. (B) Upon binding by the antibody alirocumab or evolocumab, PCSK9 is inhibited in its degradative function, leading to higher steady-state levels of the LDL receptor and greater hepatic LDL-C uptake.

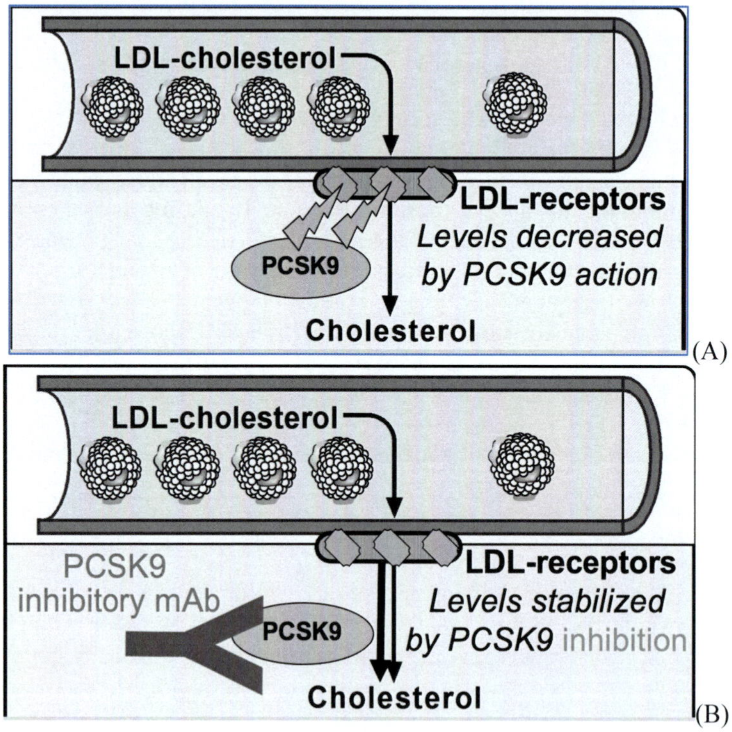

Other Dietary Agents

The increasing use of nutraceuticals by the general public warrants the serious attention of clinicians and pharmacists. Various nutraceuticals have been promoted as beneficial in lipid-lowering and reducing the risk of cardiovascular disease. These nutraceuticals are not regulated as drugs and, thus, not subject to the same standards of clinical trials testing and quality control. Fish oils rich in **omega-3 fatty acids** appear as the most efficacious of the nutraceuticals promoted for cardiovascular health benefits. In 2004, two different fish oil-inspired products (mixtures of ethyl eicosapentaenoic acid and ethyl docosahexaenoic acid) called **Omacor** (now "Lovaza") and **Omtryg** received FDA approval as licensed pharmaceuticals for the reduction of elevated triglyceride levels. While a precise molecular mechanism for the beneficial effects of omega-3 fatty acids (or their ethyl esters) remains uncertain, these particular fatty acids can modulate the activity of at least four different nuclear receptors, which are important in regulating metabolic activity. Their main effect seems to be to increase fatty acid oxidation at the expense of triglyceride storage and stimulate lipoprotein lipase activity. Omega-3 fatty acids are the only dietary supplement to carry any FDA approval, but other nutritional supplements having some benefit in lipid-lowering are also seen to be promoted. These supplements include clearesterol, garlic, green tea, policosanol and soy isoflavones. The use of such nutraceuticals for medicinal purposes should always be cautiously approached since they frequently lack strong scientific data supporting clinical benefit and are not strictly regulated as drugs (such as those summarized in **Table 12.5**).

Table 12.5 Summary of Major Drug Classes used in Hyperlipidemia Disorders

DRUG CLASS	EFFECT ON LIPIDS	PRIMARY MECHANISM	MAJOR SIDE EFFECTS
Statins atarvostatin fluvastatin lovastatin pitavastatin pravastatin rosuvastatin simvastatin	↓Total cholesterol ↓LDL ↑HDL ↓Triglycerides (Class of first choice for ↓LDL)	Inhibits HMG CoA reductase, the rate limiting step in cholesterol synthesis. Decreased synthesis increases uptake of VLDL and LDL by liver.	Myopathy, rhabdomyolysis, hepatotoxicity, GI distress, headache. Generally well tolerated.
Bile-acid resin cholestyramine colestipol colesevelam	↓Total cholesterol ↓LDL ↑HDL ↑Triglycerides	Sequesters bile acids in the intestine, preventing readsorption by causing fecal elimination. Increases demand for cholesterol in liver for bile acid synthesis leading to enhanced LDL-C uptake, but also stimulates cholesterol biosynthesis.	GI distress, bad tasting, hyperchloremic acidosis in vulnerable patients.
Absorption inhibitor ezetimibe	↓Total cholesterol ↓LDL	Inhibits absorption of cholesterol in small intestine by inhibiting activity of the sterol transporter (NPC1L1).	Liver dysfunction, myopathy, abdominal pain, fatigue, GI distress.
Niacin niacor niaspan	↓ Total cholesterol ↓ LDL ↑ HDL (most effective) ↓Triglycerides	Inhibits mobilization of free fatty acids from periphery decreasing VDLD formation. Effect on HDL less well understood.	Hepatotoxicity, cutaneous flush, pruritus, GI distress, hyperglycemia, hyperuricemia.
Fibrate fenofibrate gemfibrozil	↓Total cholesterol ↓LDL ↑HDL ↓Triglycerides (most effective)	Activates PPARα that regulates many genes involved in lipid metabolism. Triglyceride catabolism enhanced, VLDL production reduced.	GI distress, cholelithiasis, myalgia, fatigue, myopathy (especially when administered with a statin).
PCSK9 antibody alirocumab evolocumab	↓Total cholesterol ↓LDL	Inactivates the target protein Proprotein Convertase Subtilisin/Kexin type 9. Increases hepatic LDL receptor levels and LDL-C uptake.	Injection site reactions. Too new to market for definitive statement on other potential side-effects.

References

Abifadel, M., S. Elbitar, P. El Khoury, Y. Ghaleb, M. Chemaly, M. L. Moussalli, J. P. Rabes, M. Varret, and C. Boileau. 2014. Living the PCSK9 adventure: from the identification of a new gene in familial hypercholesterolemia towards a potential new class of anticholesterol drugs. *Curr Atheroscler Rep* 16 (9):439.

Cannon, C. P., M. A. Blazing, R. P. Giugliano, A. McCagg, J. A. White, P. Theroux, H. Darius, B. S. Lewis, T. O. Ophuis, J. W. Jukema, G. M. De Ferrari, W. Ruzyllo, P. De Lucca, K. Im, E. A. Bohula, C. Reist, S. D. Wiviott, A. M. Tershakovec, T. A. Musliner, E. Braunwald, R. M. Califf, and Improve-It Investigators. 2015. Ezetimibe Added to Statin Therapy after Acute Coronary Syndromes. *N Engl J Med* 372 (25):2387-2397.

Cziraky, M. J., V. J. Willey, J. M. McKenney, S. A. Kamat, M. D. Fisher, J. R. Guyton, T. A. Jacobson, and M. H. Davidson. 2013. Risk of hospitalized rhabdomyolysis associated with lipid-lowering drugs in a real-world clinical setting. *J Clin Lipidol* 7 (2):102-108.

Estruch, R., E. Ros, J. Salas-Salvado, M. I. Covas, D. Corella, F. Aros, E. Gomez-Gracia, V. Ruiz-Gutierrez, M. Fiol, J. Lapetra, R. M. Lamuela-Raventos, L. Serra-Majem, X. Pinto, J. Basora, M. A. Munoz, J. V. Sorli, J. A. Martinez, M. Fito, A. Gea, M. A. Hernan, M. A. Martinez-Gonzalez, and Predimed Study Investigators. 2018. Primary Prevention of Cardiovascular Disease with a Mediterranean Diet Supplemented with Extra-Virgin Olive Oil or Nuts. *N Engl J Med* 378 (25):e34.

Galanakis, N., T. G. Maris, N. Kontopodis, K. Tsetis, E. Kehagias, and D. Tsetis. 2022. Perfusion imaging techniques in lower extremity peripheral arterial disease. *British Journal of Radiology* 95 (1135):20211203.

Handelsman, Y. 2011. Role of bile acid sequestrants in the treatment of type 2 diabetes. *Diabetes Care* 34 Suppl 2 (Suppl 2):S244-250.

Hansson, G. K. 2005. Inflammation, atherosclerosis, and coronary artery disease. *N Engl J Med* 352 (16):1685-1695.

Investigators, Aim-High, W. E. Boden, J. L. Probstfield, T. Anderson, B. R. Chaitman, P. Desvignes-Nickens, K. Koprowicz, R. McBride, K. Teo, and W. Weintraub. 2011. Niacin in patients with low HDL cholesterol levels receiving intensive statin therapy. *N Engl J Med* 365 (24):2255-2267.

Mendes, P., P. G. Robles, and S. Mathur. 2014. Statin-induced rhabdomyolysis: a comprehensive review of case reports. *Physiother Can* 66 (2):124-132.

Raman, G., G. D. Kitsios, D. Moorthy, N. Hadar, I. J. Dahabreh, T. F. O'Donnell, D. E. Thaler, E. Feldmann, and J. Lau. 2012. In *Management of Asymptomatic Carotid Stenosis*. Rockville (MD).

Ray, K. K., H. E. Bays, A. L. Catapano, N. D. Lalwani, L. T. Bloedon, L. R. Sterling, P. L. Robinson, C. M. Ballantyne, and Clear Harmony Trial. 2019. Safety and Efficacy of Bempedoic Acid to Reduce LDL Cholesterol. *N Engl J Med* 380 (11):1022-1032.

Sadowitz, B., K. G. Maier, and V. Gahtan. 2010. Basic science review: Statin therapy--Part I: The pleiotropic effects of statins in cardiovascular disease. *Vasc Endovascular Surg* 44 (4):241-251.

Stone, N. J., J. G. Robinson, A. H. Lichtenstein, C. N. Bairey Merz, C. B. Blum, R. H. Eckel, A. C. Goldberg, D. Gordon, D. Levy, D. M. Lloyd-Jones, P. McBride, J. S. Schwartz, S. T. Shero, S. C. Smith, Jr., K. Watson, P. W. Wilson, and Guidelines American College of Cardiology/American Heart Association Task Force on Practice. 2014. 2013 ACC/AHA guideline on the treatment of blood cholesterol to reduce atherosclerotic cardiovascular risk in adults: a report of the American College of Cardiology/American Heart Association Task Force on Practice Guidelines. *Journal of the American College of Cardiology* 63 (25 Pt B):2889-2934.

Villines, T. C., A. S. Kim, R. S. Gore, and A. J. Taylor. 2012. Niacin: the evidence, clinical use, and future directions. *Curr Atheroscler Rep* 14 (1):49-59.

US Office of Disease Prevention and Health Promotion. *2015-2020 Dietary Guidelines*. 2015. health.gov/our-work/nutrition-physical-activity/dietary-guidelines/previous-dietary-guidelines/2015.

Case Study Questions

Ms. Savannah is a 53-year-old woman who reports to the clinic complaining of chest pain upon physical exertion. She does not have any known medical problems, and she is not taking any medications. Her family history is significant: her father died at age 49 of myocardial infarction. Her 77-year-old mother is still living, and her 60-year-old brother is in good health. Her social history reveals that she is divorced with two grown daughters, ages 27 and 30. She provides full-time care for her grandchildren, who are 2 and 5. She does not use tobacco or alcohol. Her diet is the typical American diet consisting of about 40% calories from fat. She does not participate in a regular exercise program and reports that "taking care of the grandkids is already a handful".

Mrs. Savannah is known to have one of the inherited hyperlipidemias listed in **Table 12.1**. Based on her history, provide a diagnosis and possible treatment plan from the options listed in **Table 12.5**.

Physical findings	Fasting blood chemistry
Height: 61 inches	Total cholesterol: 246 mg/dL
Weight: 174 pounds	LDL cholesterol: 177 mg/dL
Blood pressure: 144/98 mmHg	HDL cholesterol: 53 mg/dL
	Triglycerides: 131 mg/dL
	Glucose: 108 mg/dL

Case Study Answers

Diagnosis: Ms. Savannah's history suggests that she has a familial hyperlipidemia based on her family history of a father who died at age 49 from a myocardial infarction. Observation of her fasting blood chemistry shows that her LDL is elevated while the other components of her lipid profile are within normal limits. This suggests the patient has heterozygous familial hypercholesterolemia type IIa (see **Table 12.1**). She is also having angina, or chest pain. Her vital signs also suggest that she has hypertension as well. All of these conditions are likely exacerbated by her obesity, high-fat diet, stress, and lack of exercise.

Treatment Plan: Ms. Savannah's treatment should include medication and lifestyle changes. Based upon the criteria for initiating drug therapy for her hyperlipidemia, you decide to begin 40 mg of pravastatin daily. You also refer her to a dietician for diet and weight control advice. You counsel the patient on physical activity. You are hopeful that her hypertension will also improve with an improved lifestyle. You also refer her to a cardiologist for evaluation of her angina.

Outcomes: Two months later, you re-assess the patient. Her body weight is 163 pounds, and her LDL cholesterol is 114 mg/dL. Her blood pressure is 136/92. You are pleased that she has lost weight and her LDL has decreased. You encourage her to continue her lifestyle changes and to continue her medication. She complains about the cost of her medication.

Follow-up: The patient returns three months later for a follow-up visit. Her weight has decreased to 157 lbs, and her blood pressure continues to improve to 128/87 mm Hg. Despite these improvements, her LDL cholesterol has increased to 167 mg/dl. She says she has stopped taking her cholesterol medication due to its high cost. You explain that there is a less expensive medication called niacin but that it can cause itching and a flushing reaction. She agrees to try this medication, and you begin her on 500 mg per day of extended-release niacin. You advise her to take the niacin with aspirin after her final major meal of the day. You see her over the next several months and gradually increase the dose to 1.5 g/day. She seems to be tolerating the drug well, as her liver enzymes are unchanged, and her other blood chemistries are normal. Her LDL stabilizes to 130 mg/dL. You encourage her to continue losing weight and to exercise regularly to augment the reduction in her LDL and blood pressure.

CHAPTER 13.1

HYPERTENSION

ANTHONY SHADIACK, DO[1*] AND KEISA MATHIS, PHD[2]

[1] Grand Strand Medical Center in Myrtle Beach, South Carolina, USA
[2] University of Texas Southwestern Medical Center, Dallas, Texas, USA

Symptoms: **Cardio-Renal-Respiratory**

* *HCA Healthcare disclaimer: "This research was supported in part by HCA Healthcare and/or an HCA Healthcare affiliated entity. The views expressed in this publication represent those of the author(s) and do not necessarily represent the official views of HCA Healthcare or any of its affiliated entities."*

Drug List for Hypertension (Table 13.1.1)

Generic Name	**Mechanism of Action**
Thiazide diuretics:	
chlorthalidone chlorothiazide hydrochlorothiazide indapamide metolazone	Inhibition of sodium chloride cotransporter in the distal tubule of the nephron
Potassium-sparing diuretics:	
amiloride hydrochloride eplerenone spironolactone triamterene	Inhibition of sodium reabsorption and potassium secretion in the distal tubules and collecting ducts of the nephron
Loop diuretics:	
furosemide bumetanide	Inhibition of the sodium-potassium-2 chloride cotransporter in the ascending loop of Henle of the nephron
Combination diuretics:	
amiloride hydrochloride + hydrochlorothiazide spironolactone + hydrochlorothiazide triamterene + hydrochlorothiazide	
Beta-blockers:	
acebutolol atenolol betaxolol bisoprolol fumarate carteolol hydrochloride metoprolol tartrate metoprolol succinate nadolol nebivolol penbutolol sulfate pindolol propranolol hydrochloride solotol hydrochloride timolol maleate	Inhibition of beta-adrenergic receptors in the heart, vasculature and juxtaglomerular cells

Combination beta-blocker/diuretic: hydrochlorothiazide and bisoprolol	
ACE inhibitors: benazepril hydrochloride captopril enalapril maleate fosinopril sodium lisinopril moexipril perindopril quinapril hydrochloride ramipril trandolapril	Inhibition of the conversion of angiotensin I to angiotensin II
Angiotensin II receptor blockers: azilsartan candesartan eprosartan mesylate irbesarten losartan potassium olmesartan telmisartan valsartan	Blockade of angiotensin II receptors in the kidneys, brain, vasculature heart and vasculature
Calcium blockers: amlodipine besylate bepridil clevidipine diltiazem hydrochloride felodipine isradipine levamlodipine nicardipine nifedipine nisoldipine verapamil hydrochloride	Inhibition of calcium-induced contraction in the heart and vasculature
Alpha-blockers: doxazosin mesylate prazosin hydrochloride terazosin hydrochloride	Vasodilation of blood vessels
Alpha-2 receptor agonists: Methyldopa	Centrally-acting; suppression of sympathetic nervous system
Combined alpha and beta blockers: carvedilol labetalol hydrochloride	
Central agonists: alpha methyldopa clonidine hydrochloride guanfacine hydrochloride	Centrally-acting; vasodilation of blood vessels
Peripheral adrenergic inhibitors guanethidine monosulfate reserpine	Reduce the action of sympathetic nervous system
Blood vessel dilators: hydralazine hydrochloride minoxidil nitroprusside	Vasodilation of blood vessels

Background

Hypertension is the most common modifiable chronic risk factor for cardiovascular disease (CVD), chronic kidney disease, and cognitive impairment. It is also a leading cause of death and disability worldwide. Studies demonstrate that 34% of patients with end-stage renal disease and more than 50% of patients with coronary artery disease and stroke are attributed to hypertension.
Hypertension is arterial blood pressure that is consistently above the normal range. It affects patients of every age but is most commonly seen in adults. The prevalence of hypertension is greater in Black Americans than in White, Asian, and Hispanic Americans.

In 2017, the American College of Cardiology (ACC) along with the American Heart Association (AHA) redefined hypertension from the classic textbook value to systolic blood pressure (SBP) > 130 mmHg systolic blood pressure and diastolic blood pressure (DBP) > 80 mmHg in order to better identify those patients with the potential to develop CVD. Acute and chronically elevated blood pressure may cause a heart attack, heart failure, stroke, acute kidney injury, and sexual dysfunction. (Oparil S. Hypertension. 2018)

Presentation
Patients affected with hypertension are normally asymptomatic for many years. However, some patients may present with headache, chest pain, dyspnea, and decreased urine output, which are concerning signs of end-organ damage that should be appropriately and immediately evaluated and treated. The job of the treating physician is to assess for secondary causes of hypertension and end-organ damage, educate the patient about long-term sequela, and provide management options.

Risk Factors
Risk factors for hypertension include obesity, a high salt diet, physical inactivity, obstructive sleep apnea, and a family history of hypertension. Other risk factors less commonly considered are menopause, systemic inflammatory rheumatologic diseases, and mental stress/depression.

Pathophysiology
SBP is the value noted when cardiac contraction pushes blood into the arteries; DBP is the value noted when the heart relaxes between beats. A patient's arterial blood pressure is the product of cardiac output and peripheral vascular resistance. A patient's blood pressure is a complex process involving many organ systems working together, including the kidneys, brain, heart, and vasculature.

The renin-angiotensin-aldosterone system is an example of an interplay between systems required for proper blood pressure regulation. The juxtaglomerular (JG) cells of the kidney respond to sympathetic nervous system activation, sodium concentration reduction in the distal convoluted tubules of the nephrons, and decreased blood pressure. Upon such stimuli, JG cells release renin, which interacts with the liver-produced angiotensinogen in the bloodstream. Renin cleaves angiotensinogen into angiotensin I, which then travels to the pulmonary vessels and is converted into angiotensin II through interaction with angiotensin-converting enzyme (ACE). Angiotensin II increases arterial pressure by causing vasoconstriction and increased sodium reabsorption within the kidney tubules, leading to increased water absorption and therefore increased blood volume and blood pressure. Additionally, angiotensin II causes the release of antidiuretic hormone from the posterior pituitary gland and aldosterone from the adrenal cortex. The antidiuretic hormone increases water reabsorption in the collecting duct of the nephron, and aldosterone increases sodium reabsorption and potassium secretion in the distal convoluted tubule and collecting duct.

A patient's blood pressure is also affected by baroreceptors located in the blood vessels. Baroreceptors are mechanoreceptors that sense stretch, i.e., changes in blood pressure, and convey that information to the central nervous system. There are two types of baroreceptors: high-pressure (arterial) baroreceptors and low-pressure (volume, cardiopulmonary) baroreceptors. High-pressure baroreceptors are located in the carotid sinus and aortic arch and respond to increases in blood pressure by sending afferent signals to the medulla through the glossopharyngeal nerve and vagus nerve, respectively. Low-pressure receptors are found in the atria, ventricles, and pulmonary vasculature and transmit their signals via the vagus nerve. Elevations in blood pressure (increased stretch) increase the frequency of baroreceptor action potentials, and this results in a decrease in efferent sympathetic nerve activity and an increase in parasympathetic activity. Conversely, reductions in blood pressure (decreased stretch) decrease the frequency of baroreceptor action potentials, resulting in increased sympathetic outflow and decreased parasympathetic outflow from the CNS.

General Diagnosis
The diagnosis and management of hypertension have evolved over the past decades and are debated by several different medical agencies. In 2013, the US National Heart, Lung, and Blood Institute (NHLBI), which previously organized the Joint National Committee on Prevention, Detection, Evaluation, and Treatment of High Blood Pressure (JNC 7) to make recommendations for hypertensive management, decided to no longer be involved in the creation of

guidelines and that all future and current projects be canceled including the JNC 8. In 2014, members of the JNC 8 released the guideline that they had worked on over the previous 5 years. Later in 2017, the American College of Cardiology/American Heart Association (ACC/AHA), in collaboration with the NHLBI, released a hypertension guideline that recommended changing the definition of hypertension from 140-149/90-99 to 130-139/80-89. This change led to the US adult prevalence of hypertension increasing from 32% to 46%. Because there is one goal (<130/<80) for all adult patients regardless of age or comorbidity, the target blood pressure is now easier for practitioners and patients to remember. Importantly, these recommendations were based heavily on data from the Systolic Blood Pressure Intervention Trial (SPRINT) and the Action to Control Cardiovascular Risk in Diabetes (ACCORD) trials, which used standardized blood pressure measurement instead of routine blood pressure measurement. This is an important distinction, as a patient's blood pressure will naturally be lower when performed in a standardized fashion, and blood pressure obtained by any other means could lead to false assumptions about a patient's blood pressure and over treatment (Table 13.1.2). ACC/AHA continued to recommend stricter blood pressure goals with their 2021 Hypertension Guideline update. Other organizations including Kidney Disease: Improving Global Outcomes (KDIGO) and the American Diabetes Association (ADA) have made their recommendations based on definitions from ACC/AHA.

Table 13.1.2*. Standardized Blood Pressure Measurement
**Adapted from Drawz P et al. KDIGO Clinical Practice Guideline for the Management of Blood Pressure in CKD. 1/18/22).*
Any blood pressure not obtained with the below method is invalid.
Only blood pressure cuffs that have been calibrated and validated can be used.
Also, ensure that the cuff is appropriately sized (i.e. the bladder of the cuff would need to encircle 80% of the arm)

1. The patient should avoid caffeine, exercise, and smoking for at least 30 minutes prior to obtaining their blood pressure.
2. The patient should empty his/her bladder before the measurement.
3. The patient should sit in the exam room with the feet on the floor for >5 minutes.
4. All clothing needs to be removed from the cuff site.
5. The patient's arm needs to be supported.
6. Position the center of the cuff on the patient's upper arm at the height of the middle of the sternum which corresponds to the level of the right atrium.
7. Neither the patient nor the examiner should talk prior to nor during the measurement.
8. The recorded blood pressure is the average of ≥2 readings for systolic and diastolic blood pressures.

ACC/AHA 2017 with 2021 update

- Meta-analyses of observational studies demonstrated a linear relationship between SBP and increased cardiovascular risk (No association was found for DBP)
    a. The hazard ratio for CHD and stroke increased from 1.1 to 1.5 comparing <120 vs 120-129 mmHg.
    b. The hazard ratio for CHD and stroke increased from 1.5 to 2.0 comparing <120 vs 130-139 mmHg.
- New blood pressure goal <130/80 mmHg.
- New blood pressure categories
    a. Normal: <120 mmHg SBP and <80 mmHg DBP.
    b. Elevated: 120-129 mmHg SBP and <80 mmHg DBP.
    c. Hypertension Stage1: 130-139 mmHg SBP or 80-89 mmHg DBP.
    d. Hypertension Stage 2: ≥140 mmHg SBP or ≥90 mmHg DBP.

Examination
Once diagnosed with hypertension, proper patient care is needed to facilitate control of blood pressure and to reduce morbidity and mortality. The ultimate goal of the physical exam is to look for signs of end-organ damage, secondary hypertension, and obesity. Complete consideration of the hypertensive patient includes using standard laboratory tests and tools to assess the following:

Patient Exam
End-Organ Damage

- Ophthalmologic exam: Assess for hypertensive retinopathy, including arteriovenous nicking, cotton-wool spots, optic disc edema, arteriolar constriction, and choroidopathy.
- Cardiac exam: Assess for left ventricular hypertrophy, atrial fibrillation, arrhythmia, and signs of heart failure including pulmonary congestion, peripheral edema, and presence of a fourth heart sound (S_4).
- Carotid exam: Assess for carotid stenosis by listening for bruits.
- Pulmonary exam: Assess for pulmonary edema (seen in patients with hypertensive emergency).
- Abdomen Exam: Assess for abdominal aortic aneurysm by listening for bruit over the aorta.
- Pulses: Assess for peripheral artery disease by checking for pulses in the lower extremity.
- Neuro exam: Assess for signs of end-organ damage by checking cranial nerves and muscle strength.

Secondary Hypertension

- General: Assess for signs of Cushing's syndrome, including rounding of face and buffalo hump.
- Dermatologic exam: Assess for signs of kidney disease and neurofibromatosis, including urochrome pigmentation and neurofibromas, respectively. Patients with neurofibromatosis are at increased risk of pheochromocytoma.
- Cardiac exam: Assess for aortic stenosis.
- Thyroid exam: Assess for enlargement/nodules.
- Abdomen exam: Assess for polycystic kidney disease by evaluating the patient for kidney masses. Also, assess for renal artery stenosis by listening for bruit over renal arteries.
- Pulses: Assess for coarctation of the aorta by checking femoral pulses.

Obesity

- Assess BMI.

Laboratory and Imaging

- Complete blood count (for hemoglobin, hemoglobin A1c).
- Basic metabolic profile (for plasma sodium, potassium, serum lipid and triglyceride, and creatinine, as well as glomerular filtration rate, and fasting blood glucose).
- Urinalysis (for microalbuminuria, quantitative proteinuria).
- 12 lead electrocardiogram.
- Holter monitor.
- Carotid ultrasound.
- Abdominal ultrasound.
- Ankle-brachial index.
- Echocardiography.

Differential Diagnosis for Causes of Secondary Hypertension

- Renal parenchymal disease.
- Renovascular disease.
- Primary aldosteronism (and other forms of mineralocorticoid excess syndrome).
- Obstructive sleep apnea.
- Pheochromocytoma.
- Cushing syndrome.
- Hypothyroidism/hyperthyroidism.
- Aortic coarctation.
- Primary hyperparathyroidism.
- Congenital adrenal hyperplasia.
- Acromegaly.
- Substances including alcohol, caffeine, cocaine, bath salts.
- Medications including decongestants, amphetamines, antidepressants (monoamine oxidase inhibitors (MAOIs), serotonin and norepinephrine reuptake inhibitors (SSRI/SNRI), tricyclic antidepressants (TCA)), atypical antipsychotic (clozapine), herbal supplements (ephedra, St John's wort, licorice), immunosuppressant (cyclosporine), oral contraceptives, nonsteroidal anti-inflammatory drugs (NSAIDs), systemic corticosteroids.

General Treatment Strategies

Medical agencies agree that a heart-healthy diet is paramount in the prevention and treatment of hypertension. Patients should limit salt intake to <2000 grams/day and limit intake of foods high in omega-6 fatty acids. Instead, patients should consume foods high in magnesium, potassium, and omega-3 fatty acids. Patients should engage in 150 minutes of moderately intense physical activity weekly. They should achieve a normal BMI and treat conditions such as obstructive sleep apnea. Physicians should evaluate the patient for secondary causes of hypertension including alcohol abuse, elevated cortisol, kidney disease, etc.

Therapeutic strategy for the general adult:

- Blood pressure goal <130/80 mmHg.
- Blood pressure categories with treatments
    a. Normal: <120 mmHg SBP and <80 mmHg DBP.
    b. Elevated: 120-129 mmHg SBP and <80 mmHg DBP
        i. Recommend lifestyle intervention only.
    c. Hypertension Stage 1: 130-139 mmHg SBP or 80-89 mmHg DBP
        i. If the patient has < 10% cardiovascular risk (using the ACC atherosclerotic cardiovascular disease (ASCVD) risk calculator) for an event in the next 10 years, then recommend lifestyle

intervention for 3-6 months. If blood pressure remains uncontrolled after this period of time, consider starting pharmacologic therapy.

ii. If the patient has > 10% cardiovascular risk (using risk calculator) for an event in the next 10 years or a history of ASCVD, then advise medication management.

d. Hypertension Stage 2: ≥140 mmHg SBP or ≥90 mmHg DBP

i. For the general population (without known CVD), studies support thiazide diuretics, angiotensin-converting enzyme inhibitors (ACE inhibitors), angiotensin receptor blockers (ARB), and calcium channel blockers (CCB).

In the general population, thiazides are superior to CCB and ACE inhibitors in the prevention of heart failure. Thiazides and CCBs are superior to ACE inhibitors in preventing stroke and reducing the risk of CVD. Alpha-blockers are not first-line therapies in hypertension, as they are less effective than other agents. Studies are lacking for other drug classes, including beta blockers for hypertension in the absence of cardiovascular comorbidities. The treatment of hypertension in African American patients must be considered since studies have shown thiazides and CCBs to be superior to ACE inhibitors and ARBs in preventing heart failure and stroke.

As a caveat to the management above, there is a concern for the general elderly patient with hypertension. The American Academy of Family Physicians (AAFP) and the American College of Physicians (ACP) released a clinical practice guideline in 2017. Their recommendations were based on an analysis of the benefit vs. harm of higher or lower blood pressure targets in the treatment of adults older than 60 years of age. The analysis examined all-cause mortality, morbidity, and mortality related to stroke, major cardiac events (fatal and non-fatal myocardial infarction and sudden cardiac death), and harms resulting from lowering blood pressure to the target level.

The first recommendation of the AAFP/ACP guideline, in this patient population, was to initiate treatment if the SBP was greater than 150 mmHg, with a goal of less than 150 mmHg. In studies with lower SBP targets (<140 mmHg), low-quality evidence showed no statistically significant reduction in all-cause mortality (RR, 0.86 [CI, 0.69 to 1.06]; ARR, 0.80) or cardiac events (RR, 0.82 [CI, 0.64 to 1.00]; ARR, 0.94). However, there was moderate evidence that lower BP targets showed a reduced risk for stroke compared with higher BP targets (RR, 0.79[CI, 0.59 to 0.99]; ARR, 0.49). However, in many of these studies, targeted BP was not achieved. A review of 73,522 hypertensive patients performed by Kaiser Permanente of Northern California found worse outcomes, including cardiovascular events and electrolyte abnormalities, in patients treated to a mean SBP of 122 mmHg as compared to those treated to 132 mmHg. Cardiovascular events occurred more often because hypotension led to inadequate coronary perfusion.

The second recommendation advised lower SBP targets (<140mmHg) in patients with a history of stroke or transient ischemic attack (TIA). This was backed by moderate quality evidence that demonstrated treating to SBP of 130-140 mmHg reduced stroke recurrence (RR, 0.76 [CI, 0.66 to 0.92]; ARR, 3.02) but not cardiac events (RR, 0.78 [CI, 0.61 to 1.08]) or all-cause mortality (RR, 0.98 [CI, 0.85 to 1.19]).

The third recommendation of the AAFP/ACP noted that patients with a high cardiovascular risk, including known vascular disease, chronic kidney disease with GFR<45, some patients with diabetes mellitus, metabolic syndrome, or older age, should have an SBP goal <140 mmHg to reduce risk of stroke or cardiac events. The SPRINT trial showed that in patients without diabetes/stroke, but at high risk for CVD, targeting SBP <120 mmHg vs <140 mmHg significantly reduced all-cause mortality and fatal/nonfatal cardiovascular events. In the ACCORD trial, in patients with type 2 diabetes, there was no significant reduction in fatal/nonfatal cardiovascular events or nonfatal stroke when targeting SBP to lower targets (RR, 0.94 [CI, 0.80 to 1.11]). In ACCORD, there was a reduction in stroke (RR, 0.58[CI, 0.39 to 0.88]), but there were also more serious adverse events seen when targeting SBP<120 mmHg vs. <140 mmHg.

This organization noted that there was insufficient evidence to recommend treating blood pressure based on diastolic values.

Pharmacological Treatment Options

A plethora of prescription medications can be used to control blood pressure. It is not uncommon for patients to be treated with multiple antihypertensives; for example, resistant hypertensive patients can be prescribed three or more medications at once. Despite the many therapies available, the prevalence of hypertension continues to rise in the US and around the world. To some, this suggests other potential underlying mechanisms of hypertension need to be uncovered, so this is the focus of many funded research projects. Meanwhile, drugs that target the kidneys, brain, heart, and vasculature continue to be of benefit. A complete list of these drugs can be found in Table 13.1.1. Below we provide a description of these drugs based on their class.

Diuretics

Diuretics are useful in the treatment of hypertension because they increase urine volume, thereby reducing blood volume and blood pressure. Diuretics target transporters on the epithelial cells of the nephron, specifically in the regions of the ascending loop of Henle, collecting duct, and distal convoluted tubule. The main classes of diuretics—thiazides, loop diuretics, and potassium-sparing diuretics—can be used alone or in combination to provide additional benefits.

Thiazide diuretics act by inhibiting the Na^+-Cl^- cotransporter on the apical membrane of epithelial cells in the distal tubule. With hydrochlorothiazide therapy, Na^+ and Cl^- ions remain in the lumen of the tubule, and water accompanies them, thereby increasing urine volume. The reduction in blood volume and Na^+ concentration is believed to be responsible for reducing blood pressure. Chronic thiazide therapy can cause hypokalemia, hyponatremia, hypomagnesemia, hypochloremia, metabolic alkalosis, hyperglycemia, hyperuricemia, hyperlipidemia, and hypercalcemia. Extracellular volume depletion resulting from thiazide diuretic therapy can produce prerenal azotemia and accompanying renal dysfunction. Thiazides are also associated with erectile dysfunction.

Loop diuretics inhibit the Na^+-K^+-$2Cl^-$ cotransporter on the apical membrane of the epithelial cells of the thick ascending limb of the loop of Henle. This causes Na^+, K^+, and Cl^- to remain in the lumen of the nephron, along with water, resulting in an overall increase in urine volume, a decrease in blood volume and Na^+ concentration, and a decrease in blood pressure. Loop diuretics can produce excessive fluid loss and dehydration, producing signs of dry mouth, headaches, nausea, vomiting, and dizziness. Hypotension produced by loop diuretics can reduce renal blood flow and cause renal dysfunction, and in extreme cases, can lead to circulatory collapse. Electrolyte imbalances induced by loop diuretics can be severe, including hyponatremia, hypokalemia, hypomagnesemia, hypocalcemia, hypochloremia, and metabolic alkalosis. Patients prescribed loop diuretics are often reminded to maintain their level of dietary potassium intake by eating a banana, for example. Additional blood abnormalities such as hyperuricemia, hyperglycemia, and hyperlipidemia can also be produced. The loop diuretics are associated with ototoxicity, which most commonly results from excessively rapid IV infusion, and which is usually, but not always, reversible.

Potassium-sparing diuretics act at the level of the distal tubules to inhibit Na^+ reabsorption and K^+ secretion. These drugs produce mild diuresis and can be combined with thiazide or loop diuretics to counteract the hypokalemia caused by these drugs. Triamterene and amiloride act by blocking the epithelial Na^+ channels (ENaC) found on the luminal side of epithelial cells lining the distal tubule. Blocking these channels inhibits the reabsorption of Na^+ and consequently, the loss of K^+ in the urine. Spironolactone and eplerenone mineralocorticoid receptor antagonists; block the ability of mineralocorticoids to cause Na^+ and water retention, and K^+ and H^+ excretion. All potassium-sparing diuretics can cause adverse effects of hyperkalemia, metabolic acidosis, and gastrointestinal upset. Spironolactone is associated with gynecomastia, erectile dysfunction, and menstrual irregularity.

Beta Blockers (see also Chapters 10-11)

Beta-blockers combat hypertension through a direct action on the heart. These drugs are antagonists of β_1-adrenergic receptors on cardiomyocytes, so they decrease the effect of sympathetic nervous system activity by blocking the binding of epinephrine and norepinephrine. This results in decreased cardiac contractility, heart rate, and conduction velocity, and therefore decreases blood pressure. Specific beta-blockers (bisoprolol, carvedilol, and metoprolol) are preferred in patients with heart failure because they improve survival in this condition. Unwanted side effects of chronic beta-blocker therapy include bradycardia, exercise intolerance, weight gain, fatigue, cold appendages, AV nodal block, and in some cases, depression, and nightmares. Nonselective beta-blockers, such as propranolol, produce certain adverse effects associated with β_2 receptor blockade in non-cardiac tissues, including bronchoconstriction and impaired recovery from hypoglycemia.

ACE inhibitors

Angiotensin II affects the vasculature and the renal tubules, increasing peripheral vascular resistance and sodium reabsorption (directly and through aldosterone), respectively. Because angiotensin II increases blood pressure via several pathways, targeting the renin-angiotensin system is an ideal therapeutic approach. Angiotensin-converting enzyme (ACE) inhibitors halt the conversion of angiotensin I to angiotensin II, thereby reducing the blood pressure-enhancing effects of this hormone. ACE inhibitors also interfere with the negative feedback exerted by angiotensin II on renin release. The resultant increase in renin production increases the formation of angiotensin I, and, because it is not able to be converted to angiotensin II, angiotensin I enter alternative metabolic pathways that produce vasodilatory peptides.

ACE inhibitors have shown benefits beyond blood pressure control in certain populations. They slow the development and progression of diabetic nephropathy, and they have a similar effect on renal disease in nondiabetic patients. ACE inhibitors have also been shown to prolong survival in patients with heart failure with reduced ejection fraction (HFrEF) and to help prevent cardiac remodeling post-myocardial infarction.

Certain adverse effects of the ACE inhibitors occur because, in addition to producing angiotensin II, ACE is responsible for inactivating bradykinin and substance P; therefore, inhibition of ACE increases levels of these mediators. Adverse effects associated with elevated bradykinin and substance P include chronic dry cough, which is quite common, and angioedema, which is rare but serious. Other adverse effects of ACE inhibitors include hyperkalemia, fatigue, dizziness, headache, and loss of taste. ACE inhibitors can precipitate acute renal insufficiency in individuals with bilateral renal artery stenosis or stenosis in the renal artery of a single remaining kidney. Patients should not take this medication during pregnancy since drugs that target the renin-angiotensin system can cause renal malformations or death of the fetus.

Angiotensin II receptor blockers

Blockade of angiotensin II is also a successful therapeutic option in some hypertensive patients. Antagonizing the angiotensin type 1 receptor (AT_1) blocks the effects of angiotensin II in the kidneys, heart, and vasculature, and it does this more effectively than ACE inhibitors. Unlike ACE inhibitors, which indirectly decrease the activation of all angiotensin II receptors, angiotensin II receptor blockers (ARBs) do not antagonize angiotensin type 2 (AT_2) receptors that have vasodilatory and natriuretic effects.

Because ARBs do not inhibit ACE, they do not elevate bradykinin and substance P levels, so they are unlikely to produce the cough and angioedema that are characteristic of the ACE inhibitors. Although ARBs are highly effective at reducing blood pressure, they can produce adverse side effects including blurred vision, itching, numbness, tingling sensations, confusion, dizziness, nervousness, stomach pain, sweating, and others. Like ACE inhibitors, ARBs can cause fetal harm or death if taken during pregnancy.

Calcium channel blockers (see also Chapters 10-11)

The movement of calcium through its channels into vascular smooth muscle cells leads to contraction. Calcium channel blockers (CCB) directly reduce the contraction of vascular smooth muscle and therefore reduces peripheral vascular resistance and blood pressure. CCBs are classified as dihydropyridines or non-dihydropyridines. Dihydropyridines, such as amlodipine and nifedipine, exert their primary effect by decreasing systemic vascular resistance, thereby reducing blood pressure. Non-dihydropyridines, like verapamil and diltiazem, also decrease systemic vascular resistance, but they have additional effects on the heart. Verapamil and diltiazem decrease cardiac contractility, and they also reduce heart rate by slowing SA and AV nodal conduction. This reduces cardiac output and therefore decreases blood pressure. Long-acting and sustained-release formulations of dihydropyridines are first-line drugs for the treatment of hypertension. Non-dihydropyridines are used when individuals have comorbidities (e.g., stable angina, certain arrhythmias) that warrant the use of drugs that decrease cardiac output.

The major adverse effects of the dihydropyridine CCBs stem from their ability to cause vasodilation; these include reflex tachycardia, headache, peripheral edema, and postural hypotension. The cardiac depressant effect of the non-dihydropyridines prevents these drugs from causing tachycardia in response to vasodilation. However, they can cause bradycardia, fatigue, AV nodal depression, or AV block, and can worsen heart failure. Verapamil is known to cause constipation.

Alpha-blockers

Alpha-blockers reduce blood pressure by acting directly on the vasculature. These drugs do not allow catecholamines to bind α_1 adrenergic receptors and cause vasoconstriction, and the resulting effect is a reduction of peripheral vascular resistance and thus a reduction in blood pressure. Alpha-blockers can produce adverse effects including orthostatic hypotension, dizziness, headache, and weakness. These drugs should be initiated at low doses and gradually titrated upward to reduce the risk of hypotension and orthostatic hypotension. Labetalol, a drug with α_1-and β-blocking activity, is used to lower blood pressure in patients in hypertensive crisis.

Alpha-2 Receptor Agonists

Agonists of the α_2 adrenergic receptors reduce sympathetic nervous system activity, which can have a profound effect on heart rate, peripheral vascular resistance, renal vascular resistance, and blood pressure. Clonidine is a classic example of a centrally-acting α_2 agonist. Side effects of these drugs include anxiety, constipation, drowsiness, dry mouth, and a general feeling of discomfort or illness. Rebound hypertension can occur if clonidine is abruptly discontinued. Methyldopa is a centrally-acting α_2 agonist that has been used to treat hypertension during pregnancy because of its favorable safety profile in the mother and fetus. Its adverse effects include drowsiness, hyperprolactinemia, and a positive Coombs test.

Peripheral adrenergic inhibitors

Peripheral adrenergic inhibitors deplete catecholamines from storage vesicles in sympathetic neurons and the adrenal medulla. This slows sympathetic neurotransmission, resulting in reduced vasoconstriction and lower blood pressure. An example of these drugs is reserpine. It is seldom used in the treatment of hypertension because of its adverse effects, including dizziness, headache, anxiety, loss of appetite, nausea, vomiting, diarrhea, and dry mouth.

Vasodilators

Vasodilators increase blood flow through arteries, and this decreases peripheral vascular resistance and therefore blood pressure. Hydralazine is considered safe for use in hypertension during pregnancy, nitroprusside is used in treating hypertensive emergency, and minoxidil is a third-line therapy for chronic hypertension management. All vasodilators carry a risk of producing reflex tachycardia, which can be severe enough to cause chest pain; concomitant use of a β-blocker can counteract this effect. Other vasodilation-associated effects include headache, hypotension and orthostatic hypotension, dizziness, and edema. Nitroprusside is metabolized to cyanide and thiocyanate, both of which are toxic, so blood levels of these compounds should be monitored during prolonged infusion. Minoxidil produces a side effect of hypertrichosis, and the discovery of this feature led to its use as a topical formulation to treat alopecia.

Comorbidities and Associated Conditions

Hypertensive patients often present with symptoms and associated conditions like chronic kidney disease, diabetes, congestive heart failure, atrial fibrillation, coronary heart disease, stroke, myocardial infarction, and peripheral arterial disease. These diseases alone can cause severe morbidity and mortality and should be addressed in this conversation on hypertension.

Chronic Kidney Disease

In 2012, the KDIGO organization published an updated evidence-based practice guideline for the management of blood pressure in individuals with non-dialysis-dependent chronic kidney disease (CKD) of any stage. This report built upon the 2002 National Kidney Foundation Kidney Disease Outcome Quality Initiative (NKF-KDOQI) clinical practice guideline on CKD and the 2004 NKF-KDOQI clinical practice guideline on hypertension management. In 2021, KDIGO published updated guidelines taking into account both risk of progression to kidney failure and the risk for cardiovascular events. This group stated that albuminuria (urine albumin excretion of 30-300 mg/24 hours) is a modifiable major risk factor for CVD and CKD progression. The group recommended ACE inhibitors and ARBs in these patients to decrease the risks of doubling serum creatinine, kidney failure, or death. KDIGO recommended the following for patients with CKD and hypertension:

1. Eat less than 2000 mg of sodium per day.
2. Keep SBP goal <120 mmHg (only if obtaining blood pressure measurements in the standardized approach. If unable to obtain blood pressure in this fashion then do not treat to this goal as it will increase risk of harm).
3. Use ACE inhibitors or ARB in patients, without diabetes, but with moderate (CKD G1-4 and albuminuria category A2)-severe (CKD G1-4 and albuminuria category A3) microalbuminuria.
4. Use ACE inhibitors or ARB in patients, with diabetes, and moderate-severely increased albuminuria (CKD G1-4 and albuminuria category A2 and A3).
5. In patients with a kidney transplant, treat to SBP goal <130 mmHg and DBP goal <80 mmHg (only if obtaining blood pressure measurements in the standardized approach).
6. In patients with a kidney transplant, use dihydropyridine CCBs or ARBs as first-line therapy.
7. In children with CKD, treat 24-hour mean arterial blood pressure obtained with ambulatory blood pressure monitoring to a goal of less than or equal to 50% based on age, gender, and height.
8. In children with CKD, use an ACE inhibitor or ARB as first-line therapy.
9. Too tight control may lead to adverse effects (especially in the elderly), and looser control may improve adherence.

Diabetes (see also Chapter 15)

The 2022 ADA Standards of Care noted patients should be diagnosed with hypertension if blood pressure is ≥140/90 mmHg on multiple office visits or ≥180/110 mmHg at one visit. Patients with diabetes mellitus and elevated blood pressure (>120/80 mmHg) should start lifestyle interventions including the Dietary Approaches to Stop Hypertension (DASH) diet and increased physical activity. Patients with high cardiovascular risk (10-year ASCVD risk ≥15% or history of existing ASCVD) should target a blood pressure goal of <130/80 mmHg. Patients with a lower cardiovascular risk (10-year ASCVD risk <15%) should target a blood pressure goal of <140/90 mmHg. Pregnant patients with diabetes and pre-existing hypertension should target a blood pressure goal of 110-135/85 mmHg. Patients with diabetes and hypertension should first start ACE inhibitors, ARB, or diuretics depending on comorbid cardiovascular conditions. Patients with diabetes and hypertension with blood pressure ≥160/100 mmHg should be treated with two medications.

Heart Failure (see also Chapters 10-11)

In patients with heart failure, there is no quality evidence to guide decision-making for blood pressure goals. As a result, ACC, in their 2021 update, recommended to treat for blood pressure goals seen in their hypertension guideline for adults (<130/80 mmHg).

Stroke

In the 2021 Guideline for the Prevention of Stroke in Patients With Stroke and Transient Ischemic Attack, the American Heart Association/American Stroke Association recommended a blood pressure goal, in neurologically stable patients with cerebrovascular disease, of <130/80 mmHg, which was based on data from new randomized clinical trials and meta-analyses. This was a departure from previous concerns that lower blood pressure targets would increase the risk of stroke. The authors of this guideline recommended treating patients with hypertension and a history of stroke with diuretics, ACE inhibitors, and ARBs. The authors conceded that CCBs may be used in patients with a history of stroke who require additional medication options but should not be first-line therapies.

CHAPTER 13.2

HYPOTENSION

ANTHONY SHADIACK, DO

Grand Strand Medical Center in Myrtle Beach, South Carolina, USA

Symptoms: **Cardio-Renal-Respiratory**

HCA Healthcare disclaimer: "This research was supported in part by HCA Healthcare and/or an HCA Healthcare affiliated entity. The views expressed in this publication represent those of the author(s) and do not necessarily represent the official views of HCA Healthcare or any of its affiliated entities."

Drug List for Hypotension

- Fludrocortisone
- Pyridostigmine
- Midodrine

Background

Hypotension is arterial blood pressure that is consistently lower than the normal range. There is no standardized value to diagnose hypotension, but generally, it is accepted when values are less than 90/60 mmHg. Hypotension is a largely unrecognized condition as patients are normally asymptomatic. Hypotension becomes important when it leads to symptoms, as in the case of orthostatic hypotension (OH), also known as postural hypotension. The prevalence of OH is dependent on age, occurring in 30% of patients older than 70 and 5% of patients younger than 50. OH is an independent risk factor for mortality associated with comorbid conditions including stroke, heart failure, myocardial infarction, and atrial fibrillation. OH is the second most common cause of syncope. A 2020 meta-analysis found significant variability in how OH is diagnosed. (Saedon, 2020)

Presentation

Patients affected with hypotension are normally asymptomatic. The most common symptoms associated with hypotension are dizziness, pre-syncope, syncope, nausea, and fatigue. Rarely patients may experience chest pain, orthostatic dyspnea, and neck/shoulder pain.

Risk Factors

Risk factors for hypotension include old age, hypertension, and diabetes.

Pathophysiology

When moving from supine to standing, gravity causes 500 mL of blood to be moved from the chest to the venous system below the diaphragm. This leads to a rapid decrease in blood volume, ventricular preload, stroke volume, and mean blood pressure. Baroreceptors located in the blood vessels provide sensory input which is used in the control of blood pressure by the autonomic nervous system. High-pressure baroreceptors are located in the carotid sinus and aortic arch, and low-pressure baroreceptors are located in the atria, ventricles, and pulmonary vessels. A decrease in blood pressure produces less stretch or stimulation of the baroreceptors, resulting in a slower frequency of baroreceptor action potentials, and this produces an increase in sympathetic nervous system activity and a decrease in parasympathetic activity. Increased blood pressure enhances baroreceptor activity, resulting in decreased sympathetic and increased parasympathetic outflow. Changes in baroreceptor activity also modulate the release of antidiuretic hormone (ADH) by the posterior pituitary. Decreased baroreceptor activity (hypotension) results in an increase in the secretion of ADH, and increased baroreceptor activity (hypertension) decreases ADH secretion.

The activation of the sympathetic nervous system increases the release of renin, which converts angiotensinogen in the bloodstream to angiotensin I. Angiotensin I travels to the pulmonary vessels and is converted into angiotensin II by the angiotensin-converting enzyme (ACE). Angiotensin II increases arterial pressure by causing vasoconstriction, resulting in increased peripheral vascular resistance. It also directly stimulates sodium reabsorption within the kidney tubules, leading to increased water absorption and therefore increased blood volume and blood pressure. Angiotensin

II stimulates the release of ADH from the posterior pituitary gland, which increases water reabsorption in the collecting duct of the kidney. In addition, angiotensin II stimulates the release of aldosterone from the adrenal cortex, which causes increased sodium reabsorption and potassium excretion in the distal convoluted tubule and collecting duct of the nephron.

Examination

The goal of the physical exam is to look for signs of the underlying diagnosis.

- HEENT: Assess for anemia including pallor of conjunctiva/nail bed; diabetes insipidus or dehydration, including dry mucous membranes, delayed capillary refill, and sunken eyes; hypothyroidism including periorbital puffiness, dry coarse hair.
- Cardiac exam: Assess for cardiac arrhythmia including abnormal heart rhythm, palpitations, skipped heartbeat; myocardial infarction/myocarditis/pericarditis including chest pain, dyspnea; valvular heart disease including palpitations, venous insufficiency; heart failure including pulmonary congestion, peripheral edema and s4; diabetes insipidus including tachycardia; hypothyroidism including non-pitting edema.
- Abdominal Exam: Assess for gastroenteritis including fever, chills, diarrhea, nausea, and vomiting.
- Dermatology exam: Assess for adrenal insufficiency including hyperpigmentation of the skin; burns may lead to intravascular volume depletion.
- Psychiatry exam: Assess for anxiety/panic disorders or eating disorders.
- Neurological exam: Assess for stroke including aphasia, dysarthria, one-sided facial droop, hemiparesis, amaurosis fugax; Parkinson's disease including pill-rolling tremor, masked facies, shuffling gait; Guillain-Barre syndrome with progressive muscle weakness/atrophy; multiple sclerosis.

Labs and Imaging

Routine

- Complete blood count (evaluating for hemoglobin, white blood cells, and platelets).
- Basic metabolic profile (evaluating for sodium, potassium, creatinine, GFR, and fasting blood glucose).
- TSH.
- 12 lead EKG.
- Bedside blood pressure and heart rate taken supine and standing.

Additional testing

- Hemoglobin A1c.
- Morning serum cortisol.
- Holter monitor.
- Echocardiography.
- Abdominal ultrasound.
- CT head.
- Tilt table.
- Exercise stress test.
- Angiography if indicated.
- 24-hour blood pressure ambulatory monitor.
- Cardiac SPECT imaging for pure autonomic failure.
- MRI brain for multisystem atrophy (Shy-Drager syndrome).
- Serum and urine protein electrophoresis for primary amyloidosis.

Associated Symptoms/Conditions

Primary chronic autonomic failure with symptoms of orthostatic hypotension.

- Parkinson's disease.
- Multiple system atrophy.
- Pure autonomic failure.
- Lewy body dementia.
- Autoimmune autonomic ganglionopathy.
- Rare hereditary disorders.
- Idiopathic.

Secondary chronic autonomic failure with symptoms of orthostatic hypotension

- Drug-related.
- Diabetes mellitus.
- Cardiovascular disease.
- Renal failure.
- Autoimmune disease.

- Volume depletion.
- Venous pooling.
- Alcoholic polyneuropathy.
- Endocrine disorders.
- Amyloidosis.
- Multiple myeloma.
- Paraneoplastic syndromes.
- Cerebrovascular disease.
- Multiple sclerosis.
- Spinal cord disease.

Diagnosis

The provider needs to assess whether the patient has neurogenic OH or whether OH is the result of non-neurogenic causes. Neurogenic OH, also known as an autonomic failure, is due to impaired activation of sympathetic vasoconstrictor neurons. Although it is recommended to assess a patient's heart rate, there are no formal recommendations that inform the provider of the patient's diagnosis. Heart rate changes are seen in non-neurogenic OH and are not seen in neurogenic OH.

Bedside blood pressure and heart rate should be evaluated with the patient supine and then again after 3 minutes of standing (positive predictive value 61.7% and negative predictive value 50.2%). Classically, OH is diagnosed when there is a sustained reduction in SBP of at least 20 mmHg and/or DBP of at least 10 mmHg after 30-180 seconds of standing. Delayed OH is diagnosed with a reduction in SBP of at least 20 mmHg (30 mmHg in patients with hypertension) or a 10 mmHg decrease in DBP (15 mmHg in patients with hypertension) after between 3 and 45 minutes of standing.

Head-up tilt table testing is significantly better than the aforementioned test in diagnosing OH. Tilt table testing needs to be performed by individuals trained in advanced cardiac life support and in settings with resuscitation equipment available. This testing can help differentiate between OH and other disorders of orthostasis including dysautonomia, postural orthostatic tachycardia syndrome, and neurogenic syncope.

Treatment

Providers must treat the underlying cause of OH. All patients with OH should be instructed to move slowly from sitting to standing positions and consider isometric exercises after prolonged sitting. Additionally, patients may be instructed to take anti-hypertensives prior to sleep and possibly switch from one medication class to another. Patients should also be advised to drink adequate fluids to maintain water balance; older adults should consume a minimum of 1.25-2.5 L of fluid per day. Providers may sometimes recommend sodium replacement through salt tabs or adding salt to food. If this is necessary patients should be assessed for lower extremity swelling, weight gain, and serum sodium. If a patient does not respond to these procedures, then pharmacological therapy may be needed including fludrocortisone, midodrine, and pyridostigmine.

References and Additional Literature to Read

Shahoud JS, Sanvictores T, Aeddula NR. Physiology, Arterial Pressure Regulation. [Updated 2021 Sep 6]. In: StatPearls [Internet]. Treasure Island (FL): StatPearls Publishing; 2022.

Oparil S, Acelajado MC, Bakris GL, et al. Hypertension. *Nat Rev Dis Primers*. 2018;4:18014. Published 2018 Mar 22. doi:10.1038/nrdp.2018.14.

Modi P, Arsiwalla T. Hypertensive Retinopathy. [Updated 2021 Jul 10]. In: StatPearls [Internet]. Treasure Island (FL): StatPearls Publishing; 2022 Jan-. Available from: https://www.ncbi.nlm.nih.gov/books/NBK525980/).

Alexander M et al. Hypertension. Medscape. 2/22/2019. https://emedicine.medscape.com/article/241381-overview.

Atsma F. Hemoglobin Level is Positively Associated with Blood Pressure in Large Cohort of Health Individuals. Hypertension. 2012; 60:936-941.

Choudhury KN, Mainuddin AK, Wahiduzzaman M, Islam SM. Serum lipid profile and its association with hypertension in Bangladesh. Vasc Health Risk Manag. 2014;10:327-332. Published 2014 Jun 30. doi:10.2147/VHRM.S61019

Siddiqui M, et al. Secondary Hypertension and Complications: Diagnosis and Role of Imaging. Radiographics. 2019. 39:1036-1055.

Bird K, Chan G, Lu H, et al. Assessment of Hypertension Using Clinical Electrocardiogram Features: A First-Ever Review. Front Med (Lausanne). 2020;7:583331. Published 2020 Dec 4. doi:10.3389/fmed.2020.583331.

Lanier J. Evaluation and Management of Orthostatic Hypotension. *Am Fam Physician.* 2011 Sep 1;84(5):527-536.

Figueroa JJ, Basford JR, Low PA. Preventing and treating orthostatic hypotension: As easy as A, B, C. *Cleve Clin J Med*. 2010;77(5):298-306. doi:10.3949/ccjm.77a.09118.

Goetsch M, et al. New Guidance on Blood Pressure Management in Low-Risk Adults with Stage I Hypertension. https://www.acc.org/latest-in-cardiology/articles/2021/06/21/13/05/new-guidance-on-bp-management-in-low-risk-adults-with-stage-1-htn.

Jones DW, Whelton PK, Allen N, et al. Management of stage 1 hypertension in adults with a low 10-year risk for cardiovascular disease: filling a guidance gap: a scientific statement from the American Heart Association. *Hypertension* 2021;77:e58-e67.

Whelton PK, Carey RM, Aronow WS, et al. 2017 ACC/AHA/AAPA/ABC/ACPM/AGS/APhA/ASH/ASPC/NMA/PCNA guideline for the prevention, detection, evaluation, and management of high blood pressure in adults: a report of the American College of Cardiology/American Heart Association Task Force on Clinical Practice Guidelines. *J Am Coll Cardiol* 2018;71:e127-e248.

Wright JT Jr, Williamson JD, Whelton PK, et al. A randomized trial of intensive versus standard blood-pressure control. *N Engl J Med* 2015;373:2103-16.

Lewis CE, Fine LJ, Beddhu S, et al. Final report of a trial of intensive versus standard blood-pressure control. *N Engl J Med* 2021;384:1921-30.

Berry JD, Dyer A, Cai X, et al. Lifetime risks of cardiovascular disease. *N Engl J Med*. 2012;366:321-29.

Cheung AK, Chang TI, Cushman WC, Furth SL, Hou FF, Ix JH, Knoll GA, Muntner P, Pecoits-Filho R, Sarnak MJ, Tobe SW, Tomson CRV, Lytvyn L, Craig JC, Tunnicliffe DJ, Howell M, Tonelli M, Cheung M, Earley A, Mann JFE. Executive summary of the KDIGO 2021 Clinical Practice Guideline for the Management of Blood Pressure in Chronic Kidney Disease. Kidney Int. 2021 Mar;99(3):559-569. doi: 10.1016/j.kint.2020.10.026. PMID: 33637203.

Clark D 3rd, Hall ME, Jones DW. Dilemma of blood pressure management in older and younger adults. *Hypertension* 2020;75:35-37.

Wu S, Song Y, Chen S, et al. Blood pressure classification of 2017 associated with cardiovascular disease and mortality in young Chinese adults. *Hypertension* 2020;76:251-58.

Son JS, Choi S, Kim K, et al. Association of blood pressure classification in Korean young adults according to the 2017 American College of Cardiology/American Heart Association guidelines with subsequent cardiovascular disease events. *JAMA* 2018;320:1783.

Whelton SP, McEvoy JW, Shaw L, et al. Association of normal systolic blood pressure level with cardiovascular disease in the absence of risk factors. *JAMA Cardiol* 2020;5:1011-18.

Yano Y, Stamler J, Garside DB, et al. Isolated systolic hypertension in young and middle-aged adults and 31-year risk for cardiovascular mortality: the Chicago Heart Association Detection Project in Industry study. *J Am Coll Cardiol* 2015;65:327-35.

Yano Y, Reis JP, Colangelo LA, et al. Association of blood pressure classification in young adults using the 2017 American College of Cardiology/American Heart Association Blood Pressure guideline with cardiovascular events later in life. *JAMA* 2018;320:1774-82.

Verdecchia P. Usual vs tight control of SBP in non-diabetic patients with HTN. Lancet. 2009.

Hansson. Effects of intensive blood-pressure lowering and low-dose aspirin in patients with hypertension: principal results of the Hypertension Optimal Treatment (HOT) randomised trial. HOT Study Group. Lancet. 1998.

JATOS Study Group. Principal results of the Japanese trial to assess optimal systolic blood pressure in elderly hypertensive patients (JATOS). Hypertens Res. 2008.

Ogihara T. Valsartan in Elderly Isolated Systolic Hypertension Study Group Target blood pressure for treatment of isolated systolic hypertension in the elderly: valsartan in elderly isolated systolic hypertension study. Hypertension. 2010.

Cushman WC. ACCORD Study Group. Effects of intensive blood-pressure control in type 2 diabetes mellitus. N Engl J Med. 2010.

Wright JT. SPRINT Research Group. A randomized trial of intensive versus standard blood-pressure control. N Engl J Med. 2015.

Patel A. Effects of a fixed combination of perindopril and indapamide on macrovascular and microvascular outcomes in patients with type 2 diabetes mellitus (the ADVANCE trial): a randomised controlled trial. Lancet. 2007.

Liu L. The Felodipine Event Reduction (FEVER) Study: a randomized long-term placebo-controlled trial in Chinese hypertensive patients. J Hypertens. 2005.

White CL. Can blood pressure be lowered safely in older adults with lacunar stroke? The Secondary Prevention of Small Subcortical Strokes study experience. J Am Geriatr Soc. 2015.

PROGRESS Collaborative Group. Randomised trial of a perindopril-based blood-pressure-lowering regimen among 6,105 individuals with previous stroke or transient ischaemic attack. Lancet. 2001.

Tomson C et al. Management of blood pressure in patients with chronic kidney disease not receiving dialysis: synopsis of the 2021 kdigo clinical practice guideline.

Lewington S, Clarke R, Qizilbash N, et al; Prospective Studies Collaboration. Age-specific relevance of usual blood pressure to vascular mortality: a meta-analysis of individual data for one million adults in 61 prospective studies. Lancet. 2002;360:1903-13. [PMID: 12493255].

Bundy JD, Li C, Stuchlik P, et al. Systolic blood pressure reduction and risk of cardiovascular disease and mortality: a systematic review and network meta-analysis. JAMA Cardiol. 2017;2:775- 781. [PMID:28564682] doi:10.1001/jamacardio.2017.1421.

Ettehad D, Emdin CA, Kiran A, et al. Blood pressure lowering for prevention of cardiovascular disease and death: a systematic review and meta-analysis. Lancet. 2016;387:957-967. [PMID:26724178] doi:10.1016/S0140-6736(15)01225-8.

"Type of Blood Pressure Medications", the American Heart Association. https://www.heart.org/en/health-topics/high-blood-pressure/changes-you-can-make-to-manage-high-blood-pressure/types-of-blood-pressure-medications.

Chaudhari S, Pham GS, Brooks CD, Dinh VQ, Young-Stubbs CM, Shimoura CG, and Mathis KW. Should Renal Inflammation Be Targeted While Treating Hypertension? Frontiers in Physiology. 2022; 13: 886779.

Mancia G, Grassi G. Aggressive blood pressure lowering is dangerous: the J-curve: pro side of the argument. Hypertension. 2014;63:29-36. [PMID:24336629] doi:10.1161/01.hyp.0000441190 .09494.e9.

Verdecchia P, Angeli F, Mazzotta G, et al. Aggressive blood pressure lowering is dangerous: the J-curve: con side of the argument. Hypertension. 2014;63:37-40. [PMID:24336630] doi:10 .1161/01.hyp.0000439102.43479.43

O'Seaghdha CM, Perkovic V, Lam TH, et al; Asia Pacific Cohort Studies Collaboration. Blood pressure is a major risk factor for renal death: an analysis of 560 352 participants from the Asia-Pacific region. Hypertension. 2009;54:509-15. [PMID:19597042] doi:10 .1161/HYPERTENSIONAHA.108.128413.

Tozawa M, Iseki K, Iseki C, et al. Blood pressure predicts risk of developing end-stage renal disease in men and women. Hypertension. 2003;41:1341-5. [PMID:12707291].

American Diabetes Association; *Standards of Medical Care in Diabetes—2022* Abridged for Primary Care Providers. *Clin Diabetes* 1 January 2022; 40 (1): 10–38. https://doi.org/10.2337/cd22-as01.

Maddox T, et al. 2021 Update to the 2017 ACC Expert Consensus Decision Pathway for Optimization of Heart Failure Treatment: Answers to 10 Pivotal Issues About Heart Failure With Reduced Ejection Fraction. Journal of the American College of Cardiology. 77; 6; 772-810. 2021.

Kleindorfer D et al. 2021 Guideline for the Prevention of Stroke in Patients With Stroke and Transient Ischemic Attack: A Guideline From the American Heart Association/American Stroke Association. Stroke. 52;7;364-467. 2021.

Ricci F, De Caterina R, Fedorowski A. Orthostatic Hypotension: Epidemiology, Prognosis, and Treatment. J Am Coll Cardiol. 2015 Aug 18;66(7):848-860. doi: 10.1016/j.jacc.2015.06.1084. PMID: 26271068.

Kidney Disease Outcomes Quality Initiative (K/DOQI). K/DOQI clinical practice guidelines on hypertension and antihypertensive agents in chronic kidney disease. Am J Kidney Dis. 2004 May;43(5 Suppl 1):S1-290. PMID: 15114537.

Saedon NI, Pin Tan M, Frith J. The Prevalence of Orthostatic Hypotension: A Systematic Review and Meta-Analysis. J Gerontol A Biol Sci Med Sci. 2020 Jan 1;75(1):117-122. doi: 10.1093/gerona/gly188. PMID: 30169579; PMCID: PMC6909901.

Lanier J. Evaluation and Management of Orthostatic Hypotension. *Am Fam Physician.* 2011 Sep 1;84(5):527-536.

Ricci F, et al. Orthostatic Hypotension. JACC (Journal of the American College of Cardiology), 2015-08-18, Volume 66, Issue 7, Pages 848-860.

Andrea S Méndez, Jesús D Melgarejo, Luis J Mena, Carlos A Chávez, Alicex C González, José Boggia, Joseph D Terwilliger, Joseph H Lee, Gladys E Maestre, Risk Factors for Orthostatic Hypotension: Differences Between Elderly Men and Women, American Journal of Hypertension, Volume 31, Issue 7, July 2018, Pages 797–803, https://doi.org/10.1093/ajh/hpy050.

Norcliffe-Kaufmann L, Kaufmann H, Palma JA, et al. Orthostatic heart rate changes in patients with autonomic failure caused by neurodegenerative synucleinopathies. *Ann Neurol.* 2018;83(3):522-531. doi:10.1002/ana.25170.

Case Study Questions for Chapters 13.1-13.2

Case Study 1

A 22-year-old obese male construction worker, with a past medical history of hyperlipidemia, presents to your office with headaches. He has a family history of hypertension. He smokes cigars on occasion. He denies alcohol and drug use. His vital signs are normal except his blood pressure was 160/99 and 158/90 at the most recent office visits. The physical exam is normal. Medications currently in use are atorvastatin.

In addition to lifestyle changes, what medication would be most appropriate to start?

A Metoprolol
B Tamsulosin
C Verapamil
D Angiotensin Converting Enzyme Inhibitor
E Spironolactone

Case Study 2

A 55-year-old male, with a past medical history of hyperlipidemia and Diabetes Mellitus II, presents to your office for hypertension. He denies tobacco, alcohol, and drug use. His vital signs are normal except his systolic blood pressure was 180/99 and 170/92 at the most recent office visits. The physical exam is normal. Medications currently in use are atorvastatin. In addition to lifestyle changes, what does the 2022 ADA Standards of Care recommend for this patient?

A Angiotensin Converting Enzyme Inhibitor
B Thiazide diuretic
C Angiotensin Converting Enzyme Inhibitor and Thiazide diurectic
D Angiotensin Converting Enzyme Inhibitor and Angiotensin Receptor Blocker
E Angiotensin Converting Enzyme Inhibitor and Beta Blocker

Quiz Questions for Chapters 13.1-13.2

1. What ethnicity has the highest risk for hypertension?

A African Americans
B Caucasian
C Asian
D Hispanic
E Pacific Islanders

2. As a medical student treating a patient with hypertension your preceptor asks you what is the current definition of hypertension according to the 2017 ACC/AHA guidelines. You correctly inform your preceptor that hypertension is

A 140-149/90-99
B 130-139/80-89
C 120-129/70-79
D 150-159/100-109
E 110-119/70-79

3. You are treating an adult female patient with hypertension. According to the 2021 AHA/ACC hypertension guideline update what is the blood pressure goal for this patient?

A <130/80
B <140/80
C <150/80
D <160/80
E <120/80

4. What class of antihypertensive medications work by increasing urine volume, thereby reducing blood volume and blood pressure?

A Thiazide diuretics
B Calcium channel blocker
C Angiotensin Receptor Blocker
D Beta Blockers
E Angiotensin Converting Enzyme Inhibitor

5. What class of antihypertensive medications work by reducing the contraction of smooth muscle around the vessels and therefore reducing peripheral vascular resistance and blood pressure?

A Thiazide diuretics
B Angiotensin Receptor Blocker
C Calcium channel blocker
D Beta Blockers
E Angiotensin Converting Enzyme Inhibitor

Case Study Answers

Case Study 1

D. Metoprolol is not a first-line agent for hypertension. Tamsulosin is not a treatment for hypertension. Verapamil, a non-dihydropyridine, is used for its effects on the SA and AV node and helps with rate control and less for hypertension. Dihydropyridines, like amlodipine, act on blood vessels leading to vasodilatation and thereby reducing hypertension. Angiotensin Converting Enzyme Inhibitors are used to treat hypertension. Spironolactone is not a first-line medication for hypertension treatment.

Case Study 2

C. The 2022 ADA Standards of Care recommends that patients with diabetes and blood pressure ≥160/100 mg should be started on two anti-hypertensive medications simultaneously. When treating patients without heart failure you should never use both ACE inhibitors and ARB. Therefore, the only option is Angiotensin Converting Enzyme Inhibitor and Thiazide diuretic. Beta-blockers are not appropriate first-line agents to treat hypertension.

Quiz Answers

1. A. African Americans have the highest risk of hypertension. African Americans, as compared to Caucasians, have higher hypertension prevalence (45.3% versus 31.4%, P<0.001). Hispanic adults and Asian adults, when compared to white adults, have similar hypertension prevalence (71.1% versus 79.1%, P=0.005) and (72.5% versus 79.1%, P=0.038), respectively.
Aggarwal R, et al. Racial/Ethnic Disparities in Hypertension Prevalence, Awareness, Treatment, and Control in the United States, 2013 to 2018. Hypertension. 2021;78:1719–1726.

2. B. The AHA/ACC 2017 hypertension guideline states that the definition of HTN is 130-139/80-89.
Maddox T, et al. 2021 Update to the 2017 ACC Expert Consensus Decision Pathway for Optimization of Heart Failure Treatment: Answers to 10 Pivotal Issues About Heart Failure With Reduced Ejection Fraction. Journal of the American College of Cardiology. 77; 6; 772-810. 2021.
Whelton PK et al. 2017 ACC/AHA/AAPA/ABC/ACPM/AGS/APhA/ASH/ASPC/NMA/PCNA guideline for the prevention, detection, evaluation, and management of high blood pressure in adults: a report of the American College of Cardiology/American Heart Association Task Force on Clinical Practice Guidelines. J Am Coll Cardiol 2018;71:e127-e248.

3. A. <130/80. Hypertension remains the most modifiable risk factor for cardiovascular disease and the ACC/AHA continues to recommend stricter blood pressure goals with their 2021 Hypertension Guideline update.
Maddox T, et al. 2021 Update to the 2017 ACC Expert Consensus Decision Pathway for Optimization of Heart Failure Treatment: Answers to 10 Pivotal Issues About Heart Failure With Reduced Ejection Fraction. Journal of the American College of Cardiology. 77; 6; 772-810. 2021
Whelton PK et al. 2017 ACC/AHA/AAPA/ABC/ACPM/AGS/APhA/ASH/ASPC/NMA/PCNA guideline for the prevention, detection, evaluation, and management of high blood pressure in adults: a report of the American College of Cardiology/American Heart Association Task Force on Clinical Practice Guidelines. J Am Coll Cardiol 2018;71:e127-e248.

4. A. Diuretics target transporters on epithelial cells of the nephron, specifically in the regions of the ascending loop of Henle, collecting ducts and distal tubules. Thiazides are a class of diuretics that inhibit the Na+-Cl- cotransporter on the apical membrane of epithelial cells in the distal tubule. With hydrochlorothiazide therapy, for example, these ions remain in the lumen of the tubule and water accompanies them, thereby increasing urine volume and reducing blood pressure.
Ellison D. Clinical Pharmacology in Diuretic Use. CJASN August 2019, 14 (8) 1248-1257; DOI: https://doi.org/10.2215/CJN.09630818.

5. C. When calcium moves through its channel down the concentration gradient, into the cell, this leads to contraction. Blockade of calcium channels directly reduces the contraction of smooth muscle around the vessels and therefore reduces peripheral vascular resistance and blood pressure. These blockers also have an effect on the cardiac muscle, reducing the force and frequency of contraction.
LiverTox: Clinical and Research Information on Drug-Induced Liver Injury [Internet]. Bethesda (MD): National Institute of Diabetes and Digestive and Kidney Diseases; 2012–. Calcium Channel Blockers. 2017 Jan 11. PMID: 31643892.

SYMPTOMS 3 –

MUSCULOSKELETAL SYMPTOMS TO TREATMENT

CHAPTER 14

LOW BACK PAIN

LEAH HAMMER, PHD[1] AND RYAN SEALS, DO[2]

[1] West Virginia University, Morgantown, West Virginia, USA
[2] University of North Texas Health Science Center, Fort Worth, Texas, USA

Symptoms: **Musculoskeletal**

Drug List for Back Pain

Nonsteroidal anti-inflammatory drugs (NSAIDs):
Ibuprofen
Naproxen
Diclofenac
Indomethacin
Ketorolac
Meloxicam
Celecoxib

Corticosteroids:
Betamethasone
Dexamethasone
Prednisolone

Antidepressants - Tricyclic antidepressants (TCAs):
Nortriptyline
Amitriptyline

Antidepressants - Serotonin Norepinephrine Reuptake Inhibitors (SNRIs):
Duloxetine
Venlafaxine

Muscle Relaxants:
Cyclobenzaprine
Tizanidine
Metaxalone
Baclofen

Antiseizure drugs:
Gabapentin
Pregabalin

Local anesthetics:
Lidocaine

Opioids and Drugs with Mixed Actions

Background

Low back pain is one of the most frequent ailments of humanity and will affect 65-85% of the world's population at some point in their lives. Low back is the fifth most common reason for a physician's office visit in the United States. Additionally, back and spine impairments are among the top causes limiting activities among most age groups. Over half of low back pain resolves on its own within one week and 90% resolves within eight weeks. The remaining cases tend to linger longer than six months, and many acute cases are prone to relapse (Kelly 2021).

Pain of the lower back can arise from any pain-sensing structures such as bones, intervertebral discs, facet joints, ligaments, muscles, neural structures, and blood vessels. (Hoy et al. 2010) Pain can also be referred from internal organs such as the kidneys, bladder, aorta, ovaries, and uterus. (*Neurology in Clinical Practice* 2022) Only 5-15% of low back pain can be attributed to a specific cause such as compression fracture, neoplasm, or infection. The remainder of low back pain has a less clear "cause" and is thought to be a combination of boney, muscular, and connective tissue pain. (*Neurology in Clinical Practice* 2022; Rao et al. 2018) From a pharmacological perspective, there is overlap in the treatment approach in these groupings of non-specific/mechanical low back pain and it is helpful to distinguish acute from chronic back pain for medication selection.

Diagnosis

The most important first step when evaluating a patient with low back pain is to make a diagnosis. Although rare, several diagnoses are life-threatening (e.g. cauda equina, tumor/cancer, infection) that should be ruled out first. For infections, the physician should look for fever, chills, or other systemic signs of infection and consider the appropriate laboratory evaluation. Night pain or unexplained weight loss are suspicious for cancer and should be considered in the evaluation process. (Maher et al. 2017) A good physical examination is essential, including visualization, palpation, and motion testing of the lumbar spine, sacroiliac, and hip joints. Neurologic evaluation should always be performed for any symptoms consistent with cord or nerve root pathology. Imaging is not indicated if the pain is less than 6 weeks in duration and unless suspicion of fracture or neurologic compromise is present. Magnetic resonance imaging (MRI) is highly sensitive for identifying abnormalities of the vertebrae and discs, but these findings are not highly correlated with pain. In most cases, MRIs should be reserved for low back pain with radiculopathy that has not resolved with conservative measures within 6 weeks, unless there is suspicion of cauda equina, tumor, abscess, or a bleed. (Rao et al. 2018)

Common Causes of Low Back Pain

Types of back pain (in order of prevalence)

- Nonspecific low back pain (including myofascial pain) - 85%
- Discogenic
- Facet joint
- Spinal stenosis/myelopathy
- SI joint pain/arthritis
- Radiculopathy
- Cauda Equina
- Infection (not covered in this chapter)
- Tumors (not covered in this chapter)
- Other

Nonspecific low back pain (including myofascial pain)

Mechanical low back pain is usually caused by strain/sprain of paraspinal muscles and related ligaments and connective tissue structures. This category encompasses up to 85% of presentations of low back pain and is often a diagnosis of exclusion after ruling out more urgent/emergent causes of low back pain. (*Neurology in Clinical Practice* 2022; Urits and Burshtein 2019; Maher et al. 2017)

Presentation: Mechanical low back pain presents as localized in nature, but certain joint, ligament, and muscle pain patterns can involve radiation of the pain. Radiation of pain from muscle and ligamentous structure is non-dermatomal, dull in nature, and typically does not extend below the knee. Radiating pain from these structures is more common than radicular pain due to nerve root compression. (Kelly 2021) The pain may be triggered by physical factors such as lifting (most commonly), psychological factors such as fatigue, or a combination of both. (Barraclough 2021) However, up to one-third of patients do not recall a specific triggering event. (Maher et al. 2017)

Risk Factors: Mechanical low back pain is more common in women than men and has the highest incidence in those aged 40-69 years old, but it can impact almost all age groups. Smoking, obesity, and depressive symptoms also modestly increase the risk of developing low back pain. (Maher et al. 2017)

Pathophysiology: Pain of the lower back can arise from any pain-sensing structures such as bones, intervertebral discs, facet joints, ligaments, muscles, neural structures, and blood vessels. (Hoy et al. 2010) Non-specific low back pain is thought to be caused by irritations involving the ligaments, muscles, connective tissues, and their related nociceptive and afferent innervation.

Examination: A proper physical exam for all back pain should include inspection and palpation of the spine, paravertebral muscles, percussion of the vertebrae, range of motion of the lumbar spine and hip joints, and complete neurologic evaluation including lower extremity strength, sensation, and reflexes. A straight leg raise should also be performed, particularly if there is radiation of the pain into the lower extremity. (Kelly 2021)

Laboratory: No laboratory tests are indicated for this condition.

Imaging: No imaging is indicated during the first 4-6 weeks in the absence of concerns for fracture, systemic disease, or neurologic signs/symptoms. (Rao et al. 2018)

Diagnosis: Nonspecific low back pain is a diagnosis of exclusion based on the signs and symptoms and the absence of other underlying causative diseases.

Treatment: NSAIDs and muscle relaxants are often used (Kelly 2021; Maher et al. 2017), but combination therapy is not superior to monotherapy. (Song et al. 2018)

Management: There is no cure for chronic back pain, and any long-term management strategy should address how this pain inhibits the patient's work, social, and family roles. This can be accompanied by psychological distress and depression; therefore, the management plan should place greater emphasis on non-pharmacologic approaches with pharmacotherapy as an adjunct. (Maher et al. 2017)

Discogenic

Presentation: Discogenic pain presents in the center of the back with minimal radiation. If there is radiation, however, it is located in the buttocks or thighs. The pain is typically achy in nature and improves with standing or lying flat. Pain is typically worsened with sitting, flexion, bending, or twisting. (Urits and Burshtein 2019)

Risk Factors: Risk factors for developing problems with intervertebral discs include obesity and smoking. A higher incidence of disease is found in those with jobs involving lifting, vibration exposure, and being sedentary. (Urits and Burshtein 2019)

Pathophysiology: Disruption of the intervertebral disc is caused by the degradation of the disc and its nuclear components. Fissures can extend from the nucleus to the annulus and further complicate the integrity of the disc. (Urits and Burshtein 2019)

Examination: A proper physical exam for all back pain should include inspection and palpation of the spine, paravertebral muscles, percussion of the vertebrae, range of motion of the lumbar spine and hip joints, and complete neurologic evaluation including lower extremity strength, sensation, and reflexes. A straight leg raise should also be performed, particularly if there is radiation of the pain into the lower extremity. (Kelly 2021)

Laboratory: No laboratory tests are indicated for this condition.

Imaging: MRI can reveal disc degeneration or tears. (Urits and Burshtein 2019)

Diagnosis: The diagnosis is based on clinical symptoms consistent with discogenic pain and imaging showing evidence of disc degeneration. (Urits and Burshtein 2019) Discograms and diagnostic anesthetic blocks are sometimes used as well, but there are no universal criteria that are accepted for diagnosis. (Malik et al. 2013)

Treatment: Discogenic pain is typically managed similarly to other mechanical causes of back pain with NSAIDs and muscle relaxants in the acute phase. (Kelly 2021) Chronic pain is best treated with NSAIDs and tricyclic antidepressants with combination therapy, in general, being superior to monotherapy. (Song et al. 2018)

Management: After an initial period of 1-2 days of rest, people are encouraged to resume activities as tolerated. (Kelly 2021) There is no cure for chronic back pain, and any long-term management strategy should address how this pain inhibits the patient's work, social, and family roles. This can be accompanied by psychological distress and depression; therefore, the management plan should place greater emphasis on non-pharmacologic approaches with pharmacotherapy as an adjunct. Non-pharmacologic methods to consider include staying active, manual therapy, exercise/rehab programs, and acupuncture. (Maher et al. 2017)

Facet joint

Presentation: Facet joint pain is typically located lateral to the spine and exacerbated by extension and bending toward the affected facet joint. Pain is worsened by prolonged sitting or walking up steps. There typically are no neurologic signs or symptoms unless there is also concomitant nerve root compression. (*Neurology in Clinical Practice* 2022) Pain is frequently referred into the buttock or thigh, but usually not below the knee. (Gellhorn et al. 2013)

Risk Factors: Risk factors for developing facet joint arthritis and pain include strenuous repetitive activities, excessive weight, and abnormal posture. (*Neurology in Clinical Practice* 2022) Women also seem to be at higher risk than men. (Gellhorn et al. 2013)

Pathophysiology: In most cases, spinal degeneration begins with the degeneration of the discs. The loss of height of the discs places increased mechanical load on the facet joints and this contributes to arthritis and potential pain from these structures. (Gellhorn et al. 2013)

Examination: A proper physical exam for all back pain should include inspection and palpation of the spine and paravertebral muscles, along with percussion of the vertebrae, range of motion of the lumbar spine and hip joints, and complete neurologic evaluation including lower extremity strength, sensation, and reflexes. A straight leg raise should also be performed, particularly if there is radiation of the pain into the lower extremity. (Kelly 2021) Facet joint pain can often be reproduced with extension and bending toward the affected side. (*Neurology in Clinical Practice* 2022)

Laboratory: No laboratory tests are indicated for this condition.

Imaging: Lumbar X-rays, CTs, or MRIs can give evidence of facet arthritis.

Diagnosis: Typically, the diagnosis is based on clinical symptoms consistent with facet joint pain and imaging showing evidence of facet arthritis. Facet blocks can be done to inject anesthetic agents diagnostically, but this practice is controversial. (Gellhorn et al. 2013)

Treatment: NSAIDs are first-line agents for acute and chronic pain caused by facet joint arthritis. (*Neurology in Clinical Practice* 2022) Chronic back pain is best treated with NSAIDs and tricyclic antidepressants with combination therapy, in general, being superior to monotherapy. (Song et al. 2018)

Management: Facet joint blocks and radiofrequency neurotomy of the medial branch nerves (Urits and Burshtein 2019) can be used but the evidence is mixed and these procedures are not usually necessary. (Kelly 2021; *Neurology in Clinical Practice* 2022)

Spinal stenosis/myelopathy

Presentation: The presentation for spinal stenosis is low back, gluteal, and/or lower extremity pain and/or fatigue. These symptoms are characteristically exacerbated during upright exercise such as walking and relieved with forward flexion, sitting, or laying down. (Kreiner et al. 2013)

Risk Factors: Advanced age is the most important risk factor due to degeneration that happens over time. 20-30% of adults over 60 have evidence of spinal stenosis on imaging but are asymptomatic. (Kelly 2021)

Pathophysiology: Degenerative spinal stenosis spinal degeneration begins with degeneration of the discs. The loss of height of the discs places increased mechanical load on the facet joints and this contributes to arthritis and potential pain from these structures. (Gellhorn et al. 2013) The further degenerative changes lead to disc space narrowing, ankyloses of joints, and hypertrophy and thickening of the ligamentum flavum. (Lee et al. 2020)

Examination: A proper physical exam for all back pain should include inspection and palpation of the spine and paravertebral muscles, along with percussion of the vertebrae, range of motion of the lumbar spine and hip joints, and complete neurologic evaluation including lower extremity strength, sensation, and reflexes. A straight leg raise should also be performed, particularly if there is radiation of the pain into the lower extremity. (Kelly 2021)

Laboratory: No laboratory tests are indicated for this condition.

Imaging: MRI is the most appropriate test to confirm the presence of anatomic narrowing.

Diagnosis: A diagnosis of the clinical syndrome of lumbar spinal stenosis requires the signs and symptoms associated with this condition along with imaging confirmation of narrowing of the spinal canal. (Kelly 2021)

Treatment: Evidence for or against the use of pharmacologic treatments for spinal stenosis is lacking. (Kreiner et al. 2013) However, they can be treated similarly to other causes of acute and chronic low back pain.

Management: Epidural steroids are indicated and may provide short-term symptomatic improvement (less than six months). Lumbar spinal stenosis is the most frequent indication for spinal surgery in patients over the age of 65. Decompressive surgery may be an option for those with moderate to severe spinal stenosis. (Kelly 2021; Kreiner et al. 2013; Urits and Burshtein 2019)

SI joint pain/arthritis

Presentation: Sacroiliac (SI) joint pain presents as pain lateral to the spine where the sacrum articulates with the top of the iliac bone. Pain is usually exacerbated by movement and pressure.

Risk Factors: Patients can get SI joint pain due to degenerative arthritis, sacroiliitis, trauma, or associated with pregnancy. (Rashbaum et al. 2016)

Pathophysiology: Degeneration of the SI joint can be caused by overuse and/or excess movement of the joint. Leg length discrepancy, previous lumbar posterior fusion, and other traumas may increase the development of SI joint pain. The joint is innervated by a nerve plexus from the posterior rami of L5-S4 that picks up nociceptive information from the joint. (Rashbaum et al. 2016)

Examination: A proper physical exam for all back pain should include inspection and palpation of the spine and paravertebral muscles, along with percussion of the vertebrae, range of motion of the lumbar spine and hip joints, and complete neurologic evaluation including lower extremity strength, sensation, and reflexes. A straight leg raise should also be performed, particularly if there is radiation of the pain into the lower extremity. (Kelly 2021) To more specifically diagnose the SI joint as a cause of the pain, three of the following five special tests must be positive: distraction, compression, Gaenslen maneuver, FABER test, and high thrust. (Rashbaum et al. 2016)

Imaging: X-rays often show arthritic changes in the SI joint that support this diagnosis as the source of back pain along with the history and physical exam. (*Neurology in Clinical Practice* 2022) However, other than ruling out severe pathology and visualizing arthritic changes, imaging does not add significant value to this diagnosis beyond the physical exam criteria already noted. (Rashbaum et al. 2016)

Diagnosis: The diagnosis of SI joint pain involves understanding the patient's history and presentation of symptoms along with the physical exam and presence of 3 of the 5 physical exam special tests. Imaging can support the presence of arthritis but this information does not necessarily correlate to the primary cause of the patient's pain. (Rashbaum et al. 2016)

Treatment: Conservative care including NSAIDs, stretching, strengthening, and mobilization is typically recommended as first-line treatment for SI joint pain.

Management: If conservative approaches are not successful, then anesthetic joint injections can be performed, and radiofrequency ablation can be used to burn the nerve mediating the pain signals. Finally, SI joint fusion surgery can be offered if only temporary improvements are gained from the aforementioned procedures. (Rashbaum et al. 2016)

Radiculopathy

Presentation: Lumbosacral radiculopathy presents as pain radiating into the lower extremities secondary to nerve root compression. The compression of a spinal nerve leads to pain that has dermatomal distribution, radiates below the knee, and often has accompanying paresthesia in the same dermatome. The pain is typically described as lancinating, shooting, and sharp in quality and worsens with Valsalva, coughing, or sneezing. (Kelly 2021)

Risk Factors: The peak frequency of herniation is between the ages of 44 and 50 and then progressively declines after that. Degeneration of the spine increases with age and can also lead to the narrowing of the vertebral foramina and compression of the spinal nerve roots. (Kelly 2021)

Pathophysiology: This syndrome is caused by compression of the nerve root near the level of the vertebral foramina. Most commonly this is from a herniated disc, but in older patients, it can also be from osteophytes related to spinal degeneration. Due to the large amount of motion at the L4-5 levels (torsion motion) and L5-S1 (flexion and extension motion) over 90% of disc herniations occur at this level. (Kelly 2021; *Neurology in Clinical Practice* 2022)

Examination: A proper physical exam for all back pain should include inspection and palpation of the spine, paravertebral muscles, and areas of pain, along with percussion of the vertebrae, range of motion of the lumbar spine and hip joints, and complete neurologic evaluation including lower extremity strength, sensation, and reflexes. A straight leg raise should also be performed, particularly if there is radiation of the pain into the lower extremity. The presence of a positive straight leg raise along with neurologic findings from the same nerve root supports nerve root compression, but it is not uncommon for these signs to be absent. (Kelly 2021; *Neurology in Clinical Practice* 2022)

Imaging: MRI is the diagnostic modality of choice to visualize the neural foramina and determine the amount and cause of any compression. (*Neurology in Clinical Practice* 2022)

Diagnosis: The diagnosis is made by the clinical presentation of radiating pain along a specific dermatome along with supporting evidence from the physical exam. MRI can provide visual evidence of the compression of a nerve root involved. (*Neurology in Clinical Practice* 2022; Kelly 2021)
Treatment: Most patients can be treated conservatively initially unless they are showing symptoms of severe neurologic compromise such as severe weakness or signs/symptoms of cauda equina. Pain can be managed with drugs such as anti-inflammatory steroids, NSAIDs, and antiseizure drugs. Tricyclic antidepressants might have some slight benefits, but the evidence ranges from low to very low. (Ferreira and McLachlan 2021)

Management: There is partial to complete resolution of herniated discs in most patients and only about 10% have persistent symptoms after six weeks that then must be considered for surgical decompression. (Kelly 2021) Epidural steroid injections can provide temporary improvement for acute radicular pain. (Urits and Burshtein 2019; Song et al. 2018)

Cauda Equina
Presentation: Cauda equina syndrome is defined by the compression of the nerve roots below the termination of the spinal cord (i.e. the cauda equina). This is usually caused by an acute disc herniation at L4/L5 or L5/S1 levels, but the compression could also be caused by infection or tumor. (*Neurology in Clinical Practice* 2022; Barraclough 2021) The patient presents with either acute or chronic low back with disturbance in urinary function, saddle anesthesia, reduced anal tone, and/or bilateral sciatica. (Barraclough 2021)

Pathophysiology: Cauda equina syndrome occurs when anything mechanically compresses the cauda equina, which is the name given to the spinal nerve roots that descend distal to the apex of the spinal cord as they descend to their corresponding spinal foramina to exit peripherally. (Standring 2021) Cauda equina syndrome can occur with acute trauma, acute central disc herniation, chronic degenerative disease of the bones or discs, and infections such as abscesses, intraspinal tumors, or hematomas. (*Neurology in Clinical Practice* 2022)

Examination: A proper physical exam for all back pain should include inspection and palpation of the spine, paravertebral muscles, and areas of pain, along with percussion of the vertebrae, range of motion of the lumbar spine and hip joints, and complete neurologic evaluation including lower extremity strength, sensation, and reflexes. A straight leg raise should also be performed, particularly if there is radiation of the pain into the lower extremity. (Kelly 2021) Additionally, for suspicion of cauda equina, one should assess anal sphincter tone along with fine touch sensation of the perineum. (Barraclough 2021)
Laboratory: None indicated for diagnosis, but laboratory workup may be needed to evaluate or treat certain causes of the cord compression (e.g. spinal abscess).

Imaging: MRI is the preferred imaging approach to evaluate for compression of the cauda equina. CT scan with contrast can alternatively be used for those ineligible for MRI. (*Neurology in Clinical Practice* 2022)

Diagnosis: Presences of radiological compression of the cauda equina along with clinical features. (Barraclough 2021)

Treatment: Surgical decompression is needed emergently to remove the pressure from the nerve structures.

Pharmacologic Treatment of Back Pain

Non-steroidal anti-inflammatory drugs (NSAIDs):

- Ibuprofen
- Naproxen
- Diclofenac
- Indomethacin
- Ketorolac
- Meloxicam
- Celecoxib

Corticosteroids

- Betamethasone
- Dexamethasone
- Prednisolone

Antidepressants - Tricyclic antidepressants (TCAs):

Nortriptyline
Amitriptyline

Antidepressants - Serotonin Norepinephrine Reuptake Inhibitors (SNRIs):

Duloxetine
Venlafaxine

Muscle Relaxants:

Cyclobenzaprine
Tizanidine
Metaxalone
Baclofen

Antiseizure drugs:

Gabapentin
Pregabalin

Local anesthetics:

Lidocaine

Opioids and Drugs with Mixed Actions

Non-steroidal Anti-inflammatory Drugs (NSAIDs; see also Chapter 9)

Background and Clinical Use

NSAIDs are first-line drugs for the treatment of most types of back pain. Non-selective drugs such as **ibuprofen** and **naproxen sodium** are available without a prescription, and prescription-strength drugs are available if needed. **Aspirin**, the prototype NSAID, is rarely used for pain and inflammation today and will not be discussed here. In addition, the COX-2 selective drug, **celecoxib**, and the partially selective COX-2 drugs, **etodolac** and **meloxicam** are available for those patients who cannot tolerate the gastric effects of the non-selective drugs. The efficacy of celecoxib appears comparable to that of non-selective COX inhibitors for the treatment of low back pain.

For patients experiencing acute low back pain, NSAIDs are the first choice of pharmacotherapy. Those who cannot tolerate NSAIDs or who have contraindications to them can use **acetaminophen**, however, evidence for efficacy isn't strong. In addition, acetaminophen has no anti-inflammatory properties and is, therefore, less suitable for pain arising from inflamed tissues. For patients experiencing subacute or chronic back pain, NSAIDs can be continued if they are helpful. If they are only partially helpful, they can be continued with the addition of a second-line drug. If they have not proven helpful during the acute phase of low back pain, they should be discontinued in favor of other treatment modalities.

Acetaminophen, although not classified as an NSAID due to an absence of an anti-inflammatory effect, has a mechanism of action that is similar to NSAIDs. There is no strong data to indicate that it is efficacious in relieving low back pain and is not discussed here.

Pharmacokinetics

NSAIDs are administered orally, although parenteral administration is available for the treatment of more severe pain (e.g. **ketorolac**). Some undergo CYP450 metabolism followed by glucuronidation, while others are directly glucuronidated. Metabolites are excreted renally, although some undergo significant biliary secretion and enterohepatic recycling. Most are highly protein bound.

Mechanism of Action

All NSAIDs work by blocking the synthesis of inflammatory prostaglandins (Chapter 9). Non-selective drugs block both constitutively active COX-1 and inflammation-induced COX-2. The selective COX-2 inhibitor, celecoxib, is 10-20 times more selective for COX-2 than COX-1. Etodolac and meloxicam exhibit selectivity for COX-2 at lower doses.

Adverse Effects

The adverse effects of NSAIDs are usually extensions of their mechanism of action. Inhibition of the constitutive COX-1 enzyme results in decreased production of "housekeeping" prostaglandins such as those necessary for cytoprotection of the gut epithelium. COX-2 inhibition decreases the production of vasodilatory prostacyclin (PGI_2 from vascular endothelial cells, increasing blood pressure. Thus, non-selective drugs are irritating to the gut, COX-2 selective drugs favor coagulation, and all NSAIDs can decrease renal function.

Drug interactions
Because non-selective NSAIDs alone can result in bleeding ulcers, co-administration of drugs that are irritating to the gut (e.g. corticosteroids) should be undertaken with great caution, if at all. Chronic administration of NSAIDs can counter the antihypertensive actions of certain antihypertensive drugs. Blood pressure should be closely monitored in these patients.

Corticosteroids (see also Chapters 4 and 9)
Background and Clinical Use
Corticosteroids can be used for back pain when a stronger anti-inflammatory effect is indicated. Steroids come in many formulations that can be administered orally or parenterally, systemically, or locally. Chronic use of systemic corticosteroids can result in many dangerous adverse effects which can negate the clinical benefits. Local application of steroids can reduce the risk of systemic effects by using smaller doses. For musculoskeletal pain, injections in the area of the inflamed tissue are preferred. In the clinical settings described in this chapter, epidural injections are a common route of administration. Injectable formulations can be divided into particulate (e.g. **methylprednisolone, triamcinolone, betamethasone**), and non-particulate formulations (e.g. **dexamethasone**). Particulate formulations are comprised of larger particle sizes (larger than red blood cells), or the particles can "aggregate" to form larger particle sizes. This type of formulation is often preferred for local effects because the active drug remains at the site of action for longer periods, thus providing longer analgesia. However, when injected into the epidural space, particulate steroids have been associated with an increased risk of catastrophic injury due to blood vessel injury or embolization resulting in spinal cord ischemia. In contrast, non-particulate steroids have smaller particle sizes, are water-soluble, and are not associated with permanent injury. Because non-particulate formulations can leave the epidural space faster than particulate formulations, it is speculated that they may have less clinical efficacy. Data supporting this is inconsistent, and because of the potentially catastrophic outcomes associated with particulate steroids, risk/benefit favors using non-particulate steroids in the epidural space.

Mechanism of Action
Corticosteroids bind with intracellular glucocorticoid receptors that belong to a superfamily of nuclear receptors. When unoccupied, the glucocorticoid receptors exist in the cell's cytoplasm where they are associated with chaperone heat-shock proteins (HSP). When a corticosteroid binds to its receptor, the receptor dissociates from the HSP and forms dimers of drug-bound receptors. These dimers then enter the nucleus of the cell where they interact with DNA to regulate the transcription of genes involved in the process of inflammation.

Adverse Effects
Adverse effects of injected steroids can occur. Steroids distribute out of the epidural space and into the circulation. When administered for short periods (less than 2 weeks), adverse effects are usually limited to central nervous system stimulation (e.g. insomnia, anxiety, euphoria, mild psychosis), gastrointestinal effects (e.g. nausea/vomiting, appetite stimulation), and potentially, increased risk of infection (extension of the mechanism of action). Longer-term use, use of high potency steroids, or high doses of steroids are associated with more serious adverse effects. These include but are not limited to diabetes, iatrogenic Cushing syndrome, osteoporosis, and hypothalamic-pituitary-adrenal (HPA) axis suppression. These effects are not likely to be seen with injections used for low back pain. Similarly, hypertension or heart failure, secondary to sodium and fluid retention, is not likely to be seen when using synthetic glucocorticoids as they have little or no mineralocorticoid activity.

Antidepressants (see also Chapter 17)
Background and Clinical Use
Two classes of antidepressants are used for pain management and in certain situations, are considered first-line treatment (e.g. neuropathic pain disorders); these are the tricyclic antidepressants (TCAs, e.g. **amitriptyline, nortriptyline**) and serotonin norepinephrine reuptake inhibitors (SNRIs, e.g. **venlafaxine, duloxetine**). These are sometimes referred to as analgesic antidepressants, although evidence supporting an analgesic role is moderate at best. TCAs, compared with SNRIs, may be slightly more efficacious in the treatment of low back pain but have a worse side effect profile. Evidence for a role for antidepressants that affect only serotonin (e.g. selective serotonin reuptake inhibitors) in pain management is weak and none of them are approved for this purpose.

Pharmacokinetics
Both TCAs and SNRIs are metabolized by CYP2D6. Plasma concentrations may be altered by hepatic dysfunction, and by drugs that alter the activity of CYP2D6. Venlafaxine is metabolized to an active metabolite by CYP2D6 (desvenlafaxine). Desvenlafaxine is available commercially. Desvenlafaxine is directly conjugated and is therefore not as sensitive to changes in liver function as the other drugs.

Mechanism of Action
SNRIs and tricyclic antidepressants block both serotonin and norepinephrine reuptake. Both of these actions are believed to contribute to their antidepressant effects. However, their role in pain management seems to be more closely tied to their effect on synaptic norepinephrine levels. Within the pain circuitry, descending inhibitory nerves dampen the

afferent pain signal as it is transmitted from the primary afferent neurons at the level of the dorsal horn. The analgesic antidepressants are believed to enhance the efficacy of the descending pathways by increasing extracellular norepinephrine, potentially acting via α_2-adrenoceptors located on the nerve terminals of primary afferent nociceptive nerves.

Tricyclic antidepressants have other pharmacological effects that may contribute to pain relief. There is some evidence that their analgesic effect involves endogenous opioid systems, although the precise mechanism has not been elucidated. Roles for N-methyl-D-aspartate (NMDA) and adenosine receptors have been postulated. TCAs can block sodium channels to different degrees, with amitriptyline being the most potent. This effect may further contribute to the antinociceptive effect of these drugs.

Within the class of TCAs, different drugs interact with histamine, muscarinic, and nicotinic receptors to different degrees. It is not known if these effects contribute to the analgesic effects of TCAs but pain is often multifaceted and these effects may help reduce the perception of pain, especially if they have a positive effect on sleep. While the contribution to the clinical efficacy of this receptor blockade is not clear, it is known to contribute to many of the adverse effects of the drugs (discussed below). Depression is often present in chronic pain patients making these drug classes appropriate first choices for such patients.

Adverse Effects

Tricyclic antidepressants, due to their relatively non-specific action, cause a large number of adverse effects. In particular, the blockade of muscarinic cholinergic receptors in both the central nervous system and peripheral tissues produces a very characteristic spectrum of symptoms collectively referred to as anticholinergic or anti-muscarinic effects/syndrome. Symptoms include dry eyes, dry mouth, flushing, mydriasis, cycloplegia, urinary retention, constipation, overheating (due to suppression of thermoregulatory sweating), tachycardia, sedation, and confusion. Orthostatic hypotension can occur due to blockade of α_1-adrenoceptors. Blockade of histamine H_1 receptors can result in weight gain and sedation. In addition, tricyclic antidepressants carry a significant risk of cardiac arrhythmia, especially in overdose. Some of these effects might be considered beneficial in patients with back pain, e.g. the strong sedating effects of amitriptyline may help patients sleep at night.

SNRIs lack most of the muscarinic, histaminergic, and α_1-adrenoceptor-blocking actions of the TCAs and are therefore often preferred over TCAs for depression and pain. Adverse effects tend to be consistent with either excessive serotonergic activity (e.g. nausea, sexual dysfunction) or noradrenergic activity (e.g. hypertension, increased heart rate, CNS stimulation). Of the available SNRIs, venlafaxine has been most often associated with increases in blood pressure and arrhythmia. Liver damage is a rare effect associated with duloxetine use.

Both classes of drugs have been associated with a withdrawal syndrome and patients do better when slowly weaned off their medication than suddenly discontinuing it.

Drug Interactions

Drug interactions are typically metabolic (co-administration with a CYP2D6 inhibitor, for example) or additive (co-administration with another drug with serotonergic, anti-muscarinic, anti-histaminergic activity). Duloxetine inhibits CYP2D6 moderately, and plasma levels of TCAs can increase in the presence of CYP2D6 inhibitors, especially in patients who have a polymorphism that results in slow CYP2D6 metabolism. Drugs that lower blood pressure may potentiate the α_1-mediated orthostatic hypotension seen with some TCAs or drugs that increase blood pressure may enhance the potential hypertensive effect of venlafaxine. Men with enlarged prostates should avoid using drugs with anti-muscarinic blocking effects such as diphenhydramine with amitriptyline as this can result in severe urinary retention. Serotonin syndrome can also be a risk when taking two serotonergic drugs at the same time. The highest risk occurs when SNRIs are co-administered with monoamine oxidase inhibitors. Patients who are taking other serotonergic drugs should be advised on how to recognize serotonin syndrome.

Muscle Relaxants

This is a heterogeneous group of drugs with largely undefined mechanisms; however, those used for acute muscle pain are believed to act via central mechanisms. **Cyclobenzaprine** is the most commonly prescribed drug in this group and is structurally related to tricyclic antidepressants. It has significant anti-muscarinic activity. Other muscle relaxants available for use in the US are **metaxalone**, **baclofen**, **carisoprodol**, **chlorzoxazone**, **methocarbamol**, and **orphenadrine**. **Tizanidine** is another muscle relaxant available in the US. It is usually used to treat diseases associated with chronic spasticity but is sometimes used for low back pain. Tizanidine is an agonist of presynaptic α_2-adrenoceptors. Its muscle-relaxing effect is thought to be due to the activation of central α_2-adrenoceptors. Tizanidine is similar to the anti-hypertensive drug clonidine but is less likely to cause hypotension (see also Chapter 13). All of the centrally-acting drugs produce sedation which may contribute to their therapeutic effect, however, this may also limit their usefulness in ambulant patients, especially those who need to drive or operate heavy machinery. Night-time dosing may benefit patients who cannot tolerate the sedation. Muscle relaxants are often combined with an NSAID in the acute setting when pain relief with the NSAID alone is inadequate, but evidence for the efficacy of such combinations is limited. There is no evidence supporting the combined use of muscle relaxants with acetaminophen. Elderly patients are more sensitive to the anti-muscarinic effects of these drugs, and carisoprodol has abuse potential.

Benzodiazepines also have skeletal muscle relaxant properties, but these are generally not recommended due to their abuse liability (see Chapter 23).

Anti-seizure Drugs

Background and Clinical Use

Gabapentin and **pregabalin** were originally designed as GABA analogs for the treatment of seizures. However, their primary use today is in pain management. The only painful condition that gabapentin is FDA-approved to treat in the US is postherpetic neuralgia. Pregabalin is also approved for the treatment of postherpetic neuralgia but it is additionally approved to treat diabetic neuropathy, fibromyalgia, and neuropathic pain. Available evidence suggests a lack of efficacy for the treatment of low back pain, nonetheless, they are both used off-label in this manner.

Pharmacokinetics

An advantage of gabapentin and pregabalin over other drugs is that they are not metabolized, nor do they affect CYP450 enzymes, and they do not bind to plasma proteins. Thus, their potential for drug-drug interactions, especially via pharmacokinetic processes, is low. Absorption of gabapentin, but not pregabalin, is susceptible to saturation and thus it exhibits more patient variability in dosing requirements than pregabalin. Both are excreted via the kidney and both are available in extended-release formulations.

Mechanism of Action

Despite being structural analogs of the neurotransmitter GABA, neither produces its therapeutic effect by altering GABA neurotransmission. Their precise mechanisms are unclear, although they are known to bind to a subunit of voltage-gated calcium channels which may result in the inhibition of glutamate release.

Adverse Drug Effects

Gabapentin and pregabalin are well-tolerated. Common effects include sedation, dizziness, headache, ataxia, tremor, weight gain, and edema. The biggest concern with these drugs is that they appear to potentiate the euphoric effects of opioids and other drugs, and are thus often misused by individuals who misuse other substances. Pregabalin is a controlled substance in the US, while gabapentin remains unscheduled at the federal level. However, many states now treat gabapentin like a controlled substance which allows for prescriptions to be tracked through state prescription drug monitoring programs.

Local Anesthetics

Local anesthetics are available in injectable and topical formulations. Evidence is not strong supporting either formulation for low back pain; however, certain patients might find some relief. **Lidocaine** can be injected into "trigger points" in sore muscles. Lidocaine is commercially available in over-the-counter pain-relieving patches in the US as well as in various topical creams. The pharmacology of local anesthetics is discussed in detail elsewhere. (Becker and Reed 2012)

Opioids (see Chapter 24)

Many opioid agonists are available for treating pain; however, given the chronic nature of many types of back pain, opioids are mostly contraindicated for this purpose. The risk of misuse outweighs any temporary relief that opioids provide. Nonetheless, for patients who have failed all other treatment options (or have contraindications to other therapies) or who may benefit from the temporary relief that opioids can provide, there are many opioids to choose from. Immediate-release opioids formulated with acetaminophen have been widely used for pain. **Tramadol** and **tapentadol** may have some utility due to having additional mechanisms, but they are not devoid of abuse liability. Because opioids are not recommended for back pain they will not be discussed here.

References

Barraclough, Kevin. 2021. Easily Missed? Cauda equina syndrome. *British Medical Journal* 372 (32).

Becker, D. E., and K. L. Reed. 2012. Local anesthetics: review of pharmacological considerations. *Anesth Prog* 59 (2):90-101; quiz 102-103.

Ferreira, Giovanni, and Andrew McLachlan. 2021. Efficacy and safety of antidepressants for the treatment of back pain and osteoarthritis: a systematic review and meta-analysis. *BMJ* (372).

Gellhorn, Alfred, Jeffrey Katz, and Pradeep Suri. 2013. Osteoarthritis of the spine: the facet joints. *National Review Rheumatology* 9 (4):216-224.

Hoy, D, P Brooks, F Blyth, and R Buchbinder. 2010. The epidemiology of low back pain. *Best Practice and research Clinical Rheumatology* (24):769-781.

Kelly, Firestein and. 2021. *Textbook of Rheumatology*: Elsevier.

Kreiner, D. Scott, William Shaffer, and Jamie Baisden. 2013. An evidence-based clinical guideline for the diagnosis and treatment f degenerative lumbar spinal stenosis (update). *The Spine Journal* (13):734-743.

Lee, Byung, Seong-Hwan Moon, and Kyung-Soo Suk. 2020. Lumbar spinal stenosis: pathophysiology and treatment principle: a narrative review. *Asian Spine Journal* 14 (5):682-693.

Maher, Chris, Martin Underwood, and Rachelle Buchbinder. 2017. Non-specific low back pain. *Lancet* (389):736-747.

Malik, Khalid, Steven Cohen, David Walega, and Honorio Benzon. 2013. Diagnostic criteria and treatment of discogenic pain: a systematic review of recent clinical literature. *The Spine Journal* 13 (11):1675-1689.

Neurology in Clinical Practice. 2022. Elsevier Inc.

Rao, Dinesh, Gaelyn Scuderi, Chris Scuderi, Reetu Grewal, and Sukhwinder Sandhu. 2018. The use of imaging in management of patients with low back pain. *Journal of Clinical Imaging Science* 8 (30).

Rashbaum, Ralph, Donna Ohnmeiss, Emily Lindley, Scott Kitchel, and Vikas Patel. 2016. Sacroiliac joint pain and its treatment. *Clinical Spine Surgery* 29 (2).

Song, Liyang, Pencheng Qiu, and Jiaqi Xu. 2018. The effect of combination pharmacotherapy on low back pain: a meta-analysis. *Clinical Journal of Pain* 34 (11):1039-1046.

Standring, Susan. 2021. *Gray's Anatomy*: Elsevier Limited.

Urits, Ivan, and Aaron Burshtein. 2019. Low Back Pain, a comprehensive review: pathophysiology, diagnosis, and treatment. *Current Pain and Headache Reports* 23 (23).

Case Study Questions

Case Study 1

HPI: A 48-year-old presents with bilateral lower back pain for the last 3 weeks. The pain is located in the lower back and radiates into the gluteal region. It is described as dull at rest and sharp with twisting or flexing movements. The patient denies radiation of pain into the leg or foot, denies numbness, and denies any weakness in the lower extremities. There is no identifiable injury, but the patient was moving some furniture a few days before the pain started.
PMH: overweight, acid reflux, hypertension
PSH: Left meniscal tear, appendectomy
Social: non-smoker, married with 2 kids, works as an accountant, drinks 3-4 glasses of wine per week
Medications: Hydrochlorothiazide, omeprazole
Allergies: NKDA
Vitals: BP- 138/92; Height- 70 inches; Weight- 215 pounds; pulse- 78; pain- 4/10
Physical Exam:
Gen: Alert, Oriented, patient appears comfortable
Abdomen: Soft, non-tender, bowel sounds present
Musculoskeletal: mild pain noted with rotation of the lumbar spine bilateral; straight leg raise causes mild pain in the back, but the pain does not radiate into legs; muscle hypertonicity is noted in bilateral lumbar paraspinal muscles, and tenderness is noted to deep palpation in the muscles and ligaments.
Neuro: Reflexes 2/4 in Achilles and patella bilaterally, no weakness noted with muscle testing or when walking on heels and toes, sensation intact to pain and fine touch in lower extremity dermatomes
Skin: No rashes noted

Question 1.1: Based on this patient's history and physical exam, what is the most likely cause of back pain?

A Herniated disc
B Spinal stenosis
C Cauda equina syndrome
D Muscle strain
E Arthritis

Question 1.2: What is the best diagnostic imaging choice to confirm the suspected diagnosis?

A lumbar spine x-rays: anterior, lateral, and oblique
B lumbar spine MRI
C lumbar spine computed tomography (CT)
D DEXA scan
E No imaging is indicated

Question 1.3: What is the mechanism of action of the first-line drugs used to treat this patient?

A Inhibition of cyclooxygenase 1 and cyclooxygenase 2
B Agonist of mu-opioid receptors
C Inhibition of reuptake of norepinephrine and serotonin
D Inhibition of calcium channels
E Stimulation of GABA release

Question 1.4: Which medication is often used in addition to the first-line drug described in question 3 to treat acute musculoskeletal back pain?

A Hydrocodone plus acetaminophen
B Tramadol
C Pregabalin
D Cyclobenzaprine
E Amitriptyline
F Diazepam

Case Study 2

A 52-year-old patient presents with low back pain that came on suddenly 1 week ago. The pain is sharp, localized to the right low back, and causes radiation down the back of the right leg into the food and is described as "electric". There is some mild numbness on the outer lower right leg and foot and weakness when pushing off the right foot. There is no loss of bowel or bladder function.
PMH: hyperlipidemia
PSH: inguinal hernia repair
Social: non-smoker, divorced, works as a plumber, denies alcohol

Medications: simvastatin
Allergies: NKDA
Vitals: BP- 132/86; Height- 72 inches; Weight- 205 pounds; pulse- 78; pain- 8/10
Physical Exam:
Gen: Alert, Oriented, patient appears comfortable
Abdomen: Soft, non-tender, bowel sounds present
Musculoskeletal: straight leg raise causes electric pain down the back of the right leg; pain is reproduced with flexion and compression of the lumbar spine.
Neuro: Bilateral patellar reflex 2/4. Left Achilles reflex 2/4, right Achilles reflex absent. Weakness noted in right foot plantar flexion 3/5. Decreased fine touch sensation on right lateral foot.
Skin: No rashes noted

Question 2.1: Based on this patient's history and physical exam, what is the most likely cause of back pain?

- A Herniated disc
- B Spinal stenosis
- C Cauda equina syndrome
- D Muscle strain
- E Arthritis

Question 2.2: This patient has been self-medicating with ibuprofen since the onset of the pain a week ago. Despite taking supratherapeutic OTC doses (4 x 200 mg TID), he claims that ibuprofen is doing very little to relieve his pain. Which drug is most likely to provide him with some relief from pain?

- A Acetaminophen
- B Gabapentin
- C Cyclobenzaprine
- D Fluoxetine
- E Amitriptyline

Question 2.3: Given this patient's propensity to take more medication than recommended, what would he be placing himself at risk for if he was prescribed amitriptyline?

- A Excessive bleeding
- B Gastric irritation
- C Cardiac arrhythmias
- D Hepatotoxicity
- E Seizures
- F Respiratory depression

Case Study 3

A 72-year-old patient presents with bilateral lower back pain that has been worsening over the last six months. The pain is described as dull and achy. There is no specific radiation of the pain, but the patient endorses difficulty walking long distances, but this seems to be relieved when using a walker. The patient has a history of stress incontinence but denies any recent changes in bowel or bladder function. On physical examination, the lower extremity reflexes are symmetrically decreased. There is a mild loss of fine touch sensation in both lower extremities that does not seem to follow a specific dermatomal pattern. There is mild unsteadiness noted when observing the patient's gait. Distal pulses are present and equal.

Question 3.1: What is the pathophysiology involved in the most likely diagnosis for this patient?

- A Compression of a nerve root by the nucleus pulposus of the disc
- B Narrowing of the spinal canal causing compression on the spinal cord
- C Strain/sprain of the soft tissues of the lumbar spinal region
- D Degenerative changes of the facets and sacroiliac joints
- E Increased volume of cerebrospinal fluid causing compression in the brain

Question 3.2: What pharmacological intervention is indicated in this case?

- A Oral prednisolone
- B Oral acetaminophen
- C Oral ibuprofen
- D Epidural dexamethasone
- E Intramuscular ketorolac
- F Epidural morphine

Question 3.3: What sign or symptom, if present, would indicate a surgical emergency in a similar patient presentation?

A Bilateral sensory loss to the lower extremity.

B Positive straight leg raise

C Pain at night

D Acute loss of bowel or bladder function

E Pain worsened by spinal extension

Case Study Answers

1.1: D is correct. This is most likely muscle strain which falls under non-specific low back pain. This pain is acute onset, occurred after strenuous activity, and has no specific history or exam findings to make one suspicious of any of the other answer choices.

1.2: E is correct; no imaging is indicated at this time. This is non-specific low back pain of less than one-month duration. Without signs of trauma or evidence of neurologic impairment, imaging is not indicated and will not add to the diagnosis.

1.3: A is correct. Non-steroidal anti-inflammatory drugs such as ibuprofen are first-line agents for treating acute muscle pain. They work by inhibiting the enzyme cyclooxygenase (COX). Most NSAIDs are non-specific and block both COX-1 and COX-2. Inhibition of this enzyme subsequently inhibits the synthesis of inflammatory prostaglandins. Non-selective inhibition of prostaglandin synthesis increases acid secretion (COX-1 effect). Monitor his acid reflux. The selective COX-2 inhibitor can be used if his reflux worsens. B. describes opioid analgesics such as oxycodone. These drugs are rarely used for low back pain due to their abuse potential. C. describes the mechanism of action of tricyclic antidepressants or serotonin norepinephrine reuptake inhibitors. These two drug classes may be useful for treating chronic back pain but are not indicated for acute muscle pain. D. describes a potential mechanism of action of anticonvulsants (e.g. gabapentin) sometimes used for the management of chronic neuropathic pain. These drugs may inhibit glutamate release by inhibiting voltage-dependent calcium channels on terminals of glutamate-containing nerves. No analgesics stimulate the release of GABA.

1.4: D is correct. Cyclobenzaprine is a centrally acting muscle relaxant commonly used in the setting of acute muscle pain, in addition to a non-steroidal anti-inflammatory drug. Hydrocodone plus acetaminophen is not indicated for acute muscle pain. Like other opioid analgesics, the risks of using this drug outweigh the clinical benefit in this situation. Tramadol is also an opioid agonist with additional properties; it inhibits serotonin and norepinephrine reuptake. Like other opioid analgesics, it is not recommended for treating acute low back pain. Pregabalin is an anticonvulsant that is sometimes used for chronic neuropathic pain. It is rarely if ever, used in the acute setting. Similarly, amitriptyline is a tricyclic antidepressant used for chronic pain. Diazepam is a benzodiazepine with muscle relaxant properties but is not commonly used in this setting due to its abuse potential.

2.1: A is correct. A positive straight leg raise supports a herniated disc with radiculopathy. The pain is electric and radiates into the foot. There are neurologic findings that indicate the S1 nerve root involvement which indicates a likely disc herniation at the L5-S1 level.

2.2: B is correct. Gabapentin, steroids, and NSAIDs are typically used to manage radiating pain due to disc herniation. Tricyclic antidepressants (amitriptyline) are also sometimes used in this setting but evidence supporting efficacy is weak. No evidence supports the use of acetaminophen for low back pain. Cyclobenzaprine is a skeletal muscle relaxant that is occasionally used for low back pain but since this pain is not due to muscle spasms, it is unlikely to be effective. Fluoxetine is an antidepressant belonging to selective serotonin reuptake inhibitors. This class of antidepressants is not indicated for any type of pain.

2.3: C is correct. Tricyclic antidepressants have a place in chronic pain management, but they are dangerous in overdose. The most serious risk is cardiac toxicity. Other adverse effects include orthostatic hypotension, sedation blurred vision, and urinary retention. Excessive bleeding and gastric irritation can be adverse effects caused by NSAIDs. Hepatotoxicity is associated with acetaminophen overdose and rarely, with duloxetine use. Seizures are associated with tramadol. Respiratory depression is associated with opioids.

3.1: B is correct because this describes the pathophysiology of spinal stenosis. Key features are the pain that is relieved by leaning forward (on a walker or shopping cart) because this posture slightly elongates the spinal cord and can relieve the compression. Depending on which portion of the spinal cord is compressed there can be a variety of sensory and motor signs and symptoms.

3.2: D is correct. There is little evidence to recommend any drug treatment for spinal stenosis, however, epidural steroids are indicated and may provide temporary relief.

3.3: D is correct because this indicates compression of the cauda equina and requires urgent surgery to remove the compression from the spinal cord.

Symptoms 4 –

Neurological Symptoms to Treatment

CHAPTER 15

EXCESSIVE THIRST, HUNGER, AND URINATION IN DIABETES

NANCY S. GREGORY, RN

Palouse Medical, Pullman, WA

Symptoms: **Musculoskeletal**
Neurological
Endo-Repro-Gastrointestinal

DRUG LIST FOR TYPE 1 DIABETES
Insulin and insulin analogs

Ultra-Rapid (Duration 4-5 hours)
Aspart Niacinamide 100 u/ml
URLi 100 u/ml, 200 u/ml

Rapid (Duration 4-5 hours)
insulin Aspart 100 u/ml
insulin Glulisine 100 u/ml
insulin Lispro 100 u/ml

Short Acting (Duration 8-12 hours)
Regular insulin 100 u/ml

Intermediate (Duration 12-24 hours)
NPH 100 u/ml
Concentrated Regular 500 u/ml

LONG ACTING (Duration 18-24 hours)
Glargine 100 u/ml
Detemir 100 u/ml

ULTRA LONG ACTING (Duration 36-42 hours)
Glargine 300 u/ml
Degludec 200 u/ml

Pre-mixed
NPH/Regular 70/30
NPH/Lispro 75/25, 50/50
NPH/Aspart 70/30

DRUG LIST FOR TYPE 2 DIABETES

Insulin Response Enhancer: Decreases hepatic gluconeogenesis, Increases peripheral glucose uptake

Metformin	Biguanide

Insulin Secretagogues

Glimepiride	Sulfonylurea (2nd gen)
Glipizide	Sulfonylurea (2nd gen)
Glyburide	Sulfonylurea (2nd gen)
Nateglinide	Meglitinide
Repaglinide	Meglitinide

Glucagon-like Peptide 1 Receptor Agonist (GLP-1a)
Increases insulin secretion, inhibits glucagon secretion

Dulaglutide	Incretin Mimetic
Exenatide	Incretin Mimetic
Liraglutide	Incretin Mimetic
Semaglutide	Incretin Mimetic
Tirzepatide	Incretin Mimetic (GLP1a/GIP)

Mixed GLP-1a and Insulin Combination
Lixisenatide (GLP-1a/Glargine)

Dipeptidyl Peptidase (DPP-IV) inhibitors:
Inhibits degradation of GLP-1
Sitagliptin
Linagliptin
Saxagliptin
Alogliptin
Vildagliptin (not available in the US)
Amylin Analog
Pramlintide

Insulin Sensitizer
Pioglitazone Thiazolidinedione, PPAR-γ agonist

Sodium-Glucose Transporter-2 inhibitor (SGLT-2i)
Inhibits glucose reuptake and enhances urinary excretion
Canagliflozin
Dapagliflozin
Empagliflozin
Ertugliflozin

α-Glucosidase Inhibitors (AGIs): Inhibits carbohydrate absorption

Acarbose	poor GI absorption
Miglitol	renal clearance
Voglibose	(not available in the US)

General Background

Diabetes mellitus (DM) is clinically defined as elevated blood glucose (hyperglycemia) resulting from poor glucose metabolism and/or excess glucose production. This results in abnormal carbohydrate, protein, and fat metabolism. The word "diabetes" comes from the ancient Greek for "siphon" or "to pass through, (Hughes 2008), possibly alluding to polyuria, a cardinal symptom of the condition. The word "mellitus" comes from the Latin for "sweet," (Hughes 2008) a reference to the reported taste of urine from patients. DM consists of several different metabolic disorders with various etiologies leading to a similar range of symptoms. Despite being medically described more than 3500 years ago, (Bryan and Joachim 1930), a complete understanding of diabetes pathophysiology remains elusive. It is one of the most prevalent human diseases, with an estimated 537 million people in 2021 living with diabetes worldwide, which is projected to increase to 643 million by 2030. (Magliano and Boyko 2021) DM is thus one of the most common conditions diagnosed by family physicians and is associated with a wide range of debilitating symptoms and complications, including neuropathies, vascular disease, limb amputation, coma, and premature death.

The CDC Diabetes Statistics 2022 estimated the incidence of diabetes, both type 1 and 2, for 2019 to be 37.3 million people of all ages. This is 11.3% of the US population. Individuals unaware they have diabetes are estimated to be 8.5 million adults over the age of 18 years. Of those with pre-diabetes—96 million US adults, over one quarter, are over 65. (CDC 2022)

The estimated cost of diagnosed diabetes in 2017 was $327 billion, including $237 billion in direct medical costs and $90 billion in lost productivity. Excess medical costs associated with diabetes were $9,601 per person in 2017. (CDC 2022)

Diagnosis
The American Diabetes Association has classified diabetes into four categories. (ElSayed et al. 2023f; Garber et al. 2020)

1. Type 1 diabetes: autoimmune destruction of the β cells (including latent autoimmune diabetes). This results in absolute insulin deficiency. Multiple islet autoantibodies may be present. These may test negative over time.
2. Type 2 diabetes often begins with metabolic syndromes, insulin resistance, and gradual loss of β cell function. It may take several years before elevated blood glucose levels are apparent. Insulin resistance often starts 10-15 years before elevated serum glucose is diagnosed. In early T2DM, first-phase insulin release is lost, causing an elevated 1-hour postprandial glucose but normal or improved glucose control by 2-3 hours.
3. Other causes of diabetes include monogenic diabetes syndromes, neonatal diabetes, maturity-onset diabetes of the young (MODY), medications such as glucocorticoids, anti-psychotics, and disorders that affect the pancreas, such as cystic fibrosis and pancreatitis. Monogenic diabetes syndromes occur rarely but are essential to recognize as treatment options vary significantly.
4. Gestational diabetes occurs in the second or third trimester of pregnancy. Diabetes that occurs early in pregnancy, during the first trimester, may indicate pre-existing diabetes.

Screening

Screening for type 1 diabetes with antibody testing is recommended for children with family members with type 1 diabetes. Antibody testing can include islet cell antibodies (ICA), insulin autoantibodies (IAA), glutamic acid decarboxylase (GAD-65), insulin autoantibodies (IA-2A), and islet zinc transporter antibodies (Anti-ZnT8). These tests are available commercially. If autoantibodies are noted, the patient should be informed of the risk of developing diabetes, signs/symptoms of diabetes, and ketoacidosis. (ElSayed et al. 2023f)

Screening for type 2 Diabetes should begin at age 35 or earlier when risk factors are present. Screening for insulin resistance and type 2 diabetes risk factors should be assessed at least by age ten years and include a family history of diabetes, especially in a first-degree relative, high-risk ethnicity (people of color), history of gestational diabetes, polycystic ovarian syndrome, obesity, hypertension, sedentary lifestyle, and prediabetes. (ElSayed et al. 2023f)

Symptoms of diabetes include excessive thirst, urination, fatigue, sudden weight loss, genital infections, slow-healing cuts or wounds, and blurred vision. Signs of insulin resistance and pre-diabetes may not be readily apparent. Lab values help determine a diagnosis.

Diagnostic Criteria: (ElSayed et al. 2023f) The diagnosis of diabetes should be confirmed with two tests or on two occasions.

	Pre-Diabetes	Diabetes
Fasting (8 hours)	100-125 mg/dl	≥126 on two occasions
2 hours post prandial	140-199 mg/dl	≥200 mg/dl OGTT
Random BG		≥200 mg/dl
A1C	5.6%-6.4%	≥ 6.5%

Pre-Diabetes

Pre-diabetes is an important diagnosis, defined as fasting blood glucose between 100-125 mg/dl and/or an A1C between 5.6% and 6.4%. Patients should be informed of their risk of developing early complications and progression to diabetes. Pre-diabetes usually begins with insulin resistance. This occurs several years before hyperglycemia. Insulin resistance occurs when skeletal and adipose tissues have a decreased response to insulin. This results in hyperinsulinemia. Over 10 to 15 years, the pancreas begins to fail, resulting in elevated blood glucose levels and progression to diabetes.

Glucotoxicity is a term that refers to the process of cellular dysfunction caused by chronic hyperglycemia. Chronic hyperglycemia is an inflammatory condition. This damage may become permanent over time. The level and duration of elevated blood glucose have a profound impact on vascular tissues. Early intervention with metformin, lifestyle management, nutrition, exercise at least 150 min per week, and weight loss (7%) has the potential to reverse pre-diabetes or prevent progression to full diabetes. Reducing the risk of long-term complications is the primary goal of early intervention. (American Diabetes Association Professional Practice 2022)

Type 1 Diabetes Mellitus

Pathophysiology

Approximately 5% of individuals with diabetes have type 1 diabetes. Hyperglycemia in T1DM is caused by the loss of insulin-secreting β cells in the pancreatic islets of Langerhans. Most cases occur in childhood due to an autoimmune process with clearly defined autoimmune antibodies. Several specific autoantigens have been identified in latent autoimmune T1DM, including glutamic acid decarboxylase autoantibodies (GADA), islet cell autoantibodies (ICA), insulinoma-associated (IA-2) autoantibodies, and zinc transporter autoantibodies (ZnT8). (Magliano and Boyko 2021)
Among children with T1DM, 33% present with diabetic ketoacidosis (DKA), a serious, potentially life-threatening medical condition that requires immediate treatment. Hospitalization, rehydration, electrolyte replacement, and insulin

administration are standard treatments. In adulthood, the clinical presentation of T1DM may be more variable but still potentially life-threatening. Occasionally, within the first year of diagnosis, the individual may experience a "honeymoon phase" with a decreased need for insulin. This is only temporary. Triggers for T1DM include genetics, environmental toxins, and illness. Insulin replacement is the only effective treatment for T1DM. (ElSayed et al. 2023f; Magliano and Boyko 2021)

Presentation
Children present acutely ill to the clinic or the emergency room with increased thirst, urination, and sudden weight loss. They may or may not have nausea/vomiting. Parents may think their child has the flu when they are in diabetic ketoacidosis. Fruity-smelling breath is sometimes present.

Adults are seen complaining of increased thirst, urination, and sudden weight loss over the previous few months. Weight loss can be profound, 20-40 lbs. or more, depending on the duration of hyperglycemia.

Treatment
The only effective treatment for type 1 diabetes is insulin. Insulin can be dosed in a variety of regimens. Amylin analogs can be used in both type 1 and type 2 but are not commonly used. Screening for celiac disease and thyroid antibodies is also recommended.

Type 2 Diabetes Mellitus

Type 2 diabetes mellitus is the most common form of diabetes, affecting 90%-95% of those with diabetes. Type 2 diabetes is due to the progressive loss of beta cell function. This is usually due to insulin resistance syndromes. Type 2 diabetes was previously a disease primarily seen in the adult population over age 40 but has become more prevalent in children with the worsening of the obesity epidemic. Adults over age 65 have a higher prevalence of type 2 diabetes. This is possibly due to increased insulin resistance in aging skeletal muscle. (Shou et al., 2020)

Pathophysiology
Multiple factors are involved in the progression of diabetes. As insulin resistance worsens, hyperglycemia follows. Hyperglycemia is inflammatory to many tissues. Eventually, the beta cells cannot compensate, skeletal muscles become more resistant to insulin, and hyperglycemia results. Counterregulatory hormones increase gluconeogenesis resulting in additional hyperglycemia. Concurrently there is a loss of function of gastrointestinal incretins called glucose-dependent insulinotropic peptide GIP) and glucagon-like-peptide (GLP-1). The role of these incretins is to cause an immediate release of insulin with ingesting food. An enzyme, dipeptidyl peptidase 4 (DPP4), deactivates the hormones. (Kim and Egan 2008)

Presentation
Patients with type 2 diabetes present with various symptoms or sometimes no symptoms depending on their blood glucose level. They may or may not present with increased urination and thirst depending on their renal threshold for glucose. Typical symptoms include increased thirst, urination, and fatigue. Sometimes the complaint is a burning sensation in their feet or hands. Chronic nausea can be a symptom of gastroparesis, a neuropathic complication of diabetes. Genital mycotic infections are a common initial complaint. They may have hypertension, central obesity, or sleep apnea. Acanthosis nigricans is a velvety brownish discoloration in the folds of the skin, particularly around the neck, axilla, and groin. This is an indication of insulin resistance. Convincing patients of the seriousness of managing diabetes before they have symptoms can sometimes be challenging.

Typical lab results will show elevated glucose, elevated A1C, decreased HDL, and high triglycerides. Fructosamine levels have been used to evaluate glucose control over the previous 14-21 days (Gounden et al. 2022) though not as commonly used as A1C. A1C evaluates glucose control over the last 8-12 weeks. Patients may also have elevated transaminases related to fatty liver disease.

Multiple medications are now available to treat type 2 diabetes, both oral and parenteral.

Gestational Diabetes Mellitus (GDM)

According to the International Diabetes Federation (2021), approximately 16% of live births are associated with some form of maternal hyperglycemia, which includes preexisting diabetes mellitus. Among these cases, roughly 84% are attributed to gestational diabetes. (Magliano and Boyko 2021) Diagnostic guidelines published by the ADA indicate that diabetes diagnosed within the first trimester of pregnancy should be classified as preexisting pregestational diabetes rather than gestational diabetes. Glucose intolerance developing during the second or third trimester of pregnancy should be classified as gestational diabetes mellitus. (ElSayed et al. 2023d; ElSayed et al. 2023f) In these cases, impaired glucose tolerance is thought to be due to increased insulin demands resulting from metabolic changes during pregnancy.

Uncontrolled diabetes during pregnancy is associated with spontaneous abortions, fetal anomalies, preeclampsia, fetal demise, macrosomia, neonatal hypoglycemia, hyperbilirubinemia, and neonatal respiratory distress syndrome. (ElSayed et al. 2023d)

It is, therefore, essential for women with any form of diabetes in pregnancy (including preexisting DM or GDM) to carefully control and monitor their blood glucose levels with the support of their healthcare provider to reduce the risk of adverse outcomes. (ElSayed et al. 2023d) Ideally, pre-pregnancy counseling would identify those at risk. For those with diabetes, an A1C of <6.5% is recommended before conception. An A1C of 6% or lower during pregnancy is ideal if achievable without hypoglycemia.

Pathophysiology
Insulin resistance is the basis of gestational diabetes. This begins about week 16 and continues progressing until late in the third trimester. Insulin requirements will increase at approximately 5% per week until the last month and then stabilizes. In gestational diabetes, the pancreas cannot compensate enough to overcome insulin resistance and the need for increased insulin.

Diagnosis/Screening for gestational diabetes
Pre-pregnancy screening for insulin resistance, pre-diabetes, and undiagnosed diabetes is ideal, especially in at-risk individuals. If no pre-pregnancy screening has been done, testing may be done at less than 15 weeks gestation to determine if undiagnosed pre-diabetes or diabetes is present. This may be especially important in underserved or high-risk populations. Screening for gestational diabetes should be done between 24-28 weeks gestation with either a 75 gm glucose tolerance test or a two-step 100 gm glucose tolerance test. (ElSayed et al. 2023d)

Diagnostic Criteria for Gestational Diabetes

OGTT	75 gm	2-Step: 50 gm	100 gm
Fasting	≥ 92 mg/dl	≥130 mg/d	≥95 mg/dl
1 hour	≥180 mg/dl		≥180 mg/dl
2 hour	≥153 mg/dl		≥155 mg/dl
3 hour			≥140 mg/dl

Blood Glucose Goals of Control During Pregnancy

Fasting	<95 mg/dl
1-hour post prandial	<140 mg/dl
2-hour postprandial	<120 mg/dl
A1C	<6%

Treatment
Lifestyle management:
Nutrition: minimum of 175 g of carbohydrate, 71 gm protein, 28 g fiber
Exercise: 20-50 min per day, 2-7 days per /week, moderate intensity
Weight management

Post-partum follow up
Women who have had GMD are at a 50-60% increased lifetime risk of developing diabetes. They should be screened 4-12 weeks post-partum with a fasting 75 g oral glucose tolerance test (OGTT). An A1C may be falsely low, so it is not recommended for post-partum screening. Lifetime testing for diabetes every 1-3 years is recommended due to their increased risk of developing diabetes. (ElSayed et al. 2023d)

Medication:
Insulin for type 1 and 2 diabetes and gestational diabetes is the first-line recommendation. Glyburide and metformin have been studied in pregnancy and children exposed in-utero to these medications up to age ten. A higher incidence of macrosomia and abdominal girth was noted in neonates. A higher BMI and fat mass were noted in children 4-10 years old. (ElSayed et al. 2023d) The recommended treatment for diabetes during pregnancy is multiple daily insulin injections or insulin pump therapy.

Glucose monitoring
1. Fasting and 1-2 hour postprandial glucose if not on insulin.
2. Pre- and 1-2 hour post-prandial blood glucose if the individual is using insulin so the dosage of insulin can be adjusted with meals.
3. Both home blood glucose monitors and continuous glucose monitor devices are acceptable.

Atypical Diabetes

Atypical diabetes, such as maturity-onset diabetes of the young (MODY), affects 1-2% of the diabetes patient population worldwide and 2-3% of all cases of DM before ages 25-35. (ElSayed et al. 2023f; Naylor et al. 2018) Monogenic diabetes, a genetic malformation, results in many forms of diabetes. Genetic testing will be necessary to determine the defect so appropriate treatment can be prescribed. (Naylor et al., 2018) Diabetes is associated with several other autoimmune, genetic, endocrine, neoplastic, and post-surgical syndromes, including cystic fibrosis, hemochromatosis, Cushing syndrome, pheochromocytoma, glucagonoma, post-transplantation diabetes mellitus, and pancreatitis. Drug or chemical-induced diabetes, as with steroids and antipsychotic medications, can also trigger diabetes. (ElSayed et al. 2023; Naylor et al. 2018)

Management of Diabetes

The American Diabetes Association and the American Association of Clinical Endocrinology publish guidelines for managing diabetes. (ADA 2023; AACE 2023)

The goal of managing diabetes is to prevent complications and improve quality of life. All individuals with diabetes should receive diabetes education. Education should be client-centered, considering the client's glycemic and weight goals, risk of hypoglycemia, the complexity of the treatment regimen, affordability of medications, and the ability to access medications and health care. Education can be provided in person or through telehealth. Patients are instructed in optimal self-care behaviors, healthy coping, healthy eating, being active, taking medication, monitoring, reducing risks, and problem-solving. (Association of Diabetes et al. 2021) There are online education programs available at no cost. Some will provide online coaching as well.

Adapted from the American Diabetes Standards of Care for Diabetes 2023

1. Medical nutrition therapy (MNT) provided by a registered dietitian if available.

2. Exercise: Exercise improves insulin resistance and improves glucose control. The ADA recommends that children and those with prediabetes exercise for at least 60 minutes per day, at least three days per week. Adults should have at least 150 minutes of exercise over three days. Strength training and weight-bearing exercises that strengthen bones are important to prevent osteoporosis. Moderate intensity or vigorous exercise is recommended for all age groups. Increasing movement throughout the day and limiting sedentary time to 30 minutes at one time is also recommended.

3. Psychosocial: Diabetes is a chronic disease that can overwhelm individuals and their families. It is important to screen for depression and anxiety, stress, and coping strategies. Evaluation with a health psychologist or other mental health professional can improve quality of life. The diabetes distress scale (DDS) is a 17-question tool available online and an excellent screening tool. (DDS 2023)

4. *Smoking cessation*: Individuals should be encouraged to stop using tobacco and e-cigarettes.

5. *Sleep health*: sleep disorders and sleep apnea increase the risk of type 2 diabetes. Screening for sleep apnea with STOP-BANG and Epworth scales are simple in-office screening tools.

6. *Glycemic targets:* Blood glucose control is measured by A1C and blood glucose reports, whether using a finger stick home blood glucose monitor or continuous glucose monitor. The A1C is the glucose average over the previous 2-3 months. A1C recommendations vary based on age, comorbid conditions, risk of hypoglycemia, and pregnancy—an A1C of <7% is recommended for the general nonpregnant population. The recommendation in pregnancy is an A1C <6.5% or even lower if it can be achieved without hypoglycemia. In elderly individuals, an A1C of less than 8% may be acceptable, depending on comorbid conditions. A1C goals for children need to be individualized based on the risk of hypoglycemia. Younger children are less sensitive to hypoglycemia. An A1C goal of less than 7% is recommended in general. For children at increased risk of hypoglycemia or with hypoglycemic unawareness, an A1C of 7.5% or even <8% may be recommended. Monitoring with continuous glucose monitors has become the standard of care for those on insulin. Learning to read these reports provides valuable information regarding blood glucose control.

Metrics for understanding (CGM) Continuous Glucose Monitoring are published in ADA Standards of Care in Diabetes 2023—Abridged for Primary Care Providers, Diabetesjournals.org. Metrics include how long the CGM is worn, mean glucose, estimated A1C, standard deviation, time in range, and time above and below range. Typically, the data is evaluated for the previous two weeks.

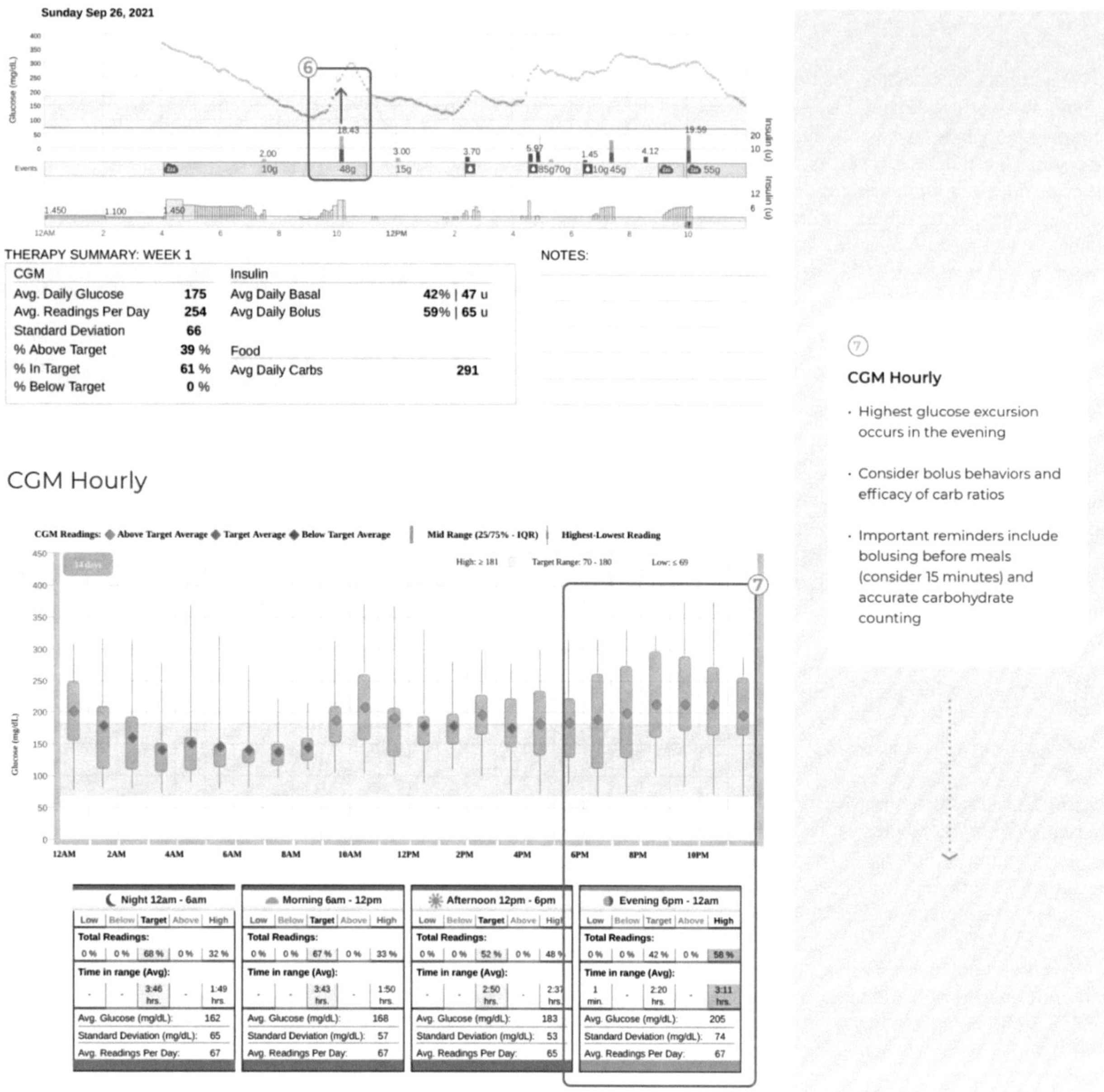

Figure 1. Tandem T slim XT2 with Control IQ paired with continuous glucose monitor to improve time in range and decrease hypoglycemia. The pump is downloaded and reviewed with the patient. It shows the average blood glucose, the time in target range, the time above target range and the time below target range. It also shows blood glucose patterns and makes recommendations for adjusting insulin dosing.

7. *Hypoglycemia: signs, symptoms, and treatment:* Hypoglycemia is defined as a blood glucose less than 70 mg/dl. Symptoms of hypoglycemia include sweating, shakiness, headache, hunger/nausea, irregular pulse or tachycardia, fatigue, irritability or anxiety, dizziness, tingling or numbness around the mouth, confusion, and possible passing out. If the individual is awake, check their blood sugar and give them juice, soda pop, or glucose tablets. 15-20 grams of simple carbohydrates is recommended if blood glucose is less than 70 mg/dl. Re-check blood glucose in 15 minutes. If it is not increasing, repeat 15-20 grams of carbohydrates. Simple carbohydrates include ½ cup juice, fruit, 5-6 hard candies, ½ cup soda pop (not diet), or standardized glucose tablets or gels. Adjustments in medications may be necessary. If the individual is not responsive, administer glucagon and call EMS. Glucagon comes in two forms, injectable pen, and nasal spray. Individuals on insulin should have either the pen or nasal spray available and have a friend or family member instructed on administering this.

8. *Technology:* Multiple devices are available to assist patients with managing their diabetes. Home blood glucose monitors require finger sticks to obtain a small amount of blood applied to a strip inserted in the device. Continuous blood glucose monitors require applying a patch (sensor) with a small wire inserted subcutaneously. These detect interstitial glucose, which may vary slightly from whole blood glucose. Glucose readings are then transmitted to a reader or phone. Some CGM devices can synchronize with insulin pumps and smart pens. CGM devices also have alarms that can alert individuals to high or low blood glucose.

Insulin can be administered with a vial and syringe or with insulin pens. Insulin pens are more convenient to use. (ElSayed et al. 2023g) Smart pens use protocols (determined by the patient and provider) to assist patients with dosing and keep track of their insulin usage. Insulin pumps have a reservoir for insulin and administer continuous rapid-acting insulin simulating basal insulin needs. (ElSayed et al. 2023g) Most insulin pumps allow for eight basal rates per 24 hours. Blood glucose targets can be set for exercise and sleep, decreasing the risk of hypoglycemia. Bolus doses are based on carbohydrates. Learning to count carbohydrates accurately improves the accuracy of the insulin pump. Insulin pumps use rapid-acting insulin only. There is no need for long-acting basal insulin as the pump administers small doses continuously. Insulin pumps can be paired with a continuous glucose monitor that allows for closed-loop technology (auto-control). The pump adjusts the basal rate and may give a small correction bolus as needed. An insulin pump is not an artificial pancreas. It requires the pump user to actively participate in managing their pump. Insulin pump users with good control do not need to remove their pumps for most surgeries. The comfort level of the nursing staff and providers caring for hospitalized patients is often a determinant in allowing patients to maintain their pumps and manage their diabetes in the hospital.

Most home blood glucose monitors can be downloaded for review with the provider and patient. Helping patients understand their trends and patterns can help them manage their diabetes. All insulin pumps, CGMs, and smart devices can be downloaded for review. The software can be obtained by contacting the device companies. The software is usually provided at no charge to medical facilities. Learning to interpret these is an essential part of managing diabetes.

9. *Obesity and weight management for preventing and treating type 2 diabetes.* Obesity continues to be a significant struggle for many patients despite controlling calories and exercising. A small to modest weight loss of 3-7% can positively affect glucose control and cardiovascular risks. More significant weight loss has greater benefits. Weight loss medications and bariatric surgery may be appropriate for selected persons unable to achieve weight loss goals with medical nutrition therapy and behavioral interventions.

Pharmacological Treatments

Type 1 Diabetes Medications: Insulins and insulin analogs

Insulin replacement therapy is the standard of care for nearly all patients with T1DM and is effective in managing T2DM for some.

Considerations for prescribing and administering insulin

Insulin is used in a variety of ways. Basal insulin is a long-acting insulin designed to control hepatic gluconeogenesis. It is dosed based on fasting blood glucose. It replicates the underlying continuous insulin release from the beta cells of the pancreas. Basal insulin is not designed to manage food or corrections. The dosage is dependent on weight and the amount of insulin resistance. Pediatric dosing can be very different from adult dosing. It may require diluting the insulin with a diluent designed to be mixed with insulin. Regular or rapid-acting insulin is used for food and corrections. Intensive control is achieved with basal insulin once or twice a day and regular or rapid-acting insulin 15-30 min before the meal 2-3 times daily. Mealtime insulin is based on the number of carbohydrates in the meal and, if needed, a correction factor to bring the blood glucose to the target range. Generally, the basal/bolus insulin ratio varies from 70% basal/30% bolus to 50% basal/50% bolus. Insulin can be administered through injection with an insulin syringe, an insulin pen, or an insulin pump. Algorithms for initiating and adjusting insulin can be found on the American Diabetes Association and the American Association of Clinical Endocrinology websites. (ADA 2023; AACE 2023)

Generic	Concentration	Onset	Peak Action	Duration	Dosage Form	Storage -opened/In-use
ULTRA-RAPID						
Aspart Niacinamide	100 u/ml	16-20 min	60 min	5-7 hours	Vial and Pen	Room temp 28 days
URLi	100 u/ml	15-17 min	2 hour	5-7 hours	Vial and Pen. Cartridge	Room temp 28 days
	200 u/ml	15-17 min	2 hours	5-7 hours	Pen only	
RAPID						
Insulin Aspart	100 u/ml	20-30 min	1-3 hours	5 hours	Vial and Pen	Room temp for 28 days
					cartridge (pen refill)	
					1/2 unit dosing pen	
Insulin Glulisine	100 u/ml	20 min	1-2 hours	5 hours	Vial and Pen	Room Temp 28 days
Insulin Lispro	100 u/ml	30 min	1-2 hours	3-5 hours	Vial and Pen	Room temp 28 days
					Cartridges-pen refill	
					1/2 unit dosing pen	
Insulin Lispro	200 u/ml	30 min	1-2 hours	3-5 hours	Pen only	Room Temp 28 days

SHORT-ACTING						
Regular	100 u/ml	0.5-2 hours	2-4 hours	8-12 hours	Vial and pen	Room temp 42 days
INTERMEDIATE-ACTING						
Regular	500 u/ml	15-30 min	4-8 hours	12-24 hours	Vial and Pen	Room Temp 31 days
NPH	100 u/ml	1-3 hours	6-8 hours	12-24 hours	Vial and Pen	Room Temp 42 days
LONG-ACTING	May take 3-5 days to reach a steady state					
Glargine	100 u/ml	4 hours	none	24 hours	Vial and Pen	Room Temp 28 days
Glargine	300 u/ml	>6 hrs	none	36 hours	Pen	Room Temp 56 days
Detemir	100 u/ml	3-4 hours	3-14 hours	18-24 hours	Vial and Pen	Room Temp 42 days
Degludec	100 u/ml	>6 hours	none	42 hours	Vial and Pen	Room Temp 56 days
Degludec	200 u/ml	>6 hours	none	42 hours	Pen only	Room Temp or Refrigerated for 8 weeks
PRE-MIXED						
NPH/Regular	70/30	30-90 min	1.5-6 hours	18-24 hrs	Vial and pen	Vial 31-42 days pen 10 days
NPH/lispro	75/25, 50/50	15-30 min	5-8 hours	14-24 hrs	Vial and pen	Vial 28 days pen 28 days
NPH/Aspart	70/30	10-20 min	1-3 hours	12-24 hrs	Vial and pen	Vial 42 days pen 14 days

Type 2 Diabetes Mellitus Medications

The American Diabetes Association and the American Association of Clinical Endocrinology have algorithms for the use of diabetes medications. (ADA 2023; AACE 2023)

Insulin Response Enhancer

Biguanides

Metformin is in a class by itself. It does not cause hypoglycemia. Its primary mechanism of action is to reduce hepatic gluconeogenesis and increase glucose uptake and utilization in skeletal muscle. It is cleared primarily through the kidney. Individuals with reduced renal function have delayed clearance. Metformin is contraindicated in individuals with GFR <30ml/min. Metformin is usually well tolerated but can cause gastrointestinal upset, nausea, and diarrhea. Starting with a low dose and titrating it or using extended-release formulations can sometimes ameliorate the side effects. Metformin is considered the first-line medication for pre-diabetes and type 2 diabetes. (NIH 2023) B12 deficiencies have been noted with the use of Metformin.

Insulin Secretagogues

Sulfonylureas

These organic compounds primarily function by eliciting insulin release from pancreatic β cells. They bind to and inhibit ATP-dependent potassium (KATP) channel complexes formed from an octameric assembly of inward-rectifier potassium channels and the sulfonylurea receptor (SUR). This, in turn, depolarizes the cell membrane, resulting in the activation of voltage-gated calcium channels (VGCCs) and calcium-dependent secretion of the endogenously produced insulin. As such, they are ineffective in treating patients with T1DM, including those with DM secondary to pancreatectomy. Furthermore, they increase the risk of hypoglycemia, so prescribers and patients must pay careful attention to recommended dosing regimens. While initial administration of sulfonylureas leads to detectable increases in plasma insulin levels, chronic treatment ultimately results in circulating insulin levels similar to those measured before treatment. This is thought to be due to the downregulation of KATP channels. However, these drugs remain effective in lowering blood glucose levels in many patients with T2DM. Hypoglycemia is the most significant risk. Prolonged hypoglycemia can lead to death which has led to recommendations to either avoid use in the elderly population or use with caution.

Sulfonylureas are inexpensive and readily available, often making them the first or second choice for prescribers. However, professional guidelines list these as the last options due to the increased risk of hypoglycemia, weight gain, and possibly contributing to cardiovascular disease. Glyburide and Glimepiride are on the Beers Criteria list and are not recommended due to extended hypoglycemia. (Croke 2020) They may be a reasonable option for financial reasons for some individuals.

Meglitinide Analogs

Repaglinide and Nateglinide are oral medications infrequently used to treat type 2 diabetes. These medications increase the secretion of insulin. Peak insulin levels occur within an hour of dosing and return to baseline by 4 hours. They are dosed immediately before the meal. They must be taken with food. They are generally safer than sulfonylureas as they are associated with less hypoglycemia. Metabolism is through the cytochrome P450 isozyme CYP2C9 (70%) and CYP3A4 (30%). Concerning side effects are hypoglycemia, weight gain, and elevation of uric acid. (Novartis 2013)

Glucagon-Like Peptide 1 Receptor Agonists
GLP-1a drugs are all parenteral except semaglutide, which has both a parenteral and oral formulation. They are recommended as a second-line medication because they reduce heart failure and improve blood glucose and weight loss. GLP-1 is a hormone (incretin) produced in the gastrointestinal tract in response to eating. It binds with specific receptors on pancreatic beta cells and increases insulin secretion. GLP-1 and GIP (gastric inhibitory peptide) incretins have a rapid and short duration. (Bonadio 2013) The GLP-1 receptor agonists delay gastric emptying, suppress glucagon secretion, and increase satiety. They can cause nausea/vomiting, especially with high-fat meals, which also slow gastric motility. Constipation or diarrhea can also occur. They are generally well tolerated. Weight loss is a strong motivator for many patients to use these medications. Combined with diet and exercise, weight loss can be substantial. They can reduce A1C by 1-3%.

Oral semaglutide is taken once daily. Exenatide has both a twice-a-day formulation and a weekly formulation. Liraglutide is once a day. The other formulations are dosed once weekly. The injectable formulations come as either multidose pens or auto-inject pens. While the benefits are clear, they are expensive, and cost may be a factor for patients. GLP-1a's are contraindicated in patients with gastrointestinal disorders, a history of bowel obstructions, gastroparesis, and inflammatory bowel disorders. They are also contraindicated in individuals who have had thyroid cancer or pancreatitis. It is essential to start at the lowest dose and follow the manufacturer's instructions to titrate the dose. Rapid titration can result in severe GI complications, nausea, vomiting, and bowel obstructions. (ElSayed et al. 2023h; Kim and Egan 2008)

Dipeptidyl Peptidase (DPP-IV) inhibitors:
DPP-IV is an enzyme that binds to the incretins and inactivates them. DPP-IV inhibitors improve glucose control by slowing the degradation of GLP-1. The DPP-IV inhibitors are oral agents taken once a day. They can be combined with most other medications. Concomitant use with GLP-1 receptor agonists should be avoided due to a similar mechanism of action. In general, they lower A1C by about 0.5%. They are very well tolerated.

Insulin Sensitizers
Pioglitazone is an oral agent used in the treatment of type 2 diabetes. Its primary effect is to lower blood glucose by improving the sensitivity to endogenous insulin. Pioglitazone is a (PPAR)-gamma agonist. This improves insulin sensitivity by increasing circulating adiponectin levels. It may take up to 12 weeks to get the full effect and should not be used in type 1 diabetes. It is recommended as a fifth-line treatment. It can be used with other antihyperglycemics, such as metformin and sulfonylurea. If combined with insulin use, lower doses of insulin may be needed. Weight gain is a common side effect due to increased adipose tissue and fluid retention. Caution is recommended in individuals with congestive heart failure. It is not indicated for those with NYHA Class III or IV heart failure. It is also contraindicated in those with bladder cancer. Studies have shown an increased risk of non-vertebral fractures and macular edema. (NIH 2023)

Sodium Glucose Transporter-2 Inhibitor (SGLT-2)
SGLT-2 inhibitors are once-daily oral medications recommended as the second or third line in treating type 2 diabetes. They block glucose reabsorption in the proximal tubule of the nephron, where 90% of glucose is normally reabsorbed. Glucose is excreted in the urine with the equivalent of approximately one-half cup of sugar per day. This also leads to weight loss, lower blood glucose levels, and decreased glucotoxicity. SGLT-2 inhibitors promote mild diuresis without loss of electrolytes. Blood pressure, arterial stiffness, and plasma volume are reduced, improving hemodynamic effects on the heart. They are indicated for cardiovascular disease, heart failure with or without diabetes, and type 2 diabetes. They are contraindicated in type 1 diabetes as they can cause euglycemic diabetic ketoacidosis. Maintaining good hydration is important when using these medications. (Stamatouli and Inzucchi 2016) Warnings and indications for use should be reviewed per the manufacturer's recommendations.

All SGLT-2 inhibitors are associated with increased perineal mycotic infections, increased urinary tract infections, and necrotizing fasciitis of the perineum (Fournier's gangrene). Canagliflozin has a black box warning for lower limb amputations in individuals with diabetes and cardiovascular disease. Dapagliflozin is approved for the reduction of chronic kidney disease and end-stage kidney disease. Dapagliflozin can be initiated per the package insert with a GFR as low as 25 ml/min. The benefit is to preserve renal function, but at this level, it has little effect on lowering glucose. (Stamatouli and Inzucchi 2016)

Alpha-glucosidase inhibitors
AGIs are oral medications used alone or with other agents. They work primarily by inhibiting the absorption of complex carbohydrates in the small intestine. This reduces the post-prandial rise in glucose. AGIs prevent the enzymes that convert non-absorbable carbohydrates into absorbable carbohydrates. It does not cause hypoglycemia. The

medication should be started with the lowest dose, given before meals, and titrated every 4-8 weeks as tolerated. Many patients discontinue the medication due to gastrointestinal complaints, increased gas, diarrhea, and abdominal pain. A low-carbohydrate diet can help reduce side effects. (Akmal and Wadhwa 2022)

Medication options:
Metformin has long been considered the cornerstone of treatment for type 2 diabetes and is recommended for pre-diabetes and insulin resistance. As diabetes progresses, other medications are added. Managing type 2 diabetes often requires 2-4 antihyperglycemic drugs, and in some cases, insulin is indicated. A change or adjustment of medication is warranted if the patient does not reach their goal within three months. Persons at high risk for cardiovascular disease should start a GLP-1a with proven cardiovascular benefits. SGLT-2i should be started in those with heart failure and/or chronic kidney disease. These are expensive medications, and many individuals cannot afford them. TZDs, AGIs, and sulfonylureas may be less desirable depending on patient goals but affordable. If the A1C is still not to goal, the addition of basal insulin and, eventually, bolus insulin should be started. (Lizzo et al., 2022)

Complications of Diabetes

The goal of diabetes education and management is to reduce the risk and occurrence of complications. Unfortunately, many individuals with diabetes are seen with complications already in process. This can result from a lack of access to care, education, and understanding of the diabetes process or not knowing they have diabetes. Socioeconomic factors have been shown to impact long-term complications. (ElSayed et al. 2023e)

Complications of diabetes can be divided into acute metabolic emergencies and chronic end-organ complications. Acute complications include diabetic ketoacidosis (DKA), hyperosmotic hyperglycemic nonketotic state (HHNK), and hypoglycemia.

Diabetic ketoacidosis is a medical emergency and can be life-threatening. It most commonly occurs in type 1 diabetes but also in type 2 diabetes. DKA causes seventy percent of diabetes-related deaths in children. (Stamatouli and Inzucchi 2016) DKA can occur within hours to days in some individuals. Pediatric DKA should be managed in the hospital. Mild adult DKA can be controlled in an outpatient setting. DKA is characterized by severe insulin deficiency, volume depletion, and metabolic acidosis. Illness, trauma, steroids, new-onset diabetes, and inadequate insulin administration are the leading causes. Insufficient insulin can be due to eating disorders (especially in teens), insulin pump or insulin device failure, and non-adherence. Insulin deficiency and increased counter-regulatory hormones lead to increased gluconeogenesis and decreased glucose utilization by peripheral tissues, worsening hyperglycemia. Hyperglycemia triggers osmotic diuresis leading to dehydration. Increased counterregulatory hormones cause the breakdown of adipose tissue and ketone formation. (Lizzo et al., 2022)

Presentation
Patients are seen with excessive thirst and urination, but as they become more dehydrated, they will have decreased urine output. They may experience dry mouth, loss of appetite, nausea, vomiting, abdominal pain, and weight loss. Confusion, headache, and change in the level of consciousness in severe DKA due to cerebral edema may be present. Hypotension indicates a more severe disease. The patient may experience Kussmaul breathing and tachypnea. (Lizzo et al., 2022)

Evaluation
If possible, a thorough medical history, medication use, and substance use should be obtained. Individuals using SGLT-2 inhibitors or alcohol may have minimally elevated blood glucose (<300mg/dl).

Labs: blood glucose >250 mg/dl
Arterial pH <7.3
Serum bicarbonate <15 mEq/l
Anion gap >14-15 mEq/l
Serum sodium is falsely low (correct by adding 1.6 mEq to the measured serum sodium for each 100 mg/dl of glucose above 100 mg/d)
Serum potassium elevated (decreases rapidly with the administration of insulin)
Magnesium low
Elevation in lipids

Treatment
Most institutions have protocols in place to manage ketoacidosis. Protocols for adults and children differ. Use caution with children, because if they rehydrate too quickly it can precipitate cerebral edema. Some recommend hydrating for an hour before administering insulin to children. Hydration alone will reduce blood glucose levels. (Bonadio 2013)

General adult guidelines:
Most institutions have protocols for managing diabetic ketoacidosis. General guidelines are reviewed here.

Replace fluids with normal saline, 15-20 ml/Kg in the first hour and 1 liter/hour for 4 hours. Slower rates of hydration are equally effective. (Lizzo et al., 2022) Potassium and magnesium should also be added to the infusion when appropriate.

Regular Insulin is continuously administered intravenously. An initial bolus of 0.1 u/kg, then 0.1 u/kg per hour until plasma glucose reaches 200-250 mg/dl. Dextrose is typically added when the blood glucose approaches 200-250 mg/dl to avoid hypoglycemia. (Lizzo et al, 2022) Treatment should continue until DKA has resolved and the anion gap has normalized.

Monitoring: Point of care (fingerstick) glucose every hour
Every 2 hours: serum glucose and electrolyte levels until stable, then every 4 hours
BUN, creatinine
Venous blood gas or arterial blood gas
Mental status and neurologic exam (Lizzo et al. 2022)

Evaluate for other causes: infection, myocardial infarction, pancreatitis, hyperosmotic hyperglycemic nonketotic state, alcoholic ketoacidosis, lactic acidosis, uremia, and toxins.

Hyperosmotic Hyperglycemic Nonketotic State (HHNK), also known as hyperosmolar hyperglycemic state (HHS), occurs primarily in obese individuals with type 2 diabetes. HHS has twice the mortality rate of DKA, up to 20%, but fortunately is rare. (Adeyinka and Kondamudi 2022) DKA and HHS have similar underlying pathophysiology, with some exceptions. Insulin resistance leading to poor glucose utilization in the peripheral muscles and inadequate insulin secretion is the underlying cause. Counterregulatory hormones and hyperglycemia trigger osmotic diuresis and dehydration. Serum glucose is usually over 600 mg/ml. Ketones are normal or slightly elevated as insulin is still produced in insufficient quantities. HHS has a higher risk of cerebral edema, so glucose levels should be corrected slowly. Specific ethnic populations are at higher risk: Native Americans, Hispanics, and African Americans.

Presentation
The clinical picture is consistent with hyperglycemia, increased thirst and urination, weakness, fatigue, dry mucosa, and dry skin. Decreased level of consciousness or coma may be present. Neurological signs are most concerning and result from decreased cerebral blood flow secondary to severe dehydration. (Adeyinka and Kondamudi 2022)

Evaluation
Detailed history, if possible, and a physical exam

Labs
Blood glucose (>600-1200 mg/dl); Monitor hourly
A1C determines glycemic control over the previous 8-12 weeks
Serum Osmolarity >290 mOsm/kg (standard 320-400 mOsm/kg)
Comprehensive metabolic panel
Sodium falsely low
Potassium may be high or low
Bicarbonate levels are usually low
Anion gap is normal or near normal
Magnesium low
Phosphorus elevated
Ketones with minimal or no elevation
Arterial blood gases: pH $\geq$7.3 Monitor every 2-3 hours
BUN/Creatinine elevated
WBC may be elevated
Serum enzymes elevated
UA specific gravity high, glucosuria, ketonuria

Treatment: Adults
An initial isotonic fluid bolus of 15 to 20 ml/kg followed by an infusion rate of 200 to 250 ml/hour. Rehydration alone can lower serum glucose by 75-100 mg/hour. Maintain a glucose level of about 300 mg/dl to prevent cerebral edema. (Adeyinka and Kondamudi 2022)

Hypoglycemia is addressed under "Management of diabetes."

Chronic end-organ complications: Microvascular and macrovascular complications are the primary cause of end-organ damage. Microvascular disorders secondary to long-term diabetes include retinopathy, nephropathy, and neuropathy. Macrovascular complications include stroke, myocardial infarction, and peripheral vascular disease. The correlation between A1C and long-term complications has been well documented. Persons with diabetes should be assessed for the risk of developing long-term complications. Controlling hypertension, lipids, glucose, and smoking cessation can significantly reduce microvascular and macrovascular complications. The risk calculator to evaluate for increased cardiovascular risks is available online. (ASCVD 2023) This is an excellent tool for assessing at-risk persons and providing guidance for lipid management, blood pressure, lifestyle, smoking cessation, and aspirin. Risks should be reassessed yearly. (ElSayed et al. 2023a)

Blood Pressure: Hypertension is often a precursor to heart failure, a leading cause of morbidity and mortality. (ElSayed et al. 2023a; ElSayed et al. 2023b) It should be measured at every visit. A goal of <130/80 is recommended. Hypertension is defined as ≥130/80. Antihypertensive medications are advised when the blood pressure persists over this. Home blood pressure monitoring helps reduce the impact of white coat syndrome and correlates better with ASCVD. The ADA recommends lifestyle interventions for individuals with BP greater than 120/80, reducing sodium intake, increasing physical activity, and weight control. (ElSayed et al. 2023b) ACEIs or ARBs are the recommended first-line treatments. Renal function should be monitored at least yearly.

Lipid Management: Multiple studies have shown significant primary and secondary benefits to using statins in individuals with diabetes. The meta-analyses of 14 RCTs show a 13% decrease in vascular mortality for every 39 mg/dl reduction in LDL cholesterol. (ElSayed et al. 2023b) Various medications are available to treat lipid abnormalities, but statins remain the cornerstone of treatment. Ezetimibe can be added to statins to augment the lipid-lowering effect. Monoclonal antibodies (PCSK9 inhibitors) and bempedoic acid, an adjunct to statins and diet, are newer treatments for hyperlipidemia. Icosapent ethyl is used for moderate hypertriglyceridemia. Fibrates can be added to statin for severe hypertriglyceridemia. (ElSayed et al. 2023b)

A lipid panel should be part of the initial lab studies. If the patient is not on a statin, the lipid panel can be checked every five years if under 40. If they are older, more frequent monitoring may be needed based on their other risk factors. Individuals on a statin should have an initial lipid panel before starting medication, 4-12 weeks after, and then yearly. (ElSayed et al. 2023a; ElSayed et al. 2023b)

Goals for lipid management:(ElSayed et al. 2023h)

Diabetes + ASCVD	All ages	High-intensity statin	LDL Target <55 mg/dl
Diabetes+Risk factors	All ages	Moderate-high intensity statin	LDL Target <70 mg/dl ≥50% reduction LDL
Diabetes w/o ASCVD	≥40 years	Moderate intensity statin	LDL Target <70 mg/dl
Diabetes	≥75 year	Moderate intensity statin	LDL Target based on risk and benefit

Anti-platelet therapy: Aspirin is recommended for people with a history of cardiovascular events as secondary prevention. The benefit of primary prevention without a history of cardiovascular events is less clear. Its use should be balanced with the increased risk of bleeding. (ElSayed et al. 2023b)

Microvascular complications: Hyperglycemia increases the transfer of glucose through the polyol pathway. Sorbitol accumulates in the cells and the resulting osmotic stress damages cells. (Fowler 2008; ElSayed et al. 2023c) The tissues most susceptible to damage from this are the kidneys, eyes, and nerves.

Retinopathy may develop several years before the diagnosis of diabetes. Advanced glycosylated end products and growth factors also play a role in the development of retinopathy. (Fowler 2008; ElSayed et al. 2023c) All persons with type 1 diabetes should have an eye exam within five years of diagnosis and every 1-2 years following. Type 2 individuals should have an exam at diagnosis after their blood sugars stabilize, then every 1-2 years. For those with diabetes who are pregnant, an eye exam should be performed during the first trimester.

Nephropathy: There is a strong correlation between chronic kidney disease (CKD) and cardiovascular disease. Hypertension and hyperglycemia are primary underlying causes that are treatable and, when well-managed, reduce the risk of nephropathy. CKD classification is based on etiology, glomerular filtration rate (GFR), and albuminuria. Treatment of CKD starts with controlling blood glucose and blood pressure. Diets low in sodium can further reduce blood pressure and cardiovascular risks. Plant proteins are preferred over animal proteins. ACEI or ARB antihypertensives are recommended but not for primary prevention. Creatinine, GFR, and potassium levels should be closely monitored. SGLT-2 inhibitors are now recommended for treating CKD with or without diabetes. Empagliflozin can be used with a GFR as low as 20 ml/min/1.73. Other SGLT2 inhibitors are approved with higher GFR. Manufacturer guidelines should be reviewed before prescribing. Adding a GLP-1a in type 2 diabetes with CKD can further reduce cardiovascular risks. Finerenone is a non-steroidal mineralocorticoid antagonist which has improved renal failure and progression of CKD. (ElSayed et al. 2023i)

Neuropathy should be screened for in all persons with diabetes. Peripheral neuropathy is often present on initial screening as neuropathy may have been insidiously occurring during the pre-diagnosis phase. Peripheral neuropathy should be evaluated annually with a ten g-monofilament testing of the feet. Identifying peripheral neuropathy and counseling on foot protective measures can reduce the risk of ulcerations and amputations.

Autonomic neuropathy is evidenced by orthostatic hypotension, resting tachycardia, syncope, sexual dysfunction, gastroparesis, exercise intolerance, constipation, diarrhea, urinary retention, urinary incontinence, or changes in sweat function, or dry, cracked skin of the extremities. Neuropathy can be improved with good glucose and lipid control, but at this time, there is no cure. Several medications are used to treat neuropathy, such as Gabapentin, Pregabalin, Duloxetine, Tri-cyclic antidepressants, and Lidocaine ointment or patches. (ElSayed et al. 2023c)

Choosing the right medication

This can be a daunting task considering all the options available to treat type 2 diabetes, risk factors, and complications. It is common for these patients to be on 4-8 medications. When choosing medications, consider comorbidities and medications that may address both diabetes and co-morbidities. Most antihyperglycemics (except insulin) lower A1C by 0.4-1.5%. Each drug class added to another will reduce blood glucose by varying degrees. Insulin will lower A1C to the necessary goal but requires monitoring to avoid hypoglycemia. Glucose control goals should be individualized based on the person's willingness to use medications, affordability, and ability to manage their medications. Other considerations include age (children and elderly are at higher risks of hypoglycemia), co-morbid conditions, life expectancy, duration of diabetes, and a person's support system. Insurance companies may have limitations on certain medications and may require pre-authorization or have specific criteria for them to be covered.

Case Study

Dr. CG is a 55-year-old Latina female who has generally been healthy. She does not know of any significant health issues but has not had lab work for many years. She is seen for her yearly physical. She is a department chair at a local university and feels she is under much stress. She has joined a local gym and works out four days weekly for 45 minutes each time. She complains of being thirsty all the time and increased urination. She has not lost any weight in the last year.

Family history:
Mother with type 2 diabetes
Brother living, age 60, MI at age 45
Sister: living, age 56, HTN

Current medications: Multiple vitamins, Aspirin 81 mg

Physical exam:
Vitals:
BP 152/88, P. 76, regular
Wt. 184, BMI 32.3
Ht. 64"

EXAM: Pleasant, well-developed female with central obesity
COR: HRRR, no rubs or murmurs.
Lungs: No wheezing rales, rhonchi
Abdomen soft, obese, no masses or tenderness
Extremities: warm, dry, 1+ pitting edema of the lower extremities.
Foot exam: no deformities, no ulcerations,
Loss of sensation with 10 gm monofilament of the toes.
Vibratory sensation present at the ankles
Skin: Soft velvety area of increased pigmentation along the back of her neck and axilla.

What is the most likely diagnosis? What would you recommend for further evaluation and treatment?
Her risk factors, age, ethnicity, central obesity, family history, and acanthosis nigricans are typical for type 2 diabetes. Acanthosis nigricans is a velvety discoloration of skin folds, especially around the neck, axilla, and groin, and is an indicator of insulin resistance. Pancreatic function declines over time, leading to type 2 diabetes.
Comprehensive labs, including CBC, Chem 26, lipids, TSH, UA, and Microalbumin, are ordered to determine her diagnosis and other risk factors, as diabetes has many comorbid conditions. Diabetes can be diagnosed with either an A1C of 6.5% or higher or fasting blood glucose > 126 mg/dl on two occasions. A random blood glucose of ≥200 mg/dl Glucose or a 2-hour 75 gm glucose tolerance testing can also diagnose diabetes. A 75 gm OGTT test requires an 8-hour fast. A fasting blood glucose is obtained, then 75 grams of glucose is consumed, followed by a two-hour blood glucose. Blood glucose over 200 mg/dl is diagnostic of diabetes. Blood glucose between 140 mg/dl and 200 mg/dl is diagnostic of "pre-diabetes." C-Peptide helps determine the difference between type 1 and type 2 diabetes. If you suspect she has type 1 diabetes, this would be appropriate.

Lab results

CMP:	Glucose	219 mg/dl (70-100 mg/dl)
	Na+	141 mmol/l (136-145 mmol/l)
	K+	3.6 mmol/l (3.5-5.1 mmol/l)
	Cl	100 mmol/l (98-107 mmol/l)
	ALT	64 U/L (14-59 U/L)
	AST	48 U/L (15-37 U/L)
	Alk Phos	103 U/L (46-116 U/L)
	Creatinine	0.6 mg/dl (0.6-1.3 mg/dl)
	BUN	11 mg/dl (7-18 mg/dl)
	GFR	123.62 ml/min/1.73m2 (>60 ml/min/1.73m2)
Lipids:	Cholesterol	313 mg/dl (<200 mg/dl)
	HDL	40 mg/dl (>39 mg/dl)
	LDL	213 mg/dl (0-100 mg/dl)
	Triglycerides	268 mg/dl (<150 mg/dl)
C-Peptide		2.25 ng/ml (1.10-4.40 ng/ml)
TSH:		0.98 μIU (0.36-3.74μIU/ml)

A1C	11.7% (estimated avg glucose 289 mg/dl)
Microalbumin ratio	6.2 mg/g (<30 mg/g)
Urine microalbumin	8.3 mg/l (<16.0 mg/l)

Her fasting labs confirm type 2 diabetes and hyperlipidemia. Her elevated ALT and AST indicate she may have fatty liver disease. Her C-peptide is normal, indicating she is secreting insulin, but her glucose is high.

Treatment Plan: Discussion regarding her lab studies and the benefit of lifestyle changes, weight loss, and nutrition. Person-centered goals are established. She is active, continues to work in a high-stress job, and is relatively young. She is motivated to manage her diabetes, improve her symptoms, and prevent long-term complications.

Goals: 1. A1C <7%, In her case lower, would be recommended if she can do so without hypoglycemia.

2. Monitor blood glucose, fasting, and 1-2 hours after meals. If her insurance covers a CGM, this can be very helpful for understanding glucose patterns. She is given a sample meter and strips and instructed on using the monitor to check her blood glucose.

3. Fasting blood glucose target 70-130 mg/dl, 2-hour postprandial BG of <180 mg/dl. She would likely benefit from lower targets (Fasting 70-110 mg/dl, 2 hours postprandial <140 mg/dl, and an A1C of 6-6.5%). Many glucometer companies and CGM companies will send meters to provider offices to dispense to clients at no charge if requested.

4. Blood pressure goal of <130/80 mm Hg

5. Cholesterol <200 mg/dl, LDL < 70 mg/dl

Education. She is referred to the diabetes educator and nutritionist for further nutrition and lifestyle management information. It is essential that persons with diabetes and their families also understand the consequences of uncontrolled diabetes in a non-threatening but informative manner. Family member support contributes to successful diabetes management. In communities that do not have a certified diabetes educator or nutritionist available, online programs are available. Some are free to the patient and provide a health coach.

Medication: Her A1C is 11.7%. It is unlikely that one medication alone will reduce her A1C to target. She has been prescribed metformin 500 mg once daily for 4-5 days, then twice daily, titrating over the next few weeks as tolerated to a maximum dose of 1000 mg twice daily. Her family history of early cardiovascular disease and her diagnosis of diabetes would make her a good candidate for a GLP-1a that has cardiovascular benefits.

Hypertension: Starting an ACEi or ARB is appropriate. She is started on Lisinopril 10 mg daily. Home blood pressure monitoring is recommended.

Hyperlipidemia: She is started on Atorvastatin 40 mg. She is at higher risk due to her family history, hyperlipidemia, and her diagnosis of diabetes. A high-intensity statin will reduce her LDL by approximately 50%.

Outcomes: She calls in 1 month and reports her average blood sugar is now less than 200 most of the time. But she still has excursions sometimes after meals over 220. She attributes this to her food choices. She has met with the nutritionist and has changed some of her high-carbohydrate ethnic foods to lower-carbohydrate options.

She is seen back in three months. Her A1C is now 8%. She has continued to exercise and eat a lower carbohydrate diet. She is feeling well. She denies excessive urination and thirst. However, her A1C is still not to target. She is started on semaglutide 0.25 mg SQ weekly. Semaglutide may lower A1C up to 3%. The dose should be titrated once a month. Over the next three months, she titrated the dose to 0.50 mg weekly for four weeks then 1 mg SQ weekly. She returned to the clinic. Her A1C was 6.8%. She lost 10 lbs. and was feeling well. She continued to see the nutritionist once a month for additional three months.

Follow-up (American Diabetes Association recommendations for follow-up):

- Visit with provider every three months, A1C every three months, Foot exam at least yearly
- eye exam every 1-2 years or per ophthalmology
- Continued regular home monitoring of blood glucose

  Routine preventive care, immunizations, labs

References

AACE. 2023. *Diabetes Resource Center* 2023 [cited 2-5-2023 2023]. Available from https://pro.aace.com/disease-state-resources/diabetes.

ADA. 2023. *Diabetes Pro* 2023 [cited 2-5-2023 2023]. Available from https://professional.diabetes.org/.

Adeyinka, A., and N. P. Kondamudi. 2022. Hyperosmolar Hyperglycemic Syndrome. In *StatPearls*. Treasure Island (FL).

Akmal, M., and R. Wadhwa. 2022. Alpha Glucosidase Inhibitors. In *StatPearls*. Treasure Island (FL).

American Diabetes Association Professional Practice, Committee. 2022. 3. Prevention or Delay of Type 2 Diabetes and Associated Comorbidities: Standards of Medical Care in Diabetes-2022. *Diabetes Care* 45 (Suppl 1):S39-S45.

ASCVD. 2023. *ASCVD Risk Estimator Plus*. ASCVD 2023 [cited 2-5-2023 2023]. Available from https://tools.acc.org/ASCVD-Risk-Estimator-Plus.

Association of Diabetes, Care, Specialists Education, and L. Kolb. 2021. An Effective Model of Diabetes Care and Education: The ADCES7 Self-Care Behaviors. *Sci Diabetes Self Manag Care* 47 (1):30-53.

Bonadio, W. 2013. Pediatric diabetic ketoacidosis: an outpatient perspective on evaluation and management. *Pediatr Emerg Med Pract* 10 (3):1-13; quiz 14.

Bryan, CP, and H Joachim. 1930. *The Papyrus Ebers.*: London: G. Bles.

CDC. 2023. *CDC 2022 National Diabetes Statistics Report* 2022 [cited 2-5-2023 2023]. Available from https://nationaldppcsc.cdc.gov/s/article/CDC-2022-National-Diabetes-Statistics-Report.

Croke, L. 2020. Beers Criteria for Inappropriate Medication Use in Older Patients: An Update from the AGS. *American Family Physician* 101 (1):56-57.

DDS. 2023. *About Diabetes Distress Scale (DDS)* 2023 [cited 2-5-2023 2023]. Available from https://diabetesdistress.org/dds-questions.

ElSayed, N. A., G. Aleppo, V. R. Aroda, R. R. Bannuru, F. M. Brown, D. Bruemmer, B. S. Collins, K. Cusi, M. E. Hilliard, D. Isaacs, E. L. Johnson, S. Kahan, K. Khunti, J. Leon, S. K. Lyons, M. L. Perry, P. Prahalad, R. E. Pratley, J. J. Seley, R. C. Stanton, R. A. Gabbay, and Association on behalf of the American Diabetes. 2023a. 4. Comprehensive Medical Evaluation and Assessment of Comorbidities: Standards of Care in Diabetes-2023. *Diabetes Care* 46 (Suppl 1):S49-S67.

ElSayed, N. A., G. Aleppo, V. R. Aroda, R. R. Bannuru, F. M. Brown, D. Bruemmer, B. S. Collins, S. R. Das, M. E. Hilliard, D. Isaacs, E. L. Johnson, S. Kahan, K. Khunti, M. Kosiborod, J. Leon, S. K. Lyons, M. L. Perry, P. Prahalad, R. E. Pratley, J. J. Seley, R. C. Stanton, R. A. Gabbay, and Association on behalf of the American Diabetes. 2023b. 10. Cardiovascular Disease and Risk Management: Standards of Care in Diabetes-2023. *Diabetes Care* 46 (Suppl 1):S158-S190.

ElSayed, N. A., G. Aleppo, V. R. Aroda, R. R. Bannuru, F. M. Brown, D. Bruemmer, B. S. Collins, C. H. Gibbons, J. M. Giurini, M. E. Hilliard, D. Isaacs, E. L. Johnson, S. Kahan, K. Khunti, J. Leon, S. K. Lyons, M. L. Perry, P. Prahalad, R. E. Pratley, J. J. Seley, R. C. Stanton, J. K. Sun, R. A. Gabbay, and Association on behalf of the American Diabetes. 2023c. 12. Retinopathy, Neuropathy, and Foot Care: Standards of Care in Diabetes-2023. *Diabetes Care* 46 (Suppl 1):S203-S215.

ElSayed, N. A., G. Aleppo, V. R. Aroda, R. R. Bannuru, F. M. Brown, D. Bruemmer, B. S. Collins, M. E. Hilliard, D. Isaacs, E. L. Johnson, S. Kahan, K. Khunti, J. Leon, S. K. Lyons, M. L. Perry, P. Prahalad, R. E. Pratley, J. Jeffrie Seley, R. C. Stanton, R. A. Gabbay, and Association on behalf of the American Diabetes. 2023d. 15. Management of Diabetes in Pregnancy: Standards of Care in Diabetes-2023. *Diabetes Care* 46 (Suppl 1):S254-S266.

ElSayed, N. A., G. Aleppo, V. R. Aroda, R. R. Bannuru, F. M. Brown, D. Bruemmer, B. S. Collins, M. E. Hilliard, D. Isaacs, E. L. Johnson, S. Kahan, K. Khunti, J. Leon, S. K. Lyons, M. L. Perry, P. Prahalad, R. E. Pratley, J. J. Seley, R. C. Stanton, R. A. Gabbay, and Association on behalf of the American Diabetes. 2023e. 1. Improving Care and Promoting Health in Populations: Standards of Care in Diabetes-2023. *Diabetes Care* 46 (Supple 1):S10-S18.

ElSayed, N. A., G. Aleppo, V. R. Aroda, R. R. Bannuru, F. M. Brown, D. Bruemmer, B. S. Collins, M. E. Hilliard, D. Isaacs, E. L. Johnson, S. Kahan, K. Khunti, J. Leon, S. K. Lyons, M. L. Perry, P. Prahalad, R. E. Pratley, J. J. Seley, R. C. Stanton, R. A. Gabbay, and Association on behalf of the American Diabetes. 2023f. 2. Classification and Diagnosis of Diabetes: Standards of Care in Diabetes-2023. *Diabetes Care* 46 (Suppl 1):S19-S40.

ElSayed, N. A., G. Aleppo, V. R. Aroda, R. R. Bannuru, F. M. Brown, D. Bruemmer, B. S. Collins, M. E. Hilliard, D. Isaacs, E. L. Johnson, S. Kahan, K. Khunti, J. Leon, S. K. Lyons, M. L. Perry, P. Prahalad, R. E. Pratley, J. J. Seley, R. C. Stanton, R. A. Gabbay, and Association on behalf of the American Diabetes. 2023g. 7. Diabetes Technology: Standards of Care in Diabetes-2023. *Diabetes Care* 46 (Suppl 1):S111-S127.

ElSayed, N. A., G. Aleppo, V. R. Aroda, R. R. Bannuru, F. M. Brown, D. Bruemmer, B. S. Collins, M. E. Hilliard, D. Isaacs, E. L. Johnson, S. Kahan, K. Khunti, J. Leon, S. K. Lyons, M. L. Perry, P. Prahalad, R. E. Pratley, J. J. Seley, R. C. Stanton, R. A. Gabbay, and Association on behalf of the American Diabetes. 2023h. 9. Pharmacologic Approaches to Glycemic Treatment: Standards of Care in Diabetes-2023. *Diabetes Care* 46 (Suppl 1):S140-S157.

ElSayed, N. A., G. Aleppo, V. R. Aroda, R. R. Bannuru, F. M. Brown, D. Bruemmer, B. S. Collins, M. E. Hilliard, D. Isaacs, E. L. Johnson, S. Kahan, K. Khunti, J. Leon, S. K. Lyons, M. L. Perry, P. Prahalad, R. E. Pratley, J. J. Seley, R. C. Stanton, R. A. Gabbay, and Association on behalf of the American Diabetes. 2023i. 11. Chronic

Kidney Disease and Risk Management: Standards of Care in Diabetes-2023. *Diabetes Care* 46 (Suppl 1):S191-S202.

Fowler, M.J. 2008. Microvascular and Macrovascular Complications of Diabetes. *Clinical Diabetes* 26 (2):77-82.

Garber, A. J., Y. Handelsman, G. Grunberger, D. Einhorn, M. J. Abrahamson, J. I. Barzilay, L. Blonde, M. A. Bush, R. A. DeFronzo, J. R. Garber, W. T. Garvey, I. B. Hirsch, P. S. Jellinger, J. B. McGill, J. I. Mechanick, L. Perreault, P. D. Rosenblit, S. Samson, and G. E. Umpierrez. 2020. Consensus Statement by the American Association of Clinical Endocrinologists and American College of Endocrinology on the Comprehensive Type 2 Diabetes Management Algorithm - 2020 Executive Summary. *Endocr Pract* 26 (1):107-139.

Gounden, V., M. Ngu, C. Anastasopoulou, and I. Jialal. 2022. Fructosamine. In *StatPearls*. Treasure Island (FL).

Hughes, A. M. 2008. Oxford English Dictionary. *Isis* 99 (3):586.

Kim, W., and J. M. Egan. 2008. The role of incretins in glucose homeostasis and diabetes treatment. *Pharmacological Reviews* 60 (4):470-512.

Lizzo, J. M., A. Goyal, and V. Gupta. 2022. Adult Diabetic Ketoacidosis. In *StatPearls*. Treasure Island (FL).

Magliano, D. J., and E. J. Boyko. 2021. In *IDF DIABETES ATLAS*. Brussels.

Naylor, R.N., S.A.W. Greeley, D. Carmody, J.L. Hwang, M. Sanyoura, L.R. Letourneau, G.I. Bell, and L.H. Philipson. 2018. Monogenic Diabetes: Maturity-Onset Diabetes of the Young (MODY) and Neonatal Diabetes. In *Atypical Diabetes: Pathophysiology, Clinical Presentations, and Treatment Options.*

NIH. 2023. *Pioglitazone* 2023 [cited 2-5-2023 2023]. Available from https://pubchem.ncbi.nlm.nih.gov/compound/Pioglitazone.

Novartis. *Starlix (nateglinide) tablets Rx only Prescribing Information* 2013 [cited. Available from https://www.novartis.com/us-en/sites/novartis_us/files/starlix.pdf.

Shou, J., P. J. Chen, and W. H. Xiao. 2020. Mechanism of increased risk of insulin resistance in aging skeletal muscle. *Diabetol Metab Syndr* 12:14.

Stamatouli, A. M., and S. E. Inzucchi. 2016. Implications of the EMPA-REG Trial for Clinical Care and Research. *Curr Diab Rep* 16 (12):131.

Quiz Questions

1. A 60-year-old thin gentleman is seen in the clinic complaining of increased urination, thirst, and a 30 lb. weight loss over the last 3-4 months. What is the likely cause of his symptoms?
   - A Type 1 diabetes
   - B Pre-diabetes
   - C Type 2 diabetes
   - D Maturity onset diabetes of the young
   - E Prostatic hypertrophy

2. Jane Doe is a 35-year-old Asian woman seen to establish care and for her yearly exam. She complains of weight gain despite changing her diet and eating less. You note central obesity. Her body mass index (BMI) is 30. On your exam, you also notice a soft dark velvety thickening of the skin around her neck and axilla. What diagnostic tests are used to diagnose diabetes?
   - A Iron studies, Ferritin, Serum folate
   - B A1C, fasting blood glucose
   - C Glucose tolerance testing
   - D B and C
   - E C peptide, insulin levels

3. Dr. Jay is a 76-year-old gentleman with a history of bladder cancer, renal stones, and chronic kidney disease. His GFR is 26. He also has type 1 diabetes and takes mixed insulin NPH/Aspart 70/30, 20 units with breakfast, 15 units with lunch, and 25 units with supper. What diabetes medications do you want to avoid?
   - A Metformin
   - B Canagliflozin
   - C Pioglitazone
   - D Liraglutide
   - E All of the above

4. Mrs. Mack is a 40-year-old woman with a history of type 1 diabetes since the age of 15 years old. She is using a continuous glucose monitor and an insulin pump with auto-control. (In auto-control, the pump regulates basal insulin and gives small corrections based on the CGM readings). She exercises daily. She does strength training and weightlifting for 30 minutes, then walks or bikes for at least 1 hour every morning. She is concerned that when she exercises, her "blood sugars skyrocket then plummet." What is the likely reason for her rapid spike and drop in blood sugar following exercise?
   - A Counter-regulatory hormones
   - B Weightlifting and strength training increases gluconeogenesis
   - C Walking/biking increases insulin utilization by skeletal muscles
   - D increased insulin sensitivity
   - E All of the above

5. Which medications can cause hypoglycemia?
   - A Metformin and Acarbose
   - B Pioglitazone, Sitagliptin
   - C Glipizide, Repaglinide
   - D Insulin, glyburide
   - E C & D

6. CJ is a 4-month-old infant with hyperglycemia. He likely has what type of diabetes?
   - A KIR6.2 Mutation, a monogenic form of diabetes
   - B Type 1 diabetes
   - C Type 2 diabetes
   - D MODY
   - E Type 1.5 diabetes (Latent autoimmune diabetes)

Quiz Answers

1. A. Type 1 diabetes can occur at any age. It is often misdiagnosed in adults due to the misconception that adults get type 2 diabetes and children get type 1 diabetes. While type 2 diabetes is more common in adults, type 1 DM and type 2 DM can occur in adults and children. It is important to evaluate for causes of pancreatic failure and hyperglycemia. The diagnosis should be confirmed with antibody testing and c-peptide. Testing will help confirm the diagnosis of type 1 diabetes. Pre-diabetes is more insidious, usually without acute symptoms. His body habitus and acute weight loss should cause speculation that he has type 1 diabetes. Prostatic hypertrophy can cause increased urination but does not cause increased thirst or weight loss.

2. D. The diagnostic criteria for diagnosis of diabetes is an A1C $\geq$ 6.5% or a fasting blood glucose $\geq$ 126mg/dl on two occasions. An oral glucose tolerance test with a 75 mg glucose load resulting in a glucose level over 200 mg/dl and a random blood glucose level over 200 mg/dl is also diagnostic of diabetes.

3. E. His GFR is below the recommended threshold by the manufacturers for these oral medications. GLP-1a's are not approved for use in type 1 diabetes.

4. E. Anaerobic exercise such as weightlifting initially increases blood glucose due to muscles' increased need for glucose. Anaerobic exercise triggers counterregulatory hormones (glucagon, epinephrine, norepinephrine, cortisone, and growth hormone), resulting in gluconeogenesis and hyperglycemia. Aerobic exercise increases insulin sensitivity and insulin utilization, lowering blood glucose.

5. E. Metformin does not cause hypoglycemia. It decreases gluconeogenesis and increases insulin sensitivity. Acarbose inhibits the absorption of complex carbohydrates but does not induce insulin secretion. Pioglitazone improves insulin sensitivity and does not directly affect insulin secretion. Sitagliptin is a DPP-IVi and prolongs GLP-1. It does not directly affect insulin secretion. Glipizide and Repaglinide are insulin secretagogues resulting in higher insulin levels, increasing the risk of hypoglycemia. Insulin has a direct effect on lowering blood glucose and can result in hypoglycemia. Glyburide is a sulfonylurea (insulin secretagogue) with prolonged action, increasing the risk of hypoglycemia. It is on the Beers list of medications advising against use in the elderly population.

6. A. KIR6.2 mutation is a monogenic form of neonatal diabetes that impairs the KATP channel. It can be permanent or transient. It occurs most often between 5 and 26 weeks. Islet cell antibodies are typically absent. Genetic testing should be performed. Sulfonylureas can be used to treat hyperglycemia caused by a KIR6-2 defect.

CHAPTER 16

ATAXIA, DIZZINESS AND BALANCE PROBLEMS

DANIEL A. LLANO, MD/PHD

University of Illinois at Urbana-Champaign, Illinois, USA

Symptoms: **Neurological**

DRUG LIST FOR VERTIGO

Anti-cholinergic/anti-histaminergic agents (see Chapters 4 and 8):

Dimenhydrinate	Anti-cholinergic/anti-histaminergic
Diphenhydramine	Anti-cholinergic/anti-histaminergic
Meclizine	Anti-cholinergic/anti-histaminergic
Scopolamine	Anti-cholinergic/anti-histaminergic

Sedatives (see Chapters 17 and 23):

Alprazolam	Benzodiazepine
Clonazepam	Benzodiazepine
Diazepam	Benzodiazepine
Lorazepam	Benzodiazepine

Anti-emetics (see Chapter 8):

Domperidone	Dopamine antagonist
Metoclopramide	Dopamine antagonist
Ondansetron	Serotonin (5HT3) antagonist
Prochlorperazine	Dopamine antagonist
Promethazine	Dopamine antagonist

DRUG LIST FOR VESTIBULAR NEURONITIS

Oral steroids (see Chapter 9):

Methylprednisolone	Corticosteroid
Prednisone	Corticosteroid

DRUG LIST FOR VESTIBULAR MIGRAINE

Abortive agents:

Sumatriptan	5HT1B/D antagonist
Zolmitriptan	5HT1B/D antagonist
Rizatriptan	5HT1B/D antagonist

Preventative agents (see Chapters 13 and 17):

Amitriptyline	Tricyclic antidepressant, 5HT/NE reuptake inhibitor
Nortriptyline	Tricyclic antidepressant, 5HT/NE reuptake inhibitor
Propranolol	Beta-adrenergic antagonist
Topiramate	Multiple mechanisms
Valproic acid	Multiple mechanisms
Verapamil	Calcium channel antagonist

DRUG LIST FOR MENIERE'S DISEASE

Betahistine	H1/H3 modulator

Diuretics (see Chapter 13):

Hydrochlorothiazide	Thiazide diuretic
Triamterene	Epithelial sodium channel antagonist
Furosemide	Loop diuretic
Acetazolamide	Carbonic anhydrase inhibitor

Oral steroids (see Chapter 9):

Prednisone	Corticosteroid
Methylprednisolone	Corticosteroid

Intratympanic steroids (see Chapter 9):

Dexamethasone	Corticosteroid
Methylprednisolone	Corticosteroid

Intratympanic antibiotics (see Chapter 3):

Gentamycin:	Aminoglycoside antibiotic

DRUG LIST FOR ATAXIA:

4-Aminopyridine:	Potassium channel blocker
Acetazolamide:	Carbonic anhydrase inhibitor
Carbamazepine:	Sodium channel blocker
Miglustat:	Inhibits glucosylceramide synthase and diminishes the synthesis of glycosphingolipids
Paroxetine:	Specific serotonin reuptake inhibitor
Riluzole:	Sodium channel and glutamate antagonist
Varenicline:	Alpha 4 beta 2 nicotinic partial agonist

Ataxia

Ataxia refers to the lack of coordination of movements. It typically manifests as a patient complains of difficulty with fine motor tasks or with balance. Ataxia is assessed at the bedside by using a series of motor tasks, which are typically differentiated into those that test for limb (a.k.a. appendicular) ataxia and those that test for midline (a.k.a. truncal) ataxia. For example, limb ataxia is usually assessed using finger-nose-finger testing whereby the examiner provides a target (usually their finger), and the subject is asked to alternate touching the tip of their finger to the examiner's finger and their own (the subject's) nose. The task can be made more difficult by having the subject "chase" the examiner's finger, which may reveal overshooting of the target, often with overcompensation, leading to the appearance of a tremor ("past-pointing"). An equivalent test in the lower extremities involves placing the subject's heel on the superior portion of their contralateral shin and running it down and up the anterior border of their tibia. Analogously to finger-nose-finger testing, the examiner may ask the subject to touch the examiner's finger with their toes, though in a supine patient, this maneuver often requires substantial strength of hip flexion and knee extension on the part of the patient to elevate the toe to the examiner's hand. Truncal ataxia may be assessed by simply having the patient sit unsupported with their arms folded on their chest and observing for postural sway. Lack of truncal control manifests as excessive rocking movements, analogously to past-pointing described above, often referred to as titubation, or as tipping to one side. Truncal ataxia also affects gait, usually manifesting as irregularly spaced foot placements, leading to compensatory widening of the lateral spacing of the feet to provide a more stable base, often referred to as a "wide-based gait."

Because coordinated movements require both sensory input from limb proprioceptors and motor control centers that integrate those sensory signals with motor commands, ataxia can be caused by disruptions in either sensory or motor neural structures. For example, a common cause of sensory loss is peripheral neuropathy, which is often related to diabetes or chronic alcohol use, is less common due to paraproteinemia, or may also be idiopathic. Such neuropathies are length-dependent and thus affect the feet first. In addition to the dysesthetic pain that often accompanies these disorders, patients may develop an ataxic gait due to a lack of proprioception from the lower extremities. Their gait may be wide-based and/or have exaggerated step height to enhance sensory input from feet ("steppage gait"). Patients may complain of balance problems, particularly when eyes are closed because of a lack of visual input to provide a cue to the location of the horizontal horizon. A common complaint from a patient in this scenario is that they have particular difficulty when washing their hair with their eyes closed, causing them to lose balance in the shower. At the bedside, this type of ataxia is often assessed with a Romberg test with the patient's eyes closed. A positive Romberg test is seen when the patient loses their balance quickly when asked to keep a narrow base with their feet while standing with their eyes closed, but can maintain balance with their eyes open. Another cause of sensory ataxia is loss of posterior column function, as the posterior columns of the spinal cord carry proprioceptive information to the brain. Common causes of posterior column dysfunction include vitamin B12 deficiency or multiple sclerosis, though a classic cause is tabes dorsalis caused by neuro-syphilis. One approach to examining for loss of proprioceptive inputs at the bedside is to have the patient report the position of their limbs with their eyes closed. This test is typically done by moving the patient's great toe superiorly or inferiorly and asking them to report its position. In patients with severe generalized peripheral neuropathy, this loss of sensation may not be specific to the proprioceptive pathways. Retention of pinprick sensation and/or temperature sensation in the feet (whose information is carried by spinothalamic pathways) with loss of joint position sense is highly suggestive of a posterior column deficit. Analogous testing can be done in the upper extremities if upper extremity ataxia is found on examination.

The other main cause of ataxia is loss of cerebellar function. The cerebellum receives a copy of motor commands from the motor cortex, known as "efference copy," via contralateral pontine nuclei, which relay information via the middle cerebellar peduncle. The cerebellum also receives proprioceptive inputs via the spinocerebellar tracts, which enter the cerebellum primarily via the inferior cerebellar peduncle, with the exception of ventral spinocerebellar tracts, which enter via the superior cerebellar peduncle. Thus, the cerebellum receives a copy of the intended motor action, and a copy of the actual position of limbs in space, and can thus issue corrective signals back to the motor cortex to adjust ongoing motor output. A deficit in this process due to a structural or functional lesion of the cerebellum leads to uncoordinated, or ataxic, movements. The location of the lesion in the cerebellum determines the type of ataxia seen. Lesions towards the midline of the cerebellum, particularly those impacting the anterior vermis, tend to lead to truncal ataxia, producing wide-based gait, and increased sway (or falls) with seated posture when unsupported. Lesions located more laterally, towards the cerebellar hemispheres, lead to more appendicular ataxia, resulting in finger-nose-finger and heel-to-shin past-pointing findings. Because cerebellar outflow through the superior cerebellar peduncle targets the contralateral motor cortex (via the motor thalamus) and because motor cortical fibers cross the midline en route to the spinal cord, cerebellar outflow is double-crossed, and cerebellar lesions will impact ipsilateral limbs. At the bedside, central cerebellar lesions cause gait ataxia with a resulting wide-based gait, while cerebellar hemispheric lesions lead to ipsilesional appendicular ataxia. Cerebellar sources of ataxia can be differentiated from sensory ataxia by assessing joint position sense, which should be intact if only the cerebellum is involved. In addition, Romberg testing is typically compromised with cerebellar lesions whether a person's eyes are open or closed because of the inability to integrate any sensorimotor information to support postural reflexes. Lesions of flocculo-nodular regions of the cerebellum typically lead to vertiginous symptoms, which will be discussed below.

Dizziness:

Complaints of dizziness are often challenging to sort through as a clinician because of the non-specificity of the term. Patients use the word "dizzy" to refer to a whole family of complaints, ranging from false percepts of environmental motion (vertigo) to hypoperfusion syndromes (presyncope), to the inability to coordinate movements (ataxia), to loss of perception of the horizontal meridian (disequilibrium). Even when pressed to clarify which of the above classes their dizziness falls into, patients often struggle to provide specificity about this complaint, in large part because the neural processes that are responsible for maintaining these functions typically operate outside of our conscious awareness. Thus, although a clinician should seek clarity from a patient when the term "dizzy" or equivalent is provided, it is important to use other information about symptoms, such as the triggers and timing of the dizziness, any associated symptoms, and careful examination findings, to sort through the differential diagnosis.

Vestibular system dysfunction:

The vestibular labyrinth contains detectors for linear acceleration (utricle and saccule) and angular acceleration (semicircular canals) and sends information about head movement to the brain via the eighth cranial nerve (the vestibulocochlear nerve). An imbalance in the activity of the two vestibular nerves is a signal to the brain that the head is moving and triggers compensatory movements of the eyes (via the vestibular-ocular reflex) and of the trunk (via vestibulospinal projections). If there is an asymmetry in vestibular afferent activity in the absence of actual head movement, the patient will have the percept of movement and may often have a sensation of being pulled or of falling, and may, in fact, fall. The vestibular-ocular reflex will drive slow movements of the eyes, generally away from the more active of the two vestibular nerves. In the absence of actual movement, the slow conjugate movement of the eyes generates unexpected slippage of visual images on the retina, trigging a reflexive saccadic movement in the opposite direction in awake patient (note that patients in coma may not generate a fast corrective movement). If the vestibular imbalance lasts longer than one cycle of eye movements, this cycle of slow movements away from the more active vestibular nerve followed by fast compensatory movements in the opposite direction generates a pattern of oscillatory eye movements known as "nystagmus." By convention, the direction of the fast, corrective, phase defines the directionality of the nystagmus.

There are multiple causes of vestibular dysfunction that can be placed into broad categories based on their timing and triggers. Here we will classify causes of dizziness based on their temporal patterns.

Paroxysmal dizziness:

Benign paroxysmal positional vertigo (BPPV)

- *Presentation:* BPPV presents as paroxysmal attacks of intense sensations of illusory movement and nausea that typically occur after head movement (rolling over in bed, leaning head back to reach for an object, etc.). It is important to specify here that, although all types of vertigo worsen with head movement, patients with BPPV typically have no symptoms while at rest, maximal symptoms for 30-60 seconds after head movement, and then a return back to baseline. Other forms of vertigo, such as vestibular neuritis (a.k.a. labyrinthitis), will typically involve long durations of vertiginous symptoms that somewhat worsen with head movement but do not have the staccato flavor of the symptoms in BPPV.
- *Risk Factors:* Minor head trauma may precede the symptoms by causing the release of an otolith. Older age is another risk factor.

- *Pathophysiology:* BPPV is most commonly caused by an otolith from the macula or saccule migrating into the posterior semicircular canal. Once entering the canal, movement of the head can cause greater than normal inertial waves of endolymph movement, causing increased signaling down the affected vestibular portion of the eighth cranial nerve. This movement of endolymph causes the sensation of movement, slow eye movements due to the vestibular-ocular reflex, and corrective fast movements, leading to nystagmus.
- *Examination:* The nystagmus is driven by slow movement towards the "good" ear followed by fast beating towards the affected ear with a rotatory component such that the 12 o'clock position rotates towards the affected ear. Diagnosis is characteristically made using a Dix-Hallpike test, whereby a patient is rapidly taken from a sitting to a supine position with head turned 45 degrees to one side, and ultimately dipping approximately 30 degrees below the plane of the body (with head supported by the examiner). When the head is turned towards the affected ear, the test will elicit rotary nystagmus towards the affected ear accompanied by severe nausea. The symptoms typically emerge after 10-15 seconds and abate after about one minute.
- *Laboratory:* None (should be normal)
- *Imaging:* None (should be normal)
- *Associated symptoms/conditions:* Severe nausea
- *Diagnosis:* See "Examination."
- *Treatment:* Treatment of BPPV in the posterior canal (responsible for 80-90% of all BPPV) is with the otolith repositioning maneuver, otherwise known as the Epley maneuver. This is a highly effective therapy that involves moving the patient's head and body in a series of movements to allow the otolith to fall out of the posterior semicircular canal. (Woodworth et al. 2004) Eventually, these otoliths are enzymatically digested in the labyrinth. Vestibular suppressant medications (covered in more detail below) such as anti-cholinergic drugs and benzodiazepines are not indicated in these scenarios because their time course of action is too slow to be effective, such that the patient is unlikely to derive any benefits and patients only experience the anti-cholinergic and sedating effects of these medications.
- *Management:* None other than acute treatment. Recurrences may be re-treated with the Epley maneuver.

Episodic Ataxias

- *Presentation:* Paroxysms of ataxia that can last from seconds to hours. The attacks are often brought about by stress, physical exertion, alcohol, or caffeine.
- *Risk Factors:* It is an autosomal dominant condition, so having a family history of similar symptoms (or genetic confirmation) is a significant risk factor.
- *Pathophysiology:* There are currently at least 8 forms of episodic ataxia (EA1-8), though EA1 and EA2 are by far the most common forms. EA1 is caused by a mutation in a potassium channel encoded by the KCNA1 gene. EA2 is caused by a mutation in a calcium channel encoded by CACNA1A. This gene can have slightly different mutations and can lead to hemiplegic migraine or spinocerebellar ataxia type 6.
- *Examination:* During an attack, truncal ataxia and direction-changing nystagmus can be seen. Between attacks, mild ataxia, myokymia, and direction-changing or downbeat nystagmus can be seen.
- *Laboratory:* Genetic testing for mutations, the most common being in the KCNA1 (EA1) or CACNA1A (EA2) genes.
- *Imaging:* Typically no findings, though cerebellar atrophy may be present.
- *Associated symptoms/conditions:* Myokymia can be seen in or outside of the periods of ataxia. Epilepsy can be seen in EA1. Other signs of brainstem dysfunction can be seen such as diplopia, tinnitus, and dysarthria can be seen. Migraines are also associated with episodic ataxias.
- *Diagnosis:* Via genetic testing as outlined above.
- *Treatment:* Acetazolamide, which is a carbonic anhydrase inhibitor that acidifies the bloodstream and causes mild hypokalemia, can be used in EA2, 4, 5, and 6. 4-aminopyridine, potassium channel blocker, may also be used in EA2. (Strupp et al. 2011) Carbamazepine has shown some benefit for EA1. (Orsucci et al. 2019)
- *Management:* Encourage adequate sleep, moderate exercise, and limiting overall caffeine intake.

Episodic dizziness brought on by cough or other Valsalva maneuvers, or by changes in ambient atmospheric pressure, which may be related to structural changes in the labyrinth such as canal dehiscence or perilymphatic fistula. These disorders are treated via surgical intervention and are beyond the scope of this chapter.

Acute onset, subchronic dizziness: "Subchronic" in this case refers to symptoms lasting for at least hours, but less than one month. The most worrisome cause here is posterior circulation ischemic stroke or hemorrhage. Classically, clinicians are taught that posterior circulation strokes should cause additional symptoms beyond dizziness (e.g., diplopia, dysarthria, long-tract signs such as limb weakness/numbness, etc.), but this is not a failsafe method as posterior circulation strokes, particularly those that impact the cerebellar nodule or flocculus, may not impact other cranial nerves or long tracts passing through the brainstem. Even diffusion-weighted MRI, typically considered a gold-standard test for identifying acute stroke, may miss posterior circulation strokes approximately 12% of the time in the acute setting. (Kattah et al. 2009) An approach that has been established to have high sensitivity and specificity for the evaluation of posterior circulation ischemic events in the emergency department is known as the HINTS exam. (Kattah et al. 2009) This exam consists of a head thrust test, an assessment of *N*ystagmus, and a *T*est of *S*kew deviation of the eyes. In brief, the head thrust test examines the integrity of the vestibular-ocular reflex, and if abnormal (e.g., eyes lag when the head is moved and require a catch-up saccade), is suggestive of a peripheral lesion. Peripheral lesions, such as vestibular neuritis, lead to horizontal nystagmus that obeys Alexander's law (nystagmus points away from the affected ear and is worst when looking away from the affected ear). If the direction of nystagmus changes with eye position, then a central lesion is more likely. With the test of skew, the eyes are alternately covered and uncovered. If vertical repositioning of the eyes is seen, then a central lesion is likely.

Vestibular neuritis (labyrinthitis)

- *Presentation:* Acute/subacute onset of intense vertigo lasting hours to days.
- *Risk Factors:* Preceding upper respiratory viral infection.
- *Pathophysiology:* Possibly a post-infectious (or infectious) inflammatory condition of the labyrinth. Can be seen after an upper respiratory infection.
- *Examination:* Patients will have an abnormal head thrust test and consistent-direction nystagmus that obeys Alexander's law.
- *Laboratory:* Normal.
- *Imaging:* Typically normal, though enhancement of the labyrinth can be seen on gadolinium-enhanced MRI.
- *Associated symptoms/conditions:* Severe nausea. Ataxia is generally mild. Most patients with vestibular neuritis can ambulate, though may be reluctant to do so. Other neurologic findings (other brainstem findings, long-tract signs) are absent.
- *Diagnosis:* Based on the clinical history and exam findings outlined above.
- *Treatment:* In all of these cases, drugs that globally suppress vestibular activity, such as anti-muscarinic/anti-histamine or benzodiazepines as listed above may be used. By suppressing vestibular reflexes, these drugs also inhibit central vestibular compensation for peripheral deficits and thus may impair long-term recovery from vestibular neuritis. Therefore, it is recommended that these drugs should only be used for a short period of time, typically three days, after the onset of symptoms. A short course of steroids (e.g., a 10-day tapering course of prednisone starting at 60 mg/day) or methylprednisolone has been shown to be helpful, but valacyclovir has not. (Strupp et al. 2004; Fishman et al. 2011)
- *Management:* Longer-term treatment consists of vestibular rehabilitation where patients are trained to enhance central reflexes to vestibular input and have been shown to be highly effective. (McDonnell and Hillier 2015)

Vestibular migraine:

- *Presentation:* Patients will present with vertigo lasting for hours often associated with other migrainous symptoms such as photophobia and phonophobia.
- *Risk Factors:* Past history of migraine headaches.
- *Pathophysiology:* Unknown, likely related to spreading depression phenomena, but anatomical localization has not been identified.
- *Examination:* There typically are not "hard" findings of vestibular dysfunction such as nystagmus or absent vestibular-ocular reflexes.
- *Laboratory:* Normal.
- *Imaging:* Normal.
- *Associated symptoms/conditions:* Vestibular migraine patients may have ear fullness, tinnitus, and hearing loss.
- *Diagnosis:* Based on clinical history.
- *Treatment:* Large randomized treatment trials are lacking, in part because this entity is only recently clinically recognized. Clinical experience suggests that typical abortive agents such as triptans, preventative agents, such as beta-blockers, and certain anti-seizure medicines, such as topiramate, may be helpful.
- *Management:* Migraine headaches are often brought on by poor sleep, stress, or particular food items. Patients should be instructed to keep a journal of their symptoms and lifestyle factors such as amount of sleep and foods eaten, to try to pinpoint, and subsequently avoid, triggers.

Meniere's Disease:

- *Presentation:* Meniere's Disease may also present with episodes of vertigo, often very severe, lasting hours, but is also classically associated with other signs of vestibular and cochlear dysfunction, such as hearing loss (characteristically in the low frequencies) and tinnitus as well as a sensation of ear fullness.
- *Risk Factors:* Family history of Meniere's Disease.
- *Pathophysiology:* Meniere's Disease is characterized by an overabundance of endolymph in the vestibular apparatus and/or cochlea, often referred to as "endolymphatic hydrops."
- *Examination:* Findings are consistent with those seen with unilateral vestibular loss as outlined above.
- *Laboratory:* Normal.

- *Imaging:* Generally normal, but MRI of the temporal bone may reveal abnormalities of the endolymphatic duct.
- *Associated symptoms/conditions:* Tinnitus, hearing loss, and a feeling of ear fullness.
- *Diagnosis:* Diagnosis is based on the clinical history and findings of low-frequency hearing loss, tinnitus, and unilateral vestibular dysfunction.
- *Treatment:* Treatment approaches include short-term vestibular suppressants as outlined above. However, longer-term therapy involves diuresis to attempt to diminish endolymphatic fluid. This outcome can be achieved via a sodium-restricted diet or traditional diuretic agents. In cases resistant to diuresis, intratympanic administration of steroids into the affected ear has been shown to be highly effective in diminishing Meniere's symptoms. For refractory cases, unilateral vestibular/cochlear lesions with intratympanic gentamycin can be considered, though an ablative technique should be considered as a last option. Ablation requires subsequent vestibular rehabilitation to optimize central compensation for the expected imbalance between the two ears.
- *Management:* Long-term prevention involves the maintenance of a low-sodium diet.

Chronic dizziness: "Chronic" refers to dizziness lasting greater than one month. Structural lesions, such as tumors in the posterior fossa, vestibular schwannoma, or Chiari malformation should be evaluated using an MRI brain or internal acoustic canal with gadolinium contrast. CT scan is typically suboptimal for posterior fossa lesions given the frequent presence of streak artifacts caused by dense bony structures surrounding the posterior fossa. Should a structural lesion be found, surgical management may be indicated to treat the lesion.

Multiple systems atrophy – cerebellar subtype:

- *Presentation:* Progressive ataxia with cerebellar degeneration in a subject over the age of 50. Subjects do not usually complain of "dizziness" and will commonly report frequent falls and balance problems.
- *Risk Factors:* Aging.
- *Pathophysiology:* This disorder is considered to be one of the atypical parkinsonism syndromes (formerly known as "Parkinson's Plus" syndromes) along with corticobasal syndrome/disease, progressive supranuclear palsy, and dementia with Lewy Bodies. Like Parkinson's disease and dementia with Lewy bodies, multiple systems atrophy is a synucleinopathy. In the case of the cerebellar subtype, there is an oligodendrogliopathy with alpha-synuclein accumulation (Papp–Lantos bodies) found in the olivopontocerebellar system.
- *Examination:* Signs of truncal ataxia, wide based-gait.
- *Laboratory:* None.
- *Imaging:* Pontine degeneration along with loss of pontocerebellar fibers leads to the "hot-crossed bun" sign in the pons seen on MRI brain, typically seen using T2-weighted imaging.
- *Associated symptoms/conditions:* Autonomic dysfunction, parkinsonism.
- *Diagnosis:* Based on clinical history, examination, imaging and/or skin biopsy for alpha-synuclein.
- *Treatment:* Supportive, though some data exist to support paroxetine for motor symptoms. (Friess et al. 2006)

Fragile-X ataxia syndrome:

- *Presentation:* This is seen in older males as an idiopathic progressive disorder involving bilateral action tremor and gait ataxia.
- *Risk Factors:* Males over age 50 with a younger male relative (grandson) with Fragile X syndrome.
- *Pathophysiology:* Males with a "pre"-mutation of the fragile X gene (55-200 copies of CGG repeats in the fragile X [FMR] gene), leading to pathology at the level of the middle cerebellar peduncles as well as the cerebral cortex, periventricular white matter and corpus callosum. Because the disease is X-linked, it is less commonly seen in females. Male offspring of these patients do not inherit this gene because they receive their X chromosome from their mother, but female offspring may be asymptomatic carriers. Because of genetic anticipation, as the gene is passed onto a third generation, it is likely to have an increase in the number of CGG repeats. Thus, the grandsons of the index patient are more likely to have a full mutation and therefore the full fragile X phenotype, which leads to intellectual disability, several body dysmorphisms, and an autistic behavioral phenotype.
- *Examination:* Physical examination reveals action tremor (tremor seen with movement) and/or intention tremor (tremor that grows as the patient's finger nears a target) is seen early, followed by ataxia of gait.
- *Laboratory:* No abnormalities.
- *Imaging:* Bilateral T2 hyperintensities in the middle cerebellar peduncle ("MCP sign") may be seen as well as white matter abnormalities in the periventricular regions and corpus callosum.
- *Associated symptoms/conditions:* Anxiety and depression, peripheral neuropathy, autonomic dysfunction, and parkinsonism may be seen. Typical facial dysmorphisms and macro-orchidism seen in the full mutation are not typically seen in this syndrome.
- *Diagnosis:* Diagnosis is based on genetic testing of the FMR gene, revealing the presence of 55-200 copies of CGG repeats.

- *Treatment:* No specific treatments have been approved for this disorder. General approaches for the treatment of ataxia (physical and occupational therapy) and tremors (weighted tremor compensatory devices) may be useful.
- *Management:* Genetic counseling may be helpful for younger generations of the family for reproductive planning.

Acquired cerebellar degeneration:

- *Presentation:* Subacute to chronic development of truncal ataxia, manifesting as disruption of gait.
- *Risk Factors:*
    - Long-term exposure to cerebellar toxins, the most common of which are ethanol and phenytoin.
    - Nutritional deficiencies associated with gastrointestinal pathology or alcohol use, leading to vitamin B1 deficiency leading to Wernicke-Korsakoff syndrome.
    - Malignancies (most common are lymphoma, lung, breast or ovarian) leading to paraneoplastic syndromes produced by anti-cerebellar antibodies.
- *Pathophysiology:* Unknown, but cerebellar Purkinje cells appear to be vulnerable to a number of metabolic or immune toxins, and loss of Purkinje cells is often seen in these disorders. Hemorrhagic necrosis of the mammillary bodies, midline thalamus, periaqueductal gray matter, and along the walls of the 3rd and 4th ventricles is observed in Wernicke encephalopathy.
- *Examination:* Most commonly there will be signs of truncal ataxia, including wide-based gait and inability to sit upright and unsupported with arms folded on the chest. Titubation may also be seen. In patients with ataxia associated with Wernicke syndrome, there may also be confusion as well as eye movement abnormalities (commonly a 6th nerve palsy).
- *Laboratory:* Paraneoplastic syndromes may be assessed by measuring panels of paraneoplastic antibodies from serum (most common antibodies leading to cerebellar ataxia are anti-ANNA1, PCA1, Ma2, Ri, CRMP5). Fasting vitamin B1 or red blood cell transketolase levels can be measured in Wernicke's encephalopathy, though usually this diagnosis is made clinically.
- *Imaging:* For chronic toxic cerebellar ataxia due to alcohol or phenytoin use, there is often cerebellar degeneration observed on MRI brain, most commonly seen in the vermis. Similar degeneration can be seen in paraneoplastic cases, though often less severe, depending on the duration of symptoms. Patients with Wernicke encephalopathy and ataxia often have T2 signal abnormalities seen in the mammillary bodies bilaterally as well as midline thalamus and along periventricular diencephalic/mesencephalic regions.
- *Associated symptoms/conditions:* With alcohol-related ataxia, superimposed upon the truncal ataxia is often sensory ataxia produced by the alcohol-induced peripheral neuropathy. In paraneoplastic syndromes, patients may show evidence of confusion, memory loss, and/or seizures. Patients with ataxia in the setting of thiamine deficiency will often show some degree of ophthalmoplegia, nystagmus, and confusion.
- *Diagnosis:* As outlined above.
- *Treatment:* In the case of alcohol or phenytoin toxicity, the appropriate treatment is to remove the offending agent. Ataxia due to B1 deficiency is treated with thiamine repletion. Paraneoplastic disorders are treated by identifying and treating the primary malignancy. In addition, supplemental immunosuppression with steroids, typically solu-medrol 1000mg/day IV x 5 days and/or intravenous immunoglobulin 0.4g/kg/day x 5 days or plasma exchange may be offered.
- *Management:* Counseling may be required to deal with substance dependence. If the patient has a seizure disorder that led to chronic phenytoin use, then an alternative anti-seizure medication will need to be evaluated. If paraneoplastic antibodies are positive and no primary malignancy is found, generally a repeat CT scan of the chest, abdomen, and pelvis, or whole-body FDG-PET scan should be repeated in 6-12 months.

Inherited cerebellar degeneration:

- *Presentation:* Exact presentation depends on the cause. There are many forms of inherited ataxia syndromes (over 30 autosomal dominant forms, known as spinocerebellar ataxia, as well as autosomal recessive forms such as Friedreich's ataxia). Their common clinical presentation is a progressive worsening of gait coupled with worsening appendicular ataxia. Most are present in childhood, but certain ones (SCA3 – Machado Joseph Disease and SCA6) can first be present in adults. A rare form of progressive developmental ataxia – Niemann-Pick disease, type C – can present in children or adults as a progressive ataxia syndrome, coupled with cognitive and neuropsychiatric symptoms.
- *Risk Factors:* Having a family history of developmental cerebellar ataxia.
- *Pathophysiology:* Multiple, depending on the specific cause. All involve cerebellar degeneration.
- *Examination:* Progressive truncal and appendicular ataxia.
- *Laboratory:* Genetic testing. Most commonly performed as an inherited ataxia panel. Whole-exome sequencing is typically not recommended as it will not detect trinucleotide repeats, which are often found in these disorders.
- *Imaging:* Most causes will show cerebellar degeneration.

- *Associated symptoms/conditions:* Depending on the cause, multiple associated symptoms can be seen. For example, Friedreich's ataxia is often associated with cardiac abnormalities, long-tract signs, peripheral nerve damage, as well as scoliosis. SCA-7 is often associated with macular degeneration while SCA-10 is often associated with seizures. Niemann-Pick disease, type C may also present with hepatosplenomegaly and vertical gaze palsies.
- *Diagnosis:* Diagnosis is made via clinical history, especially family history, and genetic testing.
- *Treatment:* There are no FDA-approved treatments for these disorders, but many are in development. There are randomized, double-blind placebo-controlled studies supporting the use of riluzole, or varenicline ((Ristori et al. 2010; Romano et al. 2015; Zesiewicz et al. 2012), reviewed in (Kwei and Kuo 2020)) that may warrant use. For Niemann-Pick disease, type C, though not FDA approved for this indication, miglustat has positive clinical trial data suggesting that it may slow down the illness. (Patterson et al. 2007; Wraith et al. 2010) Miglustat diminishes the production of glycosphingolipids, which accumulate in Niemann-Pick, type C, and is FDA-approved to treat Gaucher's Disease.
- *Management:* Patients and their families will need genetic counseling, which is preferably done before genetic testing. Patients will benefit from ongoing occupational, physical, and speech therapy. Orthopedic interventions may be needed for bony abnormalities (e.g., scoliosis).

Patients that recover from vestibular damage may continue to have long-lasting symptoms for unclear reasons. Chronic imbalance of vestibular inputs may lead to chronic feelings of disequilibrium. In addition, the severity and misery induced by vestibular dysfunction may create significant anxiety and a maladaptive focus on balance, which may manifest as subjective feelings of dizziness that remain chronic. In addition, bilateral vestibulopathy after toxin damage (e.g., aminoglycoside antibiotics) may cause chronic feelings of dizziness. There are not effective drug therapies to be provided. Vestibular suppressants should not be used chronically because of their tendency to suppress central compensation for peripheral deficits. The optimal treatment regime involves vestibular rehabilitation as well as the identification and treatment of potential psychiatric comorbidities.

Clinical Pharmacology

Anti-cholinergic/anti-histaminergic agents (see Chapters 4 and 8):

Dimenhydrinate:

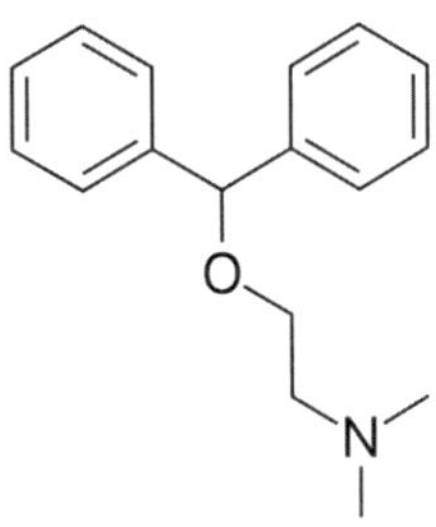

Diphenhydramine

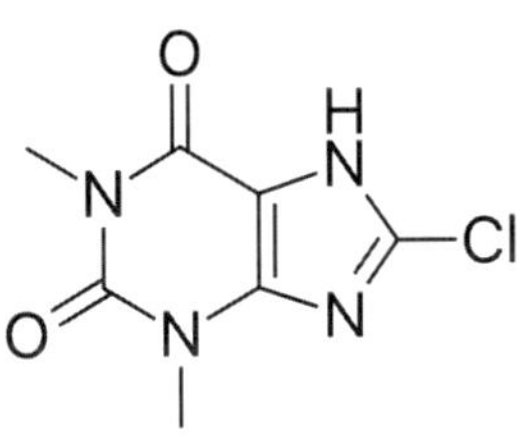

8-chlorotheophylline

Dimenhydrinate is sold as "Dramamine" over the counter and is a combination of diphenhydramine and 8-chlorotheophylline. The clinical utility of this drug is in the **diphenhydramine** ("Benadryl") which has H1-blocking and broad-spectrum antimuscarinic properties. The vestibular suppressant properties are thought to be primarily related to its antimuscarinic effects. Muscarinic receptors of various subtypes are found along the peripheral and central vestibular pathways. (Zhu et al. 2016; Ishiyama et al. 1997) Suppressing them tends to suppress vestibular function, thereby flattening imbalances between the two sides of the vestibular system and diminishing the fictive percept of motion. The H1-blocking effects of this drug tend to cause sedation, which is offset by 8-chlorotheophylline, which has stimulant properties.

Meclizine and Scopolamine:

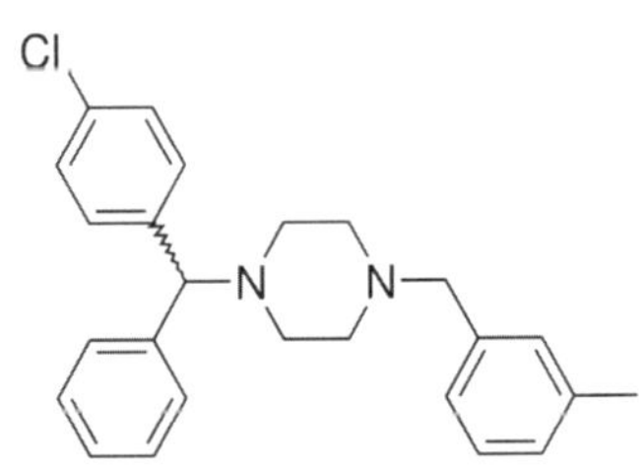

Meclizine

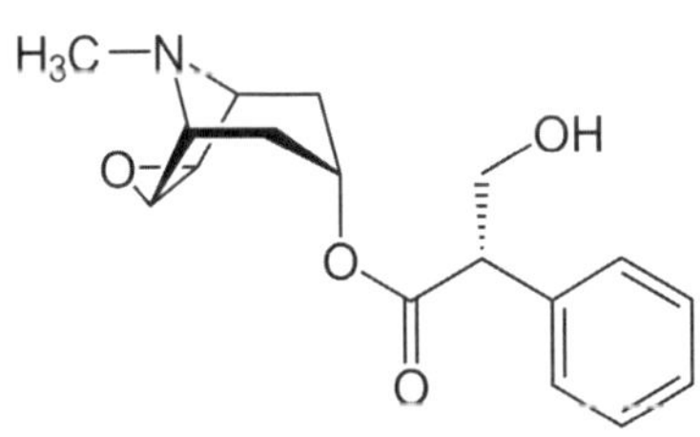

Scopolamine

Meclizine and **Scopolamine** are also anti-muscarinic/anti-histaminergic drugs whose mechanisms of action for vertigo likely derive from their antimuscarinic properties. Both are available by prescription in the U.S. Both offer similar efficacy, though the speed of onset of symptom relief may be faster and the magnitude may be greater with scopolamine. (Schmitt and Shaw 1986; Dahl et al. 1984) Scopolamine is often provided as a transdermal formulation and is commonly worn during travel (e.g., while on a cruise ship).

As with all antimuscarinic drugs, antimuscarinic side effects can be seen with these drugs. Because of muscarinic effects at post-synaptic membranes of the post-ganglionic portion of the parasympathetic pathway, many of the effects of these drugs are to functionally denervate the parasympathetic pathway, leading to diminished gastrointestinal motility (causing constipation), diminished bladder contraction (causing urinary retention), diminished salivary gland secretion (causing dry mouth) and diminished lacrimal gland secretion (causing dry eyes). In addition, diminished activity of sweat glands can lead to an increase in core temperature, leading to peripheral dilation to cool the body (causing reddening of the skin). Muscarinic receptors are important for pupillary constriction in light and accommodation. Therefore, their blockade can lead to blurred vision. Finally, muscarinic receptors are found throughout the brain and are important for learning and memory. Therefore, blockade of these receptors can cause confusion, deficits in learning and memory, and/or hallucinations. Unfortunately, it is common for elderly patients to be given "prn" meclizine (see Chapter 8) for occasional subjective dizziness (which is often transient and multifactorial), which often contributes to memory difficulties in elderly patients.

Benzodiazepines (see Chapters 17 and 23):

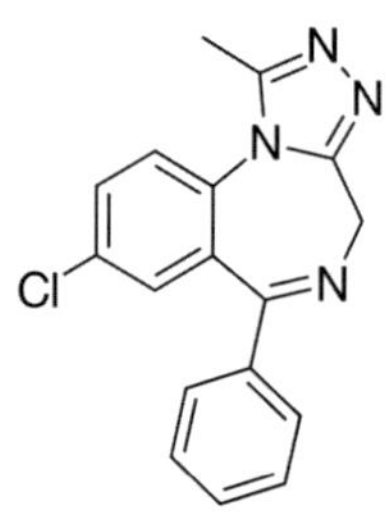

Alprazolam

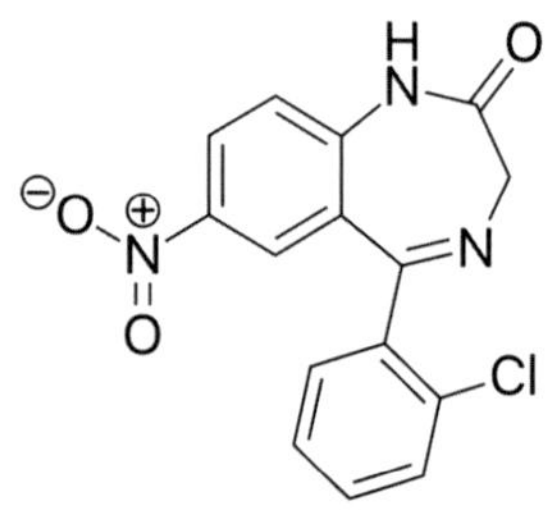

Clonazepam

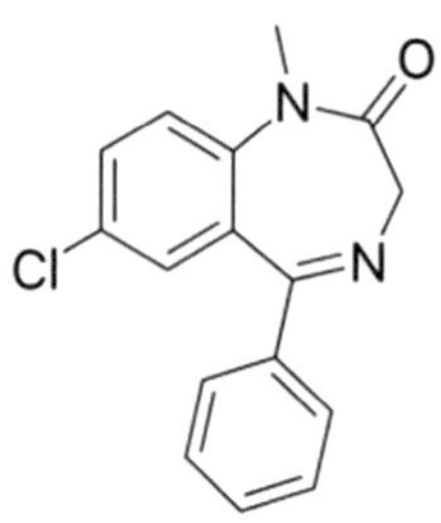

Diazepam

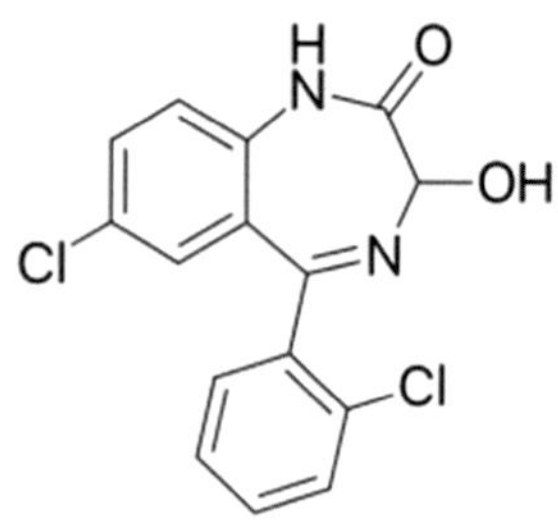

Lorazepam

Alprazolam, Clonazepam, Diazepam, and **Lorazepam** are the benzodiazepines given most commonly to treat vertigo. In theory, any benzodiazepine could be useful here, since all work by similar mechanisms, though fast-acting drugs appear to be more efficacious. (Hain and Yacovino 2005) Like anti-muscarinics, the mechanism of action is to act to suppress the central vestibular system, which expresses GABA receptors throughout its central pathways. The anxiolytic and sedating properties may also be of benefit to patients as they may help break a vicious positive feedback cycle whereby vertigo creates anxiety, which can exacerbate subjective vertiginous symptoms. Of course, with all benzodiazepines, there is a risk of dependence, and, at high doses, of worsening ataxia and respiratory suppression. These drugs are optimally provided for 1-3 days only in the acute setting, limiting the potential for dependence and toxicity, and maximizing opportunities for central compensation for peripheral vestibular dysfunction.

Antiemetic agents (see Chapter 8):
Dopamine blocking agents

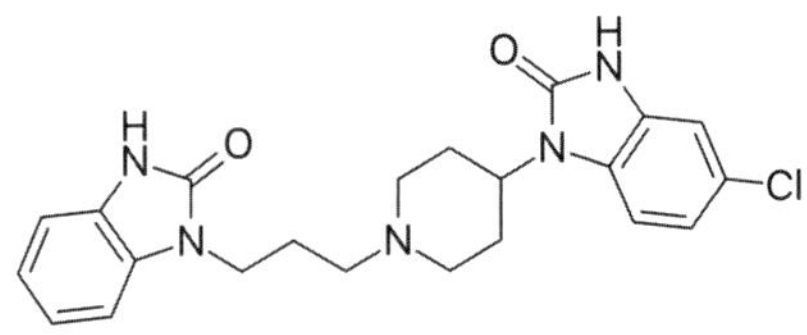

Domperidone

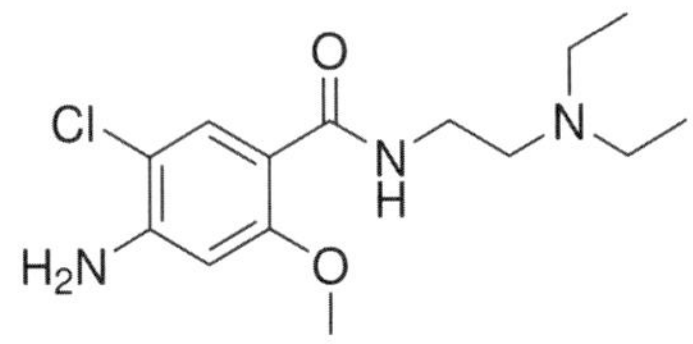

Metoclopramide

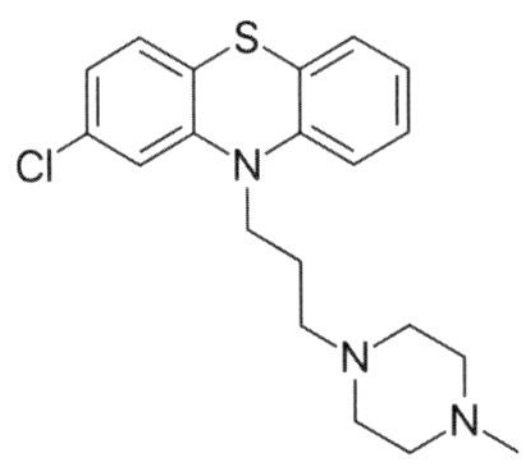

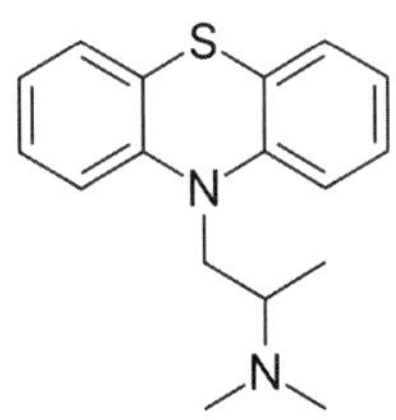

Prochlorperazine Promethazine

Domperidone, Metoclopramide, Prochlorperazine, and **Promethazine** all block D2 receptors which are found in the chemoreceptor trigger zone. Blocking these receptors diminishes the ability of the chemoreceptor trigger zone to drive emesis via the medullary vomiting center. Because these drugs block D2 receptors, their long-term use can lead to parkinsonism and/or irreversible tardive dyskinesia. These drugs should therefore be avoided in patients with known parkinsonism. Care should be taken because these drugs are often found in automated inpatient order sets as prn medications for nausea. For patients admitted for other reasons, but with a history of parkinsonism of any cause, these drugs should be replaced with 5HT3 blockers. One exception is domperidone, which has minimal penetration into the brain and works mostly via its effects on peripheral D2 receptors. Patients using these drugs should have ECG monitored because of the possibility of QT prolongation and resulting Torsades de Pointes.

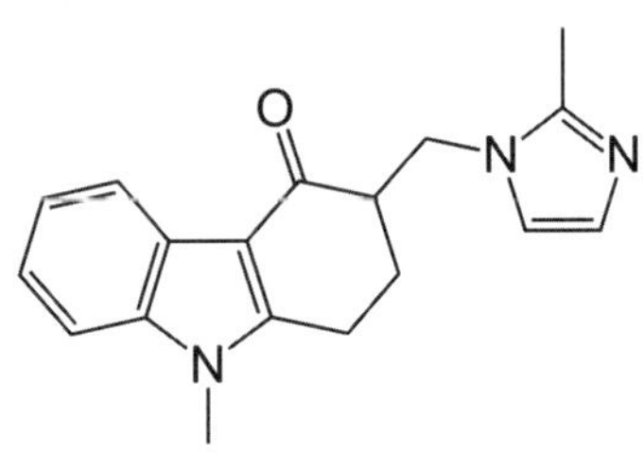

Ondansetron

Ondansetron blocks 5HT3 receptors which are also found in the chemoreceptor trigger zone in the brainstem. There are also peripheral effects at the level of the vagus nerve. It is generally well-tolerated and importantly does not cause or worsen parkinsonism, but has the potential to produce QT prolongation, so ECG monitoring is still required. Other drugs in this class may also be useful, but there is much less clinical experience with them.

Corticosteroids (see Chapter 9):

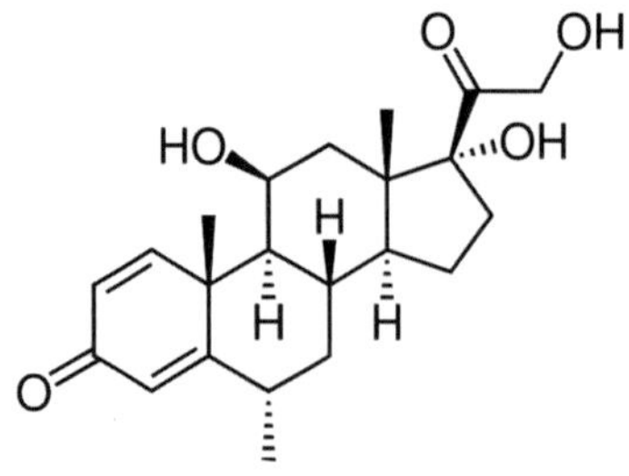

Methylprednisolone

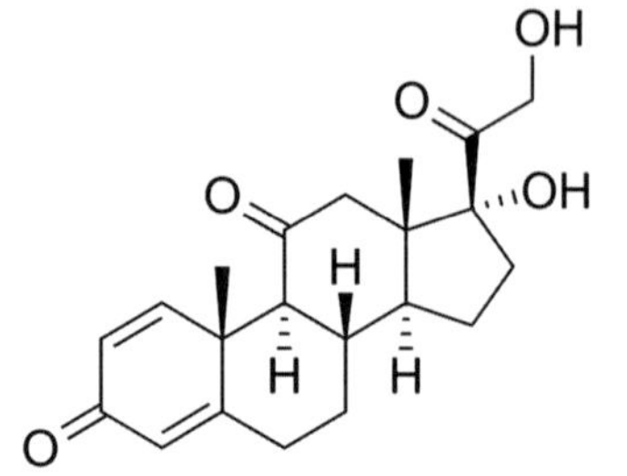

Prednisone

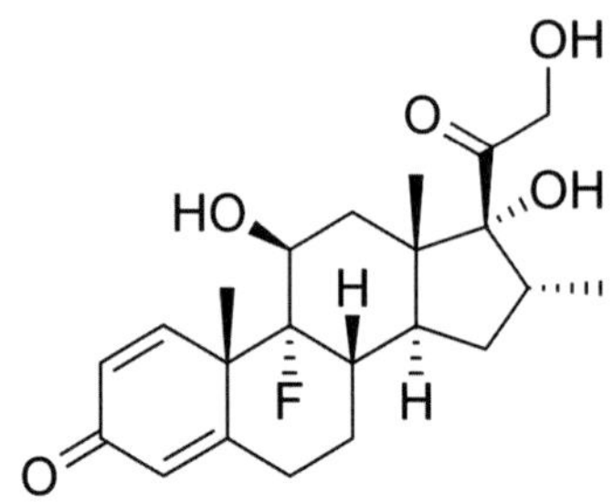

Dexamethasone

Methylprednisolone and **prednisone** are oral steroids whose main use in the treatment of vertigo is to suppress inflammation associated with vestibular neuritis. Steroids are used for a broad spectrum of disease states in clinical medicine, and their mechanisms are covered in more detail in other sections of this book. In the case of patients with vestibular neuritis, a short (< 3 weeks) tapering course of steroids is commonly used. As with the use of systemic steroids in other clinical contexts, a host of complications need to be monitored such as hyperglycemia, hypertension, euphoria/confusion, and poor wound healing. Short courses are unlikely to cause significant immunosuppression or some of the well-known body dysmorphic effects of these drugs, but avascular osteonecrosis can be seen.

Methylprednisolone or **dexamethasone** can be applied intratympanically (after application of local anesthetic) for the treatment of Meniere's disease (as well as other conditions not necessarily associated with vertigo, such as sudden onset hearing loss). The intratympanic application requires a trained practitioner (typically an otolaryngologist), avoids the systemic complications of oral use, and is generally well-tolerated with infrequent complications.

Anti-migraine agents:

Far fewer data are available on the efficacy of migraine drugs for the use of vestibular migraine compared to their use to treat the more typical cephalalgic symptoms of migraine. This lack of data is related both to the relative infrequency of vestibular migraine relative to other migraine types (~10% of all migraines are vestibular migraines) and the relative recency of recognition of vestibular migraines as a cause of vertigo. Given the likely similar pathophysiology of vestibular migraine to other forms of migraine, in this section, we consider that general migraine treatment approaches will work in the treatment of vestibular migraine, which is consistent with the relatively small amount of existing data. (Byun et al. 2021) Future work is needed to determine whether this assumption is borne out by larger studies.

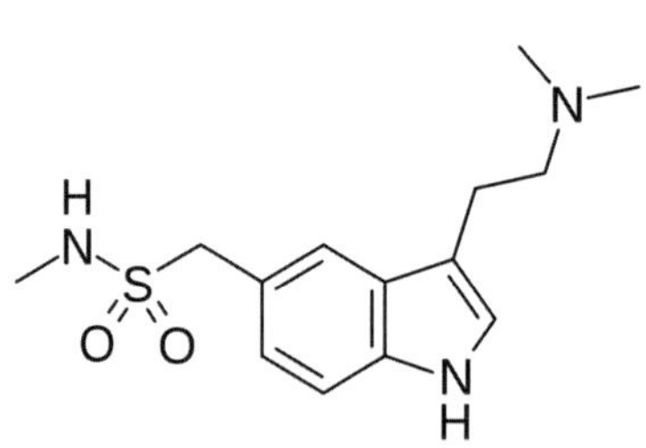

Sumatriptan

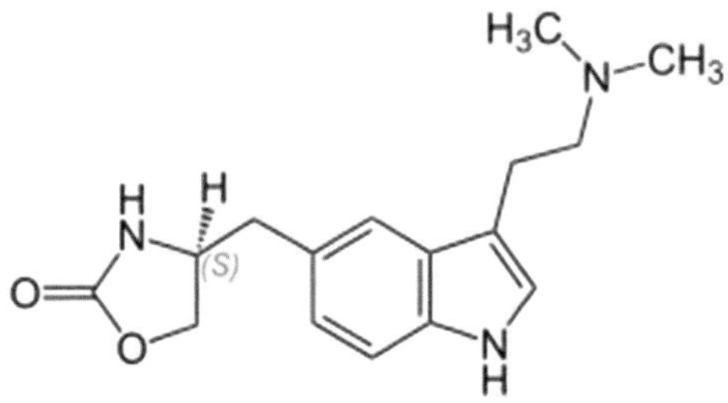

Zolmitriptan

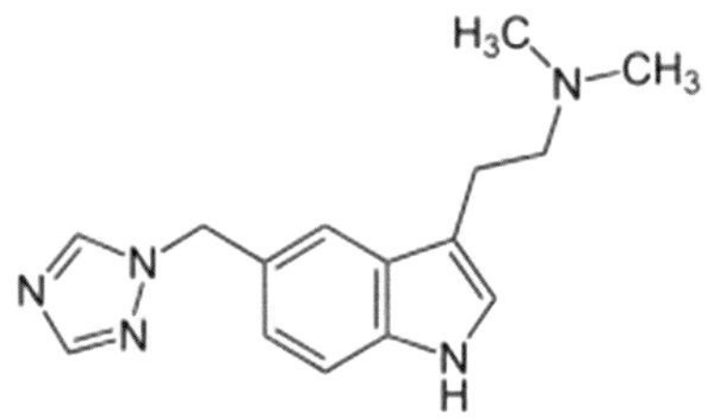

Rizatriptan

Antimigraine drugs are typically divided into abortive and prophylactic agents. Drugs in the triptan class (such as **Sumatriptan, Zolmitriptan, Rizatriptan,** and others), are thought to work by blocking 5HT1B and 1D receptors, breaking the cycle of trigeminovascular hyperactivation and inflammation leading to pain and neurological symptoms. These drugs are generally well-tolerated and should be given early in the migraine time course to have maximum benefit. Their main liability is their ability to cause vasoconstriction, leading to caution when prescribing to those which known vascular disease or a history of vasoconstrictor syndromes, though this issue has not yet been fully resolved in the literature. (Diener 2020)

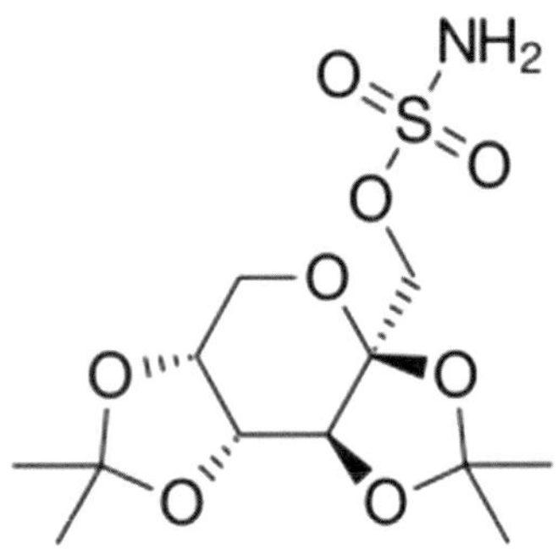

Topiramate

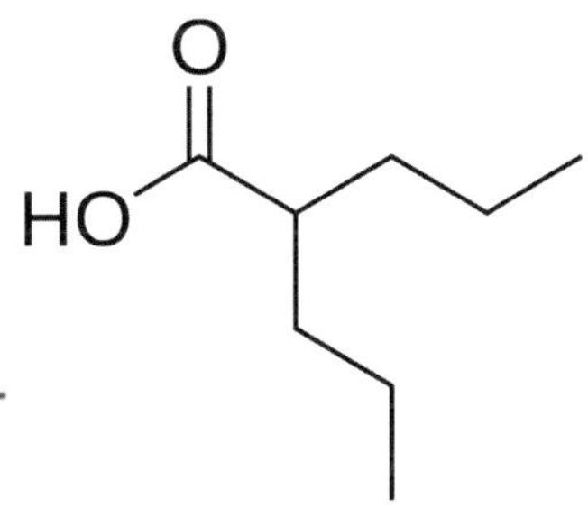

Valproic acid

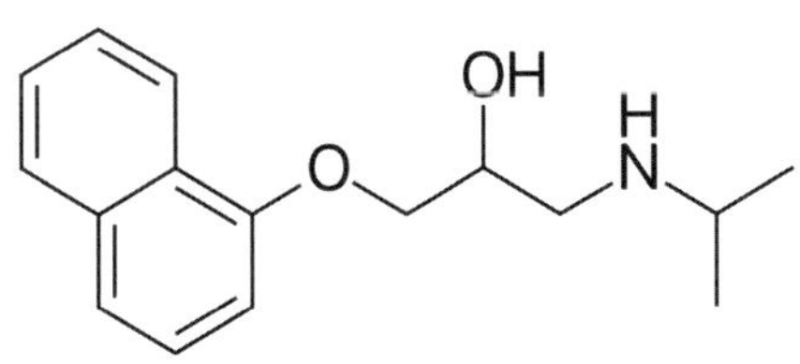

Propanolol

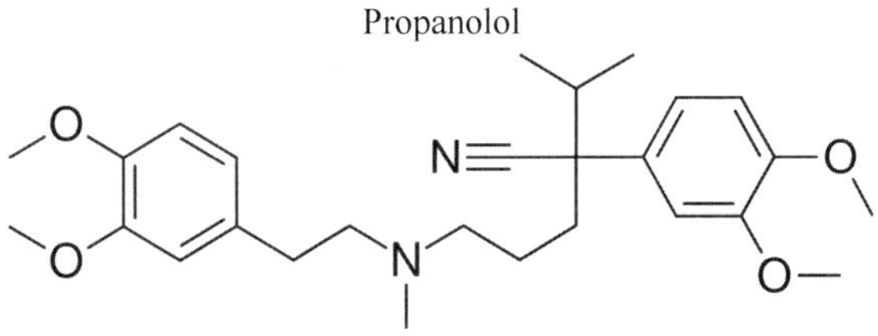

Verapamil

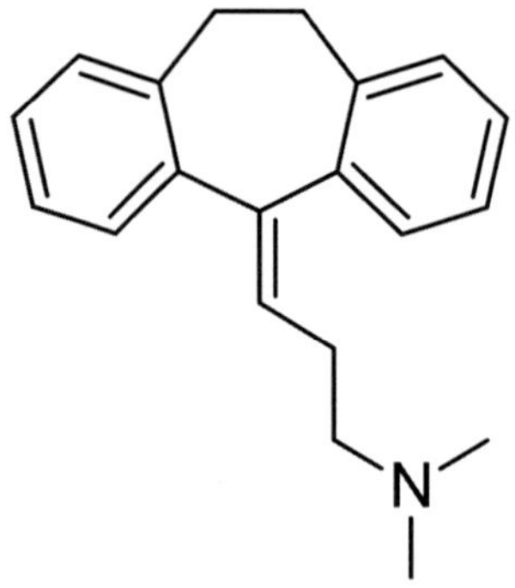

Amitriptyline

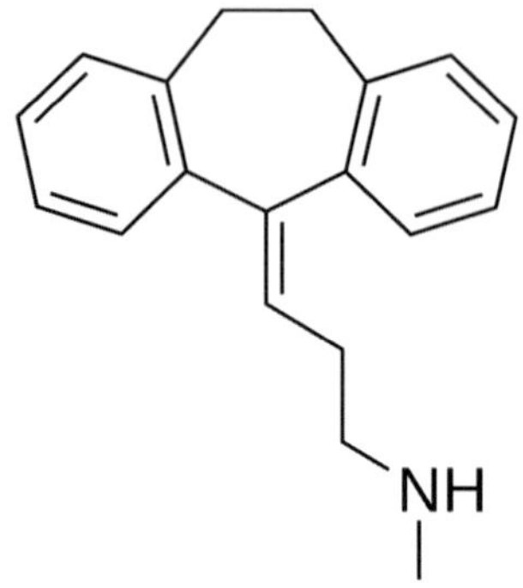

Nortriptyline

The choice of if and when to incorporate a prophylactic agent is a decision that is typically made between a clinical provider and patient based on a number of factors. Typically, once migraine frequency exceeds 2-4x per month and/or when migraines significantly impair a patient's lifestyle, a discussion of the risks and benefits of starting a daily prophylactic agent is started. Prophylactics range from anti-seizure medicines (most commonly **topiramate** and **valproic acid**), to beta blockers (most commonly **propranolol**), to calcium channel blockers (most commonly **verapamil**) or antidepressants (tricyclics such as **amitriptyline** and **nortriptyline** are most common). Topiramate is an anti-seizure medication with multiple mechanisms of action. It blocks voltage-gated sodium channels, enhances GABAergic activity, blocks glutamate receptors, and is a carbonic anhydrase inhibitor. It is generally well-tolerated but can cause cognitive symptoms (typically word-finding difficulty), weight loss, and paresthesias. Valproic acid, despite being on the market for decades, has a mechanism of action that is still poorly understood. It is a highly effective anti-seizure medication and can prevent migraines but is more poorly tolerated than topiramate. It leads to sedation, tremor, hair loss and can cause thrombocytopenia, liver toxicity and is a teratogen, so should be avoided in women of childbearing age. Propranolol and verapamil are generally well-tolerated but are both nodal blockers and can lead to bradyarrhythmias or AV block in susceptible individuals. Propranolol, by blocking beta-2 adrenergic receptors, blocks bronchodilation, which can worsen pulmonary function in patients with chronic lung disease. It can also block pancreatic insulin release. Tricyclic aromatic compounds such as amitriptyline and nortriptyline block synaptic reuptake of serotonin and norepinephrine and can block muscarinic receptors, leading to a host of side effects at high doses (see antimuscarinic side effects above) as well as cardiac arrhythmias. They are also sedating and thus are often given at bedtime.

Drug List for Meniere's Disease

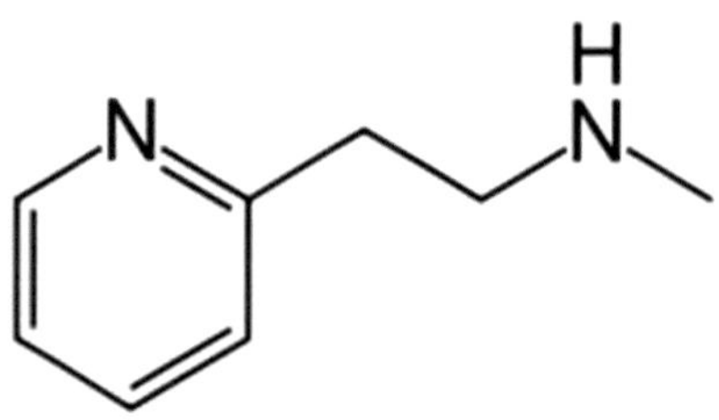

Betahistine

Drugs to treat Meniere's disease typically work by either reducing the fluid buildup in the cochlea and labyrinth or by lesioning the affected vestibular apparatus. **Betahistine** is an H1 agonist and H3 antagonist. It acts as a vasodilator at the level of the labyrinth which ultimately leads to a drop in the pressure in the labyrinth. It is generally well-tolerated, but like all vasodilators, headache is a potential side effect.

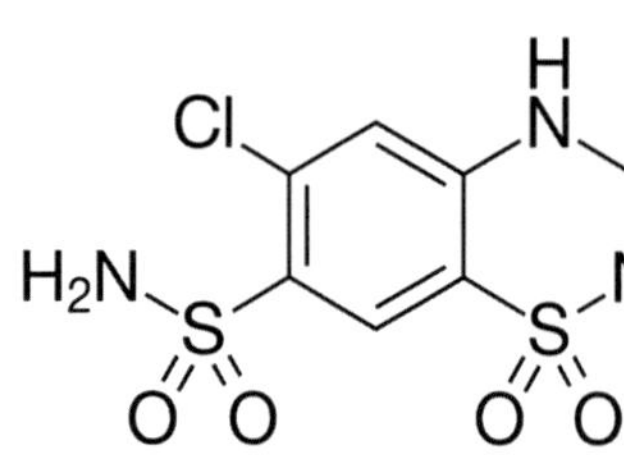

Hydrochlorothiazide

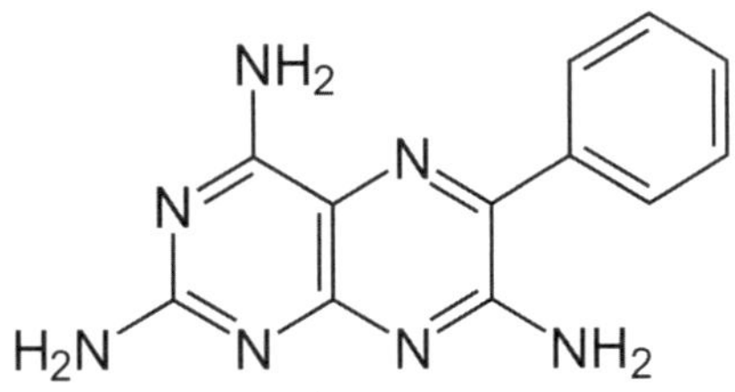

Triamterene

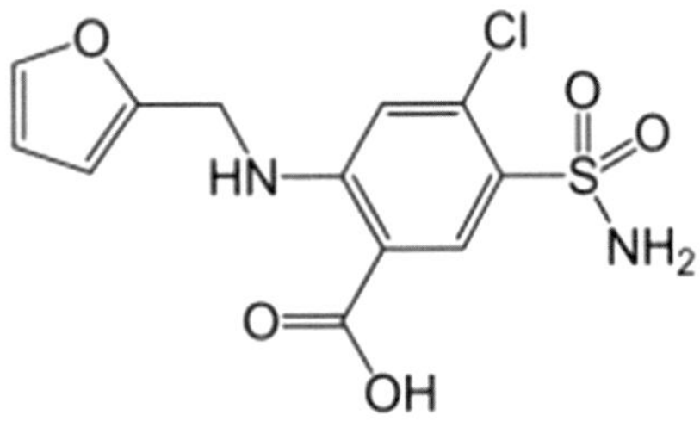

Furosemide

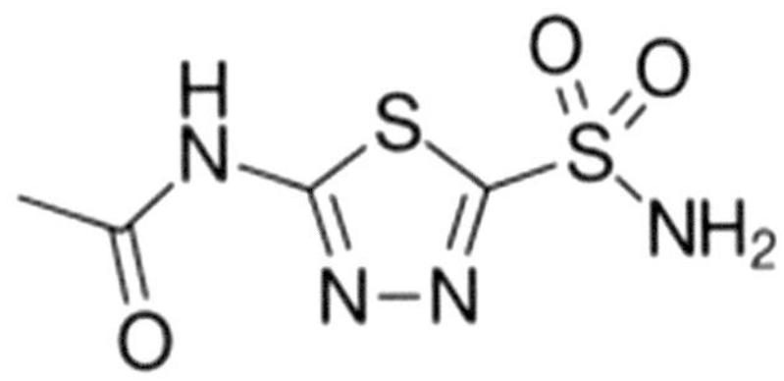

Acetazolamide

Diuretics (see Chapter 13) are intended for chronic use in Meniere's disease to diminish the buildup of endolymph in the cochlea and labyrinth. As described in other portions of this book, diuretics work at the level of the renal tubules to enhance the production of urine, lowering total blood volume. Drugs such as **hydrochlorothiazide**, **triamterene**, **furosemide,** and **acetazolamide** increase the retention of fluid within the renal tubule. They are typically used to treat hypertension, congestive heart failure, and hyperkalemia (see Chapter 13). As such, patients on these drugs should be monitored for the development of hypotension, dehydration, and hypokalemia. In the case of acetazolamide, metabolic acidosis can result from loss of bicarbonate at the level of the renal tubule.

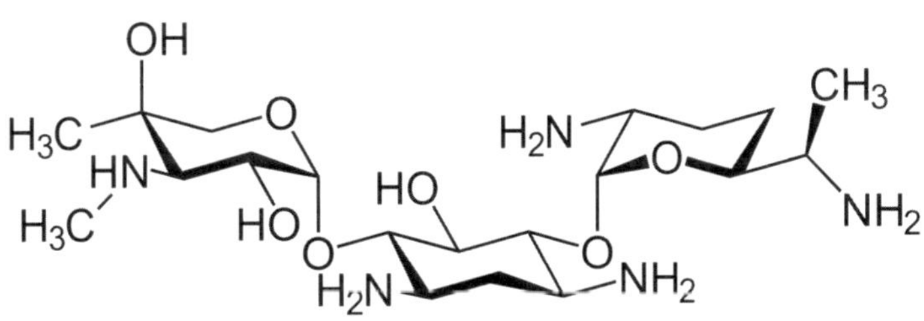

Gentamycin

Intratympanic therapy involves steroids (described above) or **gentamycin**. Aminoglycoside antibiotics are known as general vestibulotoxins that are relatively specific for the labyrinth rather than the cochlea. (Ahmed et al. 2012) This treatment is generally considered to be a last-resort approach to treating patients having severe episodes of vertigo that are refractory to the therapies outlined above. It is a destructive approach that may lead to chronic vestibular dysfunction but is intended to diminish severe and unpredictable attacks of vertigo that are disabling.

Other medications for ataxia

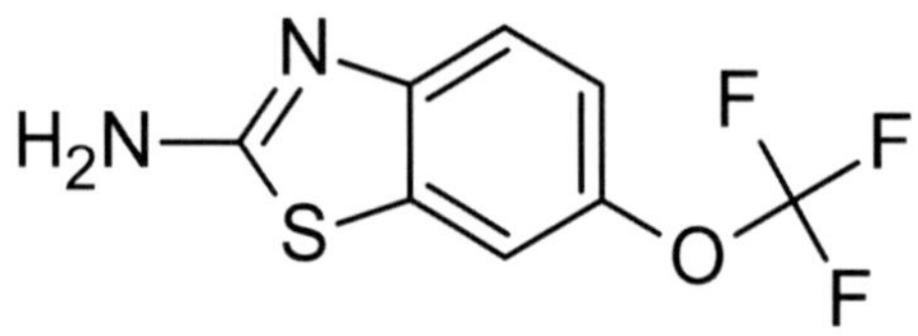

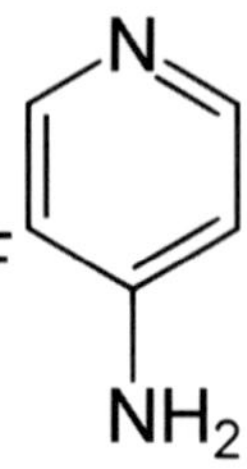

Riluzole 4-aminopyridine

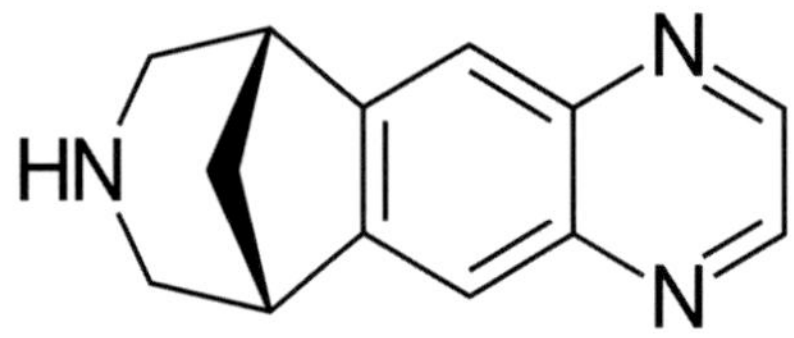

Varenicline

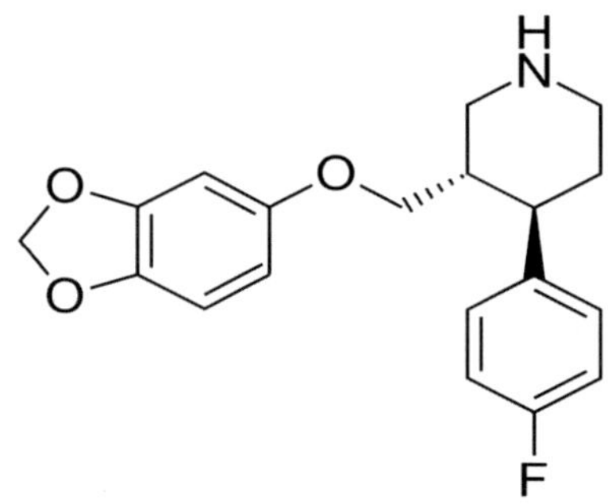

Paroxetine

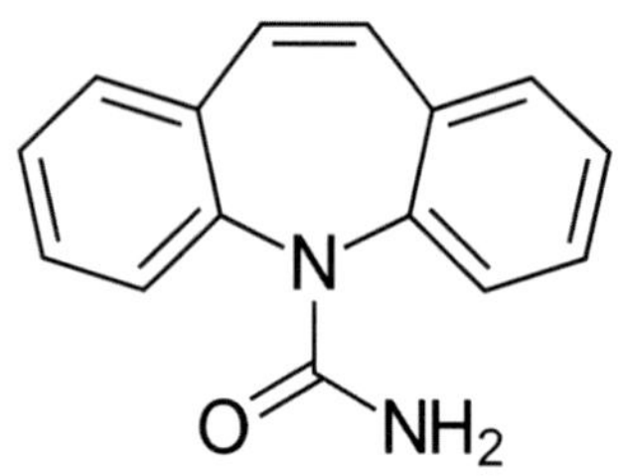

Carbamazepine

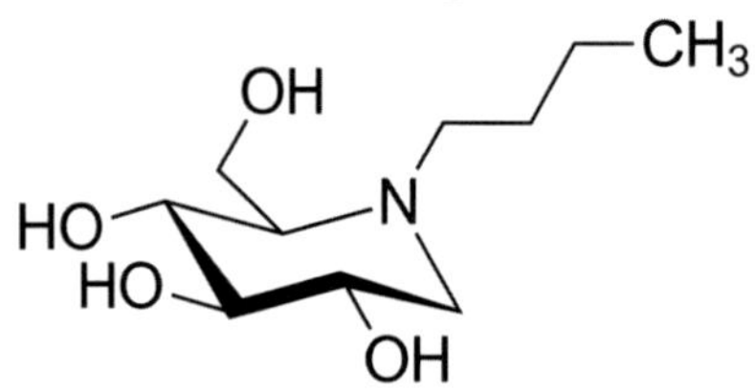

Miglustat

Although there are currently no drugs approved for the treatment of generalized ataxia, several agents have clinical trial data supporting their use for symptomatic relief of ataxia, and are summarized here. **Riluzole** is FDA-approved for the treatment of amyotrophic lateral sclerosis (ALS) and has a small impact on increasing survival in ALS patients. It is both a voltage-gated sodium channel blocker as well as an ionotropic glutamate blocker. In two randomized controlled clinical trials, it has been shown to improve speech and gait in patients with spinocerebellar ataxia and Friedreich's ataxia. (Ristori et al. 2010; Romano et al. 2015) It is generally well-tolerated, but liver function tests should be monitored in patients taking this drug. **Acetazolamide** was discussed above in the context of Meniere's disease and can significantly diminish attacks in patients with episodic ataxia type 2 (Jen et al. 2007), though the mechanism of this effect is not elucidated. As described above, major side effects are metabolic acidosis and paresthesias, which are common and can be quite disturbing to patients. **4-aminopyridine** is a potassium-channel blocker that was recently approved to treat symptoms in individuals with multiple sclerosis and has been shown to diminish the rate of attacks of ataxia in patients with episodic ataxia type 2. (Strupp et al. 2011) By blocking potassium channels, 4-aminopyridine can cause neurons to depolarize, thus facilitating excitation. It is not yet clear how this helps to treat individuals with episodic ataxia. However, this neuronal depolarizing effect also increases the likelihood of the patient having a seizure on the medication. **Varenicline** is an alpha-4-beta-2 nicotinic receptor agonist used to help individuals quit smoking. It has been shown to be effective to treat ataxia symptoms in a small randomized study of individuals with spinocerebellar ataxia type 3. (Zesiewicz et al. 2012) It is a very well-tolerated drug with its most common side effect being nausea. **Paroxetine** is a selective serotonin reuptake inhibitor (SSRI) most commonly used for the treatment of major depressive disorder as well other affective and anxiety disorders. It has been shown to diminish motor symptoms in patients with multiple systems atrophy without impacting depressive symptoms (Friess et al. 2006), suggesting that its benefit is not just an indirect effect of treating latent depression. It is generally well tolerated, but of all of the SSRIs, it is the most anti-cholinergic, so patients should be monitored for the anti-cholinergic side effects described above. **Carbamazepine** is a decades-old anti-seizure medication primarily used for partial epilepsy. It stabilizes the inactive state of voltage-gated sodium channels, diminishing the excitability of neurons. It is the treatment of choice for episodic ataxia type 1 (Orsucci et al. 2019), though the mechanism by which it works in this disorder is not clear. It carries a significant risk of hyponatremia (due to the syndrome of inappropriate antidiuretic hormone release) and thrombocytopenia and can induce its own metabolism, making it less effective over time. **Miglustat** is taken orally and is used off-label in the U.S. (but approved in the EU, Canada, and Japan) for the treatment of Niemann-Pick, type C disease. Unlike the other drugs in this section, this drug is felt to be disease-modifying, rather than only of symptomatic benefit. The most common side effects are gastrointestinal-related (e.g., diarrhea, bloating), though neuropathic pain-type symptoms (e.g. dysesthetic pain) in the distal extremities may also occur.

Case Study:
Mr. Jones is a 49-year-old man with no medical history who awoke this morning with a strong sensation of dizziness. His dizzy sensation persisted throughout the morning and he, therefore, sought treatment in the emergency department. Upon observation, the patient appears miserable. He has vomited twice since coming to the emergency department. He is lying still and reports that movement worsens his symptoms.

Pertinent negatives: Photophobia, phonophobia, hearing loss, ear fullness, or tinnitus. Vertigo is not worsened by Valsalva.

His exam findings:

Vital signs: BP = 140/90, HR = 90, RR = 24

Relevant cranial nerve findings:

- Eyes beat conjugately to the right in primary gaze.
- The right-beating nystagmus intensifies when the patient is asked to look to the right and diminishes when looking to the left.
- Head thrust test revealed that when his head was moved from a rightward position to midline (thus rotating the nose leftward or counterclockwise when observing from above) that the eyes moved past the midline and returned to center gaze with a catch-up saccade.
- The cover/uncover test revealed no shift in eye position.

The neurologic exam was otherwise normal.

What is the most likely diagnosis? How would you devise a treatment plan?

Diagnosis: This patient has acute persistent vertigo. Because of the absence of paroxysmal symptoms, BPPV is not the likely diagnosis. We should note that even though the vertiginous symptoms fluctuated with head movement, this is a non-specific finding and should not be confused as a symptom of BPPV. BPPV symptoms are brief and sudden in onset with durations of less than a minute. Because of the absence of paroxysmal symptoms, a Dix-Hallpike test would *not* be advisable. In fact, performing the Dix-Hallpike in this patient may produce quite severe symptoms, leading the examiner in the wrong diagnostic direction. Dix-Hallpike should only be performed if there is not nystagmus at rest. The finding of nystagmus at rest that does not change direction (but does change in magnitude) with changes in gaze are all suggestive of peripheral vestibular pathology. Using Alexander's Law, we can surmise that the affected ear is the left ear. This suspicion is confirmed by the finding that the head thrust test shows abnormalities (lack of maintenance of gaze) when the left ear is activated. Finally, the absence of vertical skew is reassuring for the absence of a central lesion, such as stroke.

Thus, the evaluation points to left vestibular hypofunction that is acute and has lasted several hours. The differential diagnosis of this pattern of vertigo would be vestibular neuritis, vestibular migraine, Meniere's disease, semicircular canal dehiscence, and a perilymphatic fistula. The absence of a history of migraine or photo/phonophobia makes vestibular migraine unlikely. Likewise, the absence of tinnitus, ear fullness, or hearing loss point away from a Meniere's diagnosis. The absence of worsening with Valsalva also points away from dehiscence or fistula as potential causes. Thus, vestibular neuritis, which is common, is the most likely diagnosis in this case.

Treatment Plan: Treatment should be thought of in three phases: 1) acute symptomatic, 2) etiological treatment, and 3) maintenance and recovery. Acutely, patients may benefit from vestibular suppressants such as meclizine and benzodiazepines, but these should be continued for no more than three days as they will suppress vestibular compensation. Antiemetic agents, such as 5HT3 or D2 receptor blockers can also be given in the acute phase. For treating the underlying inflammatory process, a short course (1-2 weeks) of steroids has been shown to be helpful. (Strupp et al. 2004; Fishman et al. 2011) Over the longer term, patients require vestibular rehabilitation to help speed central compensatory changes to recover lost function.

In the case of Mr. Jones, he was given IV Ativan (1 mg) and IV ondansetron (4 mg) with good relief of symptoms. He was prescribed meclizine 25mg po tid for 3 days and instructed to stop this medication if he was feeling better, and was prescribed a 10-day steroid taper starting with prednisone 60mg per day. He began vestibular occupational therapy one week after his ED visit.

Outcomes: The patient required all three days of meclizine and continued to have intermittent nausea and vertigo for about two weeks. He gradually returned to his baseline over eight weeks.

Follow-up: Mr. Jones reports that he occasionally has fleeting symptoms of nausea and vertigo, particularly if he is ill with a viral illness or trying to read on a moving train or automobile, but has returned to his baseline level of function.

References

Ahmed, Rebekah M, Imelda P Hannigan, Hamish G MacDougall, Raymond C Chan, and G Michael Halmagyi. 2012. Gentamicin ototoxicity: a 23-year selected case series of 103 patients. *Medical Journal of Australia* 196 (11):701-704.

Byun, Young Jae, Dylan A Levy, Shaun A Nguyen, Emily Brennan, and Habib G Rizk. 2021. Treatment of Vestibular Migraine: A Systematic Review and Meta-analysis. *The Laryngoscope* 131 (1):186-194.

Dahl, Eilif, Dag Offer-Ohlsen, Per Erik Lillevold, and Leiv Sandvik. 1984. Transdermal scopolamine, oral meclizine, and placebo in motion sickness. *Clinical Pharmacology & Therapeutics* 36 (1):116-120.

Diener, Hans-Christoph. 2020. The risks or lack thereof of migraine treatments in vascular disease. *Headache: The Journal of Head and Face Pain* 60 (3):649-653.

Fishman, Jonathan M, Chris Burgess, and Angus Waddell. 2011. Corticosteroids for the treatment of idiopathic acute vestibular dysfunction (vestibular neuritis). *Cochrane Database of Systematic Reviews* (5).

Friess, Elisabeth, Tania Kuempfel, Sieglinde Modell, Juliane Winkelmann, Florian Holsboer, Marcus Ising, and Claudia Trenkwalder. 2006. Paroxetine treatment improves motor symptoms in patients with multiple system atrophy. *Parkinsonism & related disorders* 12 (7):432-437.

Hain, Timothy C, and Dario Yacovino. 2005. Pharmacologic treatment of persons with dizziness. *Neurologic clinics* 23 (3):831-853.

Ishiyama, Akira, Ivan López, and Phillip A Wackym. 1997. Molecular characterization of muscarinic receptors in the human vestibular periphery. Implications for pharmacotherapy. *The American journal of otology* 18 (5):648-654.

Jen, J.C., T.D. Graves, E.J. Hess, M.G. Hanna, R.C. Griggs, R.W. Baloh, and the CINCH investigators. 2007. Primary episodic ataxias: diagnosis, pathogenesis and treatment. *Brain* 130 (10):2484-2493.

Kattah, Jorge C, Arun V Talkad, David Z Wang, Yu-Hsiang Hsieh, and David E Newman-Toker. 2009. HINTS to diagnose stroke in the acute vestibular syndrome: three-step bedside oculomotor examination more sensitive than early MRI diffusion-weighted imaging. *Stroke* 40 (11):3504-3510.

Kwei, Kimberly Tsu, and Sheng-Han Kuo. 2020. An Overview of the Current State and the Future of Ataxia Treatments. *Neurologic clinics* 38 (2):449-467.

McDonnell, Michelle N, and Susan L Hillier. 2015. Vestibular rehabilitation for unilateral peripheral vestibular dysfunction. *Cochrane Database of Systematic Reviews* (1).

Orsucci, Daniele, Laura Maria Raglione, Monica Mazzoni, and Marco Vista. 2019. Therapy of episodic ataxias: case report and review of the literature. *Drugs in context* 8:212576-212576.

Patterson, M. C., D. Vecchio, H. Prady, L. Abel, and J. E. Wraith. 2007. Miglustat for treatment of Niemann-Pick C disease: a randomised controlled study. *Lancet Neurol* 6 (9):765-772.

Ristori, G, S Romano, A Visconti, S Cannoni, M Spadaro, M Frontali, FE Pontieri, N Vanacore, and M Salvetti. 2010. Riluzole in cerebellar ataxia: a randomized, double-blind, placebo-controlled pilot trial. *Neurology* 74 (10):839-845.

Romano, Silvia, Giulia Coarelli, Christian Marcotulli, Luca Leonardi, Francesca Piccolo, Maria Spadaro, Marina Frontali, Michela Ferraldeschi, Maria Chiara Vulpiani, and Federica Ponzelli. 2015. Riluzole in patients with hereditary cerebellar ataxia: a randomised, double-blind, placebo-controlled trial. *The Lancet Neurology* 14 (10):985-991.

Schmitt, Lenore G, and Jane E Shaw. 1986. Alleviation of induced vertigo: therapy with transdermal scopolamine and oral meclizine. *Archives of Otolaryngology–Head & Neck Surgery* 112 (1):88-91.

Strupp, M, R Kalla, J Claassen, Christine Adrion, Ulrich Mansmann, T Klopstock, T Freilinger, H Neugebauer, R Spiegel, and M Dichgans. 2011. A randomized trial of 4-aminopyridine in EA2 and related familial episodic ataxias. *Neurology* 77 (3):269-275.

Strupp, Michael, Vera Carina Zingler, Viktor Arbusow, Daniel Niklas, Klaus Peter Maag, Marianne Dieterich, Sandra Bense, Diethilde Theil, Klaus Jahn, and Thomas Brandt. 2004. Methylprednisolone, valacyclovir, or the combination for vestibular neuritis. *New England Journal of Medicine* 351 (4):354-361.

Woodworth, Bradford Alan, M Boyd Gillespie, and Paul R Lambert. 2004. The canalith repositioning procedure for benign positional vertigo: a meta-analysis. *The Laryngoscope* 114 (7):1143-1146.

Wraith, James E, Darleen Vecchio, Elizabeth Jacklin, Larry Abel, Harbajan Chadha-Boreham, Cécile Luzy, Ruben Giorgino, and Marc C Patterson. 2010. Miglustat in adult and juvenile patients with Niemann–Pick disease type C: long-term data from a clinical trial. *Molecular genetics and metabolism* 99 (4):351-357.

Zesiewicz, Theresa A, PE Greenstein, Kelly L Sullivan, L Wecker, A Miller, I Jahan, R Chen, and SL Perlman. 2012. A randomized trial of varenicline (Chantix) for the treatment of spinocerebellar ataxia type 3. *Neurology* 78 (8):545-550.

Zhu, Yun, Shao-Rui Chen, and Hui-Lin Pan. 2016. Muscarinic receptor subtypes differentially control synaptic input and excitability of cerebellum-projecting medial vestibular nucleus neurons. *Journal of neurochemistry* 137 (2):226-239.

Quiz Questions

1. A 70-year-old female presents to the ED with complaints of dizziness. Upon further questioning, she reports that her symptoms were first noticed when turning over in bed, which produced severe room-spinning dizziness that subsided after several minutes. She reports that her symptoms are minimal if not moving her head, but are maximal for 1-2 minutes just after turning her head. What treatment is most likely to be effective for her?

A Meclizine
B Benzodiazepines
C Steroids
D Epley maneuver
E Riluzole

2. A 50-year-old man is brought to his physician because he is having frequent falls. On exam, he has an intention tremor and a wide-based gait. Signal abnormalities are seen in the middle cerebellar peduncle on the exam. What test is most likely to provide a specific diagnosis for this patient?

A Paraneoplastic blood panel
B Genetic testing
C HINTS testing
D Electroencephalogram
E Lumbar puncture

3. A 90-year-old man is admitted to the hospital with a urinary tract infection. He has a history of dementia with Lewy Bodies. The patient complained of nausea and dizziness and was given medication from his order set. The next morning he was found to be rigid and unable to speak. What drug was he likely given?

A Prochlorperazine
B Domperidone
C Ondansetron
D Meclizine
E Sumatriptan

4. A 30-year-old female presents with episodes of dizziness that last for several hours. She occasionally has photo- and phonophobia associated with these episodes. She has had four episodes over the past year. What is the best treatment for these episodes?

A Meclizine
B Benzodiazepines
C Steroids
D Sumatriptan
E Riluzole

5. A 40-year-old man is having severe episodes of vertigo and nausea. He complains of some trouble hearing and is found to have a 40 dB hearing loss, primarily of the low frequencies. What is the most appropriate first treatment?

A Miglustat
B Intratympanic gentamycin
C Furosemide
D Carbamazepine
E Riluzole

6. A 70-year-old man is on a cruise and is prescribed a scopolamine patch to mitigate seasickness symptoms. Which symptom is he *not* likely to experience?

A Diarrhea
B Dry mouth
C Dry eyes
D Confusion
E Urinary retention

7. A 19-year-old female is prescribed carbamazepine for episodic ataxia. What laboratory should be monitored over time?

A Potassium
B Sodium
C Bicarbonate
D Creatine
E Glucose

8. A 70-year-old with a history of hypertension, hypercholesterolemia, and brittle diabetes develops vestibular neuritis. She is prescribed a tapering course of steroids starting with prednisone 60 mg per day for the first five days. After four days of steroids, she is found on the floor of her apartment, unresponsive, but breathing. What is the likely cause of this complication?

A Hyperglycemia
B Worsening of her vestibular neuritis
C Sedation from steroids
D Anti-cholinergic side effects of steroids
E None of the above

9. A 25-year-old female is having three vestibular migraines per week. Which treatment should be considered?

A Daily acetaminophen
B Sumatriptan as needed
C Daily topiramate
D Topiramate as needed
E Daily steroids

10. A 30-year-old female is diagnosed with Meniere's disease and is prescribed betahistine. What side effect is she most likely to develop?

A Headaches
B Hypersalivation
C Abdominal pain
D Confusion
E Frequent infections

Quiz Answers

1. D. This patient likely has BPPV, which is most effectively treated with the Epley maneuver.

2. B. This patient likely has Fragile-X-ataxia syndrome, diagnosed by detecting a premutation in the Fragile X gene.

3. A. Prochlorperazine is a D2-blocker that crosses the blood-brain barrier and will significantly worsen rigidity in patients with any form of parkinsonism.

4. D. She is having vestibular migraines, best treated with a triptan. They are happening too infrequently to require a daily prophylactic.

5. C. The low-frequency hearing loss and episodes of severe vertigo are characteristic of Meniere's disease. First-line therapy is diuresis. Intratympanic gentamycin may be considered for refractory cases.

6. A. Anti-cholinergic drugs are associated with constipation, not diarrhea, as well as dry eyes, dry mouth, confusion, skin flushing, and urinary retention.

7. B. Carbamazepine can cause SIADH, thus serum sodium levels should be periodically monitored.

8. A. Steroids can cause hyperglycemia, particularly in those with brittle diabetes. Severe hyperglycemia can cause a hyperosmotic coma in those with type 2 diabetes.

9. C. Typically a daily prophylactic should be considered in cases where migraines occur more than 2-4 times per month. Topiramate is a commonly-used and effective migraine prophylactic.

10. A. Betahistine has vasodilatory properties. All vasodilating drugs can potentially cause headaches.

CHAPTER 17

MENTAL HEALTH – DEPRESSION, ANXIETY, AND SUICIDAL THOUGHTS

KATHLEEN BOTTUM, MD AND SHELLEY TISCHKAU, PHD

Southern Illinois University School of Medicine, Springfield, Illinois, USA

Symptoms: **Neurological**

Drug List

1st GENERATION ANTIDEPRESSANTS

Tricyclic Antidepressants (TCAs)
Amitriptyline
Amoxapine
Clomipramine
Desipramine
Doxepin
Imipramine
Nortriptyline
Protriptyline
Trimipramine

Monoamine oxidase inhibitors (MAOIs)
Isocarboxazid
Phenelzine
Selegiline
Tranylcypromine

2nd GENERATION ANTIDEPRESSANTS

Selective serotonin reuptake inhibitors (SSRIs)
Citalopram
Escitalopram
Fluoxetine
Fluvoxamine
Paroxetine
Sertraline

Serotonin-norepinephrine reuptake inhibitors (SNRIs)
Desvenlafaxine
Duloxetine
Levomilnacipran
Venlafaxine

Serotonin Modulators
Nefazodone
Trazodone
Vilazodone
Vortioxetine

ATYPICAL ANTIDEPRESSANTS
Brexanolone
Bupropion
Mirtazapine

ANTI-ANXIETY MEDICATION
Buspirone

Benzodiazepines (BZD)
Alprazolam
Clonazepam
Chlordiazepoxide
Clorazepate
Diazepam
Lorazepam
Oxazepam

General Background

Depressive and anxiety symptoms are relatively common in all cultures. According to the World Health Organization, depression, or a major depressive episode (MDE), is present in up to 5% of adults worldwide. (World Health Organisation 2023) A US study done in 2012-2013 found that about 10% of the population had experienced an MDE in the year before the interview, and about 20% had experienced an MDE at some point in their life. (Hasin et al. 2018) MDE is a significant cause of morbidity (loss of function at work, school, and in relationships) (Murray et al. 2013) and mortality via suicide or self-neglect.

For unclear reasons, women experience MDE more frequently than men in an approximately 2:1 ratio. (*American Psychiatric Association: Diagnostic and Statistical Manual of Mental Disorders: DSM-5-TR* 2022) This is especially true in the years between the onset of menses and menopause. Depressed women are more likely than depressed men to attempt suicide but are less likely to die by suicide. (*American Psychiatric Association: Diagnostic and Statistical Manual of Mental Disorders: DSM-5-TR* 2022) Men tend to use more lethal means in their attempts. Women respond as well as men to treatment for MDE. (*American Psychiatric Association: Diagnostic and Statistical Manual of Mental Disorders: DSM-5-TR* 2022)

Although morbidity and mortality are higher in depressive disorders, anxiety disorders are the more common mental health issue. (Bandelow et al. 2017) Anxiety disorders frequently co-occur with MDE. (*American Psychiatric Association: Diagnostic and Statistical Manual of Mental Disorders: DSM-5-TR* 2022) This can make the treatment of either disorder more complicated. Fortunately, the antidepressants listed above treat both depression and anxiety. MDE and anxiety do better when treated with both antidepressants and psychotherapy. (Chaimowitz et al. 2021)

Suicidal thoughts are most commonly thought to be from depression, and at least 50% of all suicidal people are depressed. (*American Psychiatric Association: Diagnostic and Statistical Manual of Mental Disorders: DSM-5-TR* 2022) Other qualities that increase the risk of suicide are substance abuse, psychosis, bipolar disorder, impulsivity, and tragic life circumstances. (Bachmann 2018) Although there is no specific medication for suicidal thoughts, lithium and clozapine are both associated with lower rates of suicide in people with bipolar disorder (lithium) and schizophrenia (clozapine). (Hawkins et al. 2021) Because they are older medications, these findings come from studies of adverse events from people taking these medications. These medications do not have FDA indications for suicidal thoughts. The FDA approves no medicines for suicidal ideation.

Diagnosis

The Diagnostic and Statistical Manual of Mental Disorders, 5th edition, Text Revision (DSM-5-TR) (*American Psychiatric Association: Diagnostic and Statistical Manual of Mental Disorders: DSM-5-TR* 2022) specifies symptoms for psychiatric disorders. Each disorder has a list of symptoms, which will be included in the discussion of each disease. The first DSM was published in 1952, with four other significant reversions over the years. The most current version, DSM-5-TR, was completed in 2022. The American Psychiatric Association (APA) forms working groups of its members to help design revisions.

Key Depressive Disorders:

Major Depressive Disorder (MDD)

Presentation

People afflicted with major depressive disorder (MDD) have one or more major depressive episodes (i.e., MDEs) in their lifetime and often have significant disruptions in their lives from the illness. The most common presenting symptoms are fatigue and sleep difficulty. Patients in any setting should be probed for a full MDE when seeking help with these symptoms. (*American Psychiatric Association: Diagnostic and Statistical Manual of Mental Disorders: DSM-5-TR* 2022) MDE patients have depressed mood and lack enjoyment or desire to do typical daily activities. In its extreme form, they may have difficulty getting out of bed. Elderly or malnourished patients with MDD may even develop bed sores or deep vein thrombosis because of their inactivity. (Ishida et al. 2012) MDD also contributes to malnutrition as people may either stop eating, resulting in insufficient calories, or eat comfort foods excessively, consuming inadequate micronutrients. MDD is a factor in at least 50% of suicides (*American Psychiatric Association: Diagnostic and Statistical Manual of Mental Disorders: DSM-5-TR* 2022). It significantly impacts society as a whole, as family members and coworkers often suffer along with the afflicted individual. (*American Psychiatric Association: Diagnostic and Statistical Manual of Mental Disorders: DSM-5-TR* 2022)

Risk Factors

A prior history of MDE is a strong predictor of future MDEs. Family history also influences the risk of developing MDD. (*American Psychiatric Association: Diagnostic and Statistical Manual of Mental Disorders: DSM-5-TR* 2022) However, the heritability of MDD is less than in other psychiatric disorders such as schizophrenia and bipolar disorder. (Li et al. 2021) Stressful environmental factors such as adverse childhood events, trauma, poverty, and significant loss can precipitate an episode of MDE in a predisposed person. (*American Psychiatric Association: Diagnostic and Statistical Manual of Mental Disorders: DSM-5-TR* 2022)

Pathophysiology

As is true for all psychiatric illnesses, the pathophysiology of MDE and MDD is incompletely understood. Initially, what was known about the mechanisms of antidepressant drugs produced the monoamine hypothesis of depression. (Li et al. 2021) The success of early antidepressants, which increase serotonin, norepinephrine, and dopamine (all monoamines), was taken to mean that MDD results from a deficiency of these monoamine neurotransmitters, causing brain malfunction. Later with the advent of SSRIs, which specifically elevate the levels of serotonin only, it was believed that serotonin might be the most crucial monoamine in the pathophysiology of depression. There was always an inherent problem with this theory, as the changes in monoamine levels after the administration of antidepressants take only hours, while the changes in clinical symptoms of depression take weeks. In addition, as many as 60% of patients do not adequately respond to the first trial of any given antidepressant, which is unexplainable by the monoamine hypothesis. (Li et al. 2021)

Since the late 1990s/early 2000s, it has become apparent that there is brain remodeling that happens with the treatment of depression. Antidepressants with diverse mechanisms act to increase connections between brain cells. This takes time to develop and likely partially explains why it takes antidepressants up to three months to work fully. (Duman et al. 2019)

Many other pathophysiological processes have been associated with depression. Hormonal alterations, with increases in stress hormones such as cortisol, have been found in patients with MDE. These are more pronounced in women than men, which could be related to the increased prevalence of MDE in women compared to men. (Li et al. 2021) Epigenetic changes such as decreased levels of brain-derived neurotrophic factor (BDNF, a hormone associated with increased neuroplasticity), increased levels of inflammatory cytokines (such as TNFα, IL-6, and IL-10), decreased brain GABA: glutamate ratio, and changes to the gut-brain microbiota axis are associated with MDE. (Li et al. 2021) These changes may help explain the adverse effects of stressful life events. In short, we still have a poor understanding of why some people develop MDE and others do not, but we are getting many tantalizing clues that should one day lead to a more complete picture.

Examination

A healthcare professional performs a mental status exam when assessing mental health. This is an essential part of the physical exam for mental illnesses and is conducted through careful observation of the patient. Speech and body language are crucial features, as are what the patient says about their experiences. Patients with MDD often have a quiet voice and may speak and move more slowly than non-depressed individuals. Alternately, they can be agitated and anxious, pacing the room, for example.

In interviewing psychiatric patients, listening to what they say is critically important. Symptoms elicited this way are generally more reliable than if the examiner explicitly asks about symptoms to which the patient responds yes or no. Sometimes this can take much patience, as depressed people may not spontaneously talk about what they are experiencing.

Laboratory

It is essential to rule out medical causes of depression, such as thyroid abnormalities, anemia, substance abuse/withdrawal, and vitamin deficiencies. Patients can be screened for these problems with history and laboratory tests. Since thyroid abnormalities may be the hardest to detect with history alone, all patients with new onset MDE should be screened for thyroid dysfunction. In the proper context, such as anorexia or severe alcohol use, it would be appropriate to check for deficiencies in vitamins such as vitamin B1 (thiamine), vitamin B12 (cobalamine), and folate (vitamin B9). Patients with medical comorbidity and fatigue out of proportion to their mood symptoms should have a complete blood count (CBC) and a brain natriuretic peptide (BNP) drawn to evaluate for anemia and heart failure.

Imaging

No imaging is needed to diagnose depression. Although some brain changes are found, especially with long-standing MDE, diagnosis cannot currently be made from these findings.

Associated Symptoms/Conditions

In addition to the symptoms which make up the diagnosis of MDE, other illnesses may be present. Psychiatric comorbidities include anxiety disorders, substance use disorders, and personality disorders. In addition, some medical conditions, such as irritable bowel syndrome, fibromyalgia, and chronic pain, are more common in patients with MDD.

Diagnosis

DSM-5-TR requires at least five out of nine symptoms of depression to be present nearly every day for at least two weeks to diagnose a major depressive episode (MDE). In addition, a depressed mood or anhedonia (loss of interest or pleasure in usual activities) must be present. These symptoms are:

1) Depressed mood
2) Loss of interest or pleasure in usual activities
3) Significant weight change (either gain or loss) without intentional effort or explainable cause
4) Significant sleep change (either not able to sleep or sleeping too much)
5) Psychomotor changes (either restless or not moving much) observed by others
6) Fatigue or low energy
7) Feeling worthless or having excessive and inappropriate guilt
8) Decreased ability to concentrate or make decisions
9) Recurrent thoughts of death or suicide

Symptoms clearly due to another medical disorder (for example, fatigue in a patient undergoing chemotherapy for cancer) are not counted. Similarly, symptoms attributable to substance intoxication or withdrawal (for example, fatigue in cocaine withdrawal) are not considered to be from depression.

Major depressive disorder (MDD) is diagnosed in anyone who has ever had an MDE, whether or not they are actively depressed. Some people have only one-lifetime episode of MDE, but in many patients, MDEs recur. (*American Psychiatric Association: Diagnostic and Statistical Manual of Mental Disorders: DSM-5-TR* 2022) Bipolar disorders consist of alternating MDE and hypomania or mania. If a patient has ever had a manic or hypomanic episode, the depressive episode is not considered part of MDD but bipolar disorder.

General Treatment Strategies

First-line treatment for MDE is either drug treatment with an SSRI/SNRI or psychotherapy. Patient preference between these two options usually determines which is used, although some evidence shows that combined modalities have greater efficacy than either modality alone. Drug treatment is often cheaper; psychotherapy may be more rewarding. Both therapies can have adverse events. Adverse drug reactions for pharmaceutical treatment are well understood and expected. Adverse outcomes from psychotherapies are not as well defined but include opening painful issues that the patient is not ready to deal with and developing a therapeutic relationship with the therapist that is not conducive to optimal growth (the therapist inadvertently encouraging excessive dependency, for example).

Initial treatment of MDE is usually an SSRI due to its relative safety in overdose and generally mild side effects. However, other second-generation antidepressants (SNRIs, serotonin modulators, or atypical antidepressants excluding Brexanolone) are promising alternative first-line treatments for MDE. Patients who fail to respond to SSRIs or have comorbidities might benefit from a drug that can treat depression and comorbidity. Numerous options exist for treatment in these scenarios. Tricyclic antidepressants and some SNRIs may be helpful when depression is associated with chronic pain; trazodone may benefit patients with MDE who cannot sleep. Bupropion is approved for tobacco cessation and can treat depression in patients who also wish to stop using tobacco. Drugs belonging to the MAOI class are used only when multiple other options have failed since there are much safer options. Electroconvulsive therapy (ECT) is one of the most effective treatments for depression, but it is not covered here. (Stippl et al. 2020)

Management

In addition to treating symptoms of MDD with medication and psychotherapy, psychoeducation should be provided to the patient and family. Family should be educated about the disease so they understand that many symptoms of depression are not entirely in the patient's control.

There is a higher risk of recurrence of future MDE once a person has experienced one episode. (*American Psychiatric Association: Diagnostic and Statistical Manual of Mental Disorders: DSM-5-TR* 2022) Early warning signs of a recurrent MDE should be clearly defined. While these often vary between patients, common early symptoms include problems with sleep or a lack of energy. Recurrence is higher in those who had more severe initial symptoms and are younger; it becomes progressively lower as a person maintains remission after an episode. (*American Psychiatric Association: Diagnostic and Statistical Manual of Mental Disorders: DSM-5-TR* 2022) Studies have shown that people who are maintained on antidepressants have a lower risk of recurrence than those on a placebo. (Kato et al. 2021)

Persistent depressive disorder (PDD)

Presentation

Persistent depressive disorder (PDD), previously called dysthymia, is a disease of chronic low mood that may not meet the criteria for MDE. (*American Psychiatric Association: Diagnostic and Statistical Manual of Mental Disorders: DSM-5-TR* 2022) The patient has depressed mood most of the time for at least two years, along with at least two other symptoms of depression. In children, the depressed mood must only be present for one year. (*American Psychiatric Association: Diagnostic and Statistical Manual of Mental Disorders: DSM-5-TR* 2022) An MDE can occur at any time during PDD, in which case the patient is diagnosed with PDD and MDD. (*American Psychiatric Association: Diagnostic and Statistical Manual of Mental Disorders: DSM-5-TR* 2022)

PDD often starts in childhood, earlier than MDD typically starts. (Schramm et al. 2020) Although the symptoms of depression may be less severe in PDD than in MDD, since symptoms persist over two years or more, they can cause more disability than in MDD. Similarly to MDD, PDD is twice as common in women than in men. (Schramm et al. 2020) PDD responds to antidepressant treatment but sometimes is more treatment-resistant than MDD, possibly because of the longevity of the symptoms. (Schramm et al. 2020) Both antidepressant drugs and psychotherapy are effective treatments for PDD. (Schramm et al. 2020)

Risk Factors

Risk factors for PDD are similar to those for MDD. Family history typically shows other members affected with depressive disorders. (*American Psychiatric Association: Diagnostic and Statistical Manual of Mental Disorders: DSM-5-TR* 2022) Adverse events in childhood are also thought to play a role in developing PDD.

Pathophysiology

Very little is known about the pathophysiology specific to PDD. (Schramm et al. 2020) Defects in the same pathways involved in MDD are likely present. The pathophysiological pathways differentiating PDD from MDD are unknown.

Examination

PDD is frequently unrecognized clinically because clinicians tend to focus on acute changes, and patients believe the symptoms they are experiencing are "normal," at least for them. (Schramm et al. 2020) Often the problem is not identified until an MDE develops. In assessing a patient with depressive symptoms, probing for long-standing symptoms pointing toward PDD is essential. In addition, hypomania or mania must be ruled out.

Laboratory

As is true for other depressive disorders, there is no test to diagnose PDD specifically. Instead, other causes of depressive symptoms, such as hypothyroidism, should be ruled out as appropriate.

Imaging

No imaging needs to be done for PDD.

Associated Symptoms/Conditions

Most patients with PDD also develop MDD at some point in their lifetime. Anxiety, substance use, and personality disorders are prevalent in PDD. (*American Psychiatric Association: Diagnostic and Statistical Manual of Mental Disorders: DSM-5-TR* 2022) There is a higher rate of suicidal thoughts in patients with PDD vs. MDD, likely because of the chronicity of the symptoms in PDD. (Schramm et al. 2020)

Diagnosis

According to DSM-5-TR, PDD is diagnosed when a patient has a depressed mood for most days for at least two years and at least 2 of the following symptoms:

1) Changes in appetite (either overeating or not eating enough)
2) Changes in sleep (either hypersomnia or insomnia)
3) Low energy/fatigue
4) Low self-esteem
5) Poor concentration or difficulty making decisions
6) Hopelessness

Symptoms cannot remit for more than two months during the two years. There must not be any manias or hypomanias in the patient's lifetime. (*American Psychiatric Association: Diagnostic and Statistical Manual of Mental Disorders: DSM-5-TR* 2022)

Treatment

PDD responds to antidepressant medication (Meister et al. 2016) and psychotherapy. (Konvalin et al. 2021) It typically takes longer for patients to respond, again likely explained by the chronicity of the illness. Up to 40% of patients with PDD are considered treatment-resistant. (Schramm et al. 2020) Similarly to MDD, studies suggest that PDD is best treated with combined psychotherapy and psychopharmacology. (Schramm et al. 2020)

Management

Management of PDD is similar to MDD in that educating the patient, and close family or friends about the illness is essential. Healthcare providers should emphasize that this illness is not a personality quirk and can reoccur anytime. Early identification of reoccurring symptoms is crucial to successful treatment. Patients typically do better when on maintenance medication and psychotherapy. (Schramm et al. 2020)

Premenstrual Dysphoric disorder (PMDD)

Presentation

Premenstrual dysphoric disorder (PMDD) is characterized by emotional distress and physical discomfort that begin in the luteal phase of the menstrual cycle, building up gradually after ovulation until menses. These symptoms stop at the end of the luteal phase. Emotional distress causes irritability, emotional lability, depression, and anxiety. There have even been studies that show that women are more likely to have suicidal thoughts and attempts during this time in their cycle. (Wikman et al. 2022) Premenstrual symptoms that do not reach the DSM-5-TR defined severity level are called premenstrual syndrome (PMS). As many as 30% of menstruating women have PMS, and up to 5% have PMDD. (Yonkers and Simoni 2018)

Risk Factors

Stress and trauma, especially adverse childhood events, can increase the risk of PMDD. Genetic factors play a role as well. As much as 50% of the risk for PMDD is heritable. (*American Psychiatric Association: Diagnostic and Statistical Manual of Mental Disorders: DSM-5-TR* 2022)

Pathophysiology

PMDD does not occur in the absence of ovulation and the rising levels of progesterone in the luteal phase, followed by a rapid fall in the late luteal phase. One hypothesis is that some women are susceptible to the progesterone metabolite allopregnanolone, which can bind to the $GABA_A$ receptor and mediate mood and anxiety symptoms. (Yonkers and Simoni 2018)

Another theory, supported by the efficacy of SSRIs and SNRIs, is that a serotonin deficiency causes the symptoms. In contrast to the actions of SSRIs and SNRIs in depressive disorders, these drugs work quickly in PMDD. This may be because treatment of PMDD does not require the neuroplasticity that is believed to contribute to the therapeutic effect of these drugs in depressive disorders. Alternatively, SSRIs and SNRIs are known to affect allopregnanolone levels, which may contribute to their therapeutic effect on PMDD. (Yonkers and Simoni 2018)

Examination

Women with PMDD may demonstrate mood symptoms if seen during the luteal phase. It is essential to ask about suicidal thoughts and plans. In establishing the diagnosis of PMDD, getting prospective data on mood symptoms is important. Ideally, patients would record their PMDD symptoms in relation to their cycle for at least two consecutive months.

Laboratory

No specific laboratory tests are required for PMDD. Appropriate labs should be ordered if there is any concern about thyroid or other medical issues.

Imaging

No imaging is needed in the evaluation or treatment of PMDD.

Associated Symptoms/Conditions

Many disorders, such as migraine, seizures, asthma, MDD, anxiety disorders, bipolar disorder, and eating disorders, may worsen during the luteal phase of the menstrual cycle. (*American Psychiatric Association: Diagnostic and Statistical Manual of Mental Disorders: DSM-5-TR* 2022) To distinguish this phenomenon from PMDD, it is essential to assess for a symptom-free period immediately after the menses in the follicular stage of the cycle. For example, symptoms of MDE will not go away entirely in the follicular phase, but symptoms of PMDD will be completely absent during this time.

Diagnosis

DSM-5-TR defines PMDD as having five or more symptoms out of two symptom groups during the luteal phase of the menstrual cycle. These symptoms start to get better when the menses begin and resolve by the start of the cycle's follicular phase. (*American Psychiatric Association: Diagnostic and Statistical Manual of Mental Disorders: DSM-5-TR* 2022) There must be at least one symptom from each group. The groups are as follows:

Mood Symptoms:

1) Mood swings, increased sensitivity to rejection.
2) Irritability and anger, with increased interpersonal conflicts.
3) Depressed mood, feelings of hopelessness, and worthlessness.
4) Anxiety, feeling keyed up or on edge.

Functional Symptoms:

1) Loss of interest in usual activities (anhedonia).
2) Difficulty concentrating.
3) Fatigue, low energy.
4) Either overeating or loss of appetite.
5) Sleeping too much or too little.
6) Feeling overwhelmed or out of control.
7) Breast tenderness, bloating, weight gain, joint or muscle pain.

Ideally, these symptoms are elicited prospectively, with the patient recording symptoms and menses on a calendar for at least two months. The diagnosis is considered provisional if this still needs to be done. (*American Psychiatric Association: Diagnostic and Statistical Manual of Mental Disorders: DSM-5-TR* 2022)

Treatment

First-line treatment for PMDD is SSRIs. Fluoxetine, paroxetine, and sertraline are the FDA-approved treatments of PMDD in the United States, but there is evidence that other SSRIs, such as escitalopram, are also effective. Other serotonergic drugs, such as nefazodone (a serotonin modulator) and nortriptyline (a TCA), are sometimes used off-label to treat PMDD.

Management

Medicines to treat PMDD can be given at the start of the luteal phase or when symptoms become bothersome. They are stopped after menses begin and symptoms stop. Alternatively, the medications can be given throughout the menstrual cycle for convenience, but this does not increase effectiveness. (Lanza di Scalea & Pearlstein 2019) Serotonergic agents must be provided for 4 – 12 weeks for other disorders before the medications are effective. PMDD is the only depressive disorder in which they have effectiveness in the short term.

The second-line treatment for PMDD is stopping ovulation and preventing hormonal changes in the luteal phase. (Tiranini and Nappi 2022) This can be done with oral contraceptives, gonadotropin-releasing hormone (GnRH) agonists, or bilateral oophorectomy. (Tiranini and Nappi 2022)

In addition to pharmacological treatment of PMDD, many women benefit from simply understanding what is happening. Recognizing that uncomfortable emotions are biologically caused and time-limited can help women learn not to act on them. Family and friends may also benefit from this understanding.

Key Anxiety Disorders:

Generalized Anxiety Disorder (GAD)

Presentation

Patients with generalized anxiety disorder (GAD) have persistent, excessive anxiety about everyday events that are disproportionate to these events. They cannot control their anxiety which causes significant distress or difficulty functioning. GAD may begin at any time, but the median age of onset is 30 years. (*American Psychiatric Association: Diagnostic and Statistical Manual of Mental Disorders: DSM-5-TR* 2022) The lifetime prevalence of GAD is 3 – 6% of the population. (Gomez et al. 2018)

Risk Factors

Prior history of anxiety not meeting the criteria for GAD is a risk factor for GAD. A family history of anxiety disorders also increases the chance of a person developing GAD. Adverse life events further increase the risk of developing GAD.

Pathophysiology

Our understanding of the pathophysiology of anxiety disorders is still incomplete. We know that stress pathways involving the hippocampus and fear pathways involving the amygdala are essential. (Tafet and Nemeroff 2020) Serotonergic systems in the raphe nuclei communicate with the prefrontal cortex and help to determine which stimuli to respond to and other executive functions. (Tafet and Nemeroff 2020) It is thought that the overactivation of these pathways contributes to anxiety disorders. The inhibitory effects of $GABA_A$ receptor activation help lessen anxiety. (Tafet and Nemeroff 2020)

Examination

The mental status examination may reveal signs of anxiety, such as pressured speech, restlessness, frequent extra movements, and cognitive complaints of excessive worry and anxiety.

Laboratory

There are no laboratory tests specific to anxiety. Medical conditions that can cause anxiety, such as hyperthyroidism or hypoxemia, should be looked for when appropriate.

Imaging

There is currently no imaging that is used clinically to detect anxiety disorders.

Associated Symptoms/Conditions

Patients with GAD often have other anxiety disorders or depressive disorders. They may also have substance use disorders. (*American Psychiatric Association: Diagnostic and Statistical Manual of Mental Disorders: DSM-5-TR* 2022)

Diagnosis

The diagnosis of GAD is made when a patient has had excessive anxiety and worry almost every day for the last six months. The anxiety is out of proportion to the triggering issue. The anxiety is focused on several different problems. The patient cannot control the anxiety. There must be at least 3 of the following symptoms associated with anxiety:

Physical symptoms:

1) Feeling internally restless or on edge
2) Muscle tension
3) Fatigue

Emotional/cognitive symptoms:

1) Irritability
2) Difficulty concentrating
3) Insomnia

Treatment

The first-line treatment for GAD is either an SSRI or an SNRI. Benzodiazepines (BZDs; see below and Chapter 23) are at least as effective as SSRIs or SSNRIs, but because of risks of substance abuse and tolerance, they are recommended to be used short-term only. (Gomez et al. 2018) They can offset the increased anxiety often experienced when SSRIs and SNRIs are first started. However, it can be challenging to get the patient to stop the benzodiazepine. Other agents such as tricyclic antidepressants, buspirone, and anticonvulsants such as pregabalin can be used as second or third-line agents.

Treatment of GAD frequently requires 6 – 12 weeks or longer for full effectiveness. Once stabilized on medication for GAD, patients should be continued on therapy for at least one year. Evidence indicates that this strategy reduces the risk of symptom relapse. (Strawn et al. 2018)

Management

Psychotherapy can be very effective for anxiety disorders. Cognitive behavioral treatment (CBT) has been specifically studied for this, but other forms of psychotherapy can also be effective. The best results in treating GAD usually come from combining medication with psychotherapy, as long as the patient accepts both types of therapy.

Panic Disorder (PD)

Presentation

Patients with panic attacks frequently present to emergency rooms because of the physical symptoms they are experiencing. In the disorder's early stages, panic attacks are often perceived as symptoms of a significant medical issue such as a heart attack or stroke. All medical causes must be ruled out before attributing the symptoms to a panic attack, as people with panic disorder can also have or develop emergent conditions such as heart attacks or strokes. Panic disorder occurs about twice as frequently in women than in men. (*American Psychiatric Association: Diagnostic and Statistical Manual of Mental Disorders: DSM-5-TR* 2022) The lifetime prevalence of panic disorder is about 4%. (Goddard 2017)

To meet the diagnosis of panic disorder, at least some of the panic attacks need to occur out of the blue, with no associated trigger. (*American Psychiatric Association: Diagnostic and Statistical Manual of Mental Disorders: DSM-5-TR* 2022) A typical example is waking up from sleep in a panic attack. Other panic attacks can occur in response to a specific environmental trigger. In panic attacks, the anxiety peaks within minutes of the start of the episode. (*American Psychiatric Association: Diagnostic and Statistical Manual of Mental Disorders: DSM-5-TR* 2022)

Panic attacks are common in many psychiatric conditions, such as MDD, post-traumatic stress disorder, and psychosis. To be considered for panic disorder, the patient must have significant anxiety about having panic attacks. Typically, the panic disorder will cause the patient to avoid going places or being in circumstances that might prompt a panic attack or make it difficult to escape should a panic attack occur unexpectedly. The diagnosis of panic disorder also requires more than one panic attack that occurs without any known trigger.

Risk Factors

The main risk factors for PD are genetic predisposition, chronic stress, and temperament. People who, by temperament, are uncomfortable with new situations (this quality is termed behavioral inhibition) are more likely to develop PD. (Goddard 2017) For example, having excessive fear of or difficulty with things such as moving to a new city, starting a new school or job, or being around new people are examples of behavioral inhibition. Although many genes have been evaluated in PD, only a polymorphism in the catechol-O-methyltransferase has withstood the test of replication. (Goddard 2017) Chronic stress in childhood from trauma, abuse, or other adverse events increases the risk of developing PD. (*American Psychiatric Association: Diagnostic and Statistical Manual of Mental Disorders: DSM-5-TR* 2022) In addition, many people with PD first develop symptoms during a period of high emotional or physical stress. (*American Psychiatric Association: Diagnostic and Statistical Manual of Mental Disorders: DSM-5-TR* 2022) These stresses likely cause epigenetic changes in the genome, which increase the risk of PD. (Goddard 2017)

Pathophysiology

Our understanding of the pathophysiology of panic disorder is still incomplete. We know that stress pathways involving the hippocampus and fear pathways involving the amygdala are essential. Serotonergic systems in the raphe nuclei communicate with the prefrontal cortex determining which stimuli to respond to and other executive functions. (Tafet and Nemeroff 2020) It is thought that the overactivation of these pathways contributes to anxiety disorders. The inhibitory effects of $GABA_A$ receptor activation help lessen anxiety. (Tafet and Nemeroff 2020)

Examination

There is no specific physical examination for PD other than a focused physical examination to rule out respiratory, cardiac, or neurological causes of the symptoms. The mental status exam may show a very anxious patient who is fidgety and restless during a panic attack, but may also appear completely normal when the patient is not in the midst of a panic attack.

Laboratory

Laboratory testing is governed by the physical symptoms the patient is experiencing, especially new symptoms. All patients with PD should have a recent TSH performed, as hyperthyroidism can precipitate panic attacks. An EKG and cardiac enzymes might be appropriate for a patient with chest pain.

Imaging

Imaging in PD is governed by the physical symptoms the patient is experiencing, especially recent symptoms. With shortness of breath, it is appropriate to check a chest x-ray if one has not been recently done. A CT or MRI of the brain might be warranted if neurological symptoms are prominent.

Associated Symptoms/Conditions

PD is often associated with anxiety, mood, and substance use disorders. (*American Psychiatric Association: Diagnostic and Statistical Manual of Mental Disorders: DSM-5-TR* 2022) Sometimes alcohol use disorder starts as an attempt to treat panic attacks. Agoraphobia (the fear of leaving home, being in a crowd, being on public transportation, etc.) is the highest comorbid condition with PD. Sometimes the agoraphobia seems to develop from the PD. In other cases, they develop separately. Often agoraphobia worsens when the person stops working.

Medical conditions are also commonly comorbid with PD. (*American Psychiatric Association: Diagnostic and Statistical Manual of Mental Disorders: DSM-5-TR* 2022) Again, sometimes the medical condition comes first, and other times they co-occur. Medical conditions sometimes bring out PD; for example, hyperthyroidism increases anxiety and panic attacks. Cardiac disease and COPD can also precipitate PD as the cause of chest pain, and dyspnea can be difficult to distinguish – is the chest pain from ischemia or PD? Is the dyspnea from a COPD exacerbation or PD? These patients must be carefully evaluated, as it is essential not to miss an acute cardiac or pulmonary problem.

Diagnosis

Recurrent panic attacks, at least some unexpected or untriggered, are the hallmark of PD. In addition, the panic attacks must be followed by at least one month of persistent worry about developing another panic attack and maladaptive life changes to avoid having panic attacks. Development of agoraphobia or failure to exercise are just two examples of potential maladaptive life changes in response to panic attacks.

Panic attacks are defined as acute fear or anxiety that peaks in intensity within a few minutes of onset. These attacks are accompanied by four or more of 13 symptoms. (*American Psychiatric Association: Diagnostic and Statistical Manual of Mental Disorders: DSM-5-TR* 2022)

Physical symptoms:

1) Palpitations, racing heart
2) Shortness of breath
3) Chest pain
4) Nausea or abdominal pain
5) Sweating

Neurological symptoms:

6) Feelings of being choked
7) Chills or feeling hot
8) Trembling or shaking
9) Feeling dizzy, light-headed or unsteady
10) Paresthesia (numbness or tingling sensations)

Psychological symptoms:

11) Derealization (feelings of unreality) or depersonalization (being detached from oneself)
12) Fear of losing control or “going crazy”
13) Intense fear of dying

Treatment

PD is treated with SSRIs or SNRIs as first-line therapy. These medications may take 4 to 6 weeks before the patient notices the benefit. The full effect can take 12 weeks or longer. According to a Cochrane review, (Bighelli et al. 2018) patients need to be treated for an average of 7 weeks with antidepressants for a clinically significant effect to be achieved between treatment and placebo. The data were not robust, however. Tricyclic antidepressants are also effective but are associated with more adverse effects than SSRIs or SNRIs.

Benzodiazepines (BZDs) effectively treat PD and work more quickly than antidepressants. Patients need to be treated for an average of 4 weeks with BZDs for a clinically significant effect to be achieved between treatment and placebo. (Bighelli et al. 2018) Again, the data quality was poor. While BZDs work very well for the short term, many patients find them addictive and have difficulty stopping therapy. As people age, the likelihood of adverse events from BZD increases, including falls, memory impairment, and unintentional overdose. Hence, BZDs are usually considered second-line therapy for PD.

Psychotherapy is also effective for the treatment of PD. Another Cochrane review found no differences in outcome between psychotherapy and medication (either antidepressant or BZD) in treating PD. (Imai et al. 2016) As with other Cochrane reviews for PD, the data was of poor quality. Thus, the choice of therapy is primarily left to the patient's preferences.

Management

Since many types of therapy are available for PD (as described above), the patient's preference must be considered when prescribing antidepressants, benzodiazepines, or psychotherapy for patients with PD. Often patients benefit from more than one type of therapy. The most common example is psychotherapy, especially cognitive behavioral therapy, combined with an SSRI.

Social Anxiety Disorder (SAD)

Social anxiety disorder (SAD, previously referred to as social phobia) is characterized by extreme fear or anxiety when in a position to potentially be judged by others. It can be fear induced by all social circumstances or fear specifically for performance issues. (*American Psychiatric Association: Diagnostic and Statistical Manual of Mental Disorders: DSM-5-TR* 2022; Stein et al. 2017)

SAD affects up to 7% of the population in the US during any year. It is prevalent worldwide but to a lesser extent than in the US. Areas with the lowest 12-month prevalence of SAD are Africa and the Eastern Mediterranean. (Stein et al. 2017) In all countries, SAD usually starts in childhood or adolescence but can be first recognized at any age. It often resolves as individuals age.

Presentation

Women are more likely to have SAD but less likely to seek help than men. (*American Psychiatric Association: Diagnostic and Statistical Manual of Mental Disorders: DSM-5-TR* 2022) The reasons for this are unclear but may relate to different social expectations for men and women. Patients seek help for SAD when it interferes with their lives, often when it makes it harder for them to work or when they are not able to socialize with others. They also may seek help for other disorders, only to have it become obvious that SAD contributes to the problem. (Koyuncu et al. 2019) For example, a patient with underlying SAD seeks help for alcohol use disorder and believes he cannot interact with others socially without a drink.

Risk Factors

A predisposition to SAD can be inherited; first-degree relatives of SAD patients are 2 – 6 times more likely to have SAD than the general population. (*American Psychiatric Association: Diagnostic and Statistical Manual of Mental Disorders: DSM-5-TR* 2022) People who are afraid of new situations are more likely to develop SAD. A history of being bullied or a specific condition that marks one as different can sometimes lead to the development of SAD.

Pathophysiology

Our understanding of the pathophysiology of SAD is very incomplete. The autonomic nervous system is likely involved with excessive fight or flight response activation. We know that specific brain regions, such as the amygdala, hippocampus, and prefrontal cortex, are likely involved. Serotonergic agents are beneficial in SAD, but we don't know precisely how they work to help the patient feel better.

Examination

A mental status examination for a patient with SAD may often seem completely normal unless they are acutely in the midst of social anxiety. It is necessary to ask and then rely on what the patient says about their anxiety in social circumstances. It is essential to ask how this impacts the person's life functioning.

Laboratory

No laboratory tests are necessary to diagnose SAD. If there is concern about a thyroid condition, thyroid stimulating hormone (TSH) levels should be measured. If any other medical illnesses are suspected, they should be assessed as appropriate.

Imaging

No imaging is called for in evaluating SAD unless other medical conditions are suspected which require it.

Associated Symptoms/Conditions

SAD has a high rate of psychiatric co-morbidity. (Koyuncu et al. 2019) Major depressive disorder (MDD) occurs in up to 70% of SAD patients, and as many as 50% have alcohol use disorder (AUD). (Koyuncu et al. 2019) Usually, SAD occurs first. MDD may be a response to the life consequences of SAD. Alcohol use may initially be an attempt at coping with SAD symptoms in social situations but then lead to AUD. It is vital to ask SAD patients about co-existing psychiatric symptoms.

Diagnosis

SAD is characterized by extreme fear or anxiety when in a position where others may potentially be judgemental. The patient is afraid that others will think badly of them. They know that this fear is irrational but have difficulty controlling their anxiety. This may occur in a social setting, with strangers, while eating in public, and when performing. (*American Psychiatric Association: Diagnostic and Statistical Manual of Mental Disorders: DSM-5-TR* 2022) As a result of these fears, the patient avoids these situations, which cause problems in their life, such as difficulty working, shopping, or interacting with friends or family. These fears must be present for at least six months.

Suppose the patient's fear is limited to specific performance situations, such as giving a speech or participating in an artistic performance. In that case, the problem is diagnosed as SAD, performance only, and may not impact their life as severely.

Treatment

SSRIs are usually the first-line treatment for SAD. This is primarily because of their low side-effect profile and effectiveness. Other antidepressants can be used instead, and SNRIs are frequent choices. Paroxetine, sertraline (both SSRIs), and venlafaxine (an SNRI) are the only drugs that are specifically FDA-approved for SAD. These medicines will take up to 16 weeks for full effect, and the patient may not even become aware that they are helping at all for the first 4 to 6 weeks. Patients should be educated about this to manage expectations. They should be encouraged to try what would have been a fear-invoking situation after they start to feel the medication's effects.

BZDs may also be used to treat SAD. They are considered second-line drugs because of the risks of addiction and adverse effects such as sedation, falls, and unintentional overdose. An unintentional overdose occurs when a patient does not mean to take more medication but does because they are still anxious and forget they already took it. No BZDs have FDA approval for SAD.

For the performance-only subtype of SAD, it is best to use meds only as needed before performances. A small dose of BZD can be used in this way. The patient must be warned about the risks, including sedation and addiction. The first dose they take should be a test dose, not before a performance.

Management

Psychotherapy can be used along with medications to help manage SAD. This may help provide immediate relief while the medication's full benefit develops.

Suicidal Ideation (SI)

Thoughts of suicide are referred to as "suicidal ideations (SI)" in psychiatry. They do not constitute a specific diagnosis but are a common symptom in many people with psychiatric disorders. They also occur in people without a specific psychiatric disorder.

Most people with SI will never attempt suicide, but all people who die by suicide have had SI, often for a very long period before their death. Thus, all SI needs to be taken seriously. It indicates that something is seriously wrong in the person's life, and their situation needs to be addressed. SI should not be dismissed as "attention seeking." The person may be seeking attention, but this does not negate that something is very wrong if SI is present.

Many people who have never experienced SI feel uncomfortable directly asking about SI. They may believe these questions will "plant the seed" or influence someone to think about and potentially act on SI. This is rarely the case. Usually, a person with previously unvoiced SI feels relief that these thoughts can be out in the open. Having another person listen nonjudgmentally to these thoughts and emotions can also be therapeutic.

Presentation

Patients with SI may be in obvious distress from mental illness, substance abuse, life tragedies, or chronic feelings of rejection. They may also feel hopeless about their life and incapable of improving things. It is essential to ask about SI, as many patients will not volunteer their struggles with SI. Assessing suicide risk is an integral part of any psychiatric interview.

Risk Factors

A family history of suicide and a previous suicide attempt are some of the strongest risk factors for suicide. (Fazel and Runeson 2020) Drug or alcohol abuse and psychiatric disorders also have strong associations with suicide. (Fazel and Runeson 2020) Lesser risk factors include access to lethal means of suicide, a history of adverse childhood experiences, and stressful life events. (Fazel and Runeson 2020)

Pathophysiology

As with much in psychiatry, the exact pathophysiology of SI, suicide attempts, and death by suicide are poorly understood. Various studies have compared autopsy information from people who have died by suicide vs. other means of death. Researchers have also looked at living people who have attempted suicide or are at high risk of suicide. These studies have suggested roles for serotonin, cortisol, and the HPA axis. (Melhem et al. 2022)

Examination

No specific examination finding should concern a clinician about suicide other than what the patient says. It is crucial to ask each patient about SI in a psychiatric interview.

Laboratory

No laboratory findings are of assistance in determining suicide risk.

Imaging

No specific imaging will help in detecting SI or predicting the risk of suicide.

Associated Symptoms/Conditions

Most, but not all, people who die by suicide have some diagnosable psychiatric illness. The most common are mood disorders and substance abuse. (Fazel and Runeson 2020)

Diagnosis

Diagnosis of SI is made by what the patient says. It is also essential to talk to family and friends about their perception of suicide risk. Specific actions by the patient may increase the risk of suicide. For example, a person who gives away possessions quits a job, or buys lethal means of suicide should be considered at high risk for suicide.

Treatment

The first step in treating someone with SI is to ensure safety. This might mean asking family or friends to remove means of suicide, such as guns, from the patient's possession. It might mean admission to a hospital. It might mean friends and family staying with the patient. Each situation needs individual assessment.

After initial stabilization, assessing for and treating any psychiatric issues is imperative. If the patient has been prescribed psychiatric meds but stopped them, it is essential to understand why and see if barriers to medication can be overcome. The involvement of supportive family and friends is necessary to assist the patient as they rebuild their life.

Lithium (the "gold standard" mood stabilizer) was developed for bipolar disorder but is also used to augment antidepressants. Clozapine (the "gold standard" antipsychotic) and lithium are the only two medicines that have been shown to decrease death by suicide. (Hawkins et al. 2021) These studies were done in people with schizophrenia (for clozapine) and those with bipolar disorder (for lithium). It is not known if they help SI in patients who do not have these disorders. Both are older medications with significant side effects. Since it is easier to die by overdose from these drugs vs. other antidepressants and antipsychotics, the fact that they have been found effective in preventing suicide is impressive.

Management

For most psychiatric disorders, psychotherapy plus drug treatment for the underlying psychiatric illness reduces SI. For patients with schizophrenia who have severe SI, clozapine can be tried; similarly, for patients with bipolar disorder and severe SI, lithium can be tried. Family therapy may be beneficial as well.

General Treatment Strategies by Drug Class:

As expressed in a Black Box Warning in the US, all antidepressants increase the risk of SI, especially early in the treatment and most commonly in children and young adults in their mid-20s or younger. (Becker & Correll 2020) This is thought to be related to increased energy and activation caused by many antidepressants and to changes in the developing brain. The stigma associated with treating mood disorders and concerns of serious adverse effects, such as in these Black Box Warnings, can prevent patients from seeking drug treatment. Most experts warn about failing to prescribe antidepressants for depression because of fear of suicide which can lead to increased suicide through untreated depression. (Becker & Correll 2020) Instead, close follow-up with the patient and frequent evaluations should be done to assess suicide risk. Patients should be warned about this potential side effect and asked to be on the watch for it.

Similarly, all antidepressants carry a risk of inducing hypomania or mania. This is especially true in patients with bipolar disorders and can sometimes be the first sign of bipolar disorder. In other people, it seems to be just an antidepressant side effect that typically won't recur with other antidepressants. The switch to hypomania or mania typically occurs early in treatment and may respond to a reduction in the dose of the antidepressant. Other options are to switch antidepressants or add a mood stabilizer. (Gill et al. 2020)

Serotonin syndrome is another adverse effect that has been associated with the use of many antidepressants. It is caused by a significant increase in the dose ingested (such as in an overdose) or the addition of a second drug that increases synaptic levels of serotonin. Symptoms of serotonin syndrome can be divided into 1) mental status changes (agitation, confusion), 2) autonomic changes (elevated temp, fluctuating blood pressure, diaphoresis), and 3) neuromuscular changes (tremor, clonus, hyperreflexia, ataxia)

1st GENERATION ANTIDEPRESSANTS

Tricyclic Antidepressants (TCAs)

Tertiary amines
Amitriptyline
Clomipramine
Doxepin
Imipramine
Trimipramine

Secondary amines
Desipramine
Nortriptyline
Protriptyline

Other
Amoxapine

Background and Clinical Use

As the name suggests, tricyclic antidepressants (TCAs) have three aromatic hydrocarbon rings. They were developed in the 1950s and were the first pharmaceutical treatment for mood disorders. TCAs have many side effects and are no longer first-line treatments for depression. However, they are still used, especially in chronic pain management. Except for amoxapine, TCAs are either tertiary or secondary amines. Tertiary amines have two methyl groups attached to the nitrogen (for a total of three carbons attached to nitrogen, including the backbone; Figure 1A, 2A-D).

Secondary amines only have one methyl group attached to the nitrogen (for two carbons attached to the nitrogen; Figure 1B, 3A, and B).

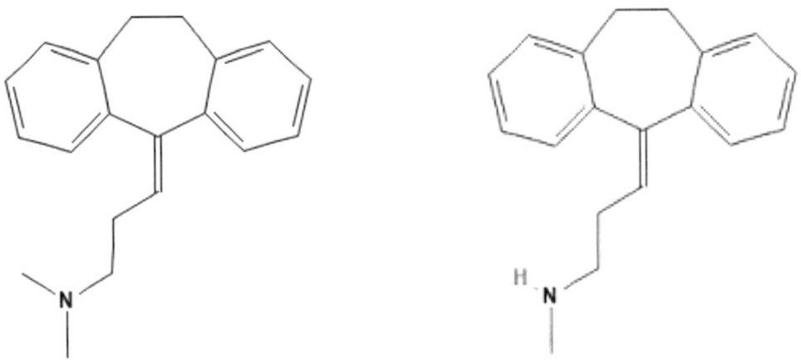

A. Amitriptyline B. Nortriptyline

Figure 1: Structures of amitriptyline (a tertiary amine) and nortriptyline (a secondary amine). (Note: The straight lines coming off the Nitrogen atoms represent bonds to Carbon atoms.)

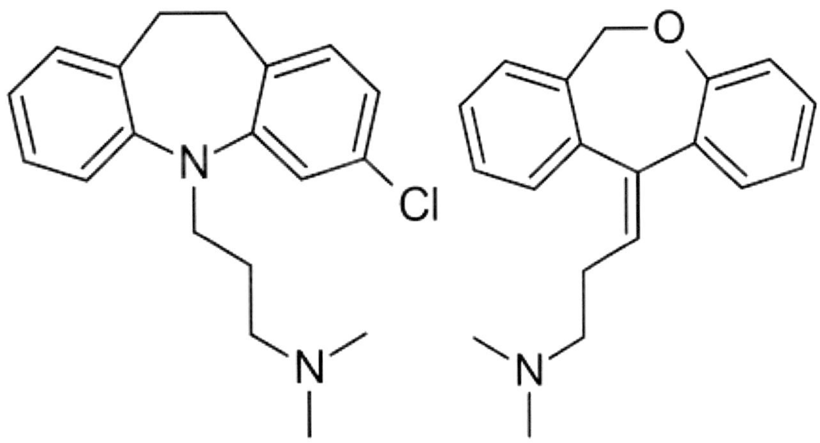

A. Clomipramine B. Doxepin

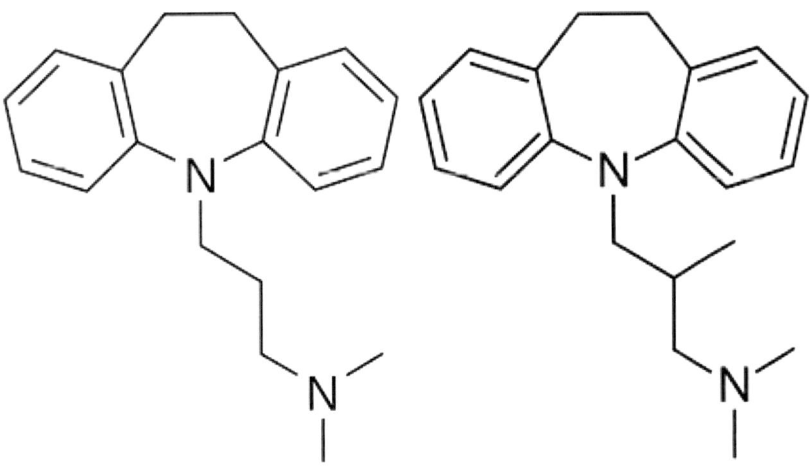

C. Imipramine D. Trimipramine

Figure 2: Structures of tertiary amines.

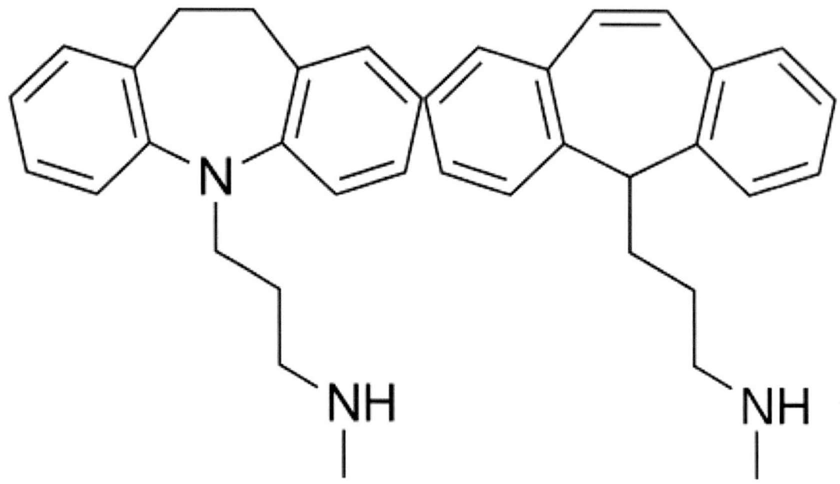

A. Desipramine B. Protriptyline

Figure 3: Structures of secondary amines

These medications have significant toxicities, and the therapeutic range of each medication is well established because it is essential to ensure that the drug level is high enough to give an effect but not too high to cause toxicities. Another advantage of the known therapeutic range of each medication is that when there is a question of whether a patient is absorbing (or taking) a TCA, it is possible to measure the blood level to confirm. When patients on TCAs experience a new adverse effect, it is often helpful to measure the level of the drug to exclude the possibility of toxicity. Unfortunately, these levels are rarely done on-site, and results are not available immediately; but they can still be helpful, especially when an unsuspected toxicity is discovered.

Pharmacokinetics

Tricyclic antidepressants undergo extensive first-pass metabolism in the liver, meaning that before the drug can go through systemic circulation, a lot of the original drug is metabolized into other compounds in the liver. (Rudorfer and Potter 1999) Many of these compounds are active; for example, nortriptyline is an active metabolite of amitriptyline, and desipramine is an active metabolite of imipramine. Once TCAs reach the systemic circulation, most drugs and metabolites are highly plasma protein bound. (Rudorfer and Potter 1999) Patients with low plasma protein levels will have a higher fraction of the free drug and hence be liable to side effects at lower doses. This can be especially significant in elderly patients.

TCAs are metabolized mainly in the liver by CYP450 enzymes. (Rudorfer and Potter 1999) Hence, the drug levels depend on genetic variations of these enzymes and other drugs' suppression or activation of these enzymes. It is always important to look at a drug-drug interaction program with information on all the medications a patient is already taking when starting all drugs. This is especially true with TCAs.

Mechanism of Action

The therapeutic effect of TCAs is thought to be due to increased serotonin and norepinephrine levels in synaptic junctions, secondary to inhibition of the transporter proteins for these neurotransmitters. Usually, these neurotransmitters are removed from the synaptic cleft by transport back into the nerve endings from which they came. Serotonin is removed from the synaptic cleft by the serotonin reuptake transporter (SERT) and norepinephrine by the norepinephrine transporter (NET). When these transporters are blocked, the neurotransmitter concentration in the synaptic cleft is elevated. While the therapeutic mechanism is not well understood, it is believed that exposure of presynaptic serotonin receptors (located on nerve terminal membranes and the somatodendritic region of nerves) to the elevated serotonin, over time, downregulates and desensitizes these receptors. This ultimately results in more serotonin being released from the terminals. Presumably, a similar effect is seen on noradrenergic neurotransmission. TCAs vary in the ratio of serotonin: norepinephrine reuptake inhibition.

Adverse Effects

Although therapeutic effects are likely from actions on serotonin and norepinephrine reuptake, the drugs bind to a wide variety of other receptors, blocking muscarinic cholinergic receptors (often referred to as anticholinergic effects), histamine receptors, and α_1-adrenoceptors. (Gillman 2007) This wide range of receptor binding is responsible for many of the adverse effects of these medications. These effects are listed below:

- Anticholinergic effects include dry mouth, constipation, confusion, urinary retention, blurry vision, and tachycardia. These are less common for secondary amines (desipramine, nortriptyline, and protriptyline)

- Sedation from blocking of histamine and muscarinic receptors in the CNS
- Weight gain from blocking of histamine receptors
- Postural hypotension from blocking of $\alpha_1$adrenoceptors
- Prolongation of QTc, which can be fatal in overdose
- Lowering of seizure threshold causing seizures
- Sexual side effects (loss of libido and delayed orgasm)
- Tremor

Safety in Overdose of Tricyclic Antidepressants

Tricyclic antidepressants can be lethal in overdose, primarily due to cardiac toxicities. Arrhythmias, QTc prolongation, seizures, electrolyte abnormalities, and hypotension must be monitored for and treated. Rarely serotonin syndrome can be seen with TCA overdose. This is most common with clomipramine, which is the most serotonergic TCA.

Drug-Specific Factors for Tricyclic Antidepressants

Certain tricyclics are commonly used, off-label, in low doses to help with sleep. Amitriptyline, nortriptyline, and doxepin are often used this way.

Amitriptyline and nortriptyline are used off-label to help with pain. They can be effective for migraine prevention, abdominal cramping, and neuropathy. The effective dose is often relatively low, bypassing most concerns about drug toxicity, except for individuals with drug-drug interactions or genetic variability.

Clomipramine has a more specific action on serotonin reuptake than the other medications. It was the first medication found to be effective for obsessive-compulsive disorder (OCD) and is considered the gold standard for treating OCD.

Amoxapine has a three aromatic hydrocarbon structure, as do the other tricyclics, but it lacks the amine chain and has other differences. Like the other tricyclics, it affects serotonin and norepinephrine levels. Unlike other TCAs, it also binds to dopamine receptors. This makes it the only antidepressant that also has some antipsychotic activity.

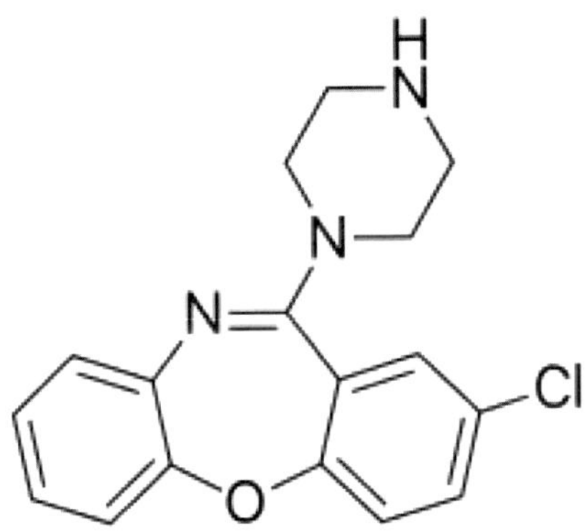

Amoxapine

Figure 4. Chemical structures of amoxapine.

Monoamine oxidase inhibitors (MAOI)

Isocarboxazid
Phenelzine
Selegiline
Tranylcypromine

Background and Clinical Use

Monoamine oxidase inhibitors (MAOIs) were initially discovered as a treatment for depression in the 1950s when an MAOI developed to treat tuberculosis failed to do so but did treat depression. They were the first antidepressants in clinical use. All have a single aromatic hydrocarbon ring, with one side chain, which varies among the drugs (see Figure 5).

MAOIs have several serious side effects, and drug-food interactions require dietary restrictions, limiting their ease of use. They are usually reserved as a last-line treatment when other medications have failed.

MAOIs have little structural similarity to each other, despite their similar mechanisms. This is demonstrated in Figure 5 below.

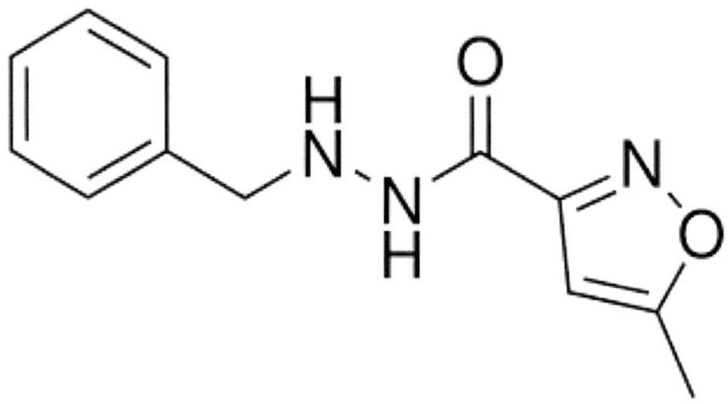

A.. Isocarboxazid

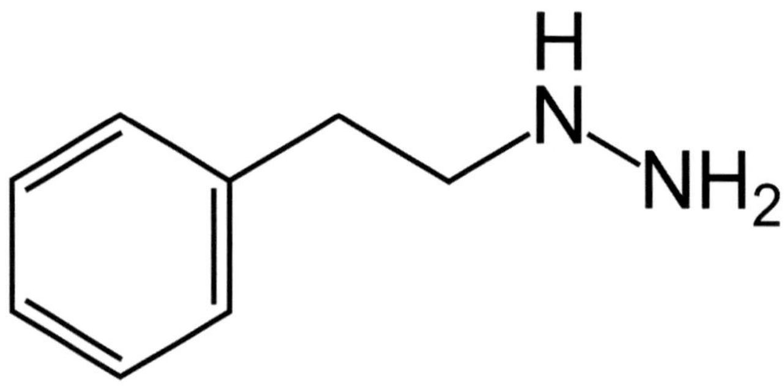

B.. Phenelzine

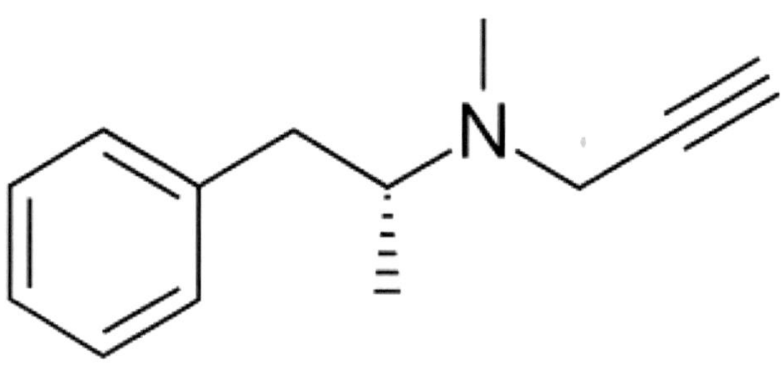

C.. Selegiline

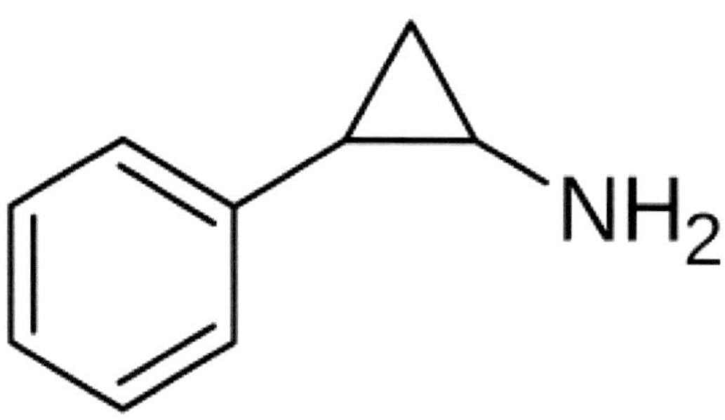

D.. Tranylcypromine

Figure 5. Chemical structures of MAOIs.

Pharmacokinetics

Monoamine oxidase inhibitors are administered orally for depression, except selegiline is administered transdermally.

All of the MAOIs available in the US are irreversible inhibitors of monoamine oxidase, the enzyme that metabolizes serotonin, norepinephrine, and dopamine. This means that the effects of the drugs will continue until a new enzyme is synthesized. This typically takes about two weeks.

Unlike many other antidepressants, MAOIs are not metabolized through the CYP450 enzyme system. Instead, they are acetylated. Genetic variability in acetylation makes some people more susceptible to elevated levels of MAOIs and increasing side effects because of slow acetylation.

Mechanism of Action

Monoamine oxidase inhibitors (MAOIs) are drugs that block the metabolism of the monoamines serotonin, norepinephrine, and dopamine, increasing their levels in synapses. It is thought that this explains the antidepressant effects of this drug class. Two isoforms of monoamine oxidases (MAOs) exist, MAO-A and MAO-B. MAO-A inhibition is required for antidepressant efficacy. (Sub Laban and Saadabadi 2022) Although selegiline is a selective MAO-B inhibitor (initially approved for use in Parkinson's disease), it loses selectivity for MAO-B at higher doses. It then inhibits MAO-A and has antidepressant properties. A transdermal patch is available and approved for treating depression in the US. Doses delivered by the patch inhibit both MAO-A and MAO-B.

Adverse Effects

Hypertensive crisis: MAOIs are rarely used because of the risk of interactions with certain foods and medicines, resulting in a severe hypertensive crisis. Tyramine is a monoamine commonly found in food which, in high enough concentrations, can raise blood pressure. Normally, MAO-A in the gut metabolizes tyramine before absorption, and plasma levels remain insignificant. MAOIs block the metabolism of tyramine, leading to elevated levels and potentially causing a hypertensive crisis. All patients being prescribed MAOIs must be given detailed diet information and counseled to adhere strictly to the diet. Aged cheeses such as cheddar, blue, and gouda, fermented foods such as sausage, pepperoni, salami and sauerkraut, soy sauce, and tap beer are very important to avoid because of their tyramine content. (Sub Laban and Saadabadi 2022)

Other side effects of MAOIs include:

- Orthostatic hypotension
- Edema
- Diaphoresis
- Weight gain
- Constipation
- Dry mouth
- Sexual dysfunction (loss of libido and delayed orgasm)
- Agitation
- Sleep disturbance
- Tremor

Drug Interactions

Drugs that are stimulants can interact with MAOIs to cause a hypertensive crisis. Sympathomimetic stimulants used to treat attention-deficit/hyperactivity disorder (ADHD) and certain cold medicines such as pseudoephedrine, phenylephrine, and phenylpropanolamine can lead to a hypertensive crisis by increasing synaptic levels of norepinephrine when combined with MAOIs.

Serotonin Syndrome: MAOIs can also cause serotonin syndrome, a potentially life-threatening condition due to excess serotonin. Monoamine oxidase commonly breaks down serotonin. Thus, when MAO is inhibited, synaptic serotonin levels increase. MAOIs can cause serotonin syndrome alone or in combination with other drugs that increase serotonin levels.

Safety in Overdose for MAOIs

MAOIs can be lethal in overdose, primarily due to the potential for hypertensive crisis and serotonin syndrome. Symptoms of MAOI overdose can worsen for as long as 48 hours after withdrawal of the offending drug due to the irreversible inhibition of MAOs.

Drug-Specific Factors for MAOIs

Selegiline is available as a transdermal patch. It is the only antidepressant available in this formulation. The patches come in 3 dose strengths, 6, 9, and 12 mg. With the 6 mg dose, the typical MAOI dietary restrictions are less critical and can be ignored. Once the dose is escalated above 6 mg, the usual MAOI diet restrictions are necessary.

2nd GENERATION ANTIDEPRESSANTS

Selective serotonin reuptake inhibitors (SSRIs)

Citalopram
Escitalopram
Fluoxetine
Fluvoxamine
Paroxetine
Sertraline

Background and Clinical Use

SSRIs were first introduced in the late 1980s and early 1990s. Compared to MAOIs and TCAs, SSRIs are much safer in overdose and have a much more favorable side effect profile. For this reason, clinicians felt comfortable prescribing them, and antidepressants became more widely used. Whereas previously antidepressants had been mainly prescribed by psychiatrists, with the SSRIs, general practitioners became comfortable treating depression. This helped decrease the stigma around mental illness as more people were being treated, and the public realized that medications could be effective.

SSRIs do not share structural similarities. There is no prototypical structure for SSRIs. Citalopram and escitalopram are related because citalopram is a racemic mixture of R and S isomers, and escitalopram is only the S isomer. The S isomer is thought to have greater activity than the R isomer.

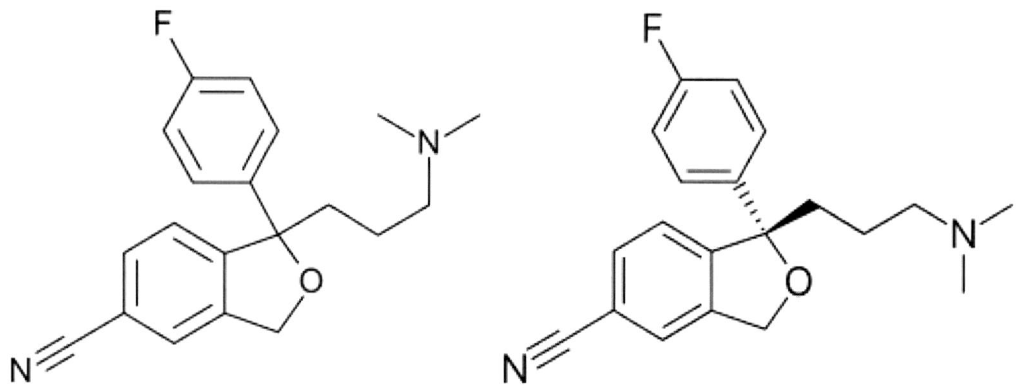

A. Citalopram (both R and S isomers) B. Escitalopram (only S isomer)

Figure 6: Chemical Structures of citalopram and escitalopram

The names of fluoxetine and fluvoxamine are similar, and they do share a tri-fluorinated aromatic ring, but otherwise, they are not related.

Sertraline is the only SSRI that is not fluorinated; instead, it has two chlorine atoms attached.

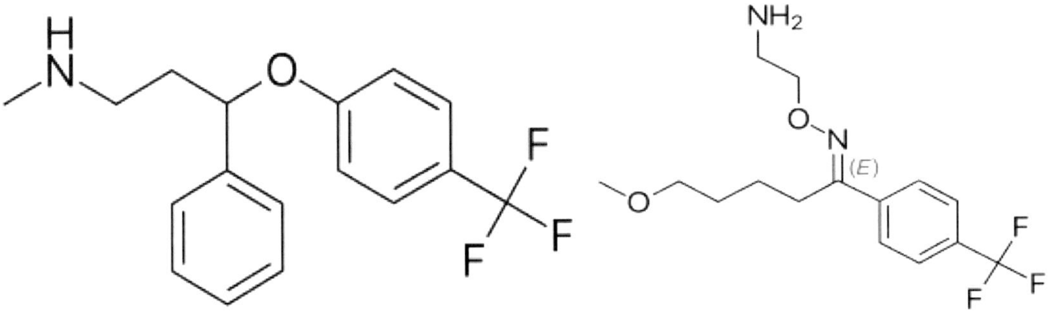

A. Fluoxetine B. Fluvoxamine

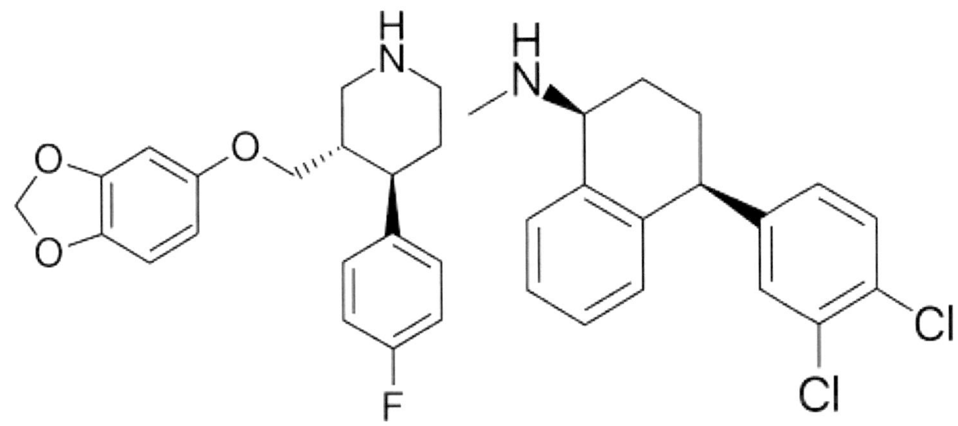

C. Paroxetine D. Sertraline

Figure 7: Chemical structures of SSRIs

Pharmacokinetics

SSRIs are well absorbed orally and only need to be taken once a day. (Preskorn 1997) Sometimes SSRIs (especially paroxetine) can cause sedation; twice daily dosing can be used if this potentially calming effect benefits the patient. Women develop higher serum SSRI levels than men at the same dose for reasons that are not entirely clear. (Preskorn 1997)

SSRIs are widely metabolized in the liver by the CYP450 enzymes. This makes drug-drug interactions a common problem when prescribing SSRIs (see Chapter 2). Sertraline, citalopram, and escitalopram have the lowest potential for drug-drug interactions. Fluvoxamine and fluoxetine have the highest potential for interactions due to their effects on CYP450 enzymes. All SSRIs, except fluvoxamine, come in liquid forms, making administration easier in people with pill swallowing issues or feeding tubes.

Mechanism of Action

As their name indicates, SSRIs inhibit the reuptake of neuronally-released serotonin by blocking SERT. This results in an increase in serotonin in the synaptic cleft. As described earlier (see TCA Mechanism of Action), this may result in the downregulation and desensitization of presynaptic receptors, leading to greater neurotransmitter release. Initially, efficacy was thought to be due to the enhanced effects of elevated serotonin on post-synaptic receptors. However, this mechanism does not entirely explain the antidepressant effects as the serotonin levels rise quickly, but the antidepressant effects take 1 – 6 weeks to start and at least 12 weeks for full effect.

Adverse Effects

SSRIs generally have fewer unwanted effects than other antidepressants, as they do not bind to as many different types of receptors.

Serotonin Syndrome: A severe side effect of SSRIs is serotonin syndrome. This occurs most frequently when the drug is first started or the dose is increased, especially if another serotonergic medication is used. Serotonin syndrome is described in more detail above.

Weight changes: SSRIs can produce both weight loss and weight gain. In general, weight gain tends to occur with higher doses and more prolonged use. The weight gained or lost is usually less than 5% of body weight.

Initial anxiety: When first started or after a dose increase, SSRIs can cause anxiety. This anxiety usually improves with time but can reoccur after further dose increases. Thus, starting at a low dose and slowly working up to a higher dose is essential. Most SSRI-induced anxiety resolves after six weeks at any given dose.

Sexual side effects: Sexual side effects are common with SSRIs. They occur in both women and men. Most commonly, they lower libido and delay orgasm. Although all SSRIs can cause sexual dysfunction, an individual patient may have more problems with one SSRI than another. Switching SSRIs because of sexual side effects sometimes solves the problem.

Hyponatremia: SSRIs can produce hyponatremia, primarily when used with other medications, such as diuretics which lead to low sodium. Hyponatremia is due to inappropriate antidiuretic hormone (ADH) secretion syndrome. It is most frequent in older adults.

Discontinuation syndrome: If SSRIs are stopped suddenly without tapering, a discontinuation syndrome occurs in about 30% of patients. Symptoms include nausea, dizziness, headache, and fatigue. Often the patient feels like they have the flu. Less common symptoms include agitation, irritability, insomnia, tremor, and an electric shock-type sensation in the head, often called "brain zaps." When these symptoms are recognized, a lower dose of the antidepressant should be restarted and slowly tapered. The discontinuation symptoms usually resolve promptly after resuming the medication.

QTc prolongation: A dose-dependent QTc prolongation has been identified with citalopram. The maximum FDA-approved dose of citalopram was lowered from 60 mg to 40 mg because of QTc concerns.

The S isomer of citalopram, escitalopram, does not have the same risk and tends to produce fewer adverse effects than the racemic mixture of S and R isomers found in citalopram. To a lesser extent, other SSRIs also cause QTc prolongation, but in isolation, this is rarely clinically significant. The risk is elevated if SSRIs are used with another medication that prolongs QTc. An EKG should be checked before initiating citalopram to be sure the patient does not already have a prolonged QTc. A different antidepressant should be started if the QTc is 500 milliseconds or more.

Other adverse effects of SSRIs include:

- Drowsiness
- Insomnia
- Nausea (usually transient)
- Headache
- Tremor
- Constipation

Safety in Overdose for SSRIs

SSRIs are the safest antidepressants in overdose. Serotonin syndrome may develop, but fatalities are rare.

Drug-Specific Factors for SSRIs

Fluoxetine has an active metabolite, norfluoxetine, with a very long half-life. It can take up to five weeks for fluoxetine to be eliminated from the body. This characteristic is taken advantage of in a once-weekly formulation containing 90 mg of fluoxetine. If a higher dose of fluoxetine is required, weekly administration is inappropriate. No other SSRIs have active metabolites.

Sertraline is better absorbed when taken with food. All other SSRIs are absorbed independently from food intake. Paroxetine is the most likely SSRI to lead to discontinuation, as it has a slightly shorter half-life and is less likely to cause discontinuation syndrome.

Serotonin-norepinephrine reuptake inhibitors (SNRIs)

Desvenlafaxine
Duloxetine
Levomilnacipran
Milnacipran
Venlafaxine

Background and Clinical Use

Antidepressant efficacy is not limited to effects on serotonin, as was initially thought when SSRIs were developed. A new class of antidepressants, acting on serotonin and norepinephrine transporters, was also effective. These SNRIs have more adverse effects and toxicity in overdose than the SSRIs and hence are not usually first-line agents. They have the added benefit of being helpful for pain, especially neurologically induced pain (e.g., peripheral neuropathy, fibromyalgia).

The SNRIs differ in their binding affinities to serotonin and norepinephrine reuptake transporters. For example, venlafaxine binds mainly to SERT at low doses but, at higher doses, binds to both SERT and NET. (Debonnel et al. 2007) At maximum doses, it still binds to SERT with 30 times its affinity for NET. (Sansone and Sansone 2014) Duloxetine shares the pattern of binding first to serotonin and then to norepinephrine reuptake pumps. Still, it has increased binding to NET, with the relative ratio of maximum binding being only 10:1 affinity for SERT: NET. (Sansone and Sansone 2014)

Milnacipran and levomilnacipran do not bind sequentially to SERT and NET; they bind immediately to both transporters. (Sansone and Sansone 2014) Milnacipran has a 1:1 SERT: NET binding and levomilnacipran has a 1:2 ratio. Hence levomilnacipran is the only SNRI that binds with greater affinity to NET than SERT. The clinical effect of these differences in relative binding to serotonin and norepinephrine transporters has yet to be fully elucidated. Still, binding to norepinephrine receptors helps the most with pain.

SNRIs have unique chemical structures, with little resemblance to each other, except for those derived from each other. Desvenlafaxine is an active metabolite of venlafaxine, formed by removing a methyl group attached to an oxygen atom and creating a hydroxyl group (Figure 8A, B). Levomilnacipran is the L isomer of milnacipran. Milnacipran occurs in 2 active isomers, but levomilnacipran is the most active form (Figure 8C, D). As is evident from the figure of these medications, there is a structural similarity between venlafaxine/desvenlafaxine and milnacipran/levomilnacipran. Duloxetine has yet another completely different structure (Figure 8E).

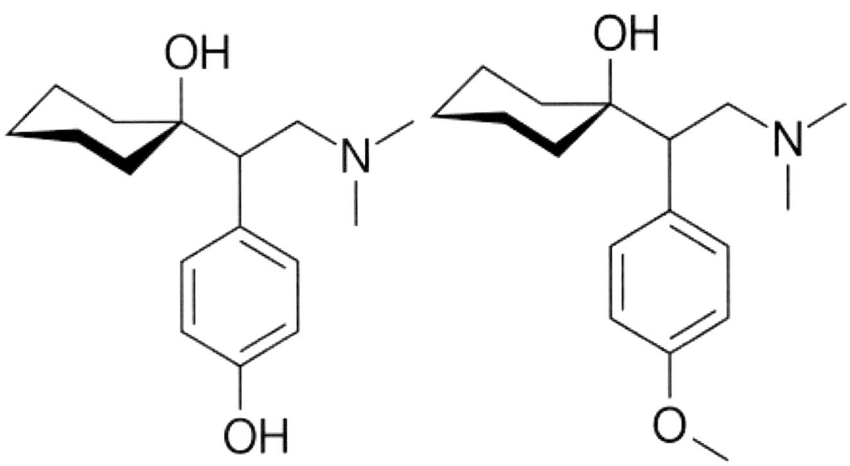

A.. Desvenlafaxine B.. Venlafaxine

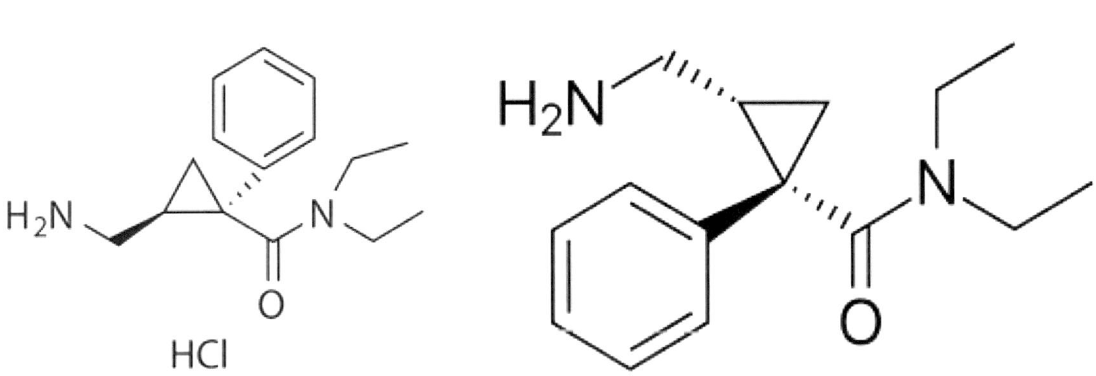

C.. Milnacipran (racemic mix of D& L isomers) D.. Levomilnacipran (L isomer only)

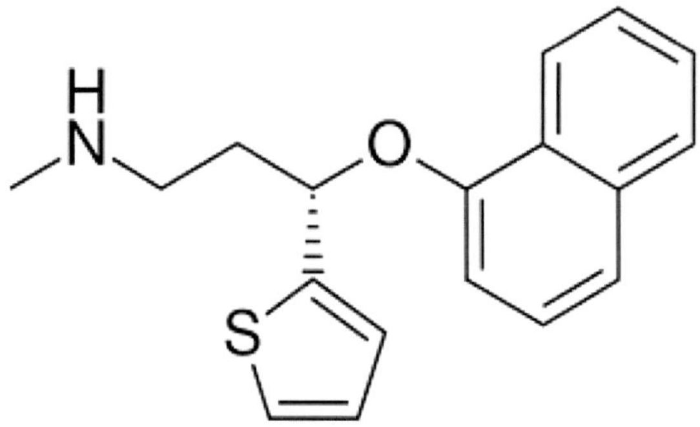

E.. Duloxetine

Figure 8. Chemical structures of SNRIs.

Pharmacokinetics/Pharmacodynamics of SNRIs

SNRIs are absorbed well after oral administration. Taking them with food can decrease the common side effect of nausea because it slows absorption and lowers the bloodstream dose. Food does not reduce the total amount of SNRI absorbed, however.

Venlafaxine, duloxetine, and, to some extent, desvenlafaxine are metabolized in the liver by CYP450 enzymes. They are liable to drug-drug interaction; caution is required when administered with CYP450 inducers and inhibitors. Duloxetine should not be used in patients with liver dysfunction or stage 4 (severe) or 5 (end-stage) kidney disease.

Both milnacipran and levomilnacipran are excreted primarily in the urine without undergoing CYP450 biotransformation. Levomilnacipran does not need any dose adjustment for liver problems. It is secreted mainly in the urine and should not be used in end-stage renal disease because it can accumulate and cause toxicity. It has a short half-life of 4 to 6 hours and is thus dosed twice daily. Similarly, milnacipran is not metabolized by CYP450 enzymes and has minimal drug interactions due to altered CYP activity. However, it does undergo some hepatic metabolism and should not be used in patients with liver failure. It is excreted by the kidneys and should be avoided in patients with kidney failure.

Adverse Effects of SNRIs

All SNRIs can cause discontinuation syndrome, also known as withdrawal syndrome. (Fava et al. 2018) SNRI discontinuation syndrome is very similar to SSRI discontinuation syndrome. Both occur in the first few days after stopping the antidepressant. Both can be treated by resuming a lower dose of the antidepressant and then tapering it more slowly. Common symptoms are nausea, dizziness, headache, insomnia, anxiety, sweating, weakness, and "brain zaps". (Fava et al. 2018) Avoiding discontinuation syndrome is an important reason to continue these medications when someone is admitted to the hospital unless the drug seems to be actively causing medical problems.

Nausea: The most commonly noted side effect for all SNRIs is nausea. Taking food with the medication will help alleviate this symptom. Nausea often improves as the patient stays on the SNRI.

BP elevation: To the extent that SNRIs increase norepinephrine levels, they are also likely to increase blood pressure. The increases are usually modest, but patients require monitoring.

Sexual dysfunction: All SNRIs can cause sexual dysfunction. Venlafaxine is the most likely to cause this unwanted effect. Switching to other SNRIs or SSRIs may help if a patient has this problem.

Serotonin syndrome: Serotonin syndrome is a risk with all the SNRIs. It occurs most frequently when the medication is first started or when doses are increased. Interactions with other drugs that increase serotonin levels, such as SSRIs and other antidepressants, tramadol, and dextromethorphan elevate the risk of serotonin syndrome.

QTc Prolongation: Venlafaxine is the only SNRI known to cause QTc prolongation.

Other side effects of SNRIs include:

- Insomnia
- Agitation
- Drowsiness
- Constipation
- Hyponatremia
- Sweating

Safety in Overdose for SNRIs

SNRIs are much more severe in overdose than SSRIs. Venlafaxine is the most dangerous in overdose, causing seizures, cardiac arrhythmias, serotonin syndrome, and sedation.

Drug-Specific Factors for SNRIs

Desvenlafaxine is the active metabolite of venlafaxine, and generally, side effects are not as severe as with venlafaxine. Sexual dysfunction is usually less. Compared to venlafaxine, desvenlafaxine has more activity at norepinephrine receptors. Desvenlafaxine is safer in overdose than venlafaxine.

Duloxetine is the SNRI that has the most FDA approvals for pain conditions. It treats depression and anxiety but is effective in pain conditions independent of depression or anxiety. It is approved for fibromyalgia, diabetic peripheral neuropathy, musculoskeletal pain, and osteoarthritis. Duloxetine is metabolized by the CYP450 enzymes in the liver and then excreted in the kidneys. It should not be used in patients with liver dysfunction or stage 4 (severe) or 5 (end stage) kidney failure.

Levomilnacipran is the L isomer of milnacipran. Of the two isomers, it is the most active. It is also the only SNRI with a higher affinity for norepinephrine than serotonin. The CYP450 enzymes do not metabolize Levomilnacipran, and thus it has fewer drug interactions. It does not need any dose adjustments for liver problems. It is secreted primarily in the urine and should not be used in end-stage renal disease because it can accumulate and cause toxicity.

Milnacipran is only FDA-approved for fibromyalgia, although it is used in other countries for depression and anxiety. It has a short half-life of 4 to 6 hours and should be dosed twice daily. CYP450 enzymes do not metabolize it, so it has minimal drug interactions. It is secreted in the kidneys. It does have some metabolism in the liver and should not be used in patients with either liver or kidney failure.

Venlafaxine is metabolized primarily through the CYP450 enzymes and is thus prone to drug interactions. It comes in an immediate-release form, which should be dosed twice daily, and an extended-release form, which is dosed daily. The immediate release form should be used with patients who have had bariatric surgery or have another cause of decreased absorption. Venlafaxine has the highest affinity for serotonin receptors compared to norepinephrine receptors of any SNRI.

Serotonin Modulators

Nefazodone
Trazodone
Vilazodone
Vortioxetine

Background and Clinical Use

Serotonin modulators are second-generation antidepressants that act at both presynaptic and postsynaptic sites, altering neurotransmitter levels and stimulating or antagonizing receptors. Different members of this class have other actions. Still, all can block serotonin reuptake (like SSRIs) at presynaptic sites and act as agonists, antagonists, or partial serotonin agonists at postsynaptic receptors. Like all other antidepressants, the exact mechanism through which these bindings yield their psychiatric effects is unclear. Specific reuptake and serotonin actions are listed in Table 1 for reference purposes:

Table 1: Mechanism of Action of Serotonin Modulators

Drug	Presynaptic Action	Postsynaptic Action
Nefazodone	Inhibits reuptake of serotonin and norepinephrine	Inhibits 5-HT 2A receptors, which causes an upregulation of 5-HT 1 A receptors
Trazodone	Inhibits serotonin reuptake	Mixed agonist (at high doses)/antagonist (at low doses) for 5-HT 2A and 2C receptors Inhibits α adrenoreceptors and H1 histamine receptors
Vilazodone	Inhibits serotonin reuptake	Partial agonist of 5-HT 1A receptors
Vortioxetine	Inhibits serotonin reuptake	Binds to: 5-HT 1A – agonist 5-HT 1B – partial agonist 5-HT 1D – antagonist 5-HT 3 – antagonist 5-HT 7 - antagonist

Serotonin modulators have no structural similarity, as seen in the pictures below.

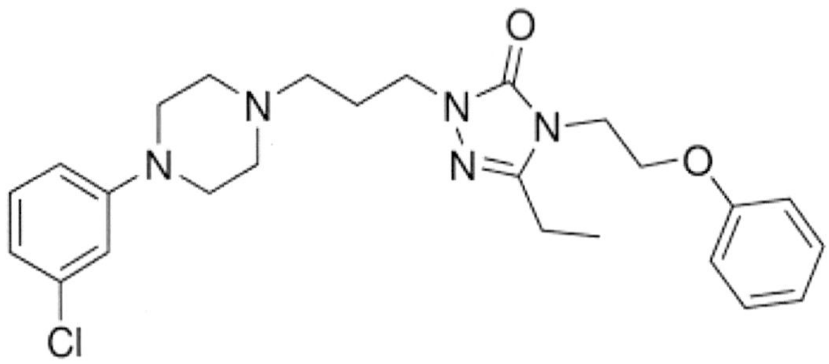

A.. Nefazodone

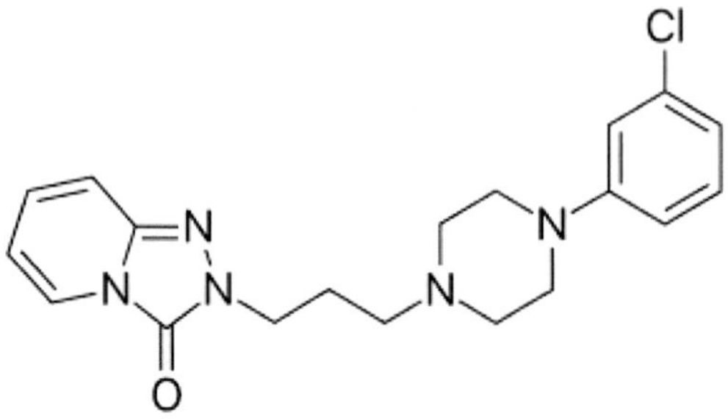

B.. Trazodone

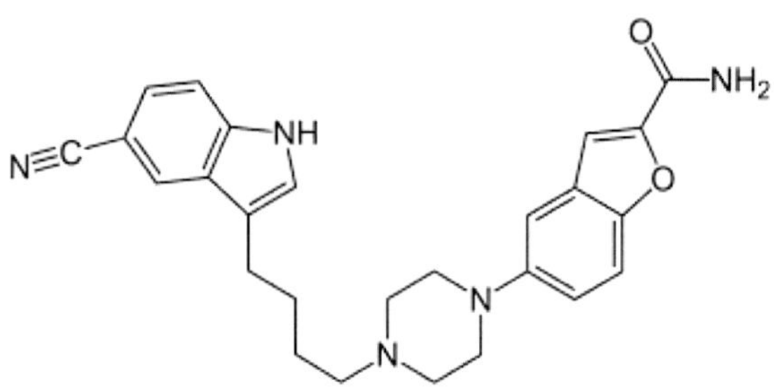

C.. Vilazodone

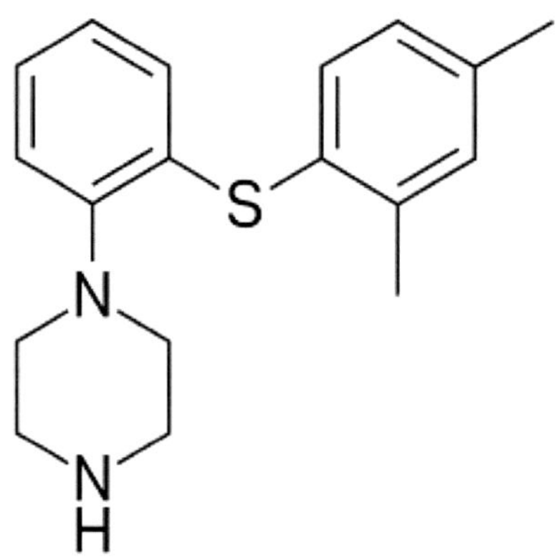

D.. Vortioxetine

Figure 9. Chemical structures of serotonin modulators

Pharmacokinetics

All serotonin modulators undergo extensive metabolism by CYP450 enzymes, making drug-drug interactions a significant concern. Trazodone has a relatively short half-life of 5 – 9 hrs. All the other serotonin modulators have half-lives of 24 hours or longer. Taking serotonin modulators with food either helps absorption or has no effect, except for nefazodone, which has decreased absorption with food.

Adverse Effects of Serotonin Modulators

Gastrointestinal issues: Gastrointestinal side effects are serotonin modulators' most common side effects. Nausea and diarrhea can be expected but usually get better with increased time on the medications. A further dose increase might exacerbate the GI symptoms, but they will improve again with time.

Sexual side effects: In general, sexual side effects are less prevalent with this class of medications than with SSRIs and SNRIs. Switching from a different class of antidepressants to a serotonin modulator may help improve antidepressant-induced sexual side effects.

Serotonin syndrome: Like other serotonin drugs, serotonin modulators can lead to serotonin syndrome. This occurs most frequently when the drug is first started, or the dose is increased, especially if another serotonergic medication is being taken. Symptoms of serotonin syndrome include altered mental status (agitation, confusion), autonomic instability (blood pressure fluctuations, fever, diaphoresis), and neuromuscular problems (tremors, clonus, hyperreflexia, ataxia). There is a spectrum of severity with serotonin syndrome. Most cases are mild, but severe cases occur, which are potentially lethal.

Other side effects of Serotonin Modulators include:

- Dizziness
- Headache
- Diarrhea
- Dry mouth
- Sedation
- Hyponatremia
- Tremor

Safety in Overdose for Serotonin Modulators

Serotonin modulators are safer in overdose than tricyclics but not as safe as SSRIs. They can lead to serotonin syndrome, cardiac arrhythmias, and liver problems.

Drug-Specific Factors for Serotonin Modulators

Nefazodone was voluntarily removed from the market by the original company that manufactured it because of rare cases of liver failure that usually occurred in the first six months of therapy. It is manufactured as a generic, but few patients are started on it, and it should never be used as a first-line therapy. (Dunner et al. 2002; Gomez et al. 2018)

Sedation is a significant side effect of trazodone. It is used primarily at a low dose (50 – 200 mg) as a sleep aid, despite being a therapeutic antidepressant at higher doses (up to 600 mg). (Fagiolini et al. 2012) Trazodone has the potential to prolong QTc, especially at higher doses. It should be used cautiously in people over 65 and with patients at an increased risk of QTc prolongation because of electrolyte imbalances, other QTc prolonging medications, or genetic problems. (Tellone et al. 2020)

Vilazodone is distinguished by a propensity to act a little more quickly than other antidepressants. Improvements in depression may be seen as early as week two of treatment. (Dawson and Watson 2009; Shi et al. 2016)

There is some evidence that vortioxetine may help more specifically with the cognitive dysfunction symptoms of depression than other antidepressants. It improved cognitive function in animal models of depression and human trials. The mechanism behind this is not known. (Sanchez et al. 2015)

ATYPICAL ANTIDEPRESSANTS

Brexanolone
Bupropion
Mirtazapine

Background and Clinical Use

These three antidepressants have unique mechanisms of action not shared by other drugs. Hence they are currently called atypical antidepressants. Brexanolone is the newest; both bupropion and mirtazapine have been around for longer. As can be seen, by the pictures below, there is no structural similarity between these drugs.

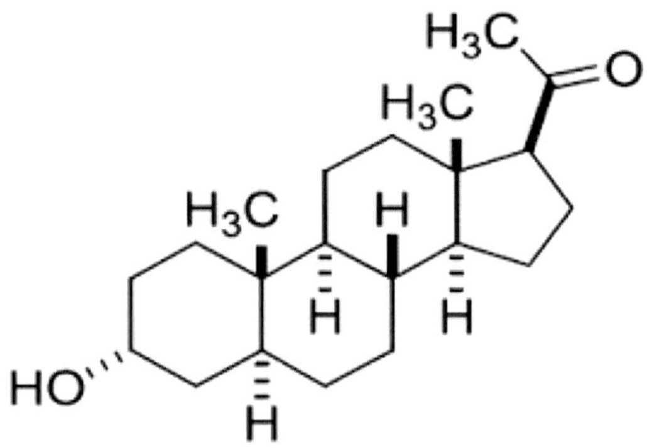

A.. Brexanolone

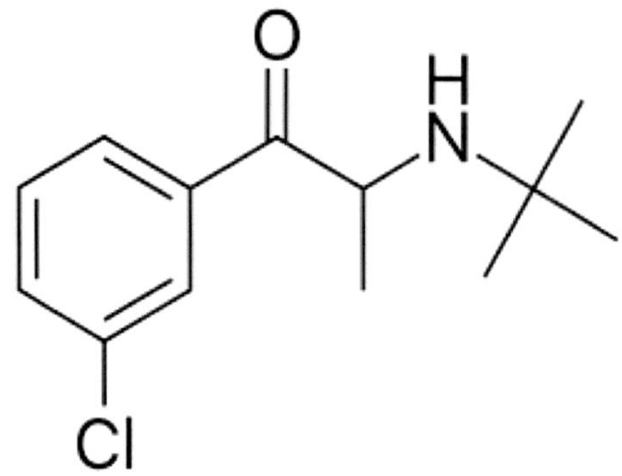

B.. Bupropion

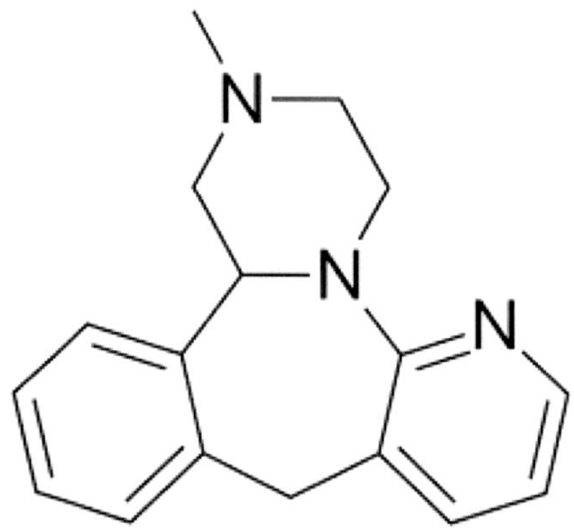

C.. Mirtazapine

Figure 10. Chemical structures of atypical antidepressants.

Since the pharmacology of each member of the group of atypical antidepressants differs, they will be dealt with individually rather than as a class.

Brexanolone

Brexanolone, the newest antidepressant, is a first of its kind in several ways. It is currently the only antidepressant given as an IV medication. Due to poor oral absorption, it is not available in pill form. (Cornett et al. 2021) Brexanolone is identical in structure to a naturally occurring hormone, allopregnanolone, which rises during pregnancy but falls quickly after delivery. (Cornett et al. 2021) Allopregnanolone (Brexanolone) is a metabolite of progesterone. Brexanolone is only used for severe postpartum depression. It cannot be given to a pregnant woman.

Postpartum depression is not a DSM-5-TR diagnosis; instead, women are considered to have a major depressive episode with peripartum onset. Peripartum depression occurs anywhere from the start of pregnancy to 4 weeks after delivery. It is common, affecting up to 10% of pregnancies. (*American Psychiatric Association: Diagnostic and Statistical Manual of Mental Disorders: DSM-5-TR* 2022) Many women have postpartum "baby blues," lasting two weeks or less. This does not meet the full criteria for a major depressive episode and is not considered a psychiatric disorder. (*American Psychiatric Association: Diagnostic and Statistical Manual of Mental Disorders: DSM-5-TR* 2022) Postpartum depression starts anywhere from the 3rd trimester of pregnancy until the first four weeks after delivery. (Cornett et al. 2021) When severe, it is included in the DSM-5-TR diagnosis of peripartum depression.

Postpartum depression ranges in severity from mild to severe. The most severe form is postpartum depression with psychosis. This is very rare (0.1 – 0.2% of deliveries) but has extremely infrequently resulted in suicide or infanticide, often triggered by psychotic hallucinations. (*American Psychiatric Association: Diagnostic and Statistical Manual of Mental Disorders: DSM-5-TR* 2022) Depressive and psychotic symptoms should always be considered in postpartum women. Women with a history of previous peripartum depression with psychosis have a higher chance of developing it again with subsequent pregnancies. (*American Psychiatric Association: Diagnostic and Statistical Manual of Mental Disorders: DSM-5-TR* 2022)

Pharmacokinetics

Brexanolone has very low bioavailability when taken orally (about 5%) and has a short half-life. (Cornett et al. 2021) It is given as an IV infusion over 60 hrs to provide a continuous steady-state serum level. Because of significant severe side effects, including excessive sedation and loss of consciousness, brexanolone can only be given through a risk evaluation and mitigation strategy (REMS) program, which requires physicians and pharmacists to have specific training to prescribe and dispense brexanolone.

Brexanolone can provide very rapid relief of symptoms. After the 60 hr infusion, many patients have no further symptoms of depression. (Cornett et al. 2021) The only study that followed the length of response went up to 30 days and found little recurrence of depression. (Cornett et al. 2021)

Mechanism of Action

Brexanolone's mechanism of action is thought to be through the stimulation of the GABAA receptor. (Cornett et al. 2021). It is an analog of allopregnanolone, an endogenous steroid hormone that increases during pregnancy and decreases rapidly after birth. The rapid decrease in allopregnanolone levels is thought to be responsible for post-partum depression in some women.

Side Effects of Brexanolone

Serious side effects: Brexanolone can cause severe sedation, hypoxia, and sudden loss of consciousness. Women receiving it need to have regular monitoring, including pulse oximetry. Brexanolone can only be given in the hospital, where patients receive regular monitoring.

Other side effects of brexanolone:

- Dizziness
- Dyspepsia
- Diarrhea
- Dry mouth
- Hot flash
- Tachycardia

Safety in Overdose of Brexanolone:

No information is available about overdoses on brexanolone. Since it is only given IV in a supervised setting, overdose is much less likely.

Bupropion

Bupropion is indicated for treating major depressive episodes, seasonal affective disorder, and smoking cessation. It is marketed separately for smoking cessation under a different trade name.

In contrast to SSRIs/SNRIs, bupropion does not cause sexual dysfunction. It also does not cause weight gain and may contribute to weight loss.

Bupropion comes in immediate-release (taken three times a day), extended-release 12 hr (taken twice a day), and extended-release 24-hour formulations (taken once a day in the morning). The immediate-release pills are helpful for people with GI problems who may not absorb the longer-acting formulations.

Pharmacokinetics

Bupropion is metabolized in the liver by multiple CYP450 enzymes and has many potential drug-drug interactions. It is excreted by the kidneys. Dose adjustments must be considered for patients with either kidney or liver impairment. Caution should be used in older adults more prone to kidney and liver impairment.

Like most antidepressants, bupropion's mechanism is not well defined. It appears not to have any effect on serotonin reuptake, but rather, its primary action is thought to be via inhibition of the reuptake of both dopamine and norepinephrine.

Adverse Effects of Bupropion

Seizures: Bupropion can induce seizures and should not be used in anyone with a history of seizure disorder. The risk of seizures is greater at higher doses. Bupropion should also not be given to people prone to electrolyte disorders, such as patients with frequent vomiting or diarrhea, as they are more likely to develop seizures.

Anxiety: Bupropion can also cause significant anxiety in susceptible patients. This is less likely to happen if the patient is also on an SSRI.

Insomnia: Bupropion can cause insomnia and should not be taken at bedtime. Ideally, the last dose should be at least 4 – 6 hrs before bedtime for the immediate- and sustained-release 12 hr formulations.

Other side effects of Bupropion include:

- Dry mouth
- Constipation
- Tremor
- Headache
- Weight loss
- Increases the risk of closed-angle glaucoma

Safety in Overdose of Bupropion

Bupropion is less safe than SSRIs in overdose but is safer than TCAs or MAOI antidepressants. By itself, bupropion rarely causes death. It can cause seizures, hallucinations, and agitation. It does not have cardiac toxicity or affect QT interval. (Lee et al. 2021)

Mirtazapine

Mirtazapine is approved only for the treatment of depression in the US.

Pharmacokinetics

CYP450 enzymes metabolize mirtazapine, so drug-drug interactions should be considered when prescribing it. Metabolism occurs in the liver and excretion via the kidney; doses must be adjusted for either hepatic or renal dysfunction. (Kaufman et al. 2016)

Mechanism of Action

Mirtazapine has a unique mechanism of action among antidepressants. (Kaufman et al. 2016) It increases serotonin and norepinephrine levels in the synaptic cleft but does not do this through reuptake inhibition. Instead, it blocks presynaptic α_2-adrenoceptors, leading to increased secretion of norepinephrine and serotonin into the synaptic cleft. This means more of these transmitters are available at the receptors on the postsynaptic neuron. (Kaufman et al. 2016) In addition, mirtazapine blocks serotonin 5-HT_2 and 5-HT_3 receptors, leaving most of serotonin to bind to 5-HT_{1A} receptors. These postsynaptic 5-HT_{1A} receptors are essential in treating depression and anxiety. (Lee et al. 2010)

Adverse Effects of Mirtazapine

Sedation and weight gain: The most significant side effects of mirtazapine are sedation and weight gain, both caused by the antagonism of histamine H1 receptors. Mirtazapine is often used for people with difficulty sleeping, especially if they need to gain weight, to take advantage of these side effects. Counterintuitively, these side effects are worse at lower doses of mirtazapine and often improve at doses of 15 mg daily or higher. (Kaufman et al. 2016) The affinity of mirtazapine for histamine H1 receptors is highest at lower doses and decreases at higher doses, which explains this observation. (Kaufman et al. 2016) In addition, at higher doses, mirtazapine has a more significant effect on norepinephrine release, which may at least partially counter the histamine-blocking effects of the drug. Patients do develop tolerance to the sedative effect of mirtazapine but often have continued weight gain on mirtazapine. Eventually, many people stop it because of weight gain. Mirtazapine can also increase cholesterol and other lipid levels.

Rare but dangerous side effects: The most life-threatening side effects of mirtazapine are cardiac arrhythmias and hematologic abnormalities, including thrombocytopenia, leukopenia, and agranulocytosis. Fortunately, arrhythmias and blood disorders are infrequent.

Sexual side effects: Even though mirtazapine increases serotonin levels, it has much lower rates of sexual side effects compared to most other serotonergic antidepressants, such as SSRIs and SNRIs. This is through the blockade of 5-HT_2 and 5-HT_3 receptors. (Gill et al. 2020)

Other side effects of mirtazapine include:

- Constipation
- Peripheral edema
- Abnormal dreams
- Dizziness
- Tremor

Safety in Overdose of Mirtazapine

Mirtazapine is not as safe as SSRIs in overdose. It can cause cardiac arrhythmias and excessive sedation. In rare cases, it can be fatal. Serotonin syndrome is another possibility.

ANTI-ANXIETY MEDICATION

Besides some serotonergic antidepressants, two other types of medications are approved for treating anxiety: Benzodiazepines and buspirone. Buspirone is currently the only medication in its class marketed in the US. There are seven benzodiazepines marketed in the US for anxiety disorders. Buspirone and benzodiazepines have no structural similarity and bind to different receptors to reduce anxiety. Benzodiazepines reduce anxiety quickly, but the anxiety returns as the drug wears off. Like antidepressants, buspirone takes weeks to work but then prevents the development of anxiety. Benzodiazepines come with a higher risk of adverse effects, including drug dependence and abuse, and a higher risk of drug interactions. As such, their clinical use is usually limited to short-term treatment. Buspirone does not present the same risks and can be used long-term.

Buspirone

Background and Clinical Use

Buspirone is the only drug in its class available in the US. It is an anti-anxiety medication that does not work through GABA or benzodiazepine receptors. It is only FDA-approved to treat generalized anxiety disorder, but it is sometimes used off-label as an augmenter of an antidepressant to help with anxiety and depression in patients with major depressive disorder. It is not used as monotherapy for major depressive disorder.

Like all antidepressants, buspirone takes weeks to months for full effectiveness and often doesn't have any effect noticeable to the patient for the first month or so. This can be quite discouraging, especially when the benzodiazepines provide immediate if temporary, anxiety relief. Often, patients on benzodiazepines first don't find buspirone effective for anxiety. This is likely because they have grown accustomed to the immediate relief provided by benzodiazepines. The advantage of buspirone is that it does not have addictive qualities or other unwanted effects of benzodiazepines.

Buspirone was developed prior to SSRIs, and in the 1980's was tested against two early benzodiazepines, diazepam and clorazepate. Buspirone's efficacy was similar to these two benzodiazepines. (Goldberg and Finnerty 1979; Eison and Temple 1986)

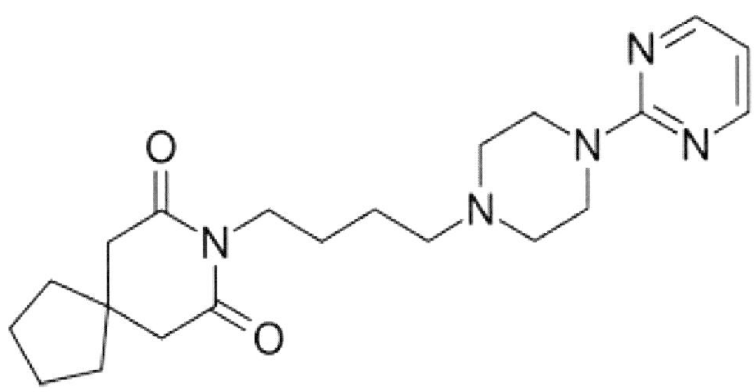

Buspirone

Figure 11. Chemical Structure of Buspirone

Pharmacokinetics

Buspirone is rapidly absorbed after oral administration, but only about 4% of the drug is bioavailable. (Mahmood and Sahajwalla 1999) CYP450 enzymes metabolize buspirone, and in liver failure, levels increase. (Dalhoff et al. 1987) It should not be used in patients with significant liver problems.

Mechanism of Action

Buspirone binds to serotonin 5-HT_{1A} and 5-HT_2 receptors eliciting an inhibitory action on serotonergic activity. It also blocks presynaptic dopamine receptors, increasing dopamine neurotransmission. (Mahmood and Sahajwalla 1999) The structure of buspirone (Figure 11) is not like any of the other psychotropic medications.

Side Effects of Buspirone

Serotonin syndrome: Buspirone can cause serotonin syndrome due to its serotonergic activity. Symptoms of serotonin syndrome are described elsewhere in this chapter.

Movement disorders: Rarely, buspirone causes movement disorders such as dyskinesia, akathisia, clonus, Parkinsonism, and dystonia. (Rissardo and Caprara 2020) Stopping buspirone can treat these problems, which resolves the symptoms. (Rissardo and Caprara 2020)

Other side effects of Buspirone include:

- Dizziness
- Diarrhea
- Nausea
- Headache
- Diaphoresis

Safety in Overdose of Buspirone

Buspirone is safer in overdose than benzodiazepines, even when mixed with alcohol. Serotonin syndrome can occur. Also, cardiac arrhythmias and seizures have been reported.

Benzodiazepines (BZD; see also Chapters 16 and 23)

Alprazolam
Clonazepam
Chlordiazepoxide
Clorazepate
Diazepam
Lorazepam
Oxazepam

Above are the benzodiazepines that are FDA-approved to treat anxiety disorders, which will be discussed in this chapter. Other benzodiazepines are FDA-approved for alcohol withdrawal, insomnia, muscle spasms, muscle rigidity, sedation, and seizures and will not be discussed here. For reference, the other benzodiazepines for use in the US are:

Alcohol withdrawal – Chlordiazepoxide, diazepam, and oxazepam
Insomnia – Estazolam, quazepam, temazepam, and triazolam
Muscle spasms and rigidity – Diazepam
Seizure disorder – Clobazam, clonazepam, clorazepate, diazepam, lorazepam, and midazolam
Sedation – Midazolam

Benzodiazepines are unique in psychopharmacology because they exert their effects quickly after ingestion. (Edinoff et al. 2021) However, their effects do not last long after the drug has left the body. This contrasts sharply with other medications discussed in this chapter, as they must build up in the body over weeks before the medication yields results. This is quite frustrating to the patient, as the drug must be taken daily for weeks without feeling much benefit. It is much more satisfying to take a benzodiazepine and feel better within minutes to hours. The problem is that the effectiveness of benzodiazepines wears off within hours, and anxiety often comes rushing back (rebound anxiety), sometimes worse than before taking the benzodiazepine.

One way to help patients and their families understand this is to compare benzodiazepines to ibuprofen/acetaminophen and antidepressants/buspirone to an antibiotic. When someone has a fever because of an infection, taking ibuprofen or acetaminophen causes the fever to go away quickly, but it will come back soon because nothing has been done to treat the infection, which is the underlying problem. When the person is given an antibiotic, it does not lower the fever immediately, but by treating the infection, in a few days, the fever is gone and does not return. Antidepressants and buspirone do not take anxiety away initially, but in the long run, they treat and prevent anxiety.

The quick effectiveness of benzodiazepines makes them all physically and psychologically addictive. The beneficial effect is quickly achieved, and then when it dissipates, it is desired again, which can lead to compulsive cravings and misuse. This is important to discuss with the patient. Before starting these medications, patients should be asked about any history of addiction or family history of addiction, as these are risk factors that increase the patient's chances of addiction. Problems with alcohol are especially important to ascertain, as alcohol and benzodiazepines both act as positive modulators of the GABA receptor. (Olsen 2018) Thus, a person may experience similar sensations to alcohol and benzodiazepines, and having a history of alcohol misuse puts them at increased risk for addiction to benzodiazepines.

Benzodiazepines have similar structures: they all have two benzenes (six-carbon aromatic rings), a seven-carbon ring containing two nitrogen atoms, and one chlorine atom attached to a benzene ring. The structures below show these similarities:

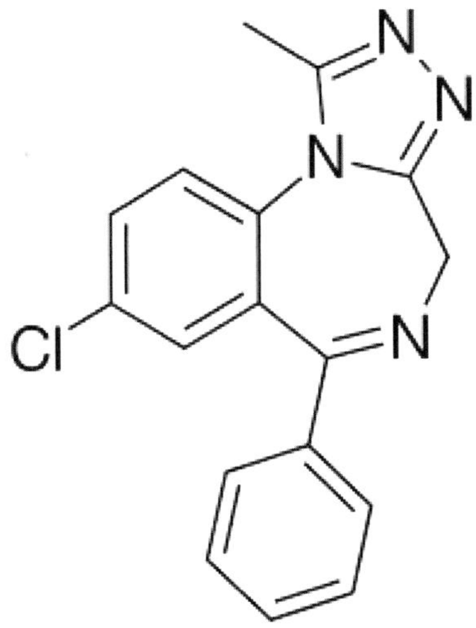

A.. Alprazolam

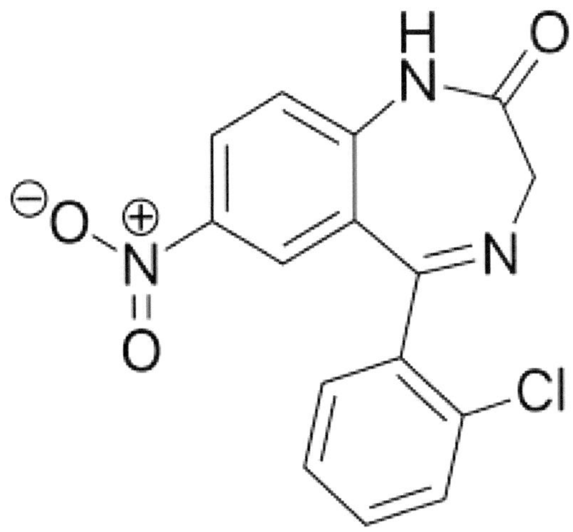

B.. Clonazepam

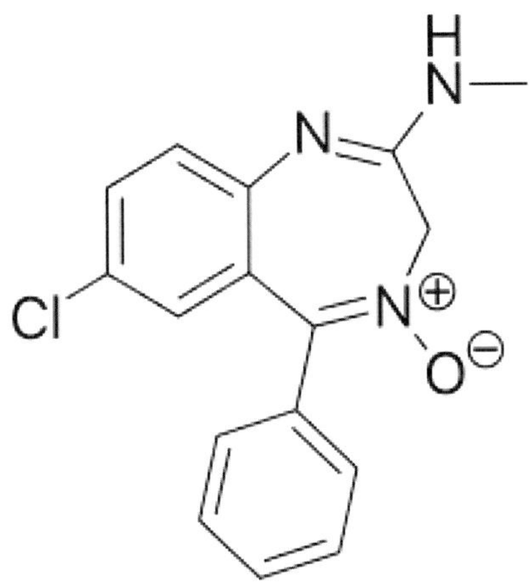

C.. Chlordiazepoxide

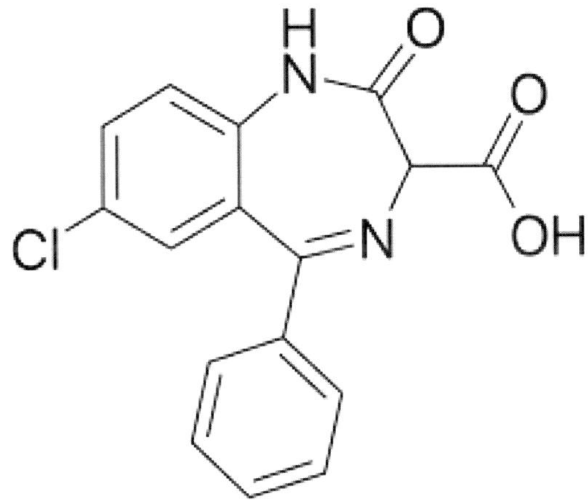

D. Clorazepate

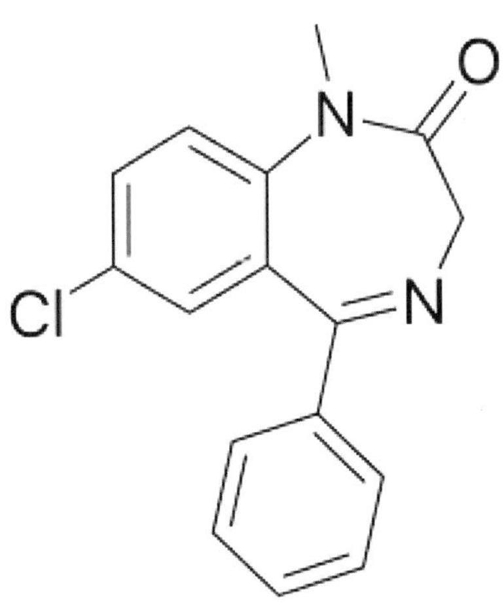

E. Diazepam

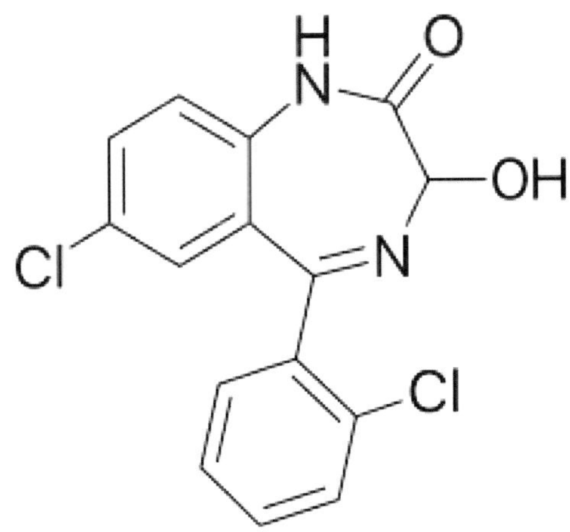

F. Lorazepam

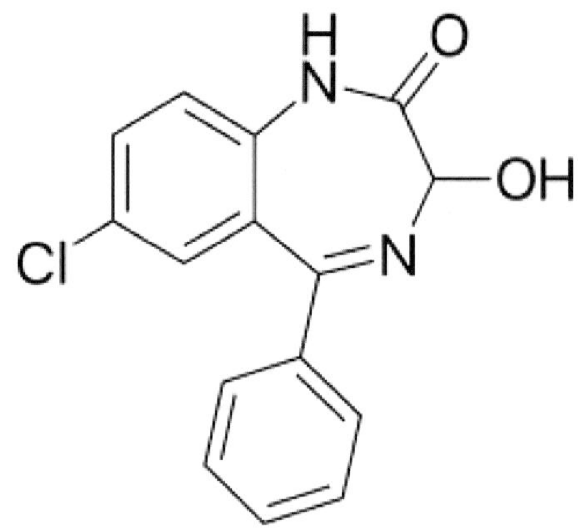

G. Oxazepam

Figure 12: Chemical structure of benzodiazepines

Pharmacokinetics

Based on their half-lives, benzodiazepines are divided into short-acting (half-life of 11 hours or less), intermediate-acting (half-life of 12 – 23 hours), and long-acting (half-life of 24 or more hours). (Greenblatt et al. 1981) By this definition, none of the benzodiazepines used for anxiety disorders are short-acting.

Another clinically significant piece of information is how quickly the drug's effect is felt (speed of onset). Speed of onset measures how quickly the compound enters the brain to exert its action. More lipophilic compounds have a faster speed of onset. The speed of onset can be classified as rapid, intermediate, or slow. (Dubovsky and Marshall 2022) Some of the pharmacokinetic properties of benzodiazepines are summarized in Table 2, and more detail about individual drugs is provided below.

Table 2 Select pharmacokinetic properties of benzodiazepines

Category of Half-life	Drug	Speed of Onset	Half-life (hours)	Active Metabolites
Intermediate	Alprazolam	Rapid	6 - 20	No
Intermediate	Lorazepam	Intermediate	10 – 20	No
Intermediate	Oxazepam	Slow	5 – 20	No
Long	Clonazepam	Intermediate	18 – 50	No
Long	Clorazepate	Slow	20- 160	Nordiazepam, Oxazepam
Long	Chlordiazepoxide	Intermediate	5-30	Nordiazepam
Long	Diazepam	Rapid	20 – 50	Nordiazepam

The addiction potential of a benzodiazepine is related to its speed of onset and its half-life. Rapid onset means the patient feels a more immediate relief of their symptoms, making the drug highly desirable. A short half-life means the drug wears off quickly, often leading to cravings for more of the drug. Note that of the benzodiazepines for anxiety, alprazolam and diazepam both have a rapid onset. Alprazolam has a shorter half-life and is most likely to cause addiction. Diazepam is also addictive because of its rapid onset, but its long half-life makes it less addictive than alprazolam.

Most benzodiazepines are metabolized in the liver by the CYP3A4 isoform of CYP450 enzymes. Some of these metabolites are active and have longer half-lives than the parent compound. Several of the benzodiazepines (chlordiazepoxide, diazepam, and clorazepate) have a common final metabolite, oxazepam, which itself is commercially available. Most benzodiazepines are dangerous in liver disease, as the drug and its metabolites build-up due to the lack of normal metabolism. Lorazepam and oxazepam are notable exceptions to this, as the CYP450 enzymes do not metabolize them. For this reason, along with its more rapid speed of onset, lorazepam is often used for treating alcohol withdrawal.

Alprazolam is very lipophilic and so has a rapid onset of action, increasing its addiction potential. It has one of the shortest half-lives of the benzodiazepines used for anxiety disorders. These two traits make it one of the most commonly abused benzodiazepines. (Edinoff et al. 2021) Falls in elderly patients are also more frequent with alprazolam than with other benzodiazepines. (Dubovsky and Marshall 2022) Because of its shorter half-life, alprazolam generally causes worse withdrawal symptoms if suddenly stopped. Alprazolam comes in an extended-release form which lasts longer and is less prone to rebound anxiety than the immediate-release form.

Clonazepam is the only long-acting benzodiazepine approved for anxiety that does not have active metabolites. This makes it easier to use, and clonazepam is generally the preferred long-acting benzodiazepine for anxiety. Because of its long half-life, it is generally less addictive and has less severe withdrawal symptoms than shorter-acting drugs. Patients withdrawing from a benzodiazepine with a shorter half-life, such as alprazolam and lorazepam, are often switched to clonazepam before tapering. Clonazepam is also FDA-approved to treat seizure disorders.

Chlordiazepoxide was the first benzodiazepine synthesized in the late 1940s. All the other benzodiazepines were designed as modifications of chlordiazepoxide. It has long-acting metabolites. It is FDA-approved for alcohol withdrawal and has been used extensively for this purpose. Its long half-life makes it ideal for a smooth withdrawal. Unfortunately, it is metabolized by CYP450 enzymes, which makes it risky to use in people with liver dysfunction (such as alcohol-induced liver disease). The liver disease will impair the synthesis of CYP450 enzymes which means drugs such as chlordiazepoxide which are substrates for these enzymes, will accumulate unpredictably to higher, potentially toxic levels.

Clorazepate has the most prolonged half-life of the benzodiazepines used for anxiety disorders. This means it can accumulate over time, increasing the risk of side effects. The CYP450 enzymes metabolize it into two active metabolites, nordiazepam, and oxazepam. In addition to anxiety disorders, it is also FDA-approved for seizures.

Oxazepam itself is commercially available. It has a slow speed of onset and an intermediate half-life, making it less addictive than other benzodiazepines. Like lorazepam, it is not metabolized by the CYP450 enzymes but is directly conjugated. It is FDA-approved for seizure disorders as well as anxiety disorders.

Diazepam has an extensive history of use over the last 60 years and is still used today. The rapid speed of onset gives patients quick relief after taking the medication but also increases the risk that it will be abused. It has an active metabolite, nordiazepam, which can accumulate over time, making side effects more apparent later in treatment. Besides anxiety disorders, it has other FDA indications, including seizures, alcohol withdrawal, and muscle spasms or rigidity.

Lorazepam has no active metabolite and is not metabolized by the CYP450 enzymes, making it helpful in treating patients with liver dysfunction. For this reason, it is often preferred in the treatment of alcohol withdrawal. Its intermediate speed of onset of action makes it less likely to be abused than Alprazolam or Diazepam. In addition to anxiety disorders, it is also approved for seizure disorders.

Mechanism of Action (see also Chapter 23)

The mechanism of action for benzodiazepines is understood much better than for any antidepressant. As mentioned above, benzodiazepines bind to benzodiazepine receptors located on the $GABA_A$ receptor complex and enhance the effect of endogenous GABA. The GABA receptor complex is a chloride ion channel comprised of 5 subunits. GABA is the major inhibitory neurotransmitter in the brain. Increased GABA activity slows down neuronal firing by allowing the central pore of the receptor complex to open and enabling the movement of chloride ions into the cell. This results in hyperpolarization of the cell and explains the calming effects of benzodiazepines and their sedative and antiseizure properties. Alcohol also binds to the $GABA_A$ receptor and increases GABA activity. Although it binds to the $GABA_A$ receptor in a slightly different location than benzodiazepines, it exerts similar effects. (Olsen 2018) Benzodiazepines are effective treatments for alcohol withdrawal, as they substitute for alcohol and can be gradually tapered.

Adverse Effects

Withdrawal: People who have taken benzodiazepines for as little as 2 – 4 weeks may experience withdrawal if they suddenly stop the drug. Factors that increase the likelihood of experiencing withdrawal include a more extended time taking the drug, a higher dose of the benzodiazepine, and a shorter half-life. (O'Brien C 2005) Symptoms of benzodiazepine withdrawal are similar to that of alcohol withdrawal – increased anxiety, tremor, muscle twitches, nausea, sweating, and sometimes tachycardia. (Edinoff et al. 2021) Benzodiazepine withdrawal can be treated by slowly tapering the benzodiazepine, switching to a longer-acting benzodiazepine and tapering it, or simply treating the symptoms themselves. (O'Brien C 2005) Benzodiazepine withdrawal is usually less severe than alcohol withdrawal, but the patient may require hospitalization for monitoring and treatment in extreme cases.

Falls: Problems with balance and gait, potentially causing falls and fractures, are one of the most dangerous side effects of benzodiazepines, especially for older people. Up to 40% of patients on alprazolam may experience this symptom. (Dubovsky and Marshall 2022) Many studies have shown that older adults on chronic benzodiazepines are at a much higher risk of falls and fractures than age-matched controls. (Dubovsky and Marshall 2022) Benzodiazepines are on Beer's list of medications that should be avoided in people over 65.

Sedation: Sedation can be a significant side effect early in treatment. Over time tolerance to this effect develops. Fortunately, although there is some controversy about this, people usually don't develop tolerance to the anti-anxiety effects of benzodiazepines. (Dubovsky and Marshall 2022; O'Brien C 2005)

Impaired driving: Because benzodiazepines can impair executive function and motor reaction times, they increase the risk of motor vehicle accidents. Several studies looking at accident records found higher rates in drivers taking benzodiazepines; driving tests and psychomotor testing confirmed that driving could be negatively affected by benzodiazepines. (Dubovsky and Marshall 2022) The risk is greatest when the drug is initiated before tolerance has developed. Elderly patients are at higher risk for driving impairment. (Dubovsky and Marshall 2022; Edinoff et al. 2021)

Other side effects of Benzodiazepines:

- Confusion
- Rash
- Constipation
- Dizziness
- Paradoxical reactions where people become agitated (rare)

Safety in Overdose of Benzodiazepines

Benzodiazepines were initially marketed as being a safer alternative to the then commonly used barbiturates, which were often fatal in overdose. Benzodiazepines are rarely fatal in overdose unless taken with other substances. (Dubovsky and Marshall 2022; Edinoff et al. 2021) Combinations of benzodiazepines and alcohol or opioid agonists have high lethality in overdose. The risk of accidental death when using opioids increases significantly when benzodiazepines are also taken, and this combination should be avoided. (Dubovsky and Marshall 2022; Edinoff et al. 2021)

Flumazenil is an antidote for benzodiazepines. It is a competitive antagonist of benzodiazepine receptors on the $GABA_A$ receptor complex. It is FDA-approved for the reversal of benzodiazepine sedation after the completion of a procedure and for benzodiazepine overdose. Since benzodiazepines by themselves are rarely fatal, it is not often used in benzodiazepine overdoses. It could be helpful if a patient is severely obtunded and not breathing well, especially if the opioid antidote naloxone is not effective. Flumazenil has a short half-life of only 60 – 80 minutes; most benzodiazepines have a longer half-life. Patients should thus be carefully observed for the need for repeated treatment. Flumazenil is somewhat risky; (An and Godwin 2016) it can cause ventricular arrhythmias. If flumazenil-induced benzodiazepine withdrawal becomes significant, seizures can develop. For these reasons, many authorities recommend not using flumazenil for benzodiazepine overdose. (An and Godwin 2016)

References

American Psychiatric Association: Diagnostic and Statistical Manual of Mental Disorders: DSM-5-TR. 2022. Fifth edition, text revision ed. Arlington, VA: American Psychiatric Association.

An, Howard, and Jesse Godwin. 2016. Flumazenil in benzodiazepine overdose. *Canadian Medical Association Journal* 188 (17-18):E537.

Bachmann, S. 2018. Epidemiology of Suicide and the Psychiatric Perspective. *Int J Environ Res Public Health* 15 (7).

Bandelow, B., S. Michaelis, and D. Wedekind. 2017. Treatment of anxiety disorders. *Dialogues Clin Neurosci* 19 (2):93-107.

Bighelli, I., M. Castellazzi, A. Cipriani, F. Girlanda, G. Guaiana, M. Koesters, G. Turrini, T. A. Furukawa, and C. Barbui. 2018. Antidepressants versus placebo for panic disorder in adults. *Cochrane Database Syst Rev* 4 (4):Cd010676.

Chaimowitz, G., P. Weerasekera, and P. Ravitz. 2021. Psychotherapy in Psychiatry. *Can J Psychiatry* 66 (11):999-1004.

Cornett, Elyse M., Lauren Rando, Austin M. Labbé, Wil Perkins, Adam M. Kaye, Alan David Kaye, Omar Viswanath, and Ivan Urits. 2021. Brexanolone to Treat Postpartum Depression in Adult Women. *Psychopharmacology bulletin* 51 (2):115-130.

Dalhoff, K., H. E. Poulsen, P. Garred, M. Placchi, R. E. Gammans, R. F. Mayol, and M. Pfeffer. 1987. Buspirone pharmacokinetics in patients with cirrhosis. *Br J Clin Pharmacol* 24 (4):547-550.

Dawson, Lee A., and Jeannette M. Watson. 2009. Vilazodone: A 5-HT1A Receptor Agonist/Serotonin Transporter Inhibitor for the Treatment of Affective Disorders. *CNS Neuroscience & Therapeutics* 15 (2):107-117.

Debonnel, Guy, Élise Saint-André, Chantal Hébert, Claude de Montigny, Normand Lavoie, and Pierre Blier. 2007. Differential physiological effects of low and high doses of venlafaxine in major depression. *International Journal of Neuropsychopharmacology* 10 (1):51-61.

Dubovsky, S. L., and D. Marshall. 2022. Benzodiazepines Remain Important Therapeutic Options in Psychiatric Practice. *Psychotherapy and Psychosomatics* 91 (5):307-334.

Duman, R. S., G. Sanacora, and J. H. Krystal. 2019. Altered Connectivity in Depression: GABA and Glutamate Neurotransmitter Deficits and Reversal by Novel Treatments. *Neuron* 102 (1):75-90.

Dunner, D. L., L. K. Laird, J. Zajecka, L. Bailey, N. Sussman, and J. L. Seabolt. 2002. Six-year perspectives on the safety and tolerability of nefazodone. *J Clin Psychiatry* 63 Suppl 1:32-41.

Edinoff, Amber N., Catherine A. Nix, Janice Hollier, Caroline E. Sagrera, Blake M. Delacroix, Tunde Abubakar, Elyse M. Cornett, Adam M. Kaye, and Alan D. Kaye. 2021. Benzodiazepines: Uses, Dangers, and Clinical Considerations. *Neurology International* 13 (4):594-607.

Eison, Arlene S., and Davis L. Temple. 1986. Buspirone: review of its pharmacology and current perspectives on its mechanism of action. *The American Journal of Medicine* 80 (3, Supplement 2):1-9.

Fagiolini, Andrea, Alessandro Comandini, Mario Catena Dell'Osso, and Siegfried Kasper. 2012. Rediscovering Trazodone for the Treatment of Major Depressive Disorder. *CNS Drugs* 26 (12):1033-1049.

Fava, G. A., G. Benasi, M. Lucente, E. Offidani, F. Cosci, and J. Guidi. 2018. Withdrawal Symptoms after Serotonin-Noradrenaline Reuptake Inhibitor Discontinuation: Systematic Review. *Psychotherapy and Psychosomatics* 87 (4):195-203.

Fazel, S., and B. Runeson. 2020. Suicide. *N Engl J Med* 382 (3):266-274.

Gill, Nav, Adam Bayes, and Gordon Parker. 2020. A Review of Antidepressant-Associated Hypomania in Those Diagnosed with Unipolar Depression—Risk Factors, Conceptual Models, and Management. *Current Psychiatry Reports* 22 (4):20.

Gillman, P. K. 2007. Tricyclic antidepressant pharmacology and therapeutic drug interactions updated. *Br J Pharmacol* 151 (6):737-748.

Goddard, A. W. 2017. The Neurobiology of Panic: A Chronic Stress Disorder. *Chronic Stress (Thousand Oaks)* 1:2470547017736038.

Goldberg, H. L., and R. J. Finnerty. 1979. The comparative efficacy of buspirone and diazepam in the treatment of anxiety. *Am J Psychiatry* 136 (9):1184-1187.

Gomez, A. F., A. L. Barthel, and S. G. Hofmann. 2018. Comparing the efficacy of benzodiazepines and serotonergic anti-depressants for adults with generalized anxiety disorder: a meta-analytic review. *Expert Opin Pharmacother* 19 (8):883-894.

Greenblatt, D. J., R. I. Shader, M. Divoll, and J. S. Harmatz. 1981. Benzodiazepines: a summary of pharmacokinetic properties. *Br J Clin Pharmacol* 11 Suppl 1 (Suppl 1):11s 16s.

Hasin, D. S., A. L. Sarvet, J. L. Meyers, T. D. Saha, W. J. Ruan, M. Stohl, and B. F. Grant. 2018. Epidemiology of Adult DSM-5 Major Depressive Disorder and Its Specifiers in the United States. *JAMA Psychiatry* 75 (4):336-346.

Hawkins, E. M., W. Coryell, S. Leung, S. V. Parikh, C. Weston, P. Nestadt, J. I. Nurnberger, Jr., A. Kaplin, A. Kumar, A. A. Farooqui, and R. S. El-Mallakh. 2021. Effects of somatic treatments on suicidal ideation and completed suicides. *Brain Behav* 11 (11):e2381.

Imai, H., A. Tajika, P. Chen, A. Pompoli, and T. A. Furukawa. 2016. Psychological therapies versus pharmacological interventions for panic disorder with or without agoraphobia in adults. *Cochrane Database Syst Rev* 10 (10):Cd011170.

Ishida, T., T. Katagiri, H. Uchida, T. Suzuki, K. Watanabe, and M. Mimura. 2012. Asymptomatic deep vein thrombosis in a patient with major depressive disorder. *Case Rep Psychiatry* 2012:261251.

Kato, M., H. Hori, T. Inoue, J. Iga, M. Iwata, T. Inagaki, K. Shinohara, H. Imai, A. Murata, K. Mishima, and A. Tajika. 2021. Discontinuation of antidepressants after remission with antidepressant medication in major depressive disorder: a systematic review and meta-analysis. *Mol Psychiatry* 26 (1):118-133.

Kaufman, Joshua, Christine DeLorenzo, Sunia Choudhury, and Ramin V. Parsey. 2016. The 5-HT1A receptor in Major Depressive Disorder. *European neuropsychopharmacology : the journal of the European College of Neuropsychopharmacology* 26 (3):397-410.

Konvalin, F., F. Grosse-Wentrup, T. Nenov-Matt, K. Fischer, B. B. Barton, S. Goerigk, E. L. Brakemeier, R. Musil, A. Jobst, F. Padberg, and M. A. Reinhard. 2021. Borderline Personality Features in Patients With Persistent Depressive Disorder and Their Effect on CBASP Outcome. *Front Psychiatry* 12:608271.

Koyuncu, A., E. İnce, E. Ertekin, and R. Tükel. 2019. Comorbidity in social anxiety disorder: diagnostic and therapeutic challenges. *Drugs Context* 8:212573.

Lee, Kyoung-Uk, Young Min Lee, Ji-Min Nam, Hae-Kook Lee, Yong-Sil Kweon, Chung Tai Lee, and Tae-Youn Jun. 2010. Antidepressant-Induced Sexual Dysfunction among Newer Antidepressants in a Naturalistic Setting. *Psychiatry investigation* 7 (1):55-59.

Lee, Wing-King, Kwok-Leung Au Yeung, Ho-Bun Lam, Chi-Keung Wong, Ting-Chi Wong, Chi-Kin Fu, Shiu-Kow Sham, Ming-Kai Au, Tat-Chung Lam, and Daniel Ki-Yan Mak. 2021. Consensus statements on the clinical understanding and use of bupropion in Hong Kong. *CNS Neuroscience & Therapeutics* 27 (S1):20-24.

Li, Z., M. Ruan, J. Chen, and Y. Fang. 2021. Major Depressive Disorder: Advances in Neuroscience Research and Translational Applications. *Neurosci Bull* 37 (6):863-880.

Mahmood, Iftekhar, and Chandra Sahajwalla. 1999. Clinical Pharmacokinetics and Pharmacodynamics of Buspirone, an Anxiolytic Drug. *Clinical Pharmacokinetics* 36 (4):277-287.

Meister, R., A. von Wolff, H. Mohr, M. Härter, Y. Nestoriuc, L. Hölzel, and L. Kriston. 2016. Comparative Safety of Pharmacologic Treatments for Persistent Depressive Disorder: A Systematic Review and Network Meta-Analysis. *PLoS One* 11 (5):e0153380.

Melhem, N. M., Y. Zhong, J. M. Miller, F. Zanderigo, R. T. Ogden, M. E. Sublette, M. Newell, A. Burke, J. G. Keilp, M. Lesanpezeshki, E. Bartlett, D. A. Brent, and J. J. Mann. 2022. Brain 5-HT1A Receptor PET Binding, Cortisol Responses to Stress, and the Familial Transmission of Suicidal Behavior. *Int J Neuropsychopharmacol* 25 (1):36-45.

Murray, C. J., C. Atkinson, K. Bhalla, G. Birbeck, R. Burstein, D. Chou, R. Dellavalle, G. Danaei, M. Ezzati, A. Fahimi, D. Flaxman, Foreman, S. Gabriel, E. Gakidou, N. Kassebaum, S. Khatibzadeh, S. Lim, S. E. Lipshultz, S. London, Lopez, M. F. MacIntyre, A. H. Mokdad, A. Moran, A. E. Moran, D. Mozaffarian, T. Murphy, M. Naghavi, C. Pope, T. Roberts, J. Salomon, D. C. Schwebel, S. Shahraz, D. A. Sleet, Murray, J. Abraham, M. K. Ali, C. Atkinson, D. H. Bartels, K. Bhalla, G. Birbeck, R. Burstein, H. Chen, M. H. Criqui, Dahodwala, Jarlais, E. L. Ding, E. R. Dorsey, B. E. Ebel, M. Ezzati, Fahami, S. Flaxman, A. D. Flaxman, D. Gonzalez-Medina, B. Grant, H. Hagan, H. Hoffman, N. Kassebaum, S. Khatibzadeh, J. L. Leasher, J. Lin, S. E. Lipshultz, R. Lozano, Y. Lu, L. Mallinger, M. M. McDermott, R. Micha, T. R. Miller, A. A. Mokdad, A. H. Mokdad, D. Mozaffarian, M. Naghavi, K. M. Narayan, S. B. Omer, P. M. Pelizzari, D. Phillips, D. Ranganathan, F. P. Rivara, T. Roberts, U. Sampson, E. Sanman, A. Sapkota, D. C. Schwebel, S. Sharaz, R. Shivakoti, G. M. Singh, D. Singh, M. Tavakkoli, J. A. Towbin, J. D. Wilkinson, A. Zabetian, Murray, J. Abraham, M. K. Ali, M. Alvardo, C. Atkinson, L. M. Baddour, E. J. Benjamin, K. Bhalla, G. Birbeck, I. Bolliger, R. Burstein, E. Carnahan, D. Chou, S. S. Chugh, A. Cohen, K. E. Colson, L. T. Cooper, W. Couser, M. H. Criqui, K. C. Dabhadkar, R. P. Dellavalle, Jarlais, D. Dicker, E. R. Dorsey, H. Duber, B. E. Ebel, R. E. Engell, M. Ezzati, D. T. Felson, M. M. Finucane, S. Flaxman, A. D. Flaxman, T. Fleming, Foreman, M. H. Forouzanfar, G. Freedman, M. K. Freeman, E. Gakidou, R. F. Gillum, D. Gonzalez-Medina, R. Gosselin, H. R. Gutierrez, H. Hagan, R. Havmoeller, H. Hoffman, K. H. Jacobsen, S. L. James, R. Jasrasaria, S. Jayarman, N. Johns, N. Kassebaum, S. Khatibzadeh, Q. Lan, J. L. Leasher, S. Lim, S. E. Lipshultz, S. London, Lopez, R. Lozano, Y. Lu, L. Mallinger, M. Meltzer, G. A. Mensah, C. Michaud, T. R. Miller, C. Mock, T. E. Moffitt, A. A. Mokdad, A. H. Mokdad, A. Moran, M. Naghavi, K. M. Narayan, R. G. Nelson, C. Olives, S. B. Omer, K. Ortblad, B. Ostro, P. M. Pelizzari, D. Phillips, M. Raju, H. Razavi, B. Ritz, T. Roberts, R. L. Sacco, J. Salomon, U. Sampson, D. C. Schwebel, S. Shahraz, K. Shibuya, D. Silberberg, J. A. Singh, K. Steenland, J. A. Taylor, G. D. Thurston, M. S. Vavilala, T. Vos, G. R. Wagner, M. A. Weinstock, M. G. Weisskopf, S. Wulf, and Murray. 2013. The state of US health, 1990-2010: burden of diseases, injuries, and risk factors. *JAMA* 310 (6):591-608.

O'Brien C, P. 2005. Benzodiazepine use, abuse, and dependence. *J Clin Psychiatry* 66 Suppl 2:28-33.

Olsen, Richard W. 2018. GABAA receptor: Positive and negative allosteric modulators. *Neuropharmacology* 136:10-22.

Preskorn, Sheldon H. 1997. Clinically Relevant Pharmacology of Selective Serotonin Reuptake Inhibitors. *Clinical Pharmacokinetics* 32 (1):1-21.

Rissardo, J. P., and A. L. F. Caprara. 2020. Buspirone-associated Movement Disorder: A Literature Review. *Prague Med Rep* 121 (1):5-24.

Rudorfer, Matthew V., and William Z. Potter. 1999. Metabolism of Tricyclic Antidepressants. *Cellular and Molecular Neurobiology* 19 (3):373-409.

Sanchez, Connie, Karen E. Asin, and Francesc Artigas. 2015. Vortioxetine, a novel antidepressant with multimodal activity: Review of preclinical and clinical data. *Pharmacology & Therapeutics* 145:43-57.

Sansone, Randy A., and Lori A. Sansone. 2014. Serotonin norepinephrine reuptake inhibitors: a pharmacological comparison. *Innovations in clinical neuroscience* 11 (3-4):37-42.

Schramm, Elisabeth, Daniel N. Klein, Moritz Elsaesser, Toshi A. Furukawa, and Katharina Domschke. 2020. Review of dysthymia and persistent depressive disorder: history, correlates, and clinical implications. *The Lancet Psychiatry* 7 (9):801-812.

Shi, L., J. Wang, S. Xu, and Y. Lu. 2016. Efficacy and tolerability of vilazodone for major depressive disorder: evidence from phase III/IV randomized controlled trials. *Drug Des Devel Ther* 10:3899-3907.

Stein, D. J., C. C. W. Lim, A. M. Roest, P. de Jonge, S. Aguilar-Gaxiola, A. Al-Hamzawi, J. Alonso, C. Benjet, E. J. Bromet, R. Bruffaerts, G. de Girolamo, S. Florescu, O. Gureje, J. M. Haro, M. G. Harris, Y. He, H. Hinkov, I. Horiguchi, C. Hu, A. Karam, E. G. Karam, S. Lee, J. P. Lepine, F. Navarro-Mateu, B. E. Pennell, M. Piazza, J. Posada-Villa, M. Ten Have, Y. Torres, M. C. Viana, B. Wojtyniak, M. Xavier, R. C. Kessler, and K. M. Scott. 2017. The cross-national epidemiology of social anxiety disorder: Data from the World Mental Health Survey Initiative. *BMC Med* 15 (1):143.

Stippl, A., F. N. Kirkgoze, M. Bajbouj, and S. Grimm. 2020. Differential Effects of Electroconvulsive Therapy in the Treatment of Major Depressive Disorder. *Neuropsychobiology* 79 (6):408-416.

Strawn, J. R., L. Geracioti, N. Rajdev, K. Clemenza, and A. Levine. 2018. Pharmacotherapy for generalized anxiety disorder in adult and pediatric patients: an evidence-based treatment review. *Expert Opin Pharmacother* 19 (10):1057-1070.

Sub Laban, T., and A. Saadabadi. 2022. Monoamine Oxidase Inhibitors (MAOI). In *StatPearls*. Treasure Island (FL): StatPearls Publishing.

Tafet, G. E., and C. B. Nemeroff. 2020. Pharmacological Treatment of Anxiety Disorders: The Role of the HPA Axis. *Front Psychiatry* 11:443.

Tellone, Valeria, Maria Teresa Rosignoli, Rossella Picollo, Patrizia Dragone, Alessandra Del Vecchio, Alessandro Comandini, Milko Radicioni, Chiara Leuratti, and Fabrizio Calisti. 2020. Effect of 3 Single Doses of Trazodone on QTc Interval in Healthy Subjects. *The Journal of Clinical Pharmacology* 60 (11):1483-1495.

Tiranini, L., and R. E. Nappi. 2022. Recent advances in understanding/management of premenstrual dysphoric disorder/premenstrual syndrome. *Fac Rev* 11:11.

Ullah, I., N. Tauqir, S. Shoib, and A. Parmar. 2022. Predicting Suicide Attempt: Is It Always Possible? *Indian J Psychol Med* 44 (1):89-90.

Wikman, A., J. Sacher, M. Bixo, A. L. Hirschberg, H. Kopp Kallner, C. N. Epperson, E. Comasco, and I. Sundström Poromaa. 2022. Prevalence and correlates of current suicidal ideation in women with premenstrual dysphoric disorder. *BMC Womens Health* 22 (1):35.

World Health Organisation. 2023. *World Health Organisation*. https://www.who.int/news-room/fact-sheets/detail/depression. Accessed: 23 May 2023.

Yonkers, Kimberly Ann, and Michael K. Simoni. 2018. Premenstrual disorders. *American Journal of Obstetrics and Gynecology* 218 (1):68-74.

Quiz Questions

1. Potential complications of a major depressive episode (MDE) include which condition?
   A Deep vein thrombosis
   B Weight loss and malnutrition
   C Work absenteeism
   D All the above

2. Which statement is NOT true about the pathophysiology of major depressive disorder (MDD)?
   A All depression symptoms can be explained by a deficiency of serotonin
   B Epigenetic chances can be involved
   C Inflammation plays a role
   D Loss of neuroplasticity is likely

3. The mental status exam of a patient with MDE could show which symptom?
   A Agitation and restlessness with increased motion
   B Slowness of motion
   C A and B
   D None of the above

4. Patients with what disorder often think their symptoms are "normal," which can delay diagnosis?
   A Generalized anxiety disorder (GAD)
   B Major depressive disorder (MDD)
   C Persistent depressive disorder (PDD)
   D Premenstrual dysphoric disorder (PMDD)

5. Which disorder is commonly seen in patients with persistent depressive disorder (PDD)?
   A Major depressive disorder (MDD)
   B Anxiety disorders
   C Substance use disorders
   D All the above

6. What is the fundamental cause of premenstrual dysphoric disorder (PMDD)?
   A Increase and then decrease in progesterone just before menstruation
   B Increase and then decrease in serotonin just before menstruation
   C Increase and then decrease In testosterone just before menstruation
   D None of the above

7. What is an example of typical anxiety/anxieties in generalized anxiety disorder (GAD)?
   A Excessive concern that an extraterrestrial will invade
   B Excessive concern that bills cannot be paid
   C Both a and b
   D Neither A nor B

8. Which parts of the brain are involved in the pathophysiology of GAD?
   A Amygdala
   B Raphe nuclei
   C Prefrontal cortex
   D All the above

9. Which quality is NOT characteristic of panic disorder (PD)?

   A Epigenetic changes may be involved in the pathophysiology behind the disease.
   B In some people, a polymorphism in Catechol-O-methyltransferase is present.
   C Panic attacks are always triggered by a stressor.
   D People more uncomfortable in new situations are more likely to have panic disorder.

10. Which is the most common comorbid condition with PD?
    A Agoraphobia
    B Alcohol use disorder
    C GAD
    D MDD

11. Which person is the least likely to have social anxiety disorder (SAD)?
    A An American teenager
    B A European in their 20s
    C A Canadian in their 40s
    D An African in their 80s

12. Which two medications have been proven to protect against suicide?
    A Lithium and amitriptyline
    B Lithium and clozapine
    C Lithium and phenelzine
    D Lithium and venlafaxine

13. Which tricyclic antidepressant (TCA) is considered the "gold standard" for treating obsessive-compulsive disorder (OCD)?
    A Amitriptyline
    B Amoxapine
    C Clomipramine
    D Doxepin

14. TCA toxicities in overdose include which symptom?
    A Seizures
    B Cardiac arrhythmias
    C Hypotension
    D All the above

15. Some common TCA side effects do not cause acute danger but are sufficiently troublesome to sometimes warrant stopping the drug. Which symptom is not usually caused by TCAs?
    A Headache
    B Weight gain
    C Dry mouth
    D Sedation

16. Which is the only TCA that binds to dopamine receptors giving it some antipsychotic activity?
    A Amitriptyline
    B Amoxapine
    C Imipramine
    D Protriptyline

17. The clinical half-life of all MAOIs commercially available in the US (isocarboxazid, phenelzine, selegiline, and tranylcypromine) is approximately how long?
    A Two hours
    B Two days
    C Two weeks
    D Two months

18. A patient on an MAOI should avoid foods with tyramine to avoid which adverse consequence?
    A Hypertensive crisis
    B Orthostatic hypotension
    C Serotonin syndrome
    D Weight loss

19. What are the symptoms of serotonin syndrome?
    A Altered mental status (agitation, confusion, etc.)
    B Autonomic instability (blood pressure, pulse, temperature, etc.)
    C Neuromuscular symptoms (tremor, hyperreflexia, clonus)
    D All the above

20. A patient complaining of electric shock sensations in his head, which he describes as "brain zaps," is likely experiencing which symptom?
    A Extreme anxiety
    B Serotonin syndrome
    C SSRI-induced headaches
    D SSRI withdrawal or discontinuation syndrome

21. Which SSRI is associated with the most significant risk of QTc prolongation?
    A Citalopram
    B Fluoxetine
    C Paroxetine
    D Sertraline

22. Which SSRI has the longest half-life?
    A Citalopram
    B Fluoxetine
    C Paroxetine
    D Sertraline

23. Which neurotransmitter is most likely responsible for the pain-relieving properties of (serotonin-norepinephrine reuptake inhibitors)?
    A Acetylcholine
    B Dopamine
    C Norepinephrine
    D Serotonin

24. A patient comes to the ER with an overdose of a large quantity of venlafaxine. Which symptom(s) might be expected?
    A Cardiac arrhythmias
    B Seizures
    C Serotonin syndrome
    D All the above

25. A patient with multiple episodes of severe MDD has done well with venlafaxine XR (extended-release) for ten years. She has chosen to remain on it long-term to avoid relapse. She is about to have bariatric surgery. What changes, if any, would you make to her treatment plan?
    A Continue current venlafaxine XR. It is working well.
    B Stop venlafaxine XR. She will probably do well with depression after her surgery.
    C Switch venlafaxine XR to the regular release form to help absorption.
    D Try an SSRI which would be better absorbed.

26. Which antidepressant has a more rapid speed of onset?
    A Citalopram
    B Nortriptyline
    C Paroxetine
    D Vilazodone

27. A patient has sexual side effects (loss of libido) on fluoxetine. Switching to which antidepressant would have the best chance of alleviating the symptoms?
    A Amitriptyline
    B Bupropion
    C Sertraline
    D Venlafaxine

28. Although it can cause QTc prolongation at higher doses, which antidepressant is often used to help with sleep?
    A Bupropion
    B Citalopram
    C Trazodone
    D None of the above

29. Which medication can be given IV?
   A Brexanolone
   B Selegiline
   C Both A and B
   D Neither A nor B

30. You see a depressed older woman who is not sleeping or eating. Based on the side effect profile, which antidepressant is most likely to help her?
   A Amitriptyline
   B Bupropion
   C Fluoxetine
   D Mirtazapine

31. In treating anxiety, what is the advantage of buspirone over benzodiazepines?
   A Buspirone acts more quickly.
   B Buspirone is less likely to lead to addiction.
   C Buspirone works better than benzodiazepines.
   D Buspirone is generic.

32. Which benzodiazepine has the longest half-life?
   A Alprazolam
   B Clonazepam
   C Lorazepam
   D Oxazepam

33. Which benzodiazepine is most likely to lead to addiction?
   A Alprazolam
   B Diazepam
   C Lorazepam
   D Clorazepate

Quiz Answers

1. D. An MDE can cause severe psychosocial and medical problems. Work absenteeism is a known problem for employers. MDE often leads to alienation in relationships. Weight loss is common in severe episodes and can cause malnutrition. Weight gain is also prevalent and can contribute to malnutrition due to the intake of excess "comfort food" lacking adequate nutrients. In extreme cases, patients with MDE stay in bed; the resulting venous stasis can lead to clot formation, especially in elderly or physically disabled people.

2. A. MDD is a complex illness affecting the brain in many ways. An increase in available synaptic serotonin is just one way that antidepressants work. Epigenetics is the mechanism whereby the environment and a person's experiences affect the brain. Inflammation is increased in MDD. Neuroplasticity is a mechanism through which the brain can heal itself. It is decreased in MDD and is improved with successful antidepressant treatment.

3. C. An MDE can affect several symptoms in two opposite ways. Along with causing either insomnia or hypersomnia and weight loss or weight gain, it can also cause agitation and restlessness with increased motion (psychomotor agitation) or decreased movement (psychomotor slowing). Just as a person cannot experience insomnia and hypersomnia or weight loss and weight gain at the same time, psychomotor agitation and psychomotor slowing do not occur simultaneously. The same patient may experience either extreme at different times, however.

4. C. PMDD often begins in youth, and the patients have felt depressed for so long that they sometimes don't remember ever feeling happy. They assume this is normal for them and may not bring it to anyone's attention. Patients with the other disorders listed are usually very aware that something is wrong.

5. D. Patients with PDD commonly have comorbid MDD, anxiety disorders, and substance use disorders. Suicidal thoughts may be higher in PDD than in patients with MDD. The chronicity of the symptoms often leads to more hopelessness.

6. A. Without ovulation and the resulting hormonal fluctuations, symptoms of PMDD do not occur. The significant increase in progesterone at the end of the luteal phase is thought to be the immediate precipitant of the disorder. Testosterone and serotonin don't significantly increase and then decrease before menstruation.

7. B. Worries in GAD are about everyday life. They are fears about things it is reasonable to worry about (such as paying bills), but the intensity and chronicity of the worry are excessive. Unless things change dramatically, extreme concern about extraterrestrial invasion is not reasonable and could be a sign of psychosis.

8. D. The amygdala is the center of the fear pathway. Serotonergic neurons in the raphe nuclei communicate with the prefrontal cortex, which integrates many incoming stimuli about events and emotions and modulates behavior as a result. The exact mechanism of these actions is incompletely understood.

9. C. By definition, a person must have at least 2 (one or more) panic attacks that come out of the blue with no identifiable trigger. Theories of causation of PD include that epigenetic changes induced by fearful experiences play a role. One polymorphism has been associated with panic disorder, the Catechol-O-methyltransferase. Behavioral inhibition, the characteristic of being very uncomfortable in new situations, is associated with PD.

10. A. Agoraphobia is very frequently seen with panic disorder. The person may be afraid of leaving their house because of panic attacks. Alcohol use disorder may start as an attempt to deal with panic PD, but it is not as commonly seen as agoraphobia. Both GAD and MDD are common comorbidities of panic disorder but are not as frequent as agoraphobia.

11. D. SAD is most prevalent in adolescents and young adults. It tends to resolve as people age, especially after age 65, so an 80-year-old would be much less likely to show SAD symptoms. In addition, the prevalence is highest in the US and lowest in Africa and the Eastern Mediterranean.

12. B. Despite having significant adverse effects in overdose, Lithium and Clozapine have an excellent track record in preventing suicide in patients with schizophrenia (Clozapine) and bipolar disorder (Lithium). Note that neither are pure antidepressants but were developed as a mood stabilizer (Lithium) and an antipsychotic (Clozapine).

13. C. Clomipramine is the gold standard drug for OCD. Clomipramine is the most potent serotonin reuptake inhibitor among tricyclics. It is probably the most effective drug for OCD, but because of side effects, SSRIs are tried first. SSRIs were developed to focus specifically on serotonin because of the effectiveness of clomipramine.

14. D. TCAs can be very dangerous in overdose and frequently require hospitalization. The patient's potential to attempt suicide by overdose should be considered before prescribing tricyclics.

15. A. TCAs do not usually cause headaches; some (especially nortriptyline and amitriptyline) are used off-label to prevent headaches and migraines. Weight gain, dry mouth, and sedation are sometimes severe enough to prompt a medication change.

16. B. Amoxapine is the only TCA with dopaminergic activity; it blocks dopamine receptors. Because of this, it does have some antipsychotic activity. It also blocks the reuptake of both serotonin and norepinephrine.

17. C. All the US MAOIs are irreversible. This means they will keep working in the body until a new monoamine oxidase (MAO) enzyme is synthesized and replaces the irreversibly inhibited enzyme. This is usually about two weeks. Before starting a new antidepressant, anyone on an MAOI available in the US must be off all antidepressants for two weeks to avoid the risk of serotonin syndrome.

18. A. Tyramine can raise blood pressure and is metabolized by MAOs. When MAOs are inhibited, severe hypertension can result. MAOIs can cause orthostatic hypotension, but this side effect is unrelated to food. Taking MAOIs along with other serotonergic agents can cause serotonin syndrome, but tyramine is not involved. MAOIs can cause weight gain, not weight loss.

19. D. Altered mental status, autonomic instability, and neuromuscular symptoms are the hallmarks of serotonin syndrome. The patient may not have all the symptoms in mild cases, but they are usually all present in severe cases. Serotonin syndrome develops quickly after an increasing serotonin load (whether from an overdose, too rapid dose increases, or taking more than one serotonergic medication).

20. D. SSRIs and other serotonergic medications may produce symptoms if stopped abruptly. "Brain zaps" are a classic description of this experience. Patients may also experience what resembles a bad case of the flu. Symptoms usually go away quickly when a lower dose of the SSRI is reintroduced and then gradually tapered off. Not all patients experience SSRI discontinuation syndrome. It is not the same as addiction; it is like rebound hypertension when suddenly stopping β blockers. Addiction requires loss of control over substance use, not just withdrawal symptoms.

21. A. Citalopram increases QTc to the greatest extent of any SSRI. This is a dose-dependent effect, and lower doses (20 mg or less) are used in older patients at greater risk of QTc problems. The other antidepressants can also prolong QTc, but the effect is milder and rarely clinically significant.

22. B. Because it has a very long-lived active metabolite, Fluoxetine has a half-life of about a week. To eliminate it from the body, such as before starting an MAO-I, the patient must be five weeks out from the last dose. This quality makes fluoxetine one of the least likely antidepressants to cause discontinuation syndrome as the body naturally tapers off fluoxetine gradually over five weeks. It also makes fluoxetine a good choice for patients prone to forgetting to take medications. Fluoxetine even comes in a 90 mg once-a-week formulation for people who are stable on fluoxetine 20 mg daily.

23. C. The effectiveness of SNRIs for neuropathic pain is related to how much norepinephrine reuptake inhibition it produces. The norepinephrine quality can also elevate blood pressure. The pain-relieving characteristic of SNRIs is not related to their treatment of depression or anxiety. People without any depression or anxiety get neuropathic pain relief from SNRIs.

24. D. SNRIs in general, and venlafaxine in particular, are more dangerous in overdose than SSRIs. Cardiac arrhythmias can be a cause of death in this situation. Seizures can occur in patients without a seizure history. Serotonin syndrome is always a concern with an overdose of a serotonergic drug.

25. C. Patients have difficulty breaking down and absorbing extended-release medications after bariatric surgery. Thus, if she stays on the current preparation, she is at risk of relapse because of inadequate dosing. Bariatric surgery is not a cure for depression, and given her history, she is likely to relapse without medication. The standard-release form will be dosed three times a day instead of once daily but should be absorbed without a problem. If standard-release venlafaxine does not work, it would be reasonable to try a switch to an SSRI. Since it is effective for the patient, it is best to remain on Venlafaxine unless it fails.

26. D. Most antidepressants take up to 12 weeks or longer for full efficacy. The patient often doesn't notice much for the first 2-6 weeks. Vilazodone more dependably has noticeable effects in the first two weeks.

27. B. Because it does not work through serotonin, bupropion is the least likely to cause sexual side effects. All serotoninergic antidepressants have some chance of causing this problem. SSRIs (e.g., sertraline), SNRIs (e.g., venlafaxine), and TCAs (e.g., amitriptyline) are especially likely to cause this problem.

28. C. Bupropion can make sleep more difficult and should be taken in the morning. Citalopram does increase QTc intervals but does not help with sleep. Trazodone is very sedating, and low doses often help with sleep. At high doses, it can increase the QTc interval.

29. A. Brexanolone is the only IV antidepressant available. It is given only to women with severe postpartum depression. It is a metabolite of the hormone progesterone and is specific to postpartum depression. It has severe side effects, including extreme sedation, hypoxia, and syncope. It is only administered in the hospital with regular observation by providers with special training through a REMS (risk evaluation and mitigation strategy) program. Selegiline is an MAOI that is available by transdermal patch. All other antidepressants must be taken orally.

30. D. The same side effects that often cause patients to stop Mirtazapine (sedation and increased appetite) can sometimes be of great advantage in severe depression. Amitriptyline also helps with sleep and stimulates appetite, but it is much more likely to cause cardiac arrhythmias than mirtazapine so it wouldn't be the first choice. Bupropion and fluoxetine can make sleep more difficult and would not help this patient. Bupropion often causes some weight loss, so it would not be appropriate for this patient.

31. B. Buspirone does not have an immediate effect when taken, so it is not addictive. A significant disadvantage of buspirone is that it acts much more slowly than benzodiazepines to relieve anxiety. It has been tested against older benzodiazepines and found to be equivalent to them in efficacy but not better. Buspirone and the benzodiazepines used for anxiety are all available in generic forms.

32. B. Alprazolam, lorazepam, and oxazepam are all intermediate-acting benzodiazepines, meaning their half-lives are all less than 24 hours. Clonazepam is a long-acting benzodiazepine with a half-life of up to 50 hours. This makes withdrawal reactions much less severe. In benzodiazepine withdrawal from an intermediate-acting drug, the patient is often first switched to clonazepam and then slowly tapered off clonazepam.

33. A. The likelihood of addiction is based on a drug's speed of onset and its half-life. Alprazolam and diazepam have a rapid onset of action, lorazepam has an intermediate onset of action, and clorazepate has a slow onset of action. Alprazolam and lorazepam have intermediate half-lives; diazepam and clorazepate have long half-lives. Thus, alprazolam with a rapid onset and intermediate half-life is the most likely to cause addiction. With a slow onset of action and a long half-life, Clorazepate is the least likely to cause addiction.

CHAPTER 18

SEIZURES

LAUREN SKALOMENOS, MD[1], CHARLES AKOS SZABO, MD[1] AND CARL L. FAINGOLD, PHD[2]

[1] University of Texas Health Science Center at San Antonio, Texas, USA
[2] Southern Illinois University School of Medicine, Springfield, Illinois, USA

Symptoms: Neurological

MEDICATION LIST FOR SEIZURES- Listed by dominant* mechanism of action

***(Many anticonvulsant drugs have more than one effect)**

$GABA_A$ ENHANCEMENT (major)

***BARBITURATES**
phenobarbital

BENZODIAZEPINES
diazepam
clonazepam
lorazepam
clobazam

OTHER GABA-enhancing Agents
***valproic acid**
tiagabine
vigabatrin
ganaxalone

SODIUM CHANNEL BLOCK
Major
phenytoin
fosphenytoin
carbamazepine
lacosamide-slow**
lamotrigine
Secondary
rufinamide
zonisamide
topiramate
oxcarbazepine

GLUTAMATE BLOCK
perampanel AMPA block
***barbiturates and congeners**
felbamate
lamotrigine

CALCIUM CHANNEL BLOCK
ethosuximide T-type
gabapentin N-type α2-δ
pregabalin N-type α2-δ

SYNAPTIC VESICLE PROTEIN SV_{2a}
levetiracetam
brivaracetam C-V

POTASSIUM CHANNEL OPENER
ezogabine (retigabine)**

AGENTS ACTING BY OTHER MECHANISMS
Serotonin enhancing agents
fenfluramine
Carbonic Anhydrase Inhibitors
acetazolamide
Cannabidiol (mechanism unknown)

MEDICATION LIST FOR TREATMENT OF STATUS EPILEPTICUS

First line therapies:
Midazolam or diazepam (intranasal)
Diazepam (intrarectal)
Lorazepam (intravenous)

Second line therapies:
Fosphenytoin
Levetiracetam
Valproic acid
Phenobarbital

Third line therapies:
Propofol
Ketamine
Pentobarbital

Seizures

Seizure is a transient occurrence of signs and/or symptoms due to abnormal excessive or synchronous neuronal activity in the brain. (Scheffer et al. 2017)

Diagnosis

Seizures are characterized by a sudden change in perception or behavior, which is associated with a synchronized discharge of cortical neurons. or A spell or ictus can represent a seizure or other phenomena. Seizures can occur in patients that are not caused by epilepsy including alcohol withdrawal, sedative-hypnotic withdrawal, fever, hyponatremia, hypomagnesemia, hypoglycemia, hyperglycemia, medications, and medication overdoses such as seen with antihistamines. Seizures due to a functional or lesion-based pathology of the brain and are classified as genetic, infectious, metabolic, immune, structural i.e., secondary to some form of brain damage such as a brain tumor or a stroke.[1] Most seizures have no known cause. In other cases, there can be more than one element involved; one example of the "two hit hypothesis" is a history of genetic predisposition followed by a structural event, such as head trauma, leading to the expression of seizures. (Perucca et al. 2020) The diagnostic work-up for as seizure typically includes an electroencephalogram (EEG), which measures changes of cortical electrical potentials over time, and neuroimaging studies, such as a head computerized tomography (CT) or brain magnetic resonance imaging (MRI) study. The ideal study for the diagnosis and characterization of seizures is the simultaneous recording of behavioral change with video and EEG, which is utilized in the setting of recurrent seizures, or epilepsy, not responding to antiseizure medications (ASMs). (Fisher et al. 2017)

There are paroxysmal changes in behavior or perception that are not seizures. (EpilepsyFoundation 2023) Seizure-like events include syncope (convulsive and non-convulsive), breath-holding, hyperventilation, psychogenic nonepileptic events, movement disorders, hypoglycemia, panic attack, transient global amnesia, transient ischemic attack even the aura associated with migraine headaches.

Common Types of Seizures

The general classification of epileptic seizures is based on the site of onset of the seizure and includes focal or partial seizures, generalized seizures, and unknown onset. (Scheffer et al. 2017) Focal-onset seizures are associated with an ictal EEG discharge originating from one region of the cerebral cortex. During focal onset seizures, person/people with epilepsy (PWE) can be initially fully aware or exhibit impaired awareness. Perceptual changes such as an epigastric rising sensation, deja vu, olfactory/gustatory symptoms, auditory or visual symptoms may help localize the seizure focus. The initial signs can also involve motor events, such as automatisms, atonic, or convulsive (clonic or tonic). Impaired awareness occurs when the ictal EEG spreads subcortical brain structures. Some people with impaired awareness can respond appropriately to questions, so the ultimate factor for determining impairment is amnesia for the episode. As the EEG activity spreads to the other hemisphere and into the brainstem, the seizure symptoms are expressed as a bilateral tonic-clonic seizure. For the generalized-onset seizures the ictal EEG discharge evolves simultaneously and often synchronized over both hemispheres. The initial signs of generalized seizures can also be motor, including tonic-clonic, tonic, and myoclonic behaviors and non-motor onset the signs include a transient loss of awareness and eyelid myoclonus (blinking) often associated with absence seizures. A PWE can exhibit more than one of these behavior patterns or seizure types at various times. As mentioned above, an EEG-based diagnosis often necessitates observation of the behavior simultaneously via video recording which often requires an overnight stay in an epilepsy monitoring unit (EMU).

Example of Generalized (onset) Seizures

Absence (French pronunciation) (petit mal*) **Seizures**

Symptoms: staring or blinking (examples available on social media). No overt convulsion

Consciousness: brief loss

Ictal Duration: up to 20 seconds, no post-ictal state

Sequelae: none

EEG: bilateral 3 Hz (cycle per second) spike and wave during the seizure

Cause: genetic

Generalized Tonic-Clonic (grand mal*) **Seizures**

Symptoms: fall, rigidity (tonic), then rhythmic jerking (clonic), with or without tongue-biting or urinary incontinence

Consciousness: lost at onset

Ictal Duration: 30 seconds to 2 min.

Sequelae: Muscle soreness, Incontinence, postictal confusion (examples available on social media)

EEG: interictal – generalized spikes and spike-and-wave discharges, ictal – bilateral generalized high amplitude and rapid abnormal activity

Cause: genetic, infectious, metabolic, immune, structural, or unknown

Examples of Focal (onset) Seizures

Focal (simple partial*) **Seizures Without Impaired Awareness**

Symptoms: variable and include lateralized clonic, tonic, dystonic motor activity, auras that are somatosensory, olfactory/gustatory, autonomic (cardiac, epigastric), visual (phosphenes in one visual quadrant) or psychic (including deja or jamais vu)

Consciousness: not impaired

Ictal Duration: variable

Sequelae: variable

EEG: focal or lateralized spikes or sharp waves interictally, at times without an EEG change, but mostly associated with a focal or unilateral rhythmical ictal discharge

May evolve to a focal seizure with impaired awareness and/or a bilateral tonic-clonic seizure

Focal (complex partial*, psychomotor*) **seizures with impaired awareness**

Consciousness: altered ("clouded")

Ictal Duration: seconds to 2-3 minutes

Symptoms: include staring, automatisms, amnesia, postictal confusion

EEG: focal or lateralized spikes or sharp waves interictally, always associated with an EEG change, mostly associated with a focal, unilateral, or asymmetrical bilateral rhythmical ictal discharge

May have an "aura" or warning

In contrast to absence seizures, there is postictal confusion, at times speech impairment and postictal focal neurological deficits

May evolve to a bilateral tonic-clonic seizure

*Older terminology

Epilepsy and Epilepsy Syndromes

Epilepsy is a disorder of the brain characterized by an enduring predisposition to generate epileptic seizures. This includes the neurobiological, cognitive, psychological, and social consequences of this condition. (Fisher et al. 2014) Similar to seizures, epilepsies are divided into focal and generalized epilepsies. The coexistence of focal and generalized epilepsy is extremely rare in people with epilepsy (PWE). Classification of epilepsy syndromes provides a more comprehensive characterization including co-morbidities and etiology; these factors inform prognosis.

Operational (Practical) Clinical Definition of Epilepsy

Epilepsy is a disease of the brain defined by any of the following conditions:

1. At least two unprovoked (or reflex) seizures occurring more than 24 hours apart.
2. One unprovoked (or reflex) seizure and a probability of further seizures similar to the general recurrence risk (at least 60%) after two unprovoked seizures occurring over the next 10 years.
3. Diagnosis of the epilepsy syndrome.

The prevalence of active epilepsy is about 1%. (EpilepsyFoundation 2023) Epilepsy can present at any age, but new-onset cases typically present in the first three decades and after the sixth decade. Generalized epilepsies present in exceptionally rare cases after the third decade, whereas focal epilepsies can present at any age. Generalized epilepsy can be familial, and often there a genetic etiology is suspected; focal epilepsies can be genetic but are more likely to be associated with developmental or structural lesion. The operational definition of epilepsy informs the decision to treat; patients with recurrent seizures or a single seizure associated with risk factors of seizure recurrence, such as interictal markers suggesting a genetic etiology or a brain MRI indicating a brain neoplasm, are at elevated risk for seizure recurrence.

Epilepsy remission is considered for individuals who had an age-dependent epilepsy syndrome but are now past the applicable age or those who have remained seizure-free for the last ten years, with no seizure medicines for the last five years. ASMs can be gradually tapered off to avoid withdrawal seizures, and EEG can be used to assess risk for interictal markers of epilepsy.

Risk factors for epilepsy include genetic abnormalities and external events, such as head trauma, brain infections, stroke, or brain tumors. In many cases there can be both a genetic and external component, i.e., a genetic abnormality can predispose to the induction of epilepsy by external factors. Genetic testing is indicated in PWE with a suspected epilepsy due to multiple affected family members, those experiencing worsening of seizures with a particular class of ASM (antiseizure medications), or those demonstrating developmental "epileptic" encephalopathies.

Examples of Generalized Epilepsies and Epilepsy Syndromes

Childhood Absence epilepsy (Park et al. 2015)

Age of onset: 4-8 years old

Seizure types: Absence, generalized myoclonic and tonic-clonic

Associated triggers: Hyperventilation

Interictal EEG Findings: Generalized 3 Hz spike-and wave discharges

Etiology: Genetic

Co-Morbidities: Attention deficit and hyperactivity, anxiety, and mood disorders

Prognosis: Remission in most cases by puberty

Juvenile Myoclonic Epilepsy (Park et al. 2015)

Age of onset: Adolescence or young adulthood, typically evolve from childhood absence epilepsy

Seizure types: Generalized myoclonic and tonic-clonic, absence

Associated triggers: Sleep deprivation, awakening, visual or cognitive stimuli

Interictal EEG Findings: Generalized 3-5 Hz spike-and wave discharges, polyspikes

Etiology: Genetic

Co-Morbidities: Anxiety and mood disorders, obsessive compulsive disorder, substance abuse

Prognosis: Lifelong, but medically controlled in most patients, remission may occur around the sixth decade

Lennox-Gastaut Syndrome (Arzimanoglou et al. 2009)

Age of onset: 3-7 years old

Seizure types: Generalized tonic and tonic-clonic, atypical absence, and atonic seizures, less frequently generalized myoclonic or focal seizures

Associated triggers: Seizures can be activated by sleep (falling asleep or awakening)

Interictal EEG Findings: Generalized slow (1.5-2.5 Hz) spike-and-wave complexes, paroxysmal fast activity, background slowing

Etiology: Developmental malformation, infection, congenital stroke, tumor or genetic

Co-Morbidities: Developmental delay, intellectual disability, behavioral abnormalities

Prognosis: Lifelong, patients rarely achieve independence

Examples of Focal Epilepsies and Epilepsy Syndromes

Mesial temporal lobe epilepsy (Guerrini and Pellacani 2012)

Age of onset: Childhood, adolescence, and early adulthood, but may emerge at any age

Seizure types: Focal seizures without (visceral, olfactory/gustatory, autonomic, and psychic auras) and with impairment of awareness, bilateral tonic-clonic seizures

Associated triggers Infrequent and variable

Interictal EEG Findings: Temporal spikes, sharp waves, intermittent or continuous temporal slowing, temporal rhythmical delta activity

Etiology: Infection, congenital strokes, status epilepticus, cortical dysplasia, trauma, genetic

Co-Morbidities: Anxiety and mood disorders, acquired memory and language deficits

Prognosis: Common cause of medically intractable epilepsy, lifelong

Benign Focal Epilepsy of Childhood (Tatum 2012)

Age of onset: 3-10 years old

Seizure types: focal motor seizures (mainly oropharynx and face) and bilateral convulsive seizures

Associated triggers: Sleep (falling asleep or awakening)

Interictal EEG Findings: repetitive spikes activated by sleep in the centrotemporal/sylvian regions

Etiology: Genetic

Co-Morbidities: typically, reversible language and cognitive dysfunction, rare long-term deficits

Prognosis: Remission in a few years, usually by puberty

Medical Approach to Treatment for Epilepsy

The major treatment strategy for epilepsy is to prevent seizures or to significantly reduce the frequency and/or intensity of the seizures. (Chong and Bazil 2010) The initial approach involves treatment with ASMs, preferably a single medication (monotherapy). However, PWE not controlled by an optimal trial of one or two medications, eventually are placed on polytherapy using a combination of two or more anti-seizure medication. In these cases, medication treatment is chronic and raises a potential concern for adverse reactions due to pharmacokinetic and pharmacodynamic interactions. The adverse effects of ASMs can be initially difficult to tolerate, so dosage is increased gradually. If an ASM is not sufficiently effective another medication may be added, and if the PWE experiences side effects of toxicity, the dose of the initial ASM can be gradually reduced to avoid seizure exacerbation. ASM levels do not need to be monitored regularly; they are indicated when PWE are not demonstrating the expected response to treatment, or they are experiencing side effects to the ASM. The choice of the ASMs is based on the seizure types, epilepsy diagnosis, and the potential for adverse effects of long-term therapies. ASM levels If PWE fail antiseizure regimens, they should be evaluated using video-EEG monitoring to ascertain the epilepsy diagnosis, rule out nonepileptic spells, and evaluate whether they would benefit from nonmedical therapies, such resective brain surgery or neurostimulation. As seizure types may change and epilepsies can evolve, AAN Practice Guidelines recommend re-evaluating people with intractable epilepsy every three years with video-EEG monitoring and brain MRI.

Note: Several drugs that are used for epilepsy are also used to treat other conditions. Carbamazepine, oxcarbazepine, and lamotrigine are commonly used to treat trigeminal neuralgia pain. Valproic acid, lamotrigine, carbamazepine, and oxcarbazepine are mood stabilizers for psychiatric conditions such as bipolar disorder. Gabapentin and pregabalin are used to treat neuropathic pain. Topiramate is a first line medication for the prevention of migraine headaches.

Surgical and Dietary Therapies

Evaluation for surgery is focused on identifying the seizure-onset zone. (Zijlmans et al. 2019; Fisher et al. 2014) This requires a multi-day 24-hour video-EEG monitoring in an Epilepsy Monitoring Unit to record ictal and interictal epileptiform activity. Magnetic resonance imaging (MRI) can be effective for identifying epileptogenic lesions in the brain, such hippocampal sclerosis, focal cortical dysplasias, low-grade tumors, scar tissue, or cavernous hemangiomas. In patients not demonstrating a lesion, functional neuroimaging studies such as ictal single photon emission computerized tomography (SPECT), interictal positron emission tomography (PET) magnetoencephalography (MEG) can be useful. If the epileptic cortex is not vital to the ability of the patient to perform normal functions, particularly movement or speech, surgical removal of the focus can lead to seizure freedom or major clinical improvement. Frequently patients undergo a second video-EEG evaluation with implanted intracranial electrodes, i.e., stereotactic EEG electrodes or subdural strip and grid electrodes to better localize the seizure onset zone and to electrocortical stimulation for functional mapping and seizure activation. The most common type of resective surgery is temporal lobectomy; selective amygdalohippocampectomies are gradually being replaced by the less invasive laser ablation therapies. The most common neurostimulation therapy is Vagal Nerve Stimulation Therapy. In addition to intermittent stimulation of the left vagal nerve, stimulation is delivered by the detection of heart rate changes typically associated with seizure activity and by magnet activation of the device. Responsive Neurostimulation stimulates the brain with intracranial electrodes once a potential ictal discharge is recognized by the device. Deep Brain Stimulation entails intermittent stimulation of the thalamic nucleus, most commonly the anterior thalamic nucleus, and is often utilized in people bi-hemispheric focal, multifocal, or generalized epilepsies. Other treatment modalities are dietary, such as the Ketogenic or Modified Atkins Diets. While these treatments demonstrate efficacy, maintaining adherence is challenging. Neurostimulation and dietary therapies may not cure epilepsy but can significantly reduce seizure frequency and intensity.

Epilepsy Co-Morbidities and Complications

The main co-morbidities of epilepsy are cognitive and/or behavioral. (Fisher et al. 2014; Tatum 2012; Guerrini and Pellacani 2012; Arzimanoglou et al. 2009; Park et al. 2015) Children with epilepsy may express attention deficit and hyperactivity or autistic spectrum disorders, which often precede the diagnosis of epilepsy. Childhood onset epilepsies can be associated with intellectual delay, learning disorders, and social dysfunction. Cognitive decline is also seen in PWE with onset of epilepsy in adolescence or young adulthood. Gradual decline in memory and language functions are well documented in medically intractable temporal lobe epilepsy. Temporal lobe epilepsy is also associated with a higher risk of mood and anxiety disorders, which have also been reported with other epilepsy syndromes. Behavioral changes may precede the onset of epilepsy even in adult-onset epilepsy. While seizure control reduces the severity of the behavioral problems and cognitive decline, treatment of the concomitant behavioral symptoms is recommended.

The most common complication of epilepsy, particularly for convulsive seizures, are seizure-related injuries. These include oral trauma, such as tongue biting, craniofacial trauma due to falls, shoulder dislocations, and rib and long bone fractures. Because of frequent head injuries due to drop attacks, specifically atonic seizures, people with Lennox-Gastaut Syndrome are relegated to wearing helmets outside of the house. Drowning and motor vehicle accidents can occur with any seizure associated with altered awareness.

Other complications of seizures and epilepsy include status epilepticus (SE) and sudden unexpected death (SUD).

Status Epilepticus (SE):

A potentially life-threatening condition presents itself in the setting of an unusually prolonged seizure or a series of seizures with recovery of awareness between them. (Glauser et al. 2016) Status epilepticus can be convulsive (in which outward signs of a seizure are observed) or nonconvulsive (which has no outward signs and is diagnosed by an abnormal EEG). Nonconvulsive status epilepticus (NCSE) is a sustained episode of confusion, agitation, loss of consciousness, or even coma. Motor activity can range from lateralized clonic or tonic movements, automatisms, and stereotypies.

Any convulsive seizure lasting more than 5 minutes is considered status epilepticus and must be treated immediately to provide the best possible outcome and prevent brain damage. (Trinka 2017) Convulsive SE is also determined by repetitive convulsive seizures for 20 minutes without regaining awareness between the seizures. NCSE is characterized by a continuous seizure or repetitive seizures without regaining consciousness for at least 20 minutes.

Similar to seizures and epilepsies, SE presents in a bimodal distribution, typically by the age of 5 years old and after the sixth decade. SE can represent the first seizure in a person developing epilepsy, and in some cases can be an isolated event. The mortality of SE is much greater in the elderly than in children, mainly because of the underlying etiologies and associated co-morbidities. The prognosis of SE is best when treated early. Factors affecting morbidity and mortality include age of onset, duration of SE, and association with stroke, brain neoplasm or severe traumatic brain injury.

Treatment of Status Epilepticus:

Acute medical management of convulsive SE includes intravenous diazepam (20 mg) or lorazepam (4 mg). (Glauser et al. 2016) The recent availability of intranasal midazolam or diazepam provides rapid alternative to intravenous administration. If seizures continue the lorazepam injection is usually repeated. Second-line therapies include fosphenytoin (20 mg/kg), valproic acid (40 mg/kg), levetiracetam 60 mg/kg, and phenobarbital (20 mg/kg). Approximately half of patients with status epilepticus will respond to one of the IV infusion anti-seizure medications, however the other half will require additional dosing of medications to control their seizures. Patients failing to respond to the first and/or second lines of therapy are intubated, and the treatment of refractory SE then shifts to anesthetics. Anesthetics with short half-lives, such as propofol or ketamine, are used initially, before commitment of the patients to long-acting anesthetics like pentobarbital.

Sudden unexpected death in epilepsy (SUDEP):

SUDEP is a common cause of death in epilepsy patients. (Lhatoo and Sander 2005; Verducci et al. 2020) SUDEP is the most common cause of death in people of epilepsy between 20 and 40 years old. Although the incidence of SUDEP is relatively low, the estimated patient years of life lost is second only to stroke among neurological disorders. (Thurman et al. 2014) The risk is greatest among people with recurrent convulsive seizures (tonic-clonic seizures with either focal or generalized onset). SUDEP occurs postictally; the mechanism is thought to be hypoxia induced by postictal respiratory arrest. Most cases are unwitnessed and occur most often nocturnally in sleep. The best current approach to SUDEP prevention is the optimization of seizure control with the anticonvulsant drugs.

References

Arzimanoglou, A., J. French, W. T. Blume, J. H. Cross, J. P. Ernst, M. Feucht, P. Genton, R. Guerrini, G. Kluger, J. M. Pellock, E. Perucca, and J. W. Wheless. 2009. Lennox-Gastaut syndrome: a consensus approach on diagnosis, assessment, management, and trial methodology. *Lancet Neurol* 8 (1):82-93.

Chong, D. J., and C. W. Bazil. 2010. Update on anticonvulsant drugs. *Curr Neurol Neurosci Rep* 10 (4):308-318.

EpilepsyFoundation. 2023 [cited. Available from www.epilepsyfoundation.org/about/statistics.cfm.

Fisher, R. S., C. Acevedo, A. Arzimanoglou, A. Bogacz, J. H. Cross, C. E. Elger, J. Engel, Jr., L. Forsgren, J. A. French, M. Glynn, D. C. Hesdorffer, B. I. Lee, G. W. Mathern, S. L. Moshe, E. Perucca, I. E. Scheffer, T. Tomson, M. Watanabe, and S. Wiebe. 2014. ILAE official report: a practical clinical definition of epilepsy. *Epilepsia* 55 (4):475-482.

Fisher, R. S., J. H. Cross, C. D'Souza, J. A. French, S. R. Haut, N. Higurashi, E. Hirsch, F. E. Jansen, L. Lagae, S. L. Moshe, J. Peltola, E. Roulet Perez, I. E. Scheffer, A. Schulze-Bonhage, E. Somerville, M. Sperling, E. M. Yacubian, and S. M. Zuberi. 2017. Instruction manual for the ILAE 2017 operational classification of seizure types. *Epilepsia* 58 (4):531-542.

Glauser, T., S. Shinnar, D. Gloss, B. Alldredge, R. Arya, J. Bainbridge, M. Bare, T. Bleck, W. E. Dodson, L. Garrity, A. Jagoda, D. Lowenstein, J. Pellock, J. Riviello, E. Sloan, and D. M. Treiman. 2016. Evidence-Based Guideline: Treatment of Convulsive Status Epilepticus in Children and Adults: Report of the Guideline Committee of the American Epilepsy Society. *Epilepsy Curr* 16 (1):48-61.

Guerrini, R., and S. Pellacani. 2012. Benign childhood focal epilepsies. *Epilepsia* 53 Suppl 4:9-18.

Lhatoo, S. D., and J. W. Sander. 2005. Cause-specific mortality in epilepsy. *Epilepsia* 46 Suppl 11:36-39.

Park, J. T., A. M. Shahid, and A. Jammoul. 2015. Common pediatric epilepsy syndromes. *Pediatr Ann* 44 (2):e30-35.

Perucca, P., M. Bahlo, and S. F. Berkovic. 2020. The Genetics of Epilepsy. *Annu Rev Genomics Hum Genet* 21:205-230.

Scheffer, I. E., S. Berkovic, G. Capovilla, M. B. Connolly, J. French, L. Guilhoto, E. Hirsch, S. Jain, G. W. Mathern, S. L. Moshe, D. R. Nordli, E. Perucca, T. Tomson, S. Wiebe, Y. H. Zhang, and S. M. Zuberi. 2017. ILAE classification of epilepsies: Position paper of the ILAE Commission for Classification and Terminology. *Epilepsia* 58 (4):512-521.

Tatum, W. O. th. 2012. Mesial temporal lobe epilepsy. *J Clin Neurophysiol* 29 (5):356-365.

Thurman, D. J., D. C. Hesdorffer, and J. A. French. 2014. Sudden unexpected death in epilepsy: assessing the public health burden. *Epilepsia* 55 (10):1479-1485.

Trinka E, Kälviäinen R. 25 years of advances in the definition, classification, and treatment of status epilepticus. Seizure. 2017 Jan; 44:65-73. doi: 10.1016/j.seizure.2016.11.001. Epub 2016 Nov 14. PMID: 27890484.

Verducci, C., D. Friedman, E. J. Donner, J. Laze, and O. Devinsky. 2020. SUDEP classification: Discordances between forensic investigators and epileptologists. *Epilepsia* 61 (11): e173-e178.

Zijlmans, M., W. Zweiphenning, and N. van Klink. 2019. Changing concepts in presurgical assessment for epilepsy surgery. *Nat Rev Neurol* 15 (10):594-606.

Case Study Questions

Case Study

A 32-year-old right-handed young man has a history of epilepsy beginning at age 13 years old. He presented with focal seizures with impaired awareness and bilateral tonic-clonic seizures. He was started on oxcarbazepine and achieved control for over 10 years. He initially experienced a few breakthrough seizures, usually focal seizures with impaired awareness. His oxcarbazepine dose gradually increased but when he turned 30 his seizures became more severe, and he started to have bilateral tonic-clonic convulsions. As he could not increase his oxcarbazepine anymore due to dizziness, his neurologist added perampanel. The convulsive seizures stopped, but the focal impaired awareness seizures continued. His dizziness worsened on the combination.

1.1 What type of tests would a neurologist order when he originally presented with recurrent seizures at age 13 years old?

A ECG
B Brain MRI
C Head CT
D EEG
E B and D
F All of the above

1.2 What should the neurologist have done when the patient presented with breakthrough seizures in his 20s?

A Ask the patient about lifestyle changes
B Ask the patient about medication adherence
C Repeat an EEG and MRI
D If adherent, increase his oxcarbazepine dose
E A and C
F All of the above

1.3 After parampanel was added the patient's seizures continued but were better controlled; however, he was experiencing dizziness. The patient was also concerned about his progressive word-finding difficulties. The neurologist ordered an MRI and identified left-sided hippocampal sclerosis, which was not noted previously. What should the neurologist do next?

A Stop the oxcarbazepine immediately
B Decrease the oxcarbazepine while increasing the parampanel
C Replace the parampanel with another anti-seizure medication
D Consider video-EEG monitoring to characterize his epilepsy and evaluate for surgery
E B and D
F All of the above

1.4 A patient with epilepsy experiences an aura consisting of an epigastric rising sensation. In the next few seconds, the patient became unresponsive. The likely behavioral change is due to the ___.

A The onset of a severe migraine headache
B Evolution of a focal seizure with impaired awareness
C Evolution of an absence seizure
D Spread of the ictal discharge to the language areas.
E B and D
F All of the above

Quiz Questions

1. A 19-year-old male presents to your clinic after having a first-time seizure. He stated he pulled an "all-nighter" to study for her finals and had a seizure in the morning as he was getting ready to leave. His roommate described it as his full body becoming stiff and then shaking all over. The patient states he is often clumsy, dropping his toothbrush and breakfast plate in the morning. His EEG showed generalized 3-5 Hz polyspike-and-wave discharges during sleep. Which medication is the most appropriate treatment?

A Valproic Acid
B Carbamazepine
C Levetiracetam
D Phenytoin
E A and C
F B and D

2. A 7-year-old girl comes to clinic for evaluation of staring spells and poor grades in school. Her mother states that she will sometimes go "into her own world" and not seem to listen to what she is saying. Afterwards she will go back to what she was doing as if nothing happened but does not remember what her mother was saying to her. She has staring spells during her classes, and her grades have started to decline recently. Her EEG showed generalized 3 Hz spike-and-wave discharges during hyperventilation. What type of epilepsy does she have?

A Juvenile myoclonic epilepsy
B Mesial temporal lobe epilepsy
C Lennox-Gastaut Syndrome
D Childhood Absence Epilepsy

3. Which condition is NOT a part of the diagnostic criteria for epilepsy?

A Two unprovoked seizures occurring more than 24 hours apart
B Two unprovoked seizures occurring less than 24 hours apart
C One unprovoked seizure with a recurrence risk of at least 60%
D The diagnosis of an epilepsy syndrome based on EEG or clinical findings

4. Convulsive status epilepticus is characterized by

A Convulsive symptoms lasting continuously for at least 5 minutes.
B Unresponsive staring for at least 20 minutes
C Convulsions occurring repeatedly for at least 20 minutes without recovery of awareness
D Convulsive symptoms lasting at least two minutes.
E A and C
F None of the above

5. Patients with epilepsy who succumb to sudden unexpected death in epilepsy (SUDEP):

A Typically die following a convulsive seizure
B Are second only to stroke among neurological disorders in terms of years of life lost
C Are only "definite" when no cause of death is identified at autopsy
D Are usually in good health when they die
E All of the above

6. Juvenile myoclonic epilepsy is characterized by

A Adult onset
B Epigastric auras prior to loss of awareness
C Myoclonic seizures upon awakening
D Remission in childhood
E A and C
F All of the above

7. Mesial temporal lobe epilepsy is associated with:

A Absence seizures
B Memory impairment
C Reflex seizures
D Increased appetite
E A and C
F All of the above

8. Which of the following are true with regards to auras?

A Auras are not seizures
B Auras have no value in characterizing the type of epilepsy
C Auras can be associated with drowning
D Auras have localizing value
E A and C
F All of the above

Case Study Answers

1.1 E. Any patient with a single seizure should be evaluated with an EEG and MRI. This can be used to confirm a diagnosis of focal or generalized epilepsy by showing generalized vs focal interictal epileptic discharges or a potentially epileptogenic lesion on neuroimaging. However, the absence of abnormalities on imaging or EEG does not exclude a diagnosis of epilepsy.

1.2 F. All of the above

1.3 E. If a new anti-seizure medication started as adjunctive therapy appears to be more effective than the first medication, the treating physician should try to optimize its dose to provide the most benefit. If the patient is not tolerating the combination therapy, then the first medication should be gradually lowered. Antiseizure medications should not be stopped suddenly, due to the risk of withdrawal seizures, but the rate of the dose reduction should take the gravity of the side effect into account. Once patients have not responded to two medications, video-EEG monitoring needs to be considered for recording the patient's seizures.

1.4 E. The epigastric rising sensation is a typical symptom for an aura, or a focal seizure without impaired awareness. Unresponsiveness can be due to loss of awareness or propagation of the ictal discharge to the primary language areas, while awareness may still be present.

Quiz Answers

1. E. Valproic acid serves as the gold standard for treating a patient with generalized epilepsy, in this case juvenile myoclonic epilepsy. However, it is rarely used in child-bearing women due to the potential for teratogenicity. Carbamazepine and phenytoin may exacerbate generalized seizure types, including myoclonic ("clumsiness") and absence seizures.

2. D. Absence seizures begin in childhood and characterized by a brief staring spell associated with a generalized 3 Hz discharge on EEG. Juvenile myoclonic epilepsy can be associated with absence seizures, but myoclonic seizures are required for that diagnosis. Lennox-Gastaut Syndrome can be associated with prolonged, atypical absence seizure seizures, but tonic seizures are required for the diagnosis. Mesial temporal lobe epilepsy is associated with focal seizures only, though focal seizures with impaired awareness may be confused with absence seizures.

3. B. Seizures, whether unprovoked or stimulation-induced, must be more than 24 hours apart for the diagnosis of epilepsy.

4. E. Non-convulsive status epilepticus is typically diagnosed in a patient with unresponsiveness lasting over 20 minutes and may include absence status or focal status epilepticus with impaired awareness. Generalized or bilateral tonic-clonic seizures typically last about 1-2 minutes.

5. E. All the choices characterize SUDEP.

6. C. Myoclonic seizures upon awakening are pathognomonic for juvenile myoclonic epilepsy (JME). JME typically begins in adolescence and early adulthood, and typically poses a lifelong risk for seizures. Remissions before the 5th decade are rare.

7. B. One of the most important cognitive consequences of mesial temporal lobe epilepsy, which typically originates or involves from the hippocampus, is short term memory impairment. Mesial temporal lobe epilepsy is not associated with generalized absence or reflex seizures. Increased appetite is not a side effect of epilepsy, but a medication effect.

8. D. Auras represent focal seizures without impaired awareness and carry potential localizing value as they often represent the symptomatogenic zone closest or most connected to the epileptic focus. While auras do not impair consciousness, and therefore are not likely to lead to accidents or drowning, they do require therapeutic intervention as they can evolve into a focal seizure with impaired awareness or even a bilateral tonic-clonic seizure.

CHAPTER 19

DRUGS FOR NEURODEGENERATIVE DEMENTIAS

MEHARVAN SINGH, PHD[1] AND DANIEL ADOLFO LLANO, MD/PHD[2]

1 Loyola University Chicago, Chicago, Illinois, USA
2 University of Illinois at Urbana-Champaign, Illinois, USA

Symptoms: **Neurological**

FDA-approved therapeutics for Alzheimer's disease (AD):

Cholinesterase inhibitors:
- Donepezil
- Galantamine
- Rivastigmine

NMDA receptor antagonist:
- Memantine

β-amyloid modifying agents:
- Aducanumab
- Lecanemab

General background

Alzheimer's disease (AD) is a progressive neurodegenerative disorder that primarily affects older adults, with females having a higher prevalence than men (Dye et al. 2012; Callahan et al. 2001). AD remains the most common cause of dementia (or major neurocognitive disorder, as defined by DSM5). AD is now the 6th leading cause of death in the United States and has an estimated financial impact on the healthcare system of approximately $321 billion (US alone) (Alzheimer's Association, n.d.). And while several mechanisms of action underlying the brain dysfunction and neuronal loss associated with AD have been described, the etiology of this syndrome is still unknown. The study of the genetics of AD has revealed that the majority of AD cases are not a result of familial inheritance, in the traditional Mendelian sense. That is to say, less than 5% of all cases of AD can be attributed to the disease-causing mutations in one or a combination of the three known "causative" genes – amyloid precursor protein (APP) gene, the presenilin-1 (PSEN1) gene, and the presenilin-2 (PSEN2) gene (Campion et al. 1999; Janssen et al. 2003). As such, the etiology of the 95% of cases of AD diagnosed are complex and multi-factorial, though certain genetic risk factors, such as having at least one copy of the APOE4 allele, have been identified.

The most prominent clinical presentation/symptoms of AD relate to selective episodic memory impairment. The ability to recall events occurring at a particular time and place (i.e., episodic memory) is significantly disrupted in AD and is consistent with the early impact of AD on such structures as the hippocampus and related medial temporal lobe regions. Another domain of cognition affected early in the progression of AD includes visuospatial deficits. In contrast, subcortical pathways that relate to procedural memory and motor learning are not typically affected until much later in the progression of the disease (Mortamais et al. 2017).

While symptomatic treatments have become available, there is no cure at this time. Moreover, it is worth noting that with the exception of the most recent drugs approved by the FDA for the treatment of AD (Aducanumab and Lecanemab), which were FDA-approved over 20 years after the last drug, all other FDA-approved drugs are for symptomatic treatment only. The following outlines the current standard of diagnostic criteria for AD, followed by a listing of pharmacological management of AD.

Diagnosis:

A detailed clinical diagnosis of probable AD has been established by the National Institute on Aging (NIA) and the Alzheimer's Association (NIA-AA) (McKhann et al. 2011). In this most recent guideline, updated from the original guidelines published by McKhann in 1984 (McKhann et al. 1984), the approach to diagnosis of AD *premortem* considers neuropsychological assessment, neuroimaging, and potentially, the use of biomarkers as means to provide the most accurate diagnosis of AD. NIA-AA criteria for probable AD dementia require the presence of cognitive symptoms and the following characteristics:

- Interference with the ability to function at work or in routine activities
- Decline (in cognitive function) from a previous level of functioning
- Symptoms not explained by delirium or major psychiatric disorder
- Demonstrable cognitive impairment as supported by history-taking from the patient and a knowledgeable informant, and objective bedside neuropsychologic testing
- Cognitive impairment involving a minimum of two of the following domains:
  -Impaired ability to acquire and remember new information
  -Impaired reasoning and handling of complex tasks, poor judgment
  -Impaired visuospatial abilities
  -Impaired language functions
  -Changes in personality, behavior, or comportment

Clinical stages of AD:

As noted above, AD is a progressive neurodegenerative disorder, and as such, its symptoms worsen over time. The rate of progression may also vary, with some patients advancing to severe impairment within 1-2 years and others that have been reported to live as many as 20 years after diagnosis. What makes effective and early diagnosis of AD an imperative to the development and application of therapeutics is the recognition that molecular and structural changes in the brain related to AD begin years before any signs of the disease. Five stages of the illness are commonly recognized: Preclinical AD, mild cognitive impairment (MCI), early (or mild) AD, middle (or moderate) AD, and advanced (or severe AD). "Preclinical AD" is often defined by biomarker measures, such as amyloid deposition seen on amyloid PET scans, diminished amyloid beta and elevated phospho-tau in the cerebrospinal fluid, biparietal hypometabolism on fluorodeoxyglucose PET scans or hippocampal atrophy. The category of preclinical AD, at this time, is largely used in research and has particular value in the context of clinical trials for early intervention strategies as well as the longitudinal study of people deemed to be at risk. According to the International Working Group, preclinical AD can be divided into two groups (Morris et al. 2014):

- Asymptomatic, where cognitively normal individuals exhibit evidence of AD molecular pathology as determined by laboratory biomarkers or imaging techniques. It is unclear, however, whether progression to symptomatic AD is a foregone conclusion in such individuals noting that data from autopsy-based analyses revealed that people whose brains exhibited pathological changes consistent with AD were not symptomatic.
- Presymptomatic, where cognitively normal and asymptomatic individuals are carriers of a dominantly inherited gene mutation are likely to develop AD over the course of their normal lifespan.

Symptomatic stages of AD:

Mild Cognitive Impairment (MCI) due to AD is an early stage of AD, typically associated with anterograde memory impairment, but with preserved instrumental activities of daily living (Petersen et al. 1999). When the primary cognitive domain affected is episodic memory, it is typically referred to as "amnestic MCI" (aMCI). aMCI patients have an increased risk of developing AD compared to baseline, but that risk is highly variable, and increases when patients have positive AD-related biomarkers.

The NIAA-AA's clinical diagnostic criteria for MCI due to AD include the following:

- A concern regarding cognition reported by the patient or observed by the clinician
- Objective evidence of impairment in one or more cognitive domains that is not explained by age or education
- Preservation of independence with regard to functional abilities
- Impairments do not meet the criteria for dementia

It is worth noting that MCI may be a prodromal state to several neurodegenerative dementias (Petersen 2004; Petersen et al. 2001), as well as non-neurodegenerative conditions (including depression), particularly when the domain of cognitive impairment is not in episodic memory. Therefore, the diagnosis of MCI due to AD is applied when the clinical symptoms are further supported by the evidence/presence of a biomarker associated with AD (to include cerebrospinal fluid testing of amyloid beta, tau/phospho-tau, or amyloid imaging) (Heister et al. 2011).

The symptomatic stages of major neurocognitive impairment due to AD can be divided into three categories: mild (early) Alzheimer's disease, moderate (middle) Alzheimer's disease, and severe (advanced) Alzheimer's disease. The distinctions between the stages are often operationalized based on office evaluations of cognition, such as the mini-mental state examination (MMSE). Using this scale, scores above 22 are generally considered early or mild, 13-21 moderate or middle, and 12 or below would be severe or advanced. More fine-grained 7- or 8-stage systems have been described, but have not been established to be clinically meaningful. It should be noted that given the continuum of AD progression, it is not always possible to place a person with AD in a specific stage as the characteristics/symptoms of the stages may overlap.

Differential diagnosis: It is worth noting, as part of the differential diagnosis, that evidence of significant cerebrovascular disease, core features of dementia with Lewy bodies (DLB), prominent features of behavioral variant frontotemporal dementia (FTD), or prominent features of semantic or nonfluent/agrammatic variants of primary progressive aphasia (PPA), or evidence of another concurrent, active neurologic or non-neurologic disease, or use of medication that could have a substantial effect on cognition, must be considered to rule out other potential diagnoses. There are no FDA-approved treatments for any of the other neurodegenerative dementias, though medications for AD are often used in an off-label fashion for these disorders. To elaborate, the following section outlines disorders whose symptoms may be confused with AD.

Disorders with similar symptoms:

The most common disorders considered in the differential diagnosis of AD are vascular dementia and other neurodegenerative dementias, which include DLB and FTD.

Vascular dementia (often referred to now as "vascular cognitive impairment") is typically caused by either ischemic or hemorrhagic strokes or small vessel cerebrovascular disease. In most series, it is the second most common cause of dementia. (Cognitive Neuropathology Group Medical Research Council, 2001) Diagnosis is relatively more specific and straightforward if there is a stroke-like course of illness, neurologic signs of stroke on examination, and imaging evidence of cerebrovascular disease. However, it is worth noting that cerebrovascular disease commonly co-occurs with AD (Schneider et al. 2007), and as such can present challenges in cleanly distinguishing vascular dementia from AD and often patients are diagnosed as having mixed dementia related to both AD and cerebrovascular disease. The most appropriate way to treat vascular cognitive impairment is to aggressively control cerebrovascular risk factors such as diabetes, hypertension, and hypercholesterolemia, as well as to address other specific risk factors for stroke, such as atrial fibrillation or valvular disease. Physicians will sometimes use AD medications off-label for the treatment of the cognitive symptoms of vascular disease.

DLB is another common type of degenerative dementia. Clinical features that help distinguish this from AD include the prominent early appearance of formed visual hallucinations, along with Parkinson-like symptoms, memory and visuospatial disturbances, dysautonomia, rapid eye movement (REM) sleep behavior disorder, and neuroleptic sensitivity (McKeith et al. 2017). No medications are approved for DLB, though given the overlap between AD and Parkinson's disease-related symptoms, AD and Parkinson's disease medicines are often used off-label. Physicians should use antipsychotic medications with caution in these patients because those with a high affinity for dopamine receptors (e.g., haloperidol) can induce severe Parkinson's-like rigidity.

FTD is a neuropathologically heterogeneous disorder characterized by focal degeneration of the frontal and/or temporal lobes. Alterations in personality, social and emotional behavior, and executive functioning are prominent early clinical characteristics of FTD (Rascovsky et al. 2007; Rascovsky et al. 2011), particularly the behavioral variant of FTD (bvFTD). bvFTD patients often show extreme levels of apathy, superimposed upon episodes of socially inappropriate behavior. They have a difficult time relating to others emotionally and may have changes in their eating habits. PPA is a notable form of FTD in which progressive language impairment is the core feature (Mesulam 2013). There are three major subtypes of FTD, with the semantic and nonfluent types being typically associated with frontotemporal lobar degeneration (FTLD) pathologies, that include the presence of tau or TDP-43 (Gorno-Tempini et al. 2011). The logopenic variant of PPA can also exhibit signs and symptoms that may confuse the diagnosis of AD. FTD has an earlier onset (typically in the 50's) than AD. There are no FDA-approved medications for FTD, though physicians often use psychotropic medications to help control behavior.

Treatment of AD:

The three classes of currently FDA-approved treatments for AD are cholinesterase inhibitors, the N-methyl-D-aspartate (NMDA) receptor antagonist, memantine, and the recently approved monoclonal antibodies targeting amyloid beta, Aducanumab, and Lecanemab.

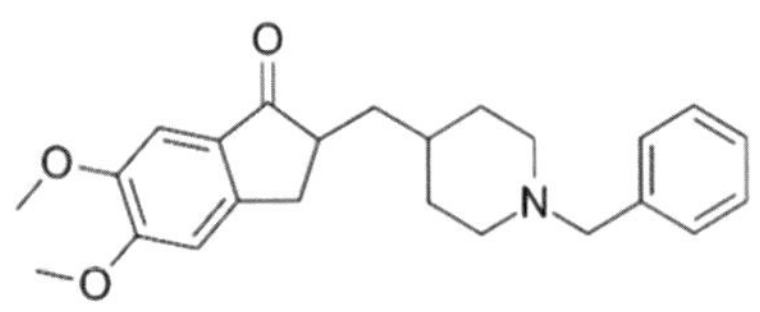

Donepezil

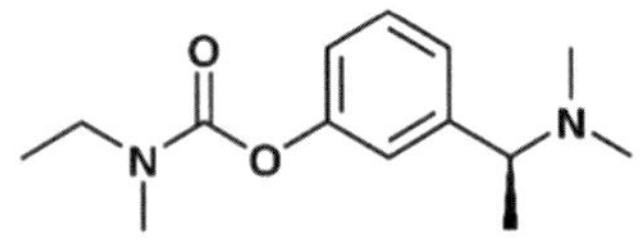

Rivastigmine

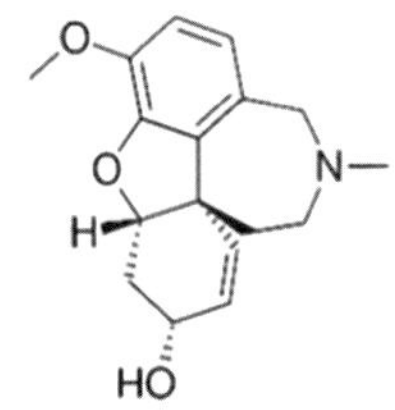

Galantamine

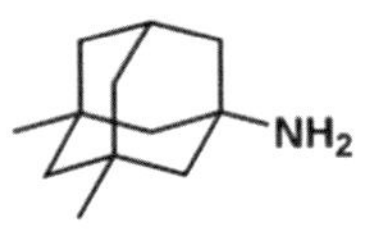

Memantine

Orally-available drugs:

Cholinesterase inhibitors include donepezil, rivastigmine, and galantamine. Mechanistically, their benefit on the symptoms of AD is to enhance cholinergic neurotransmission by reducing the degradation of acetylcholine at the synapse. It is worth noting that cholinesterase inhibitors do not appear to alter the underlying disease trajectory, but have modest effects in providing some symptomatic relief (Birks and Evans 2015; Raina et al. 2008; Trinh et al. 2003).

Donepezil was FDA-approved in 1996 and was the first of the modern slate of cholinesterase inhibitors to be FDA-approved. It is the most commonly prescribed drug for AD and is often used as a positive control in AD clinical trials. It is a highly specific blocker of acetylcholinesterase and is available orally and doses up to 23 mg/day are FDA-approved, though benefits can be seen at doses as low as 5 mg/day. It is approved for all stages of AD. It is typically dosed once per day. As a default, the short-acting version is typically dosed in the evenings, primarily so that its peak-level-related side effects (usually nausea) are experienced during sleep and are generally not noticed by patients. Its benefits relative to placebo is approximately 2-3 points on a scale known as the ADAS-Cog which is commonly employed in clinical trials. This translates into approximately 1 point on the MMSE, which is more commonly used in clinical practice. Donepezil is generally well-tolerated but can cause symptoms of cholinergic overload, such as nausea, diarrhea, and muscle cramps. For this reason, the drug is typically titrated over a 4-6 week period to desensitize patients to its side effects. It also often causes vivid dreams, which not all patients are bothered by, but can be diminished by dosing the drug in the morning. Given its cholinomimetic actions, all drugs in this class should be used with caution in patients with a history of syncope or pulmonary disease, though reports of this drug causing bradyarrhythmias or worsening pulmonary function are rare. Finally, given that weight loss is commonly seen in late-stage AD and because of the anorexia associated with the cholinergic effects of this drug, donepezil should be used with caution in patients experiencing weight loss.

Rivastigmine was FDA-approved in 2000 and is prescribed less frequently than donepezil. It is also approved for the treatment of cognitive impairment seen in Parkinson's Disease. It inhibits both acetylcholinesterase and butrylcholinesterase. The latter enzyme is found mostly in the periphery and breaks down acetylcholine as well as other related molecules, and is not thought to contribute to the pro-cognitive effects of the drug. The benefit and side-effect profiles of orally-dosed rivastigmine are similar to that seen with donepezil. A transdermal (patch) formulation was also approved in 2000 and currently is available in 4.6, 9.5, and 13.3 mg sizes. The patch should be removed and a fresh patch should be placed on a different part of the body every 24 hours. The main advantage of the transdermal formulation is its slow time course of action and consequent stable pharmacokinetics. As such, peak dose side effects, such as nausea, are seen much less commonly with this formulation. The drug may also find use in patients with advanced AD with trouble with chewing or swallowing or may be useful in patients with difficulty with adherence to oral medications. Given its use on skin, patients may develop erythema, swelling, and/or pruritis related to the presence of the patch or its adhesive.

Galantamine was FDA-approved for AD in 2001. It does not interact with butyrylcholinesterase but acts as a positive allosteric modulator of nicotinic cholinergic receptors, giving it an additional mechanism of action. Despite the additional mechanism of action, there has not been an established benefit of galantamine over the other two cholinesterase inhibitors. Generally, the benefit and side-effect profiles of galantamine match those of the orally-available formulations of the other two cholinesterase inhibitors.

Given the similarities in the mechanisms of actions of the cholinesterase inhibitors, if a patient suffers from mechanism-related side effects of one drug, there is not a clear and established benefit of switching to another drug in the same class. However, given the relatively benign side effect profile of these drugs, such a change may be considered after consultation with the patient and their caregivers. One exception here is in switching from oral cholinesterase inhibitors to patch-formulation of rivastigmine, where clear evidence for better gastrointestinal tolerability exists (Winblad et al. 2007). As such, the question may be asked whether starting with a patch may be the best strategy. In practice, this is not often done because 1) it is often easier in patients for whom medication adherence may be intrinsically challenging to incorporate another pill rather than add a daily patch, which usually involves a caregiver to put on and take off, 2) the patch may produce skin irritation and 3) there may be cost issues as the patch formulation is not yet available as a generic in the United States.

Memantine was approved in 2003 for the treatment of moderate-to-severe AD. Its mechanism of action is incompletely understood. It is typically referred to as being a low-affinity non-competitive NMDA receptor antagonist, whose intended effect is to reduce glutamate-induced excitotoxicity, and as such, has been speculated to elicit a neuroprotective effect. However, given that the NMDA receptor is also a key receptor involved in the physiological process of long-term potentiation (LTP), it is not clear if this mechanism may also exert deleterious effects on memory. Memantine also interacts with a broad portfolio of other receptor types in the brain. Thus, its mechanism of benefit may be distinct from its effects on NMDA receptors. That no follow-on drug has ever been approved for this highly commercially-successful compound supports the notion that the mechanism of action of this drug is not well understood. The magnitude of the benefit of memantine is similar to that seen with the cholinesterase inhibitors, and no long-term neuroprotective benefit has been established. Memantine is very well tolerated and is generally better tolerated than cholinesterase inhibitors. Dizziness, headache, confusion, and constipation may be seen but are rare. Memantine is generally dosed twice per day though it has a long elimination half-life (60-80hrs). Thus, in patients with challenges in medication adherence, the drug may be dosed once per day or a long-acting formulation may be used. The dose should be reduced if the patient has renal insufficiency.

Given the benefits of combination therapy in other diseases, one consideration is whether these drugs can be taken together. The benefits of memantine and cholinesterase inhibitors are additive when taken together, as determined by the registration trials cited in the memantine FDA label and subsequent meta-analyses (Chen et al. 2017; Muayqil and Camicioli 2012). Thus, the most common mode of practice in terms of oral medications for AD is to start with donepezil (or patch rivastigmine if intolerable gastrointestinal side effects occur to donepezil) and later add memantine. Given similarities in their mechanism of action to each other (and presumably distinct from that of memantine), any cholinesterase inhibitor can be combined with memantine.

Parenteral drugs:

Given the near-universal finding of amyloid deposition in the brain of AD patients, and because all three autosomal dominant forms of inherited AD involve genes that process amyloid beta, substantial interest has existed in developing drugs for AD that reduce amyloid burden. One approach that has been taken has been to use immunotherapy to attack and remove amyloid beta. A seminal study in AD model mice using active vaccination against amyloid beta was strongly suggestive of the benefit of this approach (Schenk et al. 1999). A subsequent study in humans using active vaccination against amyloid beta was halted early due to adverse effects, primarily encephalitis, but showed potential signals of efficacy (Gilman et al. 2005). Thus, a passive immunization approach of infusing antibodies against amyloid beta has been adopted by many pharmaceutical companies.

The first such drug to be approved was Aducanumab, which was approved by the FDA in 2021. Its approval was somewhat historic given that the FDA, at the time of approval for Aducanumab, had not approved a new drug for AD in approximately 26 years. It does, however, represent the first potentially disease-modifying therapeutic. Its efficacy as noted in the clinical trials for this therapeutic was less than that seen with oral medications, but showed a substantial reduction of amyloid plaque burden in the brain (McCleery and Quinn 2021). In point of fact, this therapeutic yielded positive clinical results in only one of the two Phase III trials (Budd Haeberlein et al. 2022). The drug requires monthly intravenous infusions of the antibody for one year. Side effects associated with this new therapeutic included infusion reactions and amyloid-related imaging abnormalities (ARIA), in the form of edema (ARIA-E) and/or microhemorrhage (ARIA-H), seen in up to 43% of patients and more common at higher doses and those that have at least one copy of the APOE4 gene. The high frequency of ARIA requires frequent MRI scans for monitoring. Thus, patients that cannot obtain an MRI scan are excluded from this medication medication and the drug should be used with caution in those with high intracranial bleeding risk.

The second drug in this class to be approved is Lecanemab, approved in 2023. This drug has a similar mechanism of action as Aducanumab, but is more specific for the protofibril form of amyloid beta. It is intravenously infused every two weeks and like Aducanumab leads to a significant decline in brain amyloid beta burden levels (van Dyck et al. 2022). A small signal of cognitive efficacy was seen as well. ARIA-E or ARIA-H was also seen in approximately 26.6% of patients treated. Similar to Aducanumab, the use of this drug will require frequent MRI monitoring.

Both Aducanumab and Lecanemab showed most of their efficacy at the earliest stages of AD (MCI and early AD). The use of these drugs also required confirmation of amyloid beta deposition in the brain prior to patients receiving the first infusion. Thus, it is likely that the standard of care for AD will eventually require an initial amyloid brain scan or lumbar puncture to confirm amyloid deposition and starting anti-amyloid therapy as a potential disease-modifier. At that point, the sequential addition of a cholinesterase inhibitor followed by memantine would then be used to optimize cognition.

Future opportunities:

The drug discovery efforts for AD have had a very high failure rate (Cummings et al. 2014). It has been suggested that, due to the complex etiology/pathobiology of AD, the failure of these trials may be attributed to attempts to target a single entity (Cummings et al. 2019). Indeed, as outlined above, evidence exists to support that combined treatment with memantine and a cholinesterase inhibitor was more effective at improving measures of cognition, activities of daily living (ADLs), and behavior (Tariot et al. 2004). No studies have yet evaluated whether either memantine or any of the cholinesterase inhibitors may enhance the potentially disease-modifying effects of Aducanumab or Lecanemab. Among other potential candidates as therapeutics for AD, whether used in combination with existing drugs, or as novel "stand-alone" therapeutics include the use of antioxidants (e.g., vitamin E (Farina et al. 2017), selegiline (Birks and Flicker 2003)) and anti-inflammatory compounds.

Case Study:

Mrs. Smith is an 80-year-old female that is brought to the clinic by her adult daughter because of memory concerns. The daughter notes that for the past 1-2 years, the patient will frequently repeat questions. She provides the example that on the way over to her current medical appointment, the patient asked five times where they were going and why. The patient is no longer able to manage her finances and her daughter is now helping her with this. The patient has occasionally become disoriented when driving in her neighborhood and once had to call her daughter to come to find her and guide her back home. The patient denies that she has a significant memory problem and attributes what she sees as her slight memory issues to "old age."

Pertinent negatives: No personality changes. No hallucinations or delusions. No focal weakness or tremor.

Her exam findings: Montreal Cognitive Assessment Score (MoCA) = 25/30, 4 points off on delayed recall, 1 point off on copying cube.

Neurologic exam was otherwise normal.

Additional workup: Serum TSH and vitamin B12 levels are normal. MRI of the brain showed hippocampal atrophy to 10% percentile (i.e., bottom 10% for age). Neuropsychological testing showed severe deficits in episodic memory and mild-moderate deficits in visuospatial function.

What is the most likely diagnosis? How would you devise a treatment plan?

Diagnosis: This patient meets the criteria of having dementia due to AD. She has deficits in two domains of cognition (episodic memory and visuospatial function) and has lost an instrumental activity of daily living (managing finances) and is having trouble with another (driving). Her workup does not reveal another cause, and in fact supports an AD diagnosis, given her hippocampal atrophy. Her MoCA score and the minimal level of functional impairment would put her into the early or mild (or early) category of AD.

Treatment Plan: Mrs. Smith should first be evaluated for potential treatment with anti-amyloid therapy such as Aducanumab or Lecanemab. No microhemorrhages were seen on her imaging, so there is no contra-indication to the use of these drugs. She would need confirmation of amyloid deposition in her brain, usually done with either an amyloid-PET scan or cerebrospinal fluid analysis, which would show low levels of the amyloid beta 1-42 peptide. She should also then be considered to start on donepezil and titrated to the maximum tolerated dose. Assuming that she tolerates this medication, at the moderate stage of AD, memantine can be started, again titrated to the maximum tolerated dose. Note that some practitioners will start memantine in the early stages of AD, though the FDA label supports its use in moderate and severe stages.

Outcomes and Followup: Mrs. Smith will obtain frequent MRI scans (typically 4-7 in the first year) if she starts Aducanumab or Lecanemab, as mandated on the FDA labels for these drugs. She will be followed in clinic every 3-6 months and will have ongoing cognitive assessments (either serial neuropsychological testing or serial MoCA exams) to assess her progress.

References

Alzheimer's Association. Undated. *Alzheimer's Disease and Dementia*. https://www.alz.org/.

Birks, Jacqueline, and Leon Flicker. 2003. Selegiline for Alzheimer's disease. *Cochrane Database of Systematic Reviews* (1).

Birks, Jacqueline S, and John Grimley Evans. 2015. Rivastigmine for Alzheimer's disease. *Cochrane Database of Systematic Reviews* (4).

Budd Haeberlein, Samantha, PS Aisen, F Barkhof, S Chalkias, T Chen, S Cohen, G Dent, O Hansson, K Harrison, and C von Hehn. 2022. Two randomized phase 3 studies of aducanumab in early Alzheimer's disease. *The Journal of Prevention of Alzheimer's Disease* 9 (2):197-210.

Callahan, Michael J, William J Lipinski, Feng Bian, Robert A Durham, Amy Pack, and Lary C Walker. 2001. Augmented senile plaque load in aged female β-amyloid precursor protein-transgenic mice. *The American journal of pathology* 158 (3):1173-1177.

Campion, Dominique, Cécile Dumanchin, Didier Hannequin, Bruno Dubois, Serge Belliard, Michele Puel, Catherine Thomas-Anterion, Agnes Michon, Cosette Martin, and Françoise Charbonnier. 1999. Early-onset autosomal dominant Alzheimer disease: prevalence, genetic heterogeneity, and mutation spectrum. *The American Journal of Human Genetics* 65 (3):664-670.

Chen, Ruey, Pi-Tuan Chan, Hsin Chu, Yu-Cih Lin, Pi-Chen Chang, Chien-Yu Chen, and Kuei-Ru Chou. 2017. Treatment effects between monotherapy of donepezil versus combination with memantine for Alzheimer disease: A meta-analysis. *PloS one* 12 (8):e0183586.

Cognitive Neuropathology Group Medical Research Council. 2001. Pathological correlates of late-onset dementia in a multicentre, community-based population in England and Wales. Neuropathology Group of the Medical Research Council Cognitive Function and Ageing Study (MRC CFAS). *Lancet (London, England)* 357 (9251):169-175.

Cummings, Jeffrey L, Travis Morstorf, and Kate Zhong. 2014. Alzheimer's disease drug-development pipeline: few candidates, frequent failures. *Alzheimer's research & therapy* 6 (4):1-7.

Cummings, Jeffrey, Garam Lee, Aaron Ritter, Marwan Sabbagh, and Kate Zhong. 2019. Alzheimer's disease drug development pipeline: 2019. *Alzheimer's & Dementia: Translational Research & Clinical Interventions* 5:272-293.

Dye, Richelin V, Karen J Miller, Elyse J Singer, and Andrew J Levine. 2012. Hormone replacement therapy and risk for neurodegenerative diseases. *International journal of Alzheimer's Disease* 2012.

Farina, Nicolas, David Llewellyn, Mokhtar Gad El Kareem Nasr Isaac, and Naji Tabet. 2017. Vitamin E for Alzheimer's dementia and mild cognitive impairment. *Cochrane Database of Systematic Reviews* (1).

Gilman, S, M Koller, RS Black, L Jenkins, SG Griffith, NC Fox, L Eisner, L Kirby, M Boada Rovira, and F Forette. 2005. Clinical effects of Aβ immunization (AN1792) in patients with AD in an interrupted trial. *Neurology* 64 (9):1553-1562.

Gorno-Tempini, Maria Luisa, Argye E Hillis, Sandra Weintraub, Andrew Kertesz, Mario Mendez, Stefano F Cappa, Jennifer M Ogar, Jonathan D Rohrer, Steven Black, and Bradley F Boeve. 2011. Classification of primary progressive aphasia and its variants. *Neurology* 76 (11):1006-1014.

Heister, D, James B Brewer, Sebastian Magda, Kaj Blennow, Linda K McEvoy, and Alzheimer's Disease Neuroimaging Initiative. 2011. Predicting MCI outcome with clinically available MRI and CSF biomarkers. *Neurology* 77 (17):1619-1628.

Janssen, JC, JA Beck, TA Campbell, A Dickinson, NC Fox, Richard J Harvey, H Houlden, MN Rossor, and J Collinge. 2003. Early onset familial Alzheimer's disease: mutation frequency in 31 families. *Neurology* 60 (2):235-239.

McCleery, Jenny, and Terence J Quinn. 2021. Aducanumab and the certainty of evidence: Oxford University Press, 1899-1900.

McKeith, Ian G, Bradley F Boeve, Dennis W Dickson, Glenda Halliday, John-Paul Taylor, Daniel Weintraub, Dag Aarsland, James Galvin, Johannes Attems, and Clive G Ballard. 2017. Diagnosis and management of dementia with Lewy bodies: Fourth consensus report of the DLB Consortium. *Neurology* 89 (1):88-100.

McKhann, Guy, David Drachman, Marshall Folstein, Robert Katzman, Donald Price, and Emanuel M Stadlan. 1984. Clinical diagnosis of Alzheimer's disease: Report of the NINCDS-ADRDA Work Group* under the auspices of Department of Health and Human Services Task Force on Alzheimer's Disease. *Neurology* 34 (7):939-939.

McKhann, Guy M, David S Knopman, Howard Chertkow, Bradley T Hyman, Clifford R Jack Jr, Claudia H Kawas, William E Klunk, Walter J Koroshetz, Jennifer J Manly, and Richard Mayeux. 2011. The diagnosis of dementia due to Alzheimer's disease: Recommendations from the National Institute on Aging-Alzheimer's Association workgroups on diagnostic guidelines for Alzheimer's disease. *Alzheimer's & Dementia* 7 (3):263-269.

Mesulam, M-Marsel. 2013. Primary progressive aphasia and the language network: The 2013 H. Houston Merritt Lecture. *Neurology* 81 (5):456-462.

Morris, John C, Kaj Blennow, Lutz Frölich, Agneta Nordberg, Hilkka Soininen, Gunhild Waldemar, L-O Wahlund, and B Dubois. 2014. Harmonized diagnostic criteria for Alzheimer's disease: recommendations. *Journal of internal medicine* 275 (3):204-213.

Mortamais, Marion, Jessica A Ash, John Harrison, Jeffrey Kaye, Joel Kramer, Christopher Randolph, Carine Pose, Bruce Albala, Michael Ropacki, and Craig W Ritchie. 2017. Detecting cognitive changes in preclinical Alzheimer's disease: A review of its feasibility. *Alzheimer's & Dementia* 13 (4):468-492.

Muayqil, Taim, and Richard Camicioli. 2012. Systematic review and meta-analysis of combination therapy with cholinesterase inhibitors and memantine in Alzheimer's disease and other dementias. *Dementia and geriatric cognitive disorders extra* 2 (1):546-572.

Petersen, Ronald C. 2004. Mild cognitive impairment as a diagnostic entity. *Journal of internal medicine* 256 (3):183-194.

Petersen, Ronald C, Glenn E Smith, Stephen C Waring, Robert J Ivnik, Eric G Tangalos, and Emre Kokmen. 1999. Mild cognitive impairment: clinical characterization and outcome. *Archives of neurology* 56 (3):303-308.

Petersen, Ronald C, James C Stevens, Mary Ganguli, Eric G Tangalos, Jeffrey L Cummings, and Steven T DeKosky. 2001. Practice parameter: Early detection of dementia: Mild cognitive impairment (an evidence-based review)[RETIRED]: Report of the Quality Standards Subcommittee of the American Academy of Neurology. *Neurology* 56 (9):1133-1142.

Raina, Parminder, Pasqualina Santaguida, Afisi Ismaila, Christopher Patterson, David Cowan, Mitchell Levine, Lynda Booker, and Mark Oremus. 2008. Effectiveness of cholinesterase inhibitors and memantine for treating dementia: evidence review for a clinical practice guideline. *Annals of internal medicine* 148 (5):379-397.

Rascovsky, Katya, John R Hodges, Christopher M Kipps, Julene K Johnson, William W Seeley, Mario F Mendez, David Knopman, Andrew Kertesz, Marsel Mesulam, and David P Salmon. 2007. Diagnostic criteria for the behavioral variant of frontotemporal dementia (bvFTD): current limitations and future directions. *Alzheimer Disease & Associated Disorders* 21 (4):S14-S18.

Rascovsky, Katya, John R Hodges, David Knopman, Mario F Mendez, Joel H Kramer, John Neuhaus, John C Van Swieten, Harro Seelaar, Elise GP Dopper, and Chiadi U Onyike. 2011. Sensitivity of revised diagnostic criteria for the behavioural variant of frontotemporal dementia. *Brain* 134 (9):2456-2477.

Schenk, Dale, Robin Barbour, Whitney Dunn, Grace Gordon, Henry Grajeda, Teresa Guido, Kang Hu, Jiping Huang, Kelly Johnson-Wood, and Karen Khan. 1999. Immunization with amyloid-β attenuates Alzheimer-disease-like pathology in the PDAPP mouse. *Nature* 400 (6740):173-177.

Schneider, Julie A, Zoe Arvanitakis, Woojeong Bang, and David A Bennett. 2007. Mixed brain pathologies account for most dementia cases in community-dwelling older persons. *Neurology* 69 (24):2197-2204.

Tariot, Pierre N, Martin R Farlow, George T Grossberg, Stephen M Graham, Scott McDonald, Ivan Gergel, Memantine Study Group, and Memantine Study Group. 2004. Memantine treatment in patients with moderate to severe Alzheimer disease already receiving donepezil: a randomized controlled trial. *Jama* 291 (3):317-324.

Trinh, Nhi-Ha, Jennifer Hoblyn, Subhanjoy Mohanty, and Kristine Yaffe. 2003. Efficacy of cholinesterase inhibitors in the treatment of neuropsychiatric symptoms and functional impairment in Alzheimer disease: a meta-analysis. *Jama* 289 (2):210-216.

van Dyck, Christopher H, Chad J Swanson, Paul Aisen, Randall J Bateman, Christopher Chen, Michelle Gee, Michio Kanekiyo, David Li, Larisa Reyderman, and Sharon Cohen. 2022. Lecanemab in early Alzheimer's disease. *New England Journal of Medicine*.

Winblad, B, G Grossberg, L Frölich, M Farlow, S Zechner, J Nagel, and R Lane. 2007. IDEAL: a 6-month, double-blind, placebo-controlled study of the first skin patch for Alzheimer disease. *Neurology* 69 (4 suppl 1):S14-S22.

Quiz Questions

1. A 70-year-old man presents to his primary doctor complaining of memory loss. He is able to live entirely independently. MoCA score = 28/30. Neuropsychological testing reveals a loss of episodic memory that is 1.5 standard deviations worse than age- and education-adjusted norms. MRI of the brain is normal. What is the most likely diagnosis?

A Subjective memory impairment
B Amnestic mild cognitive impairment
C Mild (early stage) AD
D Moderate (middle stage) AD
E Severe (advanced stage) AD

2. A 75-year-old woman is placed on donepezil 5mg per night to treat her AD symptoms. She and her husband report that there was no positive or negative impact of this medication. Her doctor then increases the dose to 10mg per night. She and her husband now report that she has improved memory function and is repeating herself less. Unfortunately, she is also having frequent nausea and diarrhea. What would be next most appropriate response be?

A Increase the dose of donepezil to 23 mg
B Decrease the dose of donepezil to 5 mg
C Stop all cholinesterase inhibitors and do not restart them
D Stop donepezil and start rivastigmine patch
E Stop donepezil and start oral galantamine

3. An 80-year-old man is brought to you for a memory evaluation. His score on a MoCA test is 10/30. He also has atrial fibrillation and is on an anticoagulant. MRI brain reveals numerous microhemorrhages. Which of the following drugs is contraindicated in this patient?

A Lecanemab
B Donepezil
C Memantine
D Donepezil + memantine combination therapy
E None of these drugs is contraindicated in this patient

4. An 82-year-old woman is brought to you by her daughter because she is "seeing things." The patient lives alone but reports seeing people frequently in her living room. She also reports that there is a family of goats living upstairs in her bedroom and that she often sees them jumping on her bed. Her examination reveals mild symmetric cogwheel rigidity bilaterally. MoCA score = 25/30 with 3 points taken away because of memory and 2 points because of visuospatial function. What is the most likely diagnosis?

A Frontotemporal dementia
B Alzheimer's Disease, moderate stage
C Vascular cognitive impairment
D Schizophrenia
E Dementia with Lewy Bodies

5. A 60-year-old man is referred to you by psychiatry. He was initially evaluated by psychiatry for concern about late-life depression. His wife reports that for the past year, he has lost all motivation to go to work, or even work around the house. He spends most days sitting on the couch, watching TV. He has become emotionally cold and distant from her. Recently he made some sexually inappropriate comments at a family gathering. He also started eating voraciously. She has had to put locks on the pantry as he has gained 30 pounds over the past year. His wife is fed up and she is on the brink of seeking a divorce and saw a psychiatry referral as the last chance for their marriage. What diagnosis should you be concerned about?

A Behavioral variant of frontotemporal dementia
B Alzheimer's Disease, moderate stage
C Vascular cognitive impairment
D Schizophrenia
E Dementia with Lewy Bodies

Quiz Answers

1. B. This individual has established cognitive decline beyond what would be expected from normal aging (as established by the memory score that is 1.5 SD below the mean). Hence the answer cannot be A, which implies normal cognition. However, he lives independently, so would not meet the criteria for dementia or major neurocognitive disorder, so the answer cannot be C-E. Thus the appropriate diagnosis is mild cognitive impairment. The fact that the primary cognitive domain is affected is memory makes this an amnestic disorder, thus the name amnestic mild cognitive impairment.

2. D. The patient is deriving benefits from the inhibition of acetylcholinesterase, but only at relatively high doses. So there is no point in decreasing to an ineffective dose, as in B or C. It also does not make sense to increase to 23 mg if 10mg is not tolerated as in A. Oral galantamine has the same mechanism of action as donepezil and would be expected to cause similar gastrointestinal side effects. D is the correct answer because the rivastigmine patch is better tolerated from a gastrointestinal perspective than oral cholinesterase inhibition, and allows dosing to a higher level before gastrointestinal side effects occur.

3. A. The main side effect of anti-amyloid therapy is the development of brain edema and intracranial bleeding. Thus, one would not put a patient with pre-existing brain hemorrhages and on an anticoagulant on a monoclonal antibody against amyloid-beta such as Lecanemab.

4. E. Dementia with Lewy Bodies is characterized by vivid visual hallucinations, symmetric parkinsonism, loss of episodic memory, and visuospatial function, as demonstrated by this patient. Note that patients with schizophrenia typically present at a much younger age, do not have parkinsonism in the absence of antipsychotics, and usually have auditory, rather than visual, hallucinations.

5. A. Behavioral variant of frontotemporal dementia is characterized by loss of frontal lobe function. The most common manifestations of this disorder are a combination of apathy, and emotional coldness with occasionally socially or sexually inappropriate behavior. Changes in eating habits are also often seen in this disorder, usually manifesting as voracious eating and large amounts of weight gain. It is common that this disorder is mistaken for being a psychiatric disorder, and these patients are often referred to psychiatry early in their disease course.

Symptoms 5 –

Endo-Repro-Gastrointestinal Symptoms to Treatment

CHAPTER 20

ABDOMINAL AND ESOPHAGEAL PAIN

MONTE TROUTMAN, DO[1], AND VICTOR V. UTESHEV, PHD[2]

[1] University of North Texas Health Science Center, Fort Worth, Texas, USA
[2] Epigen Biosciences Inc., San Diego, California, USA

Symptoms: **Endo-Repro-Gastrointestinal**

DRUG LIST FOR ABDOMINAL AND ESOPHAGEAL PAIN

Proton Pump Inhibitors:
Omeprazole
Esomeprazole
Pantoprazole

H2 Histamine Receptor Blockers:
Famotidine
Ranitidine
Cimetidine

Mucosal Protective Agents:
Bismuth subsalicylate
Misoprostol
Sucralfate

Antiacids:
Sodium Bicarbonate, Calcium carbonate
Magnesium/aluminum hydroxide

Pro-kinetic: D_2 Dopamine Receptor Antagonists, e.g., metoclopramide

Antibiotics: Erythromycin

Agents to Treat Irritable Bowel Syndrome (IBS):
Constipation Predominant (IBS-C): lubiprostone, linaclotide, psyllium, bran (other OTC drugs)
Diarrhea Predominant (IBS-D): rifaximin, eluxadoline, loperamide
Mixed (IBS-M): probiotics
Anti-Spasmodic Agents: dicyclomine

Agents to Treat Inflammatory Bowel Disease (IBD):
Anti-Inflammatory Agents: 5-aminosalicylic acid (5-ASA i.e., sulfasalazine=mesalamine+sulfapyridine, mesalamine)
Corticosteroids: prednisone, hydrocortisone, budesonide
Immunosuppressants, Anti-TNF/Integrin Antibodies: adalimumab, infliximab, vedolizumab
Antibiotics: metronidazole, ciprofloxacin

General Background

Abdominal pain is a frequent problem and can be challenging. It can also be caused by serious and acute problems. Pain can also present with other symptoms and complaints. Most patients have benign and self-limited problems. A thorough history and at least a focused physical are essential initially. This will identify patients needing more intense evaluation with laboratory testing and imaging studies. History needs to establish if the pain is acute or chronic. History should also include a description of the pain and other symptoms. Other aspects of the pain that need to be identified are radiation, palliative or provocative measures, and assessment of the severity of the pain.

Acute Abdominal Pain

The pain of sudden onset abdominal pain especially that of several days' duration that worsens is acute. Pain of several years' duration with minimal change is chronic. However, pain of over 3 months' duration is also classified as chronic. Subacute pain can be used to describe pain that is neither acute nor chronic. Again, as described above the historical aspects of pain that should be addressed are location, radiation, temporal events such as onset, frequency, duration, severity, nocturnal (wake from sleep), and quality such as colic, sharp, burning, gnawing or pressure. Examples of the usefulness of the historical aspects of pain are acute pancreatitis is constant with radiation to the back, perforation is sudden and severe while burning is used to describe esophageal reflux. Essential information can also be related to associated symptoms, especially other gastrointestinal symptoms such as nausea, vomiting, change in bowel habits (constipation or diarrhea), change in caliber of stools, melena, hematochezia, hematemesis, or signs of jaundice. A review of systems can often aid in establishing the cause of pain. These systems should include constitutional questions concerning fever, fatigue, weight loss, anorexia, and cardiopulmonary symptoms such as shortness of breath.

If inflammatory bowel disease (IBD) is considered, extra-intestinal manifestations of the disorders should be pursued in the history and physical exam. These include rashes, renal stones, gallstones, arthralgia, back pain, oral stomatitis, and eye disorders. Medical history, family history, and surgical history should also be reviewed. The possibility of pregnancy must always be established, especially prior to certain radiologic studies. Surgical history should include procedures such as endoscopic, laparoscopic, and cardiovascular including cardiac catheterization. The family history should focus on GI tract cancers and IBD which include Crohn's Disease and ulcerative colitis. The current and recent list of medications must be part of the person's history of taking medication. This includes over-the-counter medications including herbals and supplements. Other medications that must be reviewed are the use of anticoagulants, NSAIDs, and recent antibiotic which increases the risk of *Clostridioides difficile* (i.e., *C. difficile*) infection. All patients with abdominal pain should have current vital signs and a thorough abdominal exam. Fever should always raise the concern for sepsis with an appropriate course of evaluation. Abdominal exams include inspection, auscultation, palpation, rectal and pelvic exam when indicated. Patients with functional disorders usually have less pain on the exam when distracted. Inspection includes looking for distention, visible peristalsis which is always abnormal, hernia, and surgical incisions that should match the surgical history. Patients with peritonitis will lie still and rarely move while those with colic will writhe in pain. Auscultation of bowel sounds, or lack thereof is essential. Acute high-pitched sounds are common with early bowel obstruction. Absent bowel sounds are indicative of a more ominous situation. Sloshing sounds in the upper quadrants with the gurgling of the abdomen is a sign of gastric outlet obstruction. Bruits over the course of the abdominal vessels indicate vascular disease. Palpation can detect enlarged organs (especially the liver and spleen). Signs of peritonitis by palpation include rebound tenderness, abdominal wall muscle rigidity, and/or guarding. Palpation of the abdominal wall can detect masses, hernias, or abdominal muscular wall disorders. A rectal exam should be done on most patients with abdominal pain. Checking for fecal impaction, tenderness from a retrocecal inflamed appendix, and inspection for blood or melena. A pelvic exam should be done when indicated to exclude pelvic conditions. Patients with abdominal pain should have laboratory testing done. All female patients should have a pregnancy test especially if certain imaging is anticipated. Lab testing for acute abdominal pain should include a complete blood count (CBC), C-reactive protein (CRP), and comprehensive metabolic profile (CMP) that includes electrolytes, renal function, and liver enzymes. Lipase is always indicated with abdominal pain. Urine analysis is also routinely done.

Imaging studies are an essential aspect of the evaluation of abdominal pain especially if acute onset. Ultrasound is especially helpful for the detection of gallstones and renal stones. CT scans are useful for detection of abdominal masses, cancer, bowel obstruction, perforation, appendicitis, pelvic disease, IBD, ascites or free fluid, hernias, urinary tract obstruction as well as other disorders such as volvulus. Magnetic Resonance Imaging (MRI) and MR cholangiopancreatography (MRCP) are especially helpful for the detection of pancreatic and hepatic tumors or common bile duct pathologies such as choledocholithiasis or cholangiocarcinoma.

Endoscopic evaluation and treatment are also commonly used modalities in the assessment of abdominal pain. These include esophagogastroduodenoscopy (EGD), colonoscopy (which can also inspect the terminal ileum), and endoscopic retrograde cholangiography (ERCP). EGD and colonoscopy can detect and treat disorders such as bleeding ulcers, detect and biopsy tumors, decompress bowel, treat volvulus, dilate strictures, inset stents into the biliary and pancreatic duct, remove gallstones from the common bile duct. Advanced endoscopy such as endoscopic ultrasound (EUS) can supplement imaging as well as treat pancreatic disorders.

Patients with unstable vital signs, signs of peritonitis on an abdominal exam, or concern of life-threatening conditions or with a concern of a severe infection should be seen in an emergency department. These conditions include acute bowel obstruction, acute mesenteric ischemia or infarction, ectopic pregnancy, or bowel perforation. These conditions require prompt resuscitation, pain relief, and surgical evaluation.

A common emergency infection process that requires prompt treatment is ascending cholangitis. This presents altered vital signs and right upper quadrant pain. The patient has abnormal vital signs with a fever. The pain is associated with nausea and vomiting. Lab testing reveals abnormal liver enzymes with elevated total bilirubin typically over 4 mg/dL. Imaging demonstrates dilated bile ducts, and you may see gallstones in the gall bladder as well as in the common bile duct. Aggressive IV support, antibiotics, and pain relief are essential. The patient requires ERCP with sphincterotomy (i.e., cutting the Sphincter of Oddi which connects the bile/pancreatic duct to the duodenum) and stone removal within 12 hours to prevent overwhelming systemic sepsis and death. After recovery from sepsis, a laparoscopic cholecystectomy can be performed to remove the gallbladder.

Non-urgent evaluations with localized pain are considered by specific symptoms to guide the evaluation. Diffuse pain needs broader considerations and workup. Right upper quadrant pain frequently involves the liver and/or the biliary tree. The pain can radiate to the back, epigastrium, chest, or right shoulder. Evaluation after the history and examination should proceed with CBC, CMP, lipase, and ultrasound of the liver and gall bladder. Please refer to the comments on a common emergency in the preceding paragraph. Epigastric pain includes cardiovascular, pancreatic, gastric, or peptic ulcer disease (esophageal, gastric, or duodenal). If shortness of breath and a history of cardiac disorders are present, then cardiovascular causes should be excluded prior to any aggressive workup.

Acute pancreatitis should be suspected in patients with severe acute epigastric and/or periumbilical pain, with pain often radiating into the back. Alcohol and gallstones are by far the most common cause of acute pancreatitis. Other causes are idiopathic, autoimmune, drug-induced, and penetrating peptic ulcer disease.

A thorough history, physical exam, lab testing, and imaging (ultrasound, CT, MRI, MRCP) are the methods of diagnosis. Labs should include CBC, CMP, and lipase. Lab findings that make acute pancreatitis suspicious are elevated WBCs and lipase at least 2 times the upper limits of normal. Ultrasound of the liver and gallbladder should be done if hepatic or biliary tract concerns such as gallstones.

Liver enzymes can be elevated with acute pancreatitis. When total bilirubin is over 4.0 mg/dL and imaging shows a dilated common bile duct, then gallstone pancreatitis should be considered. This combination makes choledocholithiasis a strong possibility. History of alcohol use can also cause abnormal liver enzyme elevation as well but in a different pattern. The AST and ALT are elevated usually less than 300 IUs. The AST/ALT is usually greater than 2.

Prompt diagnosis is essential so therapy consisting of aggressive hydration and pain relief can decrease complications such as necrotizing pancreatitis and pseudocyst formation.

If peptic disease is suspected or a patient has iron deficient anemia, upper endoscopy should be performed. If the peptic disease is found, then a gastric biopsy for Helicobacter pylori should be done. If H. pylori is positive, then antibiotic treatment is indicated as well as verification of eradication. Eradication can be verified with a stool antigen test or a breath test.

Severe diffuse abdominal pain without signs of peritonitis should always be concerning. Acute mesenteric ischemia[2] is a critical problem that requires prompt diagnosis and therapy. The hallmark of the presentation is pain out of proportion to physical findings. Medical history is a significant factor as an aid to enhance suspicion. Older patients have atherosclerotic vascular disease, cardiac arrhythmias, valvular heart disease, chronic congestive heart failure, or clotting disorders.

There are no biomarkers or labs that aid in the diagnosis. The diagnostic test of choice is CT angiography. Depending on the findings treatment is surgical or vasoactive agents. A similar presentation occurs with a ruptured aortic aneurysm with surgery as the treatment. Diagnosis is made with an urgent CT scan of the abdomen. Other causes of diffuse abdominal pain are multiple and depend on the history and physical exam. These include infections or toxin-related food poisoning. A history of contact with people with similar presentations is helpful. Most presentations are self-limiting and treated with reassurance. If the etiology is not known laboratory testing includes CBC, CMP (includes liver enzymes), calcium, and lipase. Other considerations of these symptoms include IBD, diabetic ketoacidosis, hypercalcemia, and adrenal insufficiency.

Approach to Chronic Abdominal Pain

Chronic abdominal pain is common and frequently functional, such as irritable bowel syndrome. Functional abdominal pain is pain with no organic etiology. Functional pain is caused by hypersensitivity of visceral structures. These conditions can be treated with neuromodulators or other neuroactive drugs such as selective serotonin reuptake inhibitors (SSRIs; e.g., fluoxetine), selective norepinephrine inhibitors (SNRIs, e.g., duloxetine) or tricyclic antidepressants (e.g., amitriptyline).

The initial workup includes a history looking for alarm symptoms such as unintentional weight loss, fever, electrolyte disorders, GI bleeding, iron deficiency anemia, or malnutrition. Chronic abdominal pain with alarm symptoms should always consider malignancies such as esophageal, gastric, pancreatic, and colon. Iron deficiency warrants investigation for GI cancer and usually includes upper endoscopy and/or colonoscopy. Chronic abdominal pain with weight loss should always be considered pancreatic cancer with laboratory including CA19-9 and advanced imaging of the pancreas such as CT or MRI pancreatic specific.

Laboratory tests that typically performed are:
CBC
Comprehensive metabolic profile (CMP)
Lipase
C-reactive protein (CRP)

Further evaluation depends on history, physical, and lab findings:

Irritable Bowel Syndrome (IBS) is classified as IBS diarrhea-predominant (IBS-D), IBS constipation-predominant (IBS-C), or mixed (IBS-M). There is a variant that occurs after infectious diarrhea called post-infectious IBS that is treatable with probiotics and appropriate antibiotic use. The ROME criteria are a useful tool to ensure a more accurate diagnosis of IBS. ROME IV states that IBS requires:

Recurrent abdominal pain on average at least 1 day/week in the last 3 months, associated with two or more of the following criteria:

1. Related to defecation
2. Associated with a change in the frequency of stool
3. Associated with a change in the form (appearance) of stool

(Rome Foundation n.d.)

ROME IV also recognizes that some people get worsening pain with defecation.

Chronic pancreatitis in patients with excessive alcohol use or a history of recurrent episodes of calcific pancreatic depositions is a tip-off of this diagnosis. Diarrhea of exocrine pancreatic insufficiency is also possible.

If Inflammatory Bowel Disease (IBD) is suspected, then a more detailed workup is in order. Stool calprotectin is an inflammatory marker measured on a stool sample. If IBD has not already been established, imaging and endoscopy are key to diagnosis. Medication therapy includes biologics in most cases. IBD includes Crohn's Disease and chronic ulcerative colitis.

Crohn's Disease is a disease that involves the full thickness of the bowel. It can affect any part of the GI tract from the mouth to the anus. The most common symptoms are abdominal pain and diarrhea. It causes skip lesions with areas of inflammation interspersed with areas of normal mucosa. It is commonly found in the terminal ileum and the large bowel. A colonoscopy with terminal ileal inspection with biopsies is the definite diagnosis. Ulcerative colitis involves only the colon. The most common symptoms are bloody diarrhea with less pain than Crohn's Disease. It can affect only portions of the colon but can also involve the entire colon. It is superficial inflammation and is contiguous. The diagnosis is concluded through a colonoscopy with biopsy.

Celiac Disease is an underdiagnosed disorder and has varied presentations. Most notably it is associated with chronic diarrhea and iron deficiency. The anti-tissue transglutaminase is the screening test. A definitive diagnosis is duodenal biopsies obtained during upper endoscopy and should be done while the patient is eating gluten foods.

Some patients with HIV may present with unusual symptoms or unusual presentation of common disorders. An aggressive workup of infectious etiologies is indicated. Females, especially those with lower abdominal pain, should be evaluated with lab, imaging, and gynecologic evaluation for a host of possible issues such as fibroid, endometriosis, pregnancy, and ovarian or uterine carcinoma.

Gastroesophageal Reflux Disease (GERD)[3]

General Background

Reflux is a process where gastric contents move from the stomach into the esophagus. GERD is a disorder producing symptoms with symptoms of heartburn and regurgitation being the most common. Atypical symptoms are globus sensation, aspiration, middle ear disorders, hoarseness, laryngitis, and non-cardiac chest pain. Alarm symptoms are dysphagia, GI bleeding, weight loss, blood loss anemia, and melena. Complications of GERD are Barrett's esophagus, adenocarcinoma, esophageal strictures, and GI bleeding. Complications of GERD increase with advancing age, prolonged GERD, and obesity. The natural anti-reflux barrier includes healthy salivary function, esophageal motility, lower esophageal sphincter (LES) function, gastric emptying, distal esophageal barrier mechanisms, gastric anatomy including the angle of HIS and diaphragmatic crura. Estimates of GERD prevalence in the USA are based on symptom reporting. Given that some individuals may have GERD with no symptoms, such as occurs sometimes in those with Barrett's esophagus, the reported prevalence may be underrepresenting the true burden. In the USA weekly symptoms of GERD affect 20% of the population but may approach 30% in some populations. The prevalence of GERD symptoms is increasing and now over 50% of the population with at least weekly symptoms.

The most important risk factor causing the increasing incidence of GERD is obesity. Although increasing BMI is relevant, the most prevalent cause is central obesity. Other factors associated with GERD are certain medications, foods such as chocolate, mints, acid-containing foods, tobacco, alcohol, and unknown genetic factors. The most common medications that increase GERD are aspirin, NSAIDs, anticholinergics, and bronchodilators.

Common Types of GERD

- Non-erosive
- Erosive
- Functional
- Eosinophilic esophagitis (EoE) – inflammatory disorder diagnosed with an esophageal biopsy during an endoscopy that requires greater than 15 eosinophils per high power field. Note: in terms of patient presentation, there is a significant overlap of GERD and EoE.

Presentation: The diagnosis of GERD is clinical. The classic symptom is heartburn. It is generally described as a burning sensation in the substernal area and may radiate into the chest, neck, and throat. It is usually after meals that are high in fat, acid foods, spicy meals, chocolate, mints, and alcohol. Nocturnal symptoms include heartburn and regurgitation. Regurgitation is the spontaneous reflux of gastric contents into the oral pharynx with associated sleep deprivation. The diagnosis can be made when the patient complains of two or more episodes of heartburn and/or regurgitation per week or any nocturnal symptoms of heartburn or regurgitation. There are a variety of other typical and atypical symptoms. There are also symptoms described as alarm symptoms and need more urgent evaluation as to possible causes.

Atypical symptoms can also be attributed to reflux. These include hypersalivation also known as water brash, globus (lump-like sensation in the base of the neck), disorders of the ear, nose, or throat, hoarseness, aspiration pneumonia, and non-cardiac chest pain most commonly caused by esophageal spasm and atypical asthma. The chest pain experienced from reflux is due to diffuse esophageal spasms. The pain can mimic angina.

Risk factors that increase GERD are obesity, tobacco use, alcohol use, hiatal hernia, and gastroparesis.

Pathophysiology: Pathogenesis is complex and requires an understanding of normal protective mechanisms to prevent GERD:

- Saliva is basic and bathes the esophagus to neutralize residual acid not cleared by esophageal motility.
- Anatomical barriers include the intrinsic lower esophageal sphincter (LES). It is the major component of the reflux barrier system. It has a resting pressure but relaxes with a normal swallow and resumes normal resting pressure after the swallow passes.
- The diaphragmatic crura aid the anatomical structure to the LES but LES still functions if displaced by a hiatal hernia.
- The angle of HIS is the angle between the esophagus and the gastric fundus. It is an anatomical aid to prevent reflux.
- Esophageal motility sweeps food and gastric content from the esophagus into the stomach. Primary peristalsis is generated by a primary swallow. Secondary peristalsis is spontaneously generated by esophageal content such as food, and liquids, and includes acid reflux.
- The distal esophagus has mucosal defenses that resist acid damage. This mucosal defense is from tight mucosal epithelial junctions.

The mechanisms of reflux that lead to GERD are varied. The transient relaxation of the LES is a common cause of GERD. This is due to increased reflux while the LES is in its relaxed state. This transient relaxation can occur without peristalsis. Defective esophageal peristalsis can lead to prolonged exposure to spontaneous reflux. Hiatal hernia can exist without GERD. However, the hiatal hernia disrupts LES function. It acts as a reservoir of gastric content and increases reflux through a weakened LES especially if the hernia is over 3 cm in size.

Physical: Physical findings for GERD are sparse and usually minimal. Some of the findings for advanced GERD are pharyngitis including ulcerative findings. Dental erosions can also be caused by severe reflux. Asthma secondary to reflux is uncommon. It should be suspected in those over 30 years of age with no environmental exposures or genetic predisposition.

Laboratory and Imaging: Laboratory and imaging findings are low yields for the clinical diagnosis of GERD. If there is an iron deficiency anemia, this is a warning or alarm symptom, and endoscopy would be indicated. Upper endoscopy is indicated to exclude ulcerative esophagitis or esophageal adenocarcinoma. A barium esophagram is inexpensive but does not match endoscopic evaluations that include inspection and the ability to photograph, biopsy, and dilate peptic esophageal strictures. However, a barium swallow with a 13 mm barium tablet can crudely assess motility or strictures.

Other tools for esophageal evaluations are as follows:

- Wireless pH capsules attached to the esophagus endoscopically measure all forms of reflux both acid and non-acid or basic.
- Other reflux testing includes impedance with pH testing and most recently endoscopic impedance testing which are usually only performed at tertiary GI centers.
- Esophageal manometry is a measurement of LES pressure, upper esophageal sphincter pressure, and esophageal motility. A multichannel probe is passed orally into the stomach and wet swallow-initiated esophageal motility is evaluated. It will assess for conditions such as achalasia or motility disorders. This is the modality that is used to diagnose esophageal spasms. It also is a useful tool for deciding if surgical treatment for GERD is warranted.

Endoscopy is the ultimate tool for the evaluation and treatment of GERD complications. Esophagogastroduodenoscopy (EGD) is useful for diagnosis, photography, biopsy, and treatment. EGD with biopsy is the method for diagnosis of Barrett's esophagus, carcinoma, or eosinophilic esophagitis which has overlap symptoms with GERD.

Management: Behavioral modification is the basis of non-medical treatment and should be initiated prior to medical or surgical therapy. These modifications are:

- Lose weight if needed, especially central obesity
- Avoid aspirin and NSAIDs
- Avoid anticholinergic medications
- Avoid large meals and fatty, spicy, acid foods
- Do not lie down for one hour after meals
- Do not eat for 2.5 hours before bedtime
- Elevate the head of the bed 6 inches over the level of the feet
- Sleep on the left side
- Avoid tobacco, alcohol, caffeine, chocolate, or mints

Barrett's esophagus is a complication of long-standing GERD. Diagnosis is made by EGD with a biopsy of the abnormal EG junction (irregular Z line). The histology is gastric columnar epithelium with goblet cells as opposed to normal squamous cell epithelium. This is a premalignant condition and requires regular endoscopic and biopsy surveillance. The treatment of Barrett's is the same as treatment for GERD. If Barrett's biopsy reveals dysplastic changes more aggressive endoscopic surgery is indicated. Over-the-counter antacids can be used for infrequent symptoms of GERD. If symptoms continue prescription medications are indicated. When medications fail to control reflexes, surgical therapy is an option. Surgical intervention includes fundoplication and emerging and novel therapies. One of these new therapies is the magnetic sphincter which is a necklace of titanium beads with magnetic cores placed around the cardia.

Pharmacological Treatments for Abdominal and Esophageal Pain

Ulcers in the esophagus, stomach, and duodenum result from an imbalance between aggressive and protective factors. Aggressive factors include NSAIDs, gastric acid, pepsin, and *Helicobacter pylori*. Protective factors include prostaglandins, bicarbonate, and mucus secretion. The presence of *H. pylori* does not mean that the patient has an ulcer. However, most non-NSAID patients with ulcers probably have *H. pylori*. The three biggest pharmacotherapeutic problems in treating *H. pylori* are: 1) Resistance to antibiotics thus, treatment duration has been recently increased from 7 days to 14 days; 2) False-negative results (Urea Breath Test; UBT) thus, a 4-week delay after anti-*H.pylori* treatment is now recommended to confirm negative results; and 3) False-positive results (in UBT/immunoassay for *H.pylori* in stool samples) due to a lack of selectivity as other bacteria may trigger positive results.

Treatment of H. pylori ulcers: The most effective therapy (first-line regimen) for ulcers with *H. pylori* is a combination of treatments that include: one anti-secretory drug (PPI or H2 receptor blocker) and two antibiotics (e.g., clarithromycin, amoxicillin, tetracycline or metronidazole which is effective against *Clostridium difficile*). The duration of this triple therapy is 14 days. If a mucosal protective agent is added as an adjunct (e.g., bismuth subsalicylate), the treatment becomes a quadruple therapy. The risk of re-infection with *H. pylori* after a successful eradication is very low and amounts to <1 %.

1. Blockers of Gastric Acid Release (proton pump inhibitors, H2 histamine receptor blockers)

Indications: Ulcers in the esophagus, stomach & duodenum, GERD, Gastrin-producing tumors (Zollinger-Ellison syndrome).

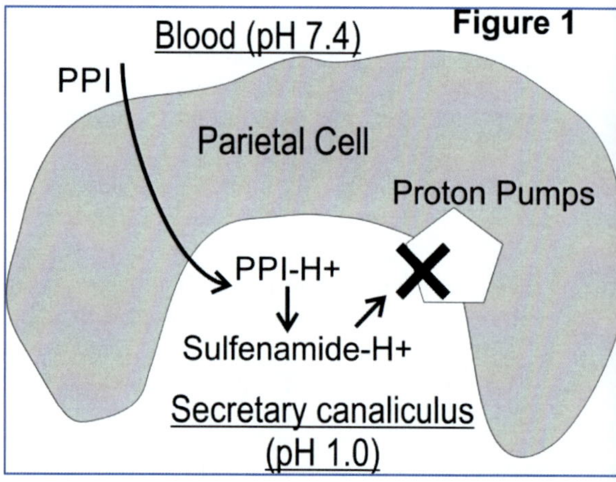

Proton Pump Inhibitors (PPIs): e.g., omeprazole (side effects due to inhibition of CYP2C19), esomeprazole, pantoprazole. PPIs are unstable at low pH and need an *enteric coating* to arrive in the intestine as pro-drugs. At neutral pH of the intestine, pro-drugs are chemically stable and lipid soluble, but inactive. PPIs are absorbed and carried by the bloodstream to parietal cells in the stomach, diffuse into secretory *canaliculi*, protonated at low pH, and trapped near the site of action. PPIs (via their prime metabolite, sulfenamide) produce a rapid irreversible blockage of proton pumps located in the secretory canaliculus of parietal cells (see **Figure 1** and an illustration in Maton PN, 1991, N Engl J Med 1991 324:965-975; PMID: 2002819, DOI: 10.1056/NEJM 199104043241406) thereby, targeting the terminal step of acid release. Note, the half-life of most PPIs is under 90 min, but their effects are much longer (>24 hours). This is because the binding of PPIs to proton pumps is irreversible and the pumps need to be replaced. The selective action of PPIs is ensured by the selective distribution of H^+/K^+-ATPase pumps in parietal cells and the so-called ionic trap near the PPIs targets because the low pH activates and traps PPIs near their targets. PPIs also exhibit antimicrobial activity against *H. pylori*. Note, PPI treatments may result in inaccurate *H. pylori* tests because PPIs are antimicrobial thus, may inhibit, but do not eradicate *H. pylori*.

Adverse effects of PPIs: PPIs are well tolerated. Occasional side effects include abdominal pain, headache, nausea, and diarrhea. PPIs increase the risk of *Clostridium difficile*-related colitis/diarrhea (treatment: metronidazole). Omeprazole (but not other PPIs) inhibits CYP2C19 and thus, reduces the metabolism of propranolol, warfarin, diazepam, and other CYP2C19-dependent drugs. Omeprazole also inhibits effects of pro-drugs: e.g., clopidogrel.

H2 Histamine Receptor Blockers (reversible effects but slower and less effective than PPIs): Famotidine (most potent), ranitidine, cimetidine (major side effects due to inhibition of multiple CYP450s e.g., CYP2C19). H2 histamine receptor blockers are less effective than PPIs because PPIs are more rapid, irreversible blockers that directly control stomach acidity as they act at the terminal step of acid release.

Adverse effects of H2 histamine receptor blockers: Famotidine and ranitidine cause occasional headache and diarrhea. Note, in 2020, the FDA requested the removal of ranitidine from the market due to contamination with N-nitroso-di-methylamine (NDMA) and the potential for cancer proliferation (see https://www.fda.gov/news-events/press-announcements/fda-requests-removal-all-ranitidine-products-zantac-market). Cimetidine inhibits multiple CYP450s (e.g., CYP2C19, CYP3A4) causing a potential for serious drug interaction and may cause headache and hormonal imbalance (e.g., gynecomastia).

2. Antibiotics (clarithromycin, amoxicillin, tetracycline, and metronidazole):

Indications: Peptic, esophageal, duodenum ulcers

Clarithromycin and amoxicillin are most effective for *H. pylori*. However, if treatments containing these antibiotics have failed, regimens that contain other antibiotics (e.g., tetracycline or metronidazole) should be used.

Adverse effects of antibiotics used for the treatment of peptic ulcer:

Clarithromycin, amoxicillin, and metronidazole may cause abdominal pain, nausea/vomiting, headache, diarrhea, anaphylaxis, and dysgeusia (loss of taste that requires discontinuation of the treatment). In addition, clarithromycin and amoxicillin may also lead to *Clostridium difficile* infection because as they target multiple types of bacteria they are ineffective against *Clostridium difficile* allowing the latter to grow unrestricted. Metronidazole is effective against *Clostridium difficile* and can be used in combination with other treatments at first symptoms of *Clostridium difficile* infection. However, metronidazole is carcinogenic in rodents (black box) and thus, its use should be avoided unless absolutely necessary.

3. Mucosal protective agents (bismuth subsalicylate, misoprostol, sucralfate):

Bismuth Subsalicylate is an insoluble salt of bismuth and salicylic acid that exhibits a broad spectrum of therapeutic effects including anti-inflammatory, mild anti-microbial, anti-motility, and anti-acid efficacies. Accordingly, it stimulates intestinal Na^+, and Cl^- absorption thus, water absorption. Salicylic acid inhibits prostaglandins and thus, motility (lower GI). Bismuth Subsalicylate exhibits a direct but mild antimicrobial activity against a variety of infections linked to Traveler's diarrhea (e.g., *Helicobacter pylori, Escherichia coli, Clostridium difficile, Campylobacter jejuni).* It also binds bacterial toxins (e.g., *Escherichia coli*). It protects mucosa and ulcer craters from acid and pepsin. It shows a weak anti-acid efficacy as it reacts with gastric acid to produce bismuth oxychloride and salicylic acid (which is quickly absorbed). In addition to being an anti-diarrheal agent, bismuth subsalicylate is an effective adjunct for the treatment and prophylaxis of duodenal and gastric ulcers and GERD.

Misoprostol (anti-NSAID) is a synthetic prostaglandin and binds to prostaglandin receptors on parietal cells inhibiting the secretion of gastric acid and pepsin. Misoprostol increases production/secretion of gastric mucus and HCO^{3-}; increases mucosal blood flow via direct vasodilation and increases intestinal electrolyte/fluid secretion and motility. It is most effective if taken 1 hour before meals and at bedtime. Misoprostol is primarily used by patients who absolutely must use NSAIDs (e.g., arthritis).

Note, selective cyclooxygenase-2 (COX-2) inhibitors (e.g., celecoxib) exhibit significantly lower GI toxicity than aspirin or other non-selective COX inhibitors and thus, are much safer for ulcer patients. However, selective COX-2 inhibitors may cause serious potentially fatal events (Black Box) by causing bleeding, ulceration, and perforation of the stomach or intestines (gastrointestinal mechanisms) and thrombotic events, myocardial infarction, and stroke (cardiovascular mechanisms). The causes of these adverse effects are as follows. COX-1 protects stomach walls and supports hemostasis by promoting the production of thromboxane A2, vasoconstriction, and coagulation. COX-1 inhibitors inhibit thromboxane A2. By contrast, prostacyclin (a.k.a. prostaglandin PGI2) supports vasodilation and inhibits coagulation by inhibiting platelet activation and aggregation. Selective COX-2 inhibitors inhibit prostacyclin and do not inhibit thromboxane A2 thereby, shifting the balance towards coagulation and vasoconstriction.

Sucralfate is an agent that at low pH polymerizes into a viscous gel protecting mucosa from acids and pepsin. It is most effective if taken 1 hour before meals and at bedtime.

Adverse effects of mucosal protective agents:

Misoprostol may cause diarrhea and abdominal pain. It should be avoided in pregnancy because it may cause serious birth defects, abortion, or premature birth due to uterine contractions (**Black Box**).

Sucralfate is exceptionally safe but may cause rare constipation.

Bismuth subsalicylate does not have side effects at therapeutic doses.

4. Antiacids (sodium bicarbonate, calcium carbonate, magnesium/aluminum hydroxide):

Indications: S*imple dyspepsia, uncomplicated GERD, adjuncts to PPI and H2 blockers.*

Antiacids neutralize the effects of gastric acid by raising the stomach pH above 4. These are over-the-counter (OTC) medicines that do not require a prescription. Both sodium bicarbonate and calcium carbonate exhibit rapid antiacid action, but may cause belching and metabolic alkalosis at higher doses. At higher doses, calcium carbonate may also cause hypercalcemia. The antiacid action of magnesium/aluminum hydroxide is slower, but these medicines do not cause similar side effects. While magnesium hydroxide is pro-kinetic and thus may cause diarrhea, aluminum hydroxide may cause constipation and thus, the combination of the two remains kinetically neutral minimizing gastrointestinal side effects and making this combination the most popular among OTC antiacid medicines. Note, antiacids elevate the stomach pH and thus, may alter the rate of absorption of other drugs. Antiacids may also reduce food digestion. Therefore, antacids should not be taken within 2 hours before or after other drugs.

5. Treatments for Inflammatory Bowel Disease (IBD)

Indications: IBD

Anti-Inflammatory Agents (inhibit inflammatory mediators, cytokines and immune cells, scavengers of reactive oxygen species):

5-aminosalicylic acid (5-ASA) and other aminosalicylate derivatives in various formulations ensure a slow release of 5-ASA or its release in the lower GI tract (from per oral to suppositories; e.g., mesalamine, sulfasalazine=mesalamine+sulfapyridine, inhibit the cyclooxygenase pathway and leukotriene formation);

Corticosteroids (prednisone, hydrocortisone, budesonide; to inhibit acute inflammation, not for chronic use because of adverse effects)

Immunosuppressants, i.e., Anti-Tumor Necrosis Factor/Integrin antibodies (the expression of TNFα is increased in IBD):

Adalimumab (anti-TNFα antibody; Black box: infections, lymphoma);

Infliximab (anti-TNFα antibody; Black box: infections, lymphoma);

Vedolizumab (anti-α4β7 integrin antibody; inhibits lymphocyte traffic; used in CD/UC patients resistant to anti-TNFα therapy);

Natalizumab (targets α4 integrins; FDA approved for CD; off-label for UC; Black box: leukoencephalopathy);

Azathioprine (off-label; Black box: lymphoma and malignancy).

Antibiotics: Metronidazole (off-label CD), ciprofloxacin (off-label CD)

Adverse effects of IBD treatments:

Sulfasalazine (due to sulfapyridine): Abdominal pain, diarrhea, nausea, headache, pain in joints (arthralgia) and muscles (myalgia); infections+hypersensitivity (fever, dermatitis, pancreatitis, pneumonitis, hepatitis, and pericarditis), inhibition of folate absorption

5-ASA and other aminosalicylates: Hypersensitivity (rare)

Corticosteroids: Increased risk of infections

6. Treatments for Irritable Bowel Syndrome (IBS)

Indications: IBS

IBS is a functional disorder and does not have diagnostic markers. A healthy diet matching GI conditions is an effective tool in the management of IBS. Drugs are used to relieve IBS symptoms.

Constipation Predominant (IBS-C): Lubiprostone, linaclotide, psyllium, bran, and other OTC products.

Diarrhea Predominant (IBS-D): Rifaximin (antibiotic, inhibits bacterial RNA synthesis; also, for Traveler's diarrhea), eluxadoline (μ agonist and δ antagonist); loperamide (peripherally restricted opioid, also, for Traveler's diarrhea), a*losetron* ($5HT_3$ blocker, women only; potentially fatal adverse effects, ischemic colitis).

Contraindications for eluxadoline: Biliary disorders, pancreatitis, patients without the gallbladder, alcoholism).

Mixed (IBS-M): Probiotics, anti-spasmodic agents (e.g., dicyclomine, a weak anti-muscarinic agent for temporary relief of IBS and GI spasms; produces only minimal anticholinergic adverse reactions).

References and Additional Literature to Read

Karkkainen, JM, Acosta, S. Acute mesenteric ischemia incidence, etiologies and how to improve early diagnosis. Best Pract Res Clinic GI. 2017: 31: 15-25.

Feldman, M, Friedman, L, Brandt, L. Sleisenger and Fordtran's Gastrointestinal and Liver Disease. 11th Edition. 2020. pp. 178, 670-692.

Feldman, M, Friedman, L, Brandt, L. Sleisenger and Fortran's Gastrointestinal and Liver Disease. 2020. 11th Edition. pp.152, 1946-865, 208-220.

Rome Foundation. Undated. *Rome IV Criteria*. https://theromefoundation.org/rome-iv/rome-iv-criteria/. Accessed 8 Jan 2023.

Case Study Questions

Case Study 1

A 65-year-old, mildly overweight, single-pack-a-day smoker has GERD relieved with a once-a-day proton pump inhibitor (PPI). The patient is very concerned about complications from PPI use.

1.1 Which statement most describes risks?

A Any dose of proton pump inhibitor for any length of time increases the risk of hip fracture
B Proton pump inhibitors confer no risk for hip fracture based on current data
C Proton pump inhibitors can increase the risk of *C. difficile* infections
D Increased risk of Barrett's esophagus.
E PPI use can increase the risk of H. pylori gastritis

Case Study 2

A 32-year-old professor in good health with no significant past medical or surgical history returned from a trip to Mexico eight months ago. The patient presents to your office complaining of symptoms that started soon after returning from the trip. For the past three months, the patient complains of epigastric abdominal pain described as burning with mild nausea, but no vomiting, as well as fatigue. The patient denies weight loss, fever, or rash, and all traveling companions are well. Despite the negative medical history, there was a history of anxiety. CBC with differential, comprehensive metabolic profile, serum lipase, CRP, and TSH are normal. A physical exam is normal except for mild epigastric tenderness. Treatment with a daily proton pump inhibitor for six weeks did not change symptoms. An EGD off the PPI was performed and was normal including a negative biopsy for H. pylori.

2.1 What would be the next step in evaluation?

A Nuclear gastric emptying test
B Increase PPI to twice daily
C Trial of low-dose neuromodulator
D H. Pylori antibody serology
E Stool antigen for H. pylori

Quiz Questions

1. A 67-year-old patient with long-standing gastroesophageal reflux now complains of crushing substernal chest pain. A cardiac workup includes a normal EKG and normal echocardiogram as well as normal cardiac enzymes. What is the most likely cause of this pain?

A Achalasia
B Barrett's esophagus
C Globus
D Diffuse esophageal spasm
E Eosinophilic esophagitis

2. What is the most common defect leading to gastroesophageal reflux disease?

A Decreased upper esophageal sphincter pressure
B Decreased lower esophageal sphincter pressure
C Hyper pulmonary insufflation
D Peptic ulcer disease
E Decreased salivation

3. Which is a premalignant disorder of the esophagus?

A Eosinophilic esophagitis
B Erosive esophagitis
C Barrett's esophagus
D Functional GERD
E Peptic esophageal stricture

4. The term to describe spontaneous gastric contents traveling from the stomach to the hypopharynx without retching is:

A Vomiting
B Reverse peristalsis
C Rumination
D Emesis
E Regurgitation

5. What medications can cause reflux symptoms?

A Aspirin
B Non-steroidal anti-inflammatory drugs
C Anticholinergics
D Peppermint oil
E All of the above

6. Pain out of proportion to physical exam findings is the hallmark of what disorder?

A Acute Mesenteric Ischemia
B Perforated duodenal ulcer
C Ectopic pregnancy
D Celiac disease
E Irritable Bowel Syndrome

7. A 27-year-old patient has chronic diarrhea. The diarrhea is non-bloody and does not affect the abdominal pain with bowel movement. A CT scan showed inflammatory changes in the terminal ileum. Colonoscopy demonstrated skip lesions with deep ulcerations and severe inflammatory changes. The terminal ileum was structured. What is the most likely diagnosis?

A Chronic ulcerative colitis
B Appendicitis
C Crohn's disease
D Severe peptic ulcer disease
E NSAID colitis

8. *Helicobacter pylori* is the leading cause of:

A Esophageal cancer
B Colon cancer
C Pancreatic cancer
D Peptic ulcer disease
E Gastroesophageal reflux disease

9. A 36-year-old female has recently been diagnosed with *H. pylori* infection. She is otherwise healthy and active. Which treatment should be used to eradicate *H. pylori* infection?

A Omeprazole
B Ranitidine + metronidazole
C Clarithromycin + amoxicillin
D Omeprazole + amoxicillin
E Omeprazole + clarithromycin + amoxicillin

10. Which is the most common cause of acute pancreatitis?

A Kidney stones
B Medications
C Marijuana
D Alcohol
E Autoimmune

11. A 57-year-old patient with acute severe right upper pain presents to the emergency department. Associated symptoms are nausea, vomiting, and fever. Serum bilirubin is 5.2 mg. Transaminases are elevated. An ultrasound of the gall bladder and liver reveals gallstones and a dilated common bile duct. You suspect.

A Peptic ulcer disease
B Ascending cholangitis
C Image negative cholecystitis
D Alcohol-induced pancreatitis
E Irritable Bowel Syndrome

12. A 35-year-old female attends a business dinner. She overeats and gets severe heartburn upon returning home. Which is the safest effective medication?

A Antiacid containing aluminum hydroxide
B Antiacid containing magnesium hydroxide
C Ranitidine
D Calcium carbonate
E A combination of A and B
F A combination of C and D

13. A 29-year-old-male complains of stomach pain and is diagnosed with non-erosive gastritis. Which drug is expected to produce an effective longest lasting suppression of stomach acidity?

A Aluminum hydroxide
B Metoclopramide
C Bismuth subsalicylate
D Pantoprazole
E Ranitidine

14. A 76-year-old-woman with Sjögren's syndrome takes 800 mg ibuprofen daily to reduce her joint pain and swelling. Which medication could be recommended as a protective agent for her gastric mucosa?

A Promethazine
B Misoprostol
C Clarithromycin
D Calcium carbonate
E Dexamethasone

15. The half-life of omeprazole is less than 90 min. Why does inhibition of proton pumps by omeprazole last for over 24h?

A Omeprazole is a prodrug with a very slow conversion rate to its active form
B Omeprazole is slowly metabolized in the liver over a 24h time window
C Omeprazole inhibits proton pumps irreversibly
D Omeprazole inhibits P-glycoproteins that take 24h to re-express
E Omeprazole is slowly absorbed in the intestine over a 24h time window

Case Study Answers

1.1 C. PPIs, especially long-term, use can alter the intestinal microbiome including the overgrowth of *C. difficile*. This can also be attributed to decrease acid production with resultant decreased defense mechanisms due to gastric acid production. Long-term PPI use may also cause osteoporosis due to a calcium decrease.

2.1 C. This history, physical exam, lab, and negative EGD with negative biopsy for H. pylori suggest functional disease. No further testing for H. pylori is necessary. Increasing the PPI dose with negative findings is not appropriate. A neuromodulator (e.g., selective serotonin reuptake inhibitor) is the best choice to treat the visceral hypersensitivity of functional disorders.

Quiz Answers

1. D. Diffuse esophageal spasm presents with pain that is hard to distinguish from cardiac angina. Achalasia and eosinophilic esophagitis are usually present with dysphagia. Barrett's esophagus is from long-standing GERD. Globus is a lump-like sensation in the back of the throat.

2. B. is the best answer. Decreased salivation occurs but is not the most common cause.

3. C. Barrett's esophagus is a pre-malignant condition for adenocarcinoma of the esophagus.

4. E. Regurgitation is what the question describes. Vomiting and emesis are the same and imply retching, not spontaneous. Rumination is voluntary and after meals.

5. E. ASA and NSAIDS can cause direct damage to the esophagus and predispose to reflux symptoms. Answer C and D can cause relaxation of the lower esophageal sphincter and increase reflux. All of the answers can cause or worsen reflux symptoms.

6. A. Pain out of proportion to a physical exam is classic for ischemia. The other choices infrequently cause severe pain or they cause an increase in pain with a physical exam.

7. C. Non-bloody chronic diarrhea in a young person with abnormal imaging and colonoscopy of deep ulcers in skip lesions and involvement of the terminal ileum is classic for Crohn's disease.

8. D. is the only correct answer.

9. E. The most effective therapy (first-line regimen) for ulcers with *H. pylori* is a combination of treatments that include: one anti-secretory drug (PPI or H2 receptor blocker) and two antibiotics (e.g. clarithromycin, amoxicillin, tetracycline or metronidazole which is effective against *Clostridium difficile*). The duration of this triple therapy is 14 days. If a mucosal protective agent is added as an adjunct (e.g. bismuth subsalicylate), the treatment becomes a quadruple therapy. The risk of re-infection with *H. pylori* after a successful eradication is very low (<1 %).

10. D. Alcohol and gallstones are by far the 2 most common causes of acute pancreatitis. Autoimmune responses and medications can cause pancreatitis, but not common.

11. B. This is a classic presentation of ascending cholangitis with RUQ pain, fever, bilirubin elevated to over 4 mg, a dilated common bile duct, and gallstones. This is most likely due to gallstones (choledocholithiasis) in the common bile duct.

12 E. Both aluminum hydroxide and magnesium hydroxide are effective antacids, but aluminum hydroxide causes constipation and magnesium hydroxide causes diarrhea. Combining these antacids in one treatment neutralizes these side effects. Calcium carbonate is effective too but may cause belching, metabolic alkalosis, and hypercalcemia. Ranitidine is an H2 histamine receptor blocker. In 2020, the FDA requested the removal of ranitidine from the market due to contamination with N-nitroso-di-methylamine (NDMA) and the potential for cancer proliferation (see https://www.fda.gov/news-events/press-announcements/fda-requests-removal-all-ranitidine-products-zantac-market).

13. D. Pantoprazole suppresses stomach acid production and is the best of all listed choices.

14. B. Misoprostol is a prostaglandin analog used as a protective agent for the gastric mucosa in patients who must take NSAIDs. Promethazine is an antihistamine medication with anticholinergic properties. The anticholinergic effects of promethazine may augment eye and mouth dryness in patients with Sjögren's syndrome. Clarithromycin is an antibiotic used in combination therapies for peptic ulcer. Calcium carbonate is an antiacid. Dexamethasone is a corticosteroid used in patients with Sjögren's syndrome to inhibit inflammation of joints, but not as a protective agent for the gastric mucosa.

15. C. Even though omeprazole (an irreversible proton pump inhibitor) is a prodrug, that is not why its effects last for over 24h. Omeprazole covalently (irreversibly) binds to proton pumps ensuring a prolonged therapeutic action (>24h) beyond its half-live (90 min) because the blocked pumps need to be replaced.

CHAPTER 21

CONSTIPATION AND DIARRHEA

MONTE TROUTMAN, DO[1], AND VICTOR V. UTESHEV, PHD[2]

[1] University of North Texas Health Science Center, Fort Worth, Texas, USA
[2] Epigen Biosciences Inc., San Diego, California, USA

Symptoms: Endo-Repro-Gastrointestinal

DRUG LIST FOR CONSTIPATION AND DIARRHEA

Anti-Diarrheal Agents:

Opioids: Loperamide
Diphenoxylate + atropine
Eluxadoline

Somatostatin Analog: Octreotide

Anti-inflammatory/anti-microbial/anti-motility/anti-acid: Bismuth Subsalicylate

Antibiotics: Ciprofloxacin
Azithromycin
Rifaximin

Anticholinergics muscarinic receptor antagonists (not commonly used due to side effects)

Laxatives:

Bulk-Forming Agents:	Methylcellulose
	Psyllium
	Ca^{2+} polycarbophil
	Bran
Stimulants:	Bisacodyl
	Senna
	Linaclotide
	Lubiprostone
Osmotic/saline Agents:	Mg^{2+} hydroxide/citrate
	Sorbitol
	Na^{+} phosphate
	Lactulose
	Polyethylene glycol-electrolyte solutions
Surfactant, Stool Softeners:	Mineral oil
	Docusate
Opioid Antagonist:	Methylnaltrexone

Constipation

- Constipation is a common gastrointestinal (GI) complaint. (Almario et al. 2018) Patients complain of multiple ways of describing their constipation including decreased frequency, hard stool, self-assisting to manually removing stools from their rectum, and excessive straining. These changes in stool may be associated with abdominal pain, cramping, and bloating. Chronic constipation is defined as when a patient has over at least one month of symptoms. (Scott et al. 2021)

Constipation is described as secondary when due to a variety of disorders. Primary constipation is from motility disorders, rectal dysfunction, or normal transit.

Because of the disparity of symptoms used to describe constipation, the ROME IV criteria were established to help standardize the actual symptoms of the causes of constipation. At least two symptoms are required 25% of the time to meet the criteria of irritable bowel syndrome. These symptoms include straining at the stool, lumpy or hard stools, the feeling of incomplete evacuation, the sensation of anal blockage, fewer than 3 stools per week, and loose stools not present without laxatives.

- Risk factors for constipation are older age, female, low socioeconomic status, use of constipating medications, low physical activity, and the standard American diet. This diet is low in fiber. Low water intake is also a contributing factor. (Forootan et al. 2018)

The adequate colonic function relies on colonic absorption of water from the stool, motor function that depends on colonic musculature, and neural intervention. The function of defecation requires other factors including a correct position with squatting being the preferred position and the complex action of anorectal function.

In patients with new-onset constipation secondary causes should be sought and excluded. These secondary causes include mechanical obstruction, medications, metabolic and endocrine disorders as well as neurologic and myopathic disorders.

The list of secondary causes of constipation includes mechanical obstruction from colon cancer, colonic strictures, and anal stenosis. Colonic strictures can be from inflammatory bowel disease (Crohn's Disease and ulcerative colitis), post-surgical complications, and diverticular disease.

Multiple medications can cause constipation. These include but are not limited to aluminum-containing antacids, anticholinergics, calcium channel blockers, non-steroidal anti-inflammatory drugs, opiates, and diuretics.

- Neurologic or myopathic disorders are also secondary causes of constipation. These are often debilitating and difficult to treat. Some of the more common disorders are diabetes especially if associated with diabetic neuropathy, thyroid disease especially hypothyroidism, electrolyte imbalance especially hypercalcemia, and heavy metal toxicity, especially lead. The neurologic or myopathic disorders that can cause constipation are autoimmune neuropathy, Chagas disease, pseudo-obstruction, multiple sclerosis, stroke, and Parkinson's disease. (Bharucha and Wald 2019)

A cause of acute constipation is colonic pseudo-obstruction. The exact cause is unknown but usually can occur after surgery. This is called Ogilvie's syndrome. Ogilvie's syndrome involves the colon. Another cause of constipation after surgery is ileus. Post-operative ileus is a more generalized problem and involves both large and small bowel. The symptoms are significant abdominal distension and hypoactive bowel sounds for both disorders. Diagnosis is usually made by radiologic imaging.

Primary constipation may be classified as normal transit, slow transit, and defecatory disorders. Normal transit is associated with psychiatric disorders or rectal dysfunction.

- Slow transit constipation is associated with abdomen pain bloating and malaise. This is associated with irritable bowel syndrome (IBS). The most severe presentation of this disorder is colonic inertia. (McCoy and Beck 2012) It has a similar presentation as IBS but does not meet all IBS ROME IV criteria.

- Defecation disorder is the term to describe the inability to evacuate stool from the rectum, it may be associated with slow transit. (Bharucha et al. 2006) This disorder includes tenesmus, dyssynergia, obstructive defecation, and outlet obstruction. This condition can also be caused by rectocele, descending perineum syndrome, and rectal prolapse.

One of the most common and well-known causes of constipation in the USA is irritable bowel syndrome (IBS). IBS can cause constipation (IBS-C), diarrhea (IBS-D), or both known as mixed (IBS-M). IBS-C should meet ROME IV criteria as described earlier. Patients often complain of bloating, abdominal distention, and dyspepsia. The ROME IV criteria are the most useful method to diagnose IBS-C. The most helpful criteria are symptoms lasting more than 6 months, abdominal pain with constipation, and relief of the pain with bowel movement.

A detailed history is essential in the approach to constipation. This history includes whether the acute or chronic, duration of symptoms, associated symptoms, palliative or provocative measures for the pain, and/or constipation. The use of the Bristol stool chart may also aid in the description of the stool.

Warning or alarm signs and symptoms are essential parts of history. Alarm symptoms are straining at the stool, unintentional weight loss, melena, severe abdominal pain, development of anemia especially iron deficiency, and rectal bleeding. A family history is a must and should include GI tract cancers, especially colorectal cancer. Medical, surgical, and obstetrical history is also essential. The history of endoscopic procedures is most important in the elderly.

A detailed history of current medications including over-the-counter medications and supplements should be recorded. A dietary history is also part of the history. Eating habits are part of this history and include if breakfast is a daily part of the diet. Finally, a psychiatric history including sexual and physical abuse will aid in the diagnosis. Questions about posturing during defecation may aid in the diagnosis of an anorectal disorder.

The physical examination of the abdomen is also important. The abdomen should be observed, auscultated, and palpated. Parts of the exam that are important are looking for distention, hernias, and palpation for masses. Inspection for previous surgical scars should match the surgical history. A rectal exam is paramount. Features of the rectal exam are inspection for prolapse, perineal descent with Valsalva, feel for masses, and inspect extracted stool for blood, melena and feel for impaction of stool in the rectum. Anal wink should be elicited to test for pudendal nerve function. A general physical including general appearance, exam of the neck for thyroid enlargement, and generalized lymphatic exam. A neurological exam will help diagnose the underlying condition when neurological disorders may be the cause of constipation.

Diagnostic Testing and Criteria

Further testing is not always necessary if conditions like IBS are obvious. For suspected secondary causes or patients with alarm symptoms, laboratory testing includes CBC, a complete metabolic profile that includes electrolytes, calcium, glucose, renal function, and inflammatory markers as serum C-reactive protein (CRP). If the CBC reveals anemia, especially if microcytic, then iron studies should be done. Iron deficient anemia counts as an alarming symptom when present. More intense laboratory testing is necessary if neoplastic, inflammatory, metabolic, or neurologic disorders are suspected.

Imaging studies including CT scans, MRI, or barium studies specifically for the colon may aid in the diagnosis. Barium enemas have dropped off dramatically due to more diagnostic studies available especially colonoscopies. Small bowel studies are at times used in constipation workups. CT or MRI enterography has all but displaced small bowel barium studies.

Colonoscopy should be used specifically if alarm symptoms are revealed. However, a colonoscopy can be performed for colorectal cancer screening at age 45 or earlier if there is a family history of colon cancer. This may aid in determining the cause of constipation.

Another more specific testing may be of use but would be done after a specialist referral. This specialized testing includes radiopaque marker testing and a wireless motility capsule. Defecography and anorectal manometry are supplemental tests useful in defecation disorders.

Diagnostic Criteria of Irritable Bowel Syndrome*

Recurrent abdominal pain on average at least 1 day/week in the last 3 months, associated with two or more of the following criteria:

1. Related to defecation;
2. Associated with a change in the frequency of stool;
3. Associated with a change in the form (appearance) of stool.

* Criteria fulfilled for the last 3 months with symptom onset at least 6 months prior to diagnosis. IBS-C: >25% of bowel movements with Bristol Stool types 1 or 2 and < 25% of bowel movements with Bristol stool types 6 or 7.

Diagnostic Criteria of Functional Constipation*

Must include two or more of the following:**

1. Straining during more than 25% of defecations;
2. Lumpy or hard stools (Bristol Stool Form Scale 1-2) more than 25% of defecations;

3. Sensation of incomplete evacuation of more than 25% of defecations;
4. Sensation of anorectal obstruction/blockage of more than 25% of defecations;
5. Manual maneuvers to facilitate more than 25% of defecations (e.g., digital evacuation, support of the pelvic floor);
6. Fewer than three SBM per week;
7. Loose stools are rarely present without the use of laxatives;
8. Insufficient criteria for irritable bowel syndrome.

*Criteria fulfilled for the last 3 months with symptom onset at least 6 months prior to diagnosis.

**For research studies, patients meeting the criteria for opioid-induced constipation (OIC) should not be given a diagnosis of FC because it is difficult to distinguish between opioid side effects and other causes of constipation. However, clinicians recognize that these two conditions may overlap.

Treatment

Non-pharmacologic treatment is the initial treatment in most cases unless a treatable secondary cause is found. The basis of this form of treatment is lifestyle changes. These include:

- Eat breakfast
- Increase physical activity
- Increase fiber in the diet to 25-30 grams per day
- Increase water intake
- Avoid constipating medications
- Improve squatting position while on the toilet
- If the trial of the above is no help, add fiber supplements and stool softeners
- Surgery is a last resort after additional medications fail

Diarrhea

Diarrhea is an alteration in bowel habits. Three or more bowel movements in a day and/or loose or liquid stool, a Bristol stool chart with the consistency of type 6 or 7 is also consistent with diarrhea. Type 6 is described as fluffy pieces of stool with ragged edges and mushy while type 7 is watery, with no solid pieces and entirely liquid. Fecal incontinence is described as diarrhea but is usually not diarrhea. It is the inability to control the bowels. It results in accidental leakage of stool or uncontrolled bowel movements. Diarrhea is a common symptom in the USA but most episodes are of short duration and resolve spontaneously without medical care.

Normally 99% of the fluid in the gastrointestinal tract is absorbed by the small and large intestines. Diarrhea results when this process is altered by inflammation from various diseases or ingestion of toxins, bacteria, or other noxious substances.

Multiple altered mechanisms lead to diarrhea. Either a decrease in absorption or an increase in secretion leads to diarrhea. Regulation of a complex communication system of extracellular and intracellular messengers can be altered resulting in diarrhea. Toxins, cytokines, drugs, and hormones are major causes of diarrhea.

Osmotic diarrhea occurs with the ingestion of poorly absorbed cations and anions or poorly absorbed sugars. This process restricts total absorption. This process restricts total fluid absorption and results in diarrhea. Some disaccharides like lactose and sucrose or fructose are common agents leading to this type of diarrhea. Another spectrum of foods that causes osmotic diarrhea is FODMAP foods. FODMAP stands for Fermentable Oligosaccharides Disaccharides Monosaccharides and Polyols. A helpful characteristic of osmotic diarrhea is that it ceases with fasting or avoidance of the offending agent.

Diarrhea due to disordered electrolyte transport is secretory but may be decreased absorption. Secretory diarrhea has many causes. The mechanism is the net secretion of anions or potassium or inhibition of sodium absorption. Infection is the most common cause of secretory diarrhea. Enterotoxins from bacteria, viruses, and parasites interact with the intestinal receptors of absorption. Peptides from endocrine tumors stimulate secretion resulting in diarrhea.

Other causes of secretory diarrhea with less well-understood mechanisms of action are small intestinal bacterial overgrowth (SIBO). Alteration in the microbiome is thought to be a major contributor.

Other disorders leading to diarrhea are alterations in the motility of the bowel and include ischemia, thyroid disorders, scleroderma, and pseudo-obstruction. The mechanism of the cause of diarrhea is not well known but secretory mechanisms are thought to play a role.

Secretory or osmotic disorders are causes of many diarrhea disorders. Unusually, they are the sole causes of diarrhea. Most causes of diarrhea are complex. The list of causes of diarrhea due to a complex array of pathophysiologic mechanisms includes inflammatory bowel disease (IBD), IBS-D, and food allergies.

Clinical classification of diarrhea has several methods which include acute versus chronic, the volume of stool, characteristics (watery, fatty, inflammatory), or epidemiologic.

Acute diarrhea of fewer than 4 weeks is usually infectious. Most infectious causes last about 7 days. Some protozoal infections last longer. Immunocompromised hosts are prone to more persistent diarrhea from these causes.

Stool volume may give a clue as to the site of the disorders. Small-volume diarrhea leans to the left colon. Large volume implies pancreas, left colon, or small bowel.

Other stool characteristics that may aid in the source include osmotic versus secretory, watery versus fatty versus inflammatory. One of the most useful approaches is epidemiologic factors. These factors include travel, camping, swimming in lakes or rivers, and exposure to ill persons with diarrhea and foods consumed. Local health department publications also list infectious agents currently prevalent in the community.

Evaluation

Taking the history of the chief complaint must be thorough. Duration, onset, intermittent or continuous, and medical factors such as medications, surgical history, or radiation treatments are some of the important factors. Alarm symptoms must be sought out as they have a bearing on the aggressiveness of the workup. These alarm symptoms are weight loss, blood in the stool, melena, fever, and level of pain. Factors that increase, set off, or relieve pain are important historical features.

Medical history and family history are paramount. A family history of IBD, celiac disease, and cancer can be helpful and critical. A thorough review of all medications both prescription and the counter are mandatory. The review of systems should include questions about extra-intestinal manifestations of IBD. These are the presence of rash, oral ulcers, kidney or gallstones, arthralgias, back pain, perianal disease, and painful red eye symptoms.

Surgical history especially abdominal surgeries is important. Some surgeries may be the cause of diarrhea. These surgeries include cholecystectomy, vagotomy, and bowel resection concentrating on the portion of the bowel removed, how much of the bowel was removed, and what portions of the bowel were removed.

Certain medical disorders can also be the cause of diarrhea. Diabetes, AIDS, IBD, multiple endocrine disorder especially hyperthyroidism, Addison's disease, and many more. Cancer of the GI tract also causes diarrhea. These diarrheas are usually chronic and watery.

A physical exam (PE) follows a thorough history and is most helpful in determining the severity of diarrhea. Volume status, and checking vital signs for fever, tachycardia, and hypotension are essential. The PE should check for edema, muscle wasting, arthritis, lymphadenopathy, and thyroid nodules or enlargement. The abdominal exam includes observation for distention and visible peristalsis, and listening for bowel sounds and bruits. Palpation for tenderness, guarding, rebound, and palpation for masses complete the abdominal exam. A rectal exam should also be done to check for blood which is considered an alarming symptom.

The basic laboratory in patients with chronic diarrhea is CBC, comprehensive metabolic profile including blood sugar, electrolytes including calcium, IgA transglutaminase (for celiac disease), and CRP. Stool studies should include fecal calprotectin, bacterial cultures including Clostridioides difficile, ova, and parasites when indicated especially Giardia, stool fat studies, stool sodium, and potassium to calculate the osmolar gap. Patients with risk factors should be tested for HIV. HIV increases the number of possible infectious agents causing diarrhea.

Acute diarrhea lasting more than 7 days or patients with warning signs warrant a more aggressive approach than a wait-and-see approach. The lab should include a CBC, a comprehensive metabolic profile, and bacterial cultures. An elevated white cell count on the CBC increases the cause as bacterial. Diarrhea that develops while in the hospital or after antibiotic treatment for other infections raises the possibility of *C. difficile* and testing should be done. Colonoscopy or sigmoidoscopy with biopsies and stool collection is an unusual part of the workup for acute diarrheas.

- The differential for chronic diarrhea is extensive and more complex. A careful history and physical exam will highlight possible causes such as radiation damage to the GI tract, a post-surgical abdomen, or IBD. Most patients with chronic diarrhea are usually not identified after history, physical, and laboratory. (Smalley et al. 2019) The lab most appropriate for chronic diarrhea includes CBC, INR (testing for vitamin K malabsorption), inflammatory markers (CRP, ESR), stool inflammatory markers (calprotectin), lipase for pancreatic evaluation, stool for ova and parasites, stool fat studies, and stool electrolytes studies (helps distinguish osmotic vs secretory diarrhea) Many of these patients with chronic diarrhea require imaging and endoscopy with biopsies for pathologic evaluation to make and/or verify the diagnosis.

Upper endoscopy is needed for the diagnosis of celiac disease. The patient cannot be on a gluten-free diet prior to the endoscopy with duodenal biopsies. Other diseases that can be identified with upper endoscopy and biopsy are amyloidosis, lymphoma, Whipple's disease, and eosinophilic gastroenteritis. Colonoscopy with stool collection and biopsies are valuable for the diagnosis of Crohn's Disease, chronic ulcerative colitis, and microscopic colitis.

No matter the method of collecting stool, especially in chronic diarrhea the osmolar gap should be calculated to help with the diagnosis of osmotic or secretory diarrhea. The formula is **290 mOsm/kg – 2 x (stool [Na^+]+ stool [K^+])**, where 290 mOsm/kg is the average stool osmolarity and the amount of cations is doubled to account for the contribution of anions. The range of 50-100 is normal, greater than 100 is osmotic, and less than 50 is secretory.

Certain imaging can be helpful and is especially helpful for chronic diarrhea. CT scanning can identify pancreatic disorders, masses, or tumors and abnormal imaging of the bowel helping to identify possible IBD. Special MRI and CT studies of the small bowel are called MR enterography or CT enterography. These are especially helpful for identifying skip lesions of the small bowel that are consistent with Crohn's Disease.

One of the more difficult causes of diarrhea to diagnose is fatty diarrhea. Chronic pancreatic insufficiency is a common cause of this. CT or MRI imaging studies of the pancreas help identify pancreatic disorders. Chronic alcohol use is a factor that will increase suspicion of pancreatic insufficiency.

Small intestinal bacterial overgrowth (SIBO) is another difficult chronic syndrome to diagnose. It should be suspected of bloating. A specialized breath test is the method of diagnosis.

Some of the other diarrheal syndromes that should be considered are:

Traveler's Diarrhea: This is elicited by a history of travel especially to endemic areas.
IBD-D or functional: Use of ROME IV criteria is most useful. This is chronic and usually without warning or alarm symptoms.
Food-induced diarrhea.
Microscopic colitis: 2 varieties exist and diagnosis can only be made by colonoscopy with biopsy of normal appearing mucosa; common in middle-aged patients; women more than men.
Bile acid-induced diarrhea. Secondary to resection of terminal ileum as in Crohn's Disease surgery. Also occurs in over 10% of post-cholecystectomy patients.
Diarrhea of obscure origin: The differential is broad but some of the most common causes are IBS, SIBO, and laxative abuse.

Pharmacological Treatment of Constipation and Diarrhea

An imbalance between water intake and absorption results in either diarrhea (intake>absorption) or constipation (intake<absorption). The GI transit time defines the outcome: slow GI kinetics translates to constipation (and nausea; see Symptoms 8: Nausea and Vomiting). By contrast, fast GI kinetics supports diarrhea (and is anti-emetic; see Symptoms 8: Nausea and Vomiting). Medications that inhibit net water absorption are defined as laxatives. By contrast, drugs that augment net water absorption are called anti-diarrheal. The mechanism of action for these effects can be peripheral, central, or combined.

Treatment of Constipation

Bulk-Forming Agents (simple constipation): e.g., Bran, Ca^{2+} polycarbophil, Psyllium, Methylcellulose. These agents are non-digestible materials also known as dietary fibers. It can be synthetically made (e.g., methylcellulose) or originate from plants (bran, whole grain). The mechanism of action is via absorbing water and thereby, softening stool and increasing its amount. Bulk-forming agents are effective within 48 hours of intake. They are safe and can be used long-term in combination with other laxatives.

Stimulants: Bisacodyl (bowel preparation before surgery; direct action). Bisacodyl directly acts on parasympathetic nerves of the guts/colon causing peristalsis and bowel evacuation. Bisacodyl is effective within 24 hours of intake. Bisacodyl should not be used chronically because it causes tolerance and Bisocodyl dependence.

Osmotic/saline agents: Mg^{2+} hydroxide, Mg^{2+} citrate, Na^+ phosphate (acute constipation), Sorbitol (occasional constipation; 5-7% in prune juice), Lactulose (chronic constipation; → lactic/acetic acids), Polyethylene glycol-electrolyte solutions (PEG; complete colon cleaning). These agents are also non-digestible. They increase osmotic pressure in the lumen and soften stool by elevating water content. Effective time is dose-dependent but always falls within 6-24 hours. Osmotic/saline laxatives are safe and can be used long-term in combination with other laxatives. Magnesium/Sodium-containing agents are very safe and can be used for a variety of needs including emptying the bowel prior to colonoscopy or surgery or clearance of poison.

Sorbitol: Prune juice contains 5% sorbitol which is a non-digestible sugar that increases osmotic pressure in the lumen. Sorbitol can also be administered rectally including enema with similar therapeutic effects.

Lactulose: intestinal bacteria break down lactulose (indigestible sugar) into lactic, acetic, and formic acids and increase acidification of the intestine (drops the pH and promotes NH3 dissociation to $NH4^+$ and OH^- and ammonium is not absorbed in intestines) and increases osmolarity thereby causing peristalsis.

Polyethylene glycol-electrolyte solutions are used for preparing the bowel for colonoscopy or colorectal surgery because PEG ensures the most complete evacuation of the GI tract. Patients are given up to 4 liters of PEG over 6 hours prior to surgical/colonoscopy procedures.

Laxatives: Linaclotide (chronic constipation, IBS-C; GC→cGMP), Lubiprostone (chronic constipation, IBS-C; Cl^- ion channel influx), senna, and other OTC products (occasional constipation).

Linaclotide is a guanylate cyclase agonist that activates guanylyl cyclase on the luminal surface of intestinal epithelium thereby increasing the cGMP level which stimulates the secretion of chloride ions and bicarbonate into the lumen followed by water and resulting in stool softening.

Lubiprostone activated chloride ion channels in the small intestine and promotes chloride influx into the intestine followed by water and resulting in stool softening. Lubiprostone does not cause tolerance, but chronic use may cause nausea.

Senna leaves contain anthraquinone derivatives with laxative effects within 6 hours after consumption.

Surfactant: Mineral oils and other surfactants reduce surface tension

Docusate (acute; reduces straining; not very effective; limited clinical use).

Opioid Antagonist: Methylnaltrexone (opioid-induced constipation). Methylnaltrexone is a peripherally-restricted μ-opioid receptor antagonist. Methylnaltrexone does not cross the blood-brain barrier and thus, does not inhibit the analgesic efficacy of prescribed opioids.

Treatment of Diarrhea

Diarrhea may result from increased: 1) Intestinal motility (rapid transit); 2) Intestinal osmolarity and water retention (osmotic); 3) Secretion of electrolytes into the intestinal lumen (secretary); and 4) Inflammation of the colon lining, mucosal injury, and reduced water absorption (inflammatory/exudative). Determining the best treatment depends on the cause of the diarrhea. For instance, hormonal therapy may be best for the treatment of diarrheas caused by endocrine tumors or AIDS, while osmotic diarrhea may require only the elimination of osmotic irritants (e.g., magnesium intake). On the other hand, Traveler's Diarrhea is caused by various infections such as *Escherichia coli, Clostridium difficile, Campylobacter jejuni* and can be treated by loperamide or bismuth subsalicylate alone or in combination with antibiotics e.g., azithromycin, ciprofloxacin or rifaximin.

Opioids: loperamide, diphenoxylate +atropine, eluxadoline. Constipation is a major side effect of opioid analgesics. This property is successfully used in developing peripherally-restricted opioids with anti-diarrheal efficacy. Agonists of μ- and δ-opioid receptors expressed in the GI tract produce potent anti-diarrheal effects by decreasing peristalsis, reducing gastric secretion, and enhancing salt and water absorption from the intestinal lumen. Because of the limited blood-brain-barrier permeability of peripherally-restricted opioids such as loperamide and eluxadoline, these agents exhibit limited potential for addiction and do not cause other major central side effects. By contrast, diphenoxylate readily crosses the brain-blood barrier and thus, can be used as anti-diarrheal only in combination with aversive agents such as atropine (to create unpleasant anticholinergic sensations). Note, the FDA has warned that eluxadoline, a μ-opioid receptor agonist and δ-opioid receptor antagonist approved in 2015 for the treatment of IBS-D, should not be used in patients without a gallbladder because of an increased risk of serious pancreatitis.

As of February 2017, the FDA had received reports of 118 cases of serious, nonfatal pancreatitis and 2 deaths associated with the use of eluxadoline. Both deaths occurred in patients without a gallbladder who developed severe abdominal pain and vomiting shortly after taking the first dose. At least 48 of the cases occurred after only 1 or 2 doses of eluxadoline. Of the 68 patients whose gallbladder status was reported, 56 did not have a gallbladder. Most of the patients without a gallbladder (44/56) were taking the reduced dosage of eluxadoline recommended for such patients (75 mg once/day).

Somatostatin analogs: Octreotide is a somatostatin analog with a much longer half-life time of 90 min as compared to 3 min for somatostatin. Octreotide inhibits GI motility and secretion by acting on somatostatin receptors. It is commonly used to treat severe diarrhea caused by endocrine tumors or AIDS.

Bismuth Subsalicylate is an insoluble salt of bismuth and salicylic acid that exhibits a broad spectrum of therapeutic effects including anti-inflammatory, mild anti-microbial, anti-motility, and anti-acid efficacies. Accordingly, it stimulates intestinal Na^+, and Cl^- absorption thus, water absorption. Salicylic acid inhibits prostaglandins and thus, motility (lower GI). Bismuth Subsalicylate exhibits a direct but mild antimicrobial activity against a variety of infections linked to Traveler's Diarrhea (e.g., *Helicobacter pylori, Escherichia coli, Clostridium difficile, Campylobacter jejuni).* It also binds bacterial toxins (e.g., *Escherichia coli*). It protects mucosa and ulcer craters from acid and pepsin. It shows a weak anti-acid efficacy as it reacts with gastric acid to produce bismuth oxychloride and salicylic acid (which is quickly absorbed). In addition to being an anti-diarrheal agent, bismuth subsalicylate is an effective adjunct for the treatment and prophylaxis of duodenal and gastric ulcers and GERD.

Antibiotics: Azithromycin (off-label for Traveler's Diarrhea and fluoroquinolone-resistant bacteria; e.g., *Campylobacter*), Ciprofloxacin, Rifaximin (severe Traveler's Diarrhea).

Treatment of IBS depends on the IBS type: constipation or diarrhea-predominant or mixed type. Agents used for the treatment of constipation/diarrhea are also used for the treatment of IBS-C/D.

Treatment of Constipation Predominant (IBS-C): Lubiprostone, Linaclotide, psyllium, bran, and other OTC products.

Treatment of Diarrhea Predominant (IBS-D): Rifaximin (antibiotic; also, for Traveler's Diarrhea), Eluxadoline, Loperamide (also, for Traveler's Diarrhea). Alosetron ($5HT_3$ blocker, women only; potentially fatal adverse effects, ischemic colitis).

Treatment of Mixed (IBS-M): Probiotics, Anti-Spasmodic Agents such as dicyclomine (weak anti-muscarinic agent).

Adverse Effects of anti-diarrheal drugs:

Opioids: Abdominal pain, nausea, constipation

Contraindications for eluxadoline: Biliary disorders, pancreatitis, patients without a gallbladder, alcoholism

Fluoroquinolones (ciprofloxacin): Black Box: Tendon inflammation/rupture; muscle weakness (warning for patients with myasthenia gravis)

Macrolides (azithromycin): Abdominal pain, nausea/vomiting, prolonged QT interval

Octreotide: Abdominal pain, nausea, headache, dizziness, arrhythmia, hyperglycemia

Bismuth Subsalicylate: No side effects at therapeutic doses

Note: *Anticholinergics inhibit parasympathetic activity:* mAChR antagonists (e.g., atropine) decrease motility, relax intestinal smooth muscle, inhibit ACh-mediated release of serotonin, and decrease secretions. However, anticholinergics exhibit serious side effects: dry mouth, dry eye, blurred vision, tachycardia, and constipation, and thus, are not commonly used. In fact, atropine is used as an adjunct to diphenoxylate to counteract its addictive potential with unpleasant anticholinergic sensations.

Adverse Effects of Laxatives:

General contraindication: GI obstruction known or suspected.

Linaclotide: Diarrhea, abdominal pain. Black Box: Contraindicated in pediatric patients <6 y.o. Avoid use in pediatric patients <18 y.o.

Lubiprostone: Diarrhea, nausea, abdominal pain.

References

Almario, C. V., M. L. Ballal, W. D. Chey, C. Nordstrom, D. Khanna, and B. M. R. Spiegel. 2018. Burden of Gastrointestinal Symptoms in the United States: Results of a Nationally Representative Survey of Over 71,000 Americans. *Am J Gastroenterol* 113 (11):1701-1710.

Bharucha, A. E., and A. Wald. 2019. Chronic Constipation. *Mayo Clin Proc* 94 (11):2340-2357.

Bharucha, A. E., A. Wald, P. Enck, and S. Rao. 2006. Functional anorectal disorders. *Gastroenterology* 130 (5):1510-1518.

Forootan, M., N. Bagheri, and M. Darvishi. 2018. Chronic constipation: A review of literature. *Medicine (Baltimore)* 97 (20):e10631.

McCoy, J. A., and D. E. Beck. 2012. Surgical management of colonic inertia. *Clin Colon Rectal Surg* 25 (1):20-23.

Scott, S. M., M. Simren, A. D. Farmer, P. G. Dinning, E. V. Carrington, M. A. Benninga, R. E. Burgell, E. Dimidi, A. Fikree, A. C. Ford, M. Fox, C. L. Hoad, C. H. Knowles, K. Krogh, K. Nugent, J. M. Remes-Troche, K. Whelan, and M. Corsetti. 2021. Chronic constipation in adults: Contemporary perspectives and clinical challenges. 1: Epidemiology, diagnosis, clinical associations, pathophysiology, and investigation. *Neurogastroenterol Motil* 33 (6):e14050.

Smalley, W., C. Falck-Ytter, A. Carrasco-Labra, S. Wani, L. Lytvyn, and Y. Falck-Ytter. 2019. AGA Clinical Practice Guidelines on the Laboratory Evaluation of Functional Diarrhea and Diarrhea-Predominant Irritable Bowel Syndrome in Adults (IBS-D). *Gastroenterology* 157 (3):851-854.

Quiz Questions

1. A 27-year-old with a history of chronic diarrhea has no weight loss or blood in the stool. The patient is treated for depression and anxiety. Patient symptoms are diarrhea with abdominal pain. Symptoms present for several years and the pain decreases with bowel movements. What criteria should be used in the diagnosis of Irritable Bowel Syndrome (IBS)?

A ROME
B MOSCOW
C CHICAGO
D PARIS
E LONDON

2. A 32-year-old patient has severe abdominal pain and non-bloody diarrhea. The patient has associated oral ulcers, rash, and arthritis in large joints. Lab reveals iron deficient anemia and stool positive for calprotectin. The patient has lost weight. Colonoscopy reveals areas of deep ulceration and marked mucosal hyperemia. There are areas of normal mucosa between these ulcerated areas. The terminal ileum also has discreetly punched-out ulcers. What is the most likely diagnosis?

A Functional diarrhea
B Infectious diarrhea
C Ulcerative colitis
D Irritable Bowel Syndrome-Diarrhea (IBS-D)
E Crohn's Disease

3. Which of the following are alarm symptoms that if present make secondary constipation likely?

A Unintentional weight loss
B Iron deficient anemia
C Change in stool caliber
D Severe abdominal pain
E All of the above

4. Patient returns from a vacation in Central America. The patient develops non-bloody diarrhea with nausea and vomiting. It lasted 4-5 days and resolved without treatment. What was the likely cause of the symptoms?

A Inflammatory Bowel Disease (IBD)
B Irritable Bowel Syndrome (IBS)
C Clostridioides difficile
D Parasitic infection
E Traveler's Diarrhea

5. A 64-year-old female cancer patient is given morphine to reduce pain. As a result, she has developed severe constipation. Which medication works by specifically addressing the pathophysiologic mechanism by which opioids produce constipation?

A Bisacodyl
B Methylnaltrexone
C Docusate
D Linaclotide
E Lubiprostone

6. A 48-year-old male and his 44-year-old wife are nearly simultaneously diagnosed with diarrhea-predominant Irritable Bowel Syndrome (IBS-D). They are prescribed the same medication to reduce abdominal discomfort. Which medication should not be prescribed to both of them?

A Eluxadoline
B Alosetron
C Loperamide
D Rifaximin
E Dicyclomine

7. Which medication is contraindicated in IBS-D patients without a gallbladder?

A Eluxadoline
B Alosetron
C Loperamide
D Rifaximin
E Dicyclomine

Quiz Answers

1. A. ROME is the correct answer. It is the city where GI societies come to establish diagnostic criteria for a multitude of functional disorders including IBS.

2. E. Crohn's Disease is the correct answer because of the symptom complex of chronic abdominal pain and diarrhea. The endoscopic finding of deep ulcer and inflammation as well as terminal ileum make Crohn's Disease the answer. Ulcerative colitis causes bloody diarrhea and has shallow colonic involvement of erosions, not deep ulcerations, and does not involve the terminal ileum. IBS-D has no mucosal damage and no extra manifestations as this case does. Likewise, functional diarrhea has no colonoscopy abnormalities.

3. E. The causes of secondary constipation include colorectal cancer. Unintentional weight loss, development of iron deficient anemia (chronic intestinal blood loss) chronic change in stool caliber (for example ribbon-shaped stool), and development of abdominal pain are all called alarm symptoms. Any or any combination of these alarm symptoms would require further urgent evaluation to exclude colorectal cancer for one of the causes of secondary constipation.

4. E. This clinical scenario is classic for Traveler's Diarrhea. It involves travel to an endemic area, is non-bloody, and resolves quickly without treatment. IBD is chronic and usually has an extra-intestinal manifestation of the disease and either abdominal pain and/or bloody diarrhea. Parasitic infection is usually chronic and does not spontaneously resolve. *C.Difficile* is also chronic and is usually associated with previous antibiotic use or recurring episode of this infection.

5. B. Methylnaltrexone is a peripherally-restricted opioid receptor antagonist and the only suitable medicine on the list to treat opioid-induced constipation.

6. B. Alosetron is ineffective in men with IBS-D.

7. A. Eluxadoline is contraindicated in patients without a gallbladder because of an increased risk of pancreatitis

CHAPTER 22

ABDOMINAL PAIN OR ABNORMAL UTERINE BLEEDING AND DRUGS FOR FEMALE REPRODUCTIVE DISORDERS AND CONTRACEPTION

SHELLEY A. TISCHKAU, PHD AND KATHLEEN M. BOTTUM, MD

Southern Illinois University School of Medicine, Springfield, Illinois, USA

Symptoms: Endo-Repro-Gastrointestinal

DRUG LIST

ESTROGENS

Oral:
Conjugated (equine) estrogen
Esterified estrogen
Estradiol

Transdermal (patches, gels, sprays):
Estradiol

Vaginal preparations for genitourinary syndrome of menopause:
Conjugated estrogen (cream)
Estradiol (creams, inserts, rings)
Estrone (cream)

Depot estrogen (oil for long-lasting intramuscular injection)
Estradiol cypionate

ESTROGEN/PROGESTIN COMBINATIONS:

Oral:
Conjugated estrogens (equine) and medroxyprogesterone acetate
Esterified estrogen and methyltestosterone
Estradiol and drospirenone
Estradiol and levonorgestrel
Estradiol and norethindrone
Estradiol and norgestimate
Ethinyl estradiol and desogestrel
Ethinyl estradiol and drospirenone
Ethinyl estradiol and levonorgestrel
Ethinyl estradiol and norethindrone

Transdermal weekly patches:
Ethinyl estradiol and levonorgestrel
Ethinyl estradiol and norelgestromin

Vaginal ring preparations:
Ethinyl estradiol etonogestrel (monthly change)
Ethinyl estradiol segesterone (yearly change)

ESTROGEN AND SELECTIVE ESTROGEN RECEPTOR MODULATOR (SERMs):

Oral:
Conjugated estrogen (equine) and bazedoxifene

PROGESTINS:

Oral:
Drospirenone
Medroxyprogesterone Acetate
Megestrol Acetate (pill form and oral suspension)
Norethindrone Acetate
Progesterone

Intramuscular Injections:
Hydroxyprogesterone caproate
Medroxyprogesterone acetate
Norethindrone enantate

Subcutaneous implants:
Etonogestrel
Levonorgestrel

Intrauterine Device (IUD)
Levonorgestrel

Vaginal preparations:
Progesterone (vaginal tablets, vaginal gels)

SELECTIVE ESTROGEN RECEPTOR MODULATORS (SERMs):

Oral:
Ospemifene
Tamoxifen (pill form and oral suspension)
Toremifene
Raloxifene

SELECTIVE ESTROGEN RECEPTOR DOWN REGULATOR (SERD):

Oral:
Fulvestrant

SELECTIVE PROGESTERONE RECEPTOR MODULATOR (SPRM):

Oral:
Mifepristone

ANTIPROGESTIN:

Oral:
Ulipristal acetate

General Background

Female reproductive disorders present most frequently as abnormal uterine bleeding, pelvic pain, or infertility. Dysfunction may occur from pathologies anywhere within the reproductive organs themselves (ovaries, fallopian tubes, uterus, vagina, breast) or within other associated organs (hypothalamus, pituitary gland, thyroid, kidney, adrenal glands, liver) (reviewed in Johnston-MacAnanny et al. 2022). Pharmaceutical treatments for female reproductive dysfunction reflect the physiological function of the naturally occurring endocrine hormones. These drugs can re-establish hormonal balance, correct dysmenorrhea, or interrupt the natural sequence of events suspending menstrual cyclicity.

We must understand physiological reproductive function to understand female reproductive dysfunction and its treatment. The pulsatile release of gonadotropin-releasing hormone (GnRH) from the hypothalamus is stimulated by estradiol and inhibited by progesterone. GnRH targets gonadotrophs of the anterior pituitary gland to secrete follicle-stimulating hormone (FSH) and luteinizing hormone (LH). Composed of a common alpha subunit and a unique beta subunit, FSH and LH act on the ovary to regulate the development of a cohort of follicles. They are necessary for selecting a dominant follicle from the cohort, ovulating a mature ovum, and producing ovarian steroids (estrogens, androgens, and progestins).

Ovarian follicles consist of a developing oocyte surrounded by granulosa and theca cells which produce estrogens and progestins. These hormones can regulate GnRH secretion through feedback mechanisms. Estrogen increases the production of FSH and LH. Another primary physiological function of estrogen, which dominates the follicular phase (1st half) of the menstrual cycle, is to increase the proliferation of the uterine endometrium. After ovulation, residual ovarian follicle cells transform into a corpus luteum, a primary progesterone source throughout the luteal phase (2nd half) of the menstrual cycle.

Progesterone acts at the hypothalamus to inhibit GnRH secretion. At the uterus, progesterone limits the proliferative effects of estrogen, transforming the endometrium through the maturation of endometrial blood vessels and stimulation of epithelial secretions necessary to support the potential implantation of an embryo. If pregnancy does not occur, the corpus luteum cannot sustain progesterone secretion sufficient to maintain the endometrial vasculature. Low levels of estrogens and progestins initiate menstruation; this endometrium sloughing marks the cycle's end.

Estrogens and progestins also act on other organs in the reproductive tract, typically opposing each other. Estrogens increase smooth muscle contractility in fallopian tubes and myometrium, whereas progestins suppress smooth muscle contraction. In the cervix, estrogens increase the water content of the cervical mucus facilitating sperm transport, while progestins thicken cervical mucus to act as a sperm barrier.

Ovarian hormones help establish and maintain homeostasis in a variety of organ systems. Thus, disorders of female reproductive function can contribute to pathologies in other tissues. Elevated estrogen and suppressed progesterone may increase the risk of endometrial cancer. Low estrogen states are associated with atrophy of estrogen-responsive tissues, leading to decreased cardiovascular compliance, osteoporosis, and atrophic vaginitis. (Johnston-MacAnanny et al. 2022)

Diagnosis:

Virtually all women experience variations in their menstrual cycle throughout their reproductive lifespan. Evaluation of menstrual cycle disturbances must consider the patient's age, the history of her menstrual cycles, and any family history of amenorrhea. Other disease states may also influence menstrual cycle function. Thyroid, adrenal gland, and pituitary dysfunction can all affect menstrual cycles and must be considered when menstrual dysfunction occurs. Many women have irregular cycles throughout their reproductive lifespan without any pathology.

Causes of reproductive cycle dysfunction can be genetic, anatomic, metabolic, endocrine, or environmental. Because pregnancy is the most common cause of amenorrhea, evaluation of amenorrhea must always include measurement of human chorionic gonadotropin (hCG) before proceeding with any further differential diagnoses.

Common Conditions for Hormonal Therapy

Menopause:

A natural decline in female reproductive system function during the 4th and 5th decades of life culminates in menopause. The mean age of natural menopause varies between 48 years (developing countries) and 51 years (industrialized nations). (Santoro et al. 2015) Age of onset varies substantially, with about 5% of women experiencing menopause between 40-45 and another approximately 5% after age 55. For nearly 90% of women, menopause occurs between ages 45-55. Age at menopause is influenced by ethnicity, genetics, shift work, reproductive history, and smoking. The perimenopausal transition period typically begins four years before the last menstrual period and is characterized by increasing irregularity of menstrual cycles with pronounced hormonal fluctuations. Menopause is defined as 12 consecutive months of amenorrhea following the last menstrual period, which is determined retrospectively.

Presentation: Women typically present in midlife for evaluation of perimenopause or menopause, with goals of either understanding menopausal changes and consequences of estrogen deficiency or seeking postmenopausal hormone therapy to alleviate symptoms. All women experience menstrual irregularity and fluctuations in hormone levels during the perimenopausal period. After menopause, women may develop the genitourinary syndrome of menopause consisting of vaginal dryness, burning, dyspareunia, and frequent urinary tract infections.

Risk Factors: Oophorectomy and age are the causes of menopause.

Pathophysiology: Menopause occurs secondary to a marked decline in the ovarian follicle reserve, significantly lowering circulating estrogen levels. Accompanied by decreased hypothalamic and pituitary sensitivity to estrogen, lowered estrogen and inhibin B production alters the normal feedback effects, resulting in elevated levels of follicle-stimulating hormone and problems with generating the ovulatory LH surge. (Talaulikar 2022)

Aging causes decreased responsiveness of the ovary to the pituitary gonadotropins FSH and LH. Reduced ovarian responsiveness to FSH shortens the follicular phase of the menstrual cycle and contributes to increased irregularity in overall cyclicity. Decreased ovarian responsiveness to LH diminishes ovulations such that each cycle may not be associated with the release of an egg. Failure to ovulate results in decreased progesterone production due to the lack of corpus luteum formation. Occasionally double ovulations and luteal-out-of-phase events occur and cause a temporary elevation in estrogen levels.

Examination: Menstrual cycle history and the appearance of menopausal symptoms are assessed. Pelvic examinations to evaluate vaginal atrophy are performed for any reports of vaginal dryness, dyspareunia, or sexual dysfunction. Evaluation of suspected menopause depends on the patient's age, which can be divided into three categories, broadly <40 years, 40-45 years, and >45 years. (Harlow et al. 2012) Women over 45 who present with menstrual irregularities and other menopausal symptoms are typically entering the menopausal transition and are not recommended for further evaluation of a new endocrine disorder. On the other hand, heavy or prolonged menses are evaluated using the same criteria as in younger women. (Casper 2022)

Laboratory: Serum FSH is often measured, although it is not considered diagnostic, and can be confusing as it may be either normal or in the elevated postmenopausal range. Anti-Mullerian hormone (AMH) and inhibin B may also be measured and will be low in the perimenopausal and menopausal periods. In women under 45, thyroid stimulating hormone (TSH) and prolactin (PRL) should also be measured. FSH has different meanings and should be interpreted very carefully in women who have had a hysterectomy or endometrial ablation, have underlying menstrual cycle irregularities, or are currently using hormonal contraceptives. Serum hCG should always be performed to exclude pregnancy.

Imaging: Although ultrasound can be used to evaluate ovarian follicle count and volume to assist in determining whether menopause has occurred, it is rare for imaging to be a part of the menopausal diagnostic process. Bone density should be measured after determining a hypoestrogenic state to evaluate the risk of osteoporosis.

Associated Symptoms/Conditions: Changes resulting from menopause that can affect the quality of life include hot flashes, sleep disturbances, depression and mood changes, cognitive changes, genitourinary syndrome of menopause, joint pain, breast pain, and menstrual migraines. 75-80% of women experience hot flashes, the most common symptom, but only 20% seek medical intervention. (Santen RJ et al. 2022) Long-term estrogen deficiency can lead to osteoporosis, cardiovascular disease, and dementia.

Diagnosis: Menopause is a clinical diagnosis that differs slightly based on a patient's age, history of menstrual cycle disorders, and contraceptive use. In women over 45, "perimenopause" is diagnosed based on changes in the menstrual cycle; the presence of associated symptoms or hormone levels is unnecessary. Menopause is diagnosed after 12 months of amenorrhea without any other physiological cause; elevated FSH is not required for diagnosis. (Casper 2022)

The criteria for diagnosis in women aged 40-45 remains the same as above, except other causes of menstrual cycle dysfunction must be excluded. Non-menopausal causes of oligo/amenorrhea include pregnancy, hyperprolactinemia, and thyroid dysfunction.

Menopause is not diagnosed in women under the age of 40. Amenorrhea in this group is diagnosed as primary ovarian insufficiency. In women with underlying menstrual cycle disorders, changes in cycle regularity are not diagnostic, and the determination of menopause is more complicated. In women with polycystic ovarian syndrome or hypothalamic amenorrhea that display menopausal symptoms, FSH levels are helpful for diagnostic purposes. Similarly, FSH concentrations can be used to diagnose menopause after a hysterectomy if one or both ovaries remain.

Clear diagnosis in women taking hormonal contraceptives requires cessation of birth control, followed by a serum FSH measurement 2-4 weeks later. It is typical to stop hormonal birth control usage at around 51 years of age. (Casper 2022)

Treatment: Many of the symptoms of menopause occur secondary to decreased estrogen levels and are responsive to estrogen therapy. The most common symptom of menopause is hot flashes; sleep disturbances, mood changes, joint pains, and genitourinary syndrome of menopause may also be relieved with estrogen treatment.

The treatment method depends on the targeted symptoms and whether the woman has an intact uterus. Genitourinary syndrome of menopause is adequately treated with low-dose vaginal estrogen. Systemic estrogen is necessary to treat hot flashes, sleep disturbances, mood, and joint pains. In patients with an intact uterus, systemic estrogen treatment should also include progestin to prevent endometrial hyperplasia, which could lead to uterine cancer. Vaginal estrogen therapies are not associated with endometrial hyperplasia; thus, no progestin is necessary. (Martin and Barbieri 2022)

Management: Although hormonal therapy for menopause has been available since the 1960s, in 2002, the Women's Health Initiative study found an increased risk of cardiovascular disease and breast cancer associated with hormonal therapy, and hormonal treatment dramatically reduced. However, further investigation demonstrated significant benefits for symptomatic women under 60, within ten years of menopause, and with a low risk of liver or thromboembolic disease ("The 2017 hormone therapy position statement of the North American Menopause Society"). (Baber et al. 2016) Menopausal management is specific to the patient's age and the severity of the symptoms; for women who are perimenopausal or early in menopause, continuous estrogen, and cyclic progestin are the preferred treatment, with the lowest effective dose of estrogen employed. Oral contraceptives can be used. In women who have had a hysterectomy, progestins are not needed. Current guidelines recommend discontinuing hormone therapy in 5 years or less or by age 60. (Martin and Manson 2008). Abrupt cessation of estrogen is associated with the return of menopausal symptoms.

Primary Ovarian Insufficiency:

Primary ovarian insufficiency is defined as the development of hypogonadotropic hypogonadism with onset before the age of 40 years in women who previously had regular menses. Ovarian insufficiency is not attributable to another cause, such as radiation or chemotherapy, hence the distinction of it being "primary" insufficiency. Approximately 1% of women spontaneously develop the condition. It is distinguished from induced ovarian insufficiency resulting from salpingo-oophorectomy or following gonadotoxic radiation or chemotherapies. (De Vos et al. 2010)

Presentation: Women present with irregular menstrual cycles, amenorrhea, or difficulty getting pregnant. Primary ovarian insufficiency may be discovered after discontinuing hormonal contraceptives or following pregnancy/lactation when menstrual cycles fail to resume. Symptoms of estrogen deficiency, such as hot flashes and vaginal dryness, may or may not be reported, as early in ovarian decline, ovaries are intermittently functional. Dry eyes, difficulty concentrating, and decreased sexual desire may also occur.

Risk Factors: Age is the primary risk factor, increasing risk after age 35. Other risk factors include a family history and ovarian surgery. Carriers of permutations of the *FMR1* gene (fragile X syndrome) also have increased risk.

Pathophysiology: The pathophysiology is essentially the same as described above for menopause. Ovarian follicle development and ovulation require tightly coordinated events within the hypothalamic-pituitary-gonadal axis. Etiologies are broad, but can be classified into two major categories, accelerated follicle depletion or decreased steroid production without depletion of ovarian reserve. It is typical for oocytes to be predominantly depleted around 51 years of age, resulting in menopause. Genetic disorders, autoimmune disorders, exposure to chemotherapy, radiation therapy, viruses, or ovarian toxins can cause early follicle depletion. Alteration of either X chromosome can affect ovarian function leading to premature follicle depletion. The most common genetic causes are Turner's Syndrome (XO), inversions, duplications and translocations of an X chromosome, and balanced X chromosome to autosome translocations. Carriers of *FMR1* permutations exhibit hormonal changes associated with premature ovarian aging but may have regular menstrual cycles. The age of menopause is dependent upon the premutation repeat length in these women.

Primary hypogonadism without follicle depletion leading to primary ovarian failure can occur through two different mechanisms. FSH receptor mutations that reduce FSH binding decrease steroid production in the ovary. Similarly, reductions in gonadotropin receptor activation within the ovary can occur in women who produce biologically inert gonadotropins, polymorphisms in the alpha subunit of inhibin, or defects in the guanine nucleotide regulatory protein of adenylate cyclase that links the receptor to activation of the downstream signaling pathway. Alternatively, alterations in steroidogenic enzymes, including steroidogenic acute regulatory protein CYP17 and aromatase, will reduce estrogen levels leading to primary hypogonadism.

Examination: Menstrual cycle history and the appearance of menopausal symptoms are assessed. A pelvic examination to evaluate vaginal atrophy is performed for any reports of vaginal dryness, dyspareunia, or sexual dysfunction. Additional laboratory studies are required for diagnostic purposes.

Laboratory: Serum hCG, TSH, and PRL are measured to rule out pregnancy, thyroid dysfunction, and hyperprolactinemia, respectively. FSH and estradiol levels are measured weekly for 2-4 weeks. Elevated FSH with low estradiol is diagnostic. (Nelson 2009) Follow-up studies to measure AMH (anti-mullerian hormone) help determine ovarian reserve. Low levels of AMH indicate diminished ovarian reserve and predict potential responsiveness to fertility treatments. Other laboratory studies to evaluate the cause of follicle depletion can be performed once a diagnosis is made. These include genetic testing for permutations in *FMR1* antibody (Elizur et al. 2019) for detecting autoimmune hypothyroidism (Bakalov et al. 2012) and evaluation of hypothalamic-pituitary-adrenal axis function to detect adrenal insufficiency. (Bakalov et al. 2005; Bakalov et al. 2002) A karyotype should also be performed to evaluate X chromosome abnormalities.

Imaging: Although ultrasound can be used to evaluate ovarian reserve, imaging is rarely a part of the diagnostic process. Bone density should be measured after determining a hypoestrogenic state to assess the risk of osteoporosis.

Associated Symptoms/Conditions: The associated changes affecting the quality of life include hot flashes, sleep disturbances, depression and mood changes, cognitive changes, genitourinary syndrome of menopause, joint pain, breast pain, and menstrual migraines. Long-term estrogen deficiency can lead to osteoporosis, cardiovascular disease, and dementia.

Diagnosis: The clinical diagnosis of primary ovarian insufficiency is made in women under 40 who present with irregular menses or amenorrhea and FSH levels in the postmenopausal range. Due to intermittent ovarian function, many women have some periods of ovarian function even years beyond their initial presentation; complete amenorrhea is not required for diagnosis. Some women may have normal FSH levels but diminished ovarian reserve, which warrants the diagnosis of "occult" primary ovarian insufficiency. AMH levels and imaging can assist in this diagnosis.

Treatment: Combined estrogen/progestin therapy can be prescribed to alleviate symptoms of estrogen deficiency, maintain bone density, and provide cardiovascular protection in women who do not desire to conceive. Progestin is necessary only if the woman has a uterus and needs protection from endometrial cancer. Assisted reproductive technologies are available to assist in developing a pregnancy. These may require hormonal treatment and an egg donor. (Welt 2022)

Management: The diagnosis of primary ovarian insufficiency can be quite traumatic as it frequently alters life plans, especially regarding family planning. Early detection may allow for fertility preservation through cryopreservation of eggs, ovarian tissue, or embryos, which can assist in prolonging fertility. Early diagnosis is also helpful in preventing osteoporosis and, perhaps, coronary artery disease. After the initial diagnosis, further evaluation should be performed to determine the underlying cause and evaluate other coexisting conditions. Management of these patients necessitates considering estrogen-deficiency symptoms, sexual function, fertility, bone density, cardiovascular health, emotional well-being, and cognitive health. Primary ovarian insufficiency can be an autoimmune condition, and evaluation for other autoimmune illnesses should be considered. Primary adrenal insufficiency is more common in women with primary ovarian insufficiency. Since adrenal failure can be fatal, it is essential to find adrenal insufficiency early.

Estrogen therapy is indicated for primary ovarian insufficiency unless there is an absolute contraindication ("Committee Opinion No. 698: Hormone Therapy in Primary Ovarian Insufficiency," 2017). Hormone therapy should mimic ovarian function as nearly as possible. Hormone replacement depends on the presentation, with treatments for primary amenorrhea differing from secondary amenorrhea. For primary amenorrhea, lower doses of unopposed estrogen are started initially to imitate changes in puberty. Progestins are added later.

In contrast, full doses of estrogen are used immediately for patients with secondary amenorrhea. Transdermal or vaginal estrogen delivery is preferable and is used in conjunction with oral or injectable forms of progestin. Hormonal treatments are continued until the woman reaches the age of natural menopause. Hormonal therapies can be used until the time of natural menopause and are commonly terminated in the early 50s. (Welt 2022)

Primary Amenorrhea:

Amenorrhea is a transient, intermittent, or permanent condition where menses fail to develop - "primary failure." It results from anatomical or hormonal dysfunction of the female reproductive tract. Primary amenorrhea is defined as the absence of menarche by age 14 in the absence of secondary sex characteristics or by the absence of menarches by age 16, regardless of the appearance of secondary sex characteristics. (Marsh and Grimstad 2014) Most commonly, primary amenorrhea results from a genetic or anatomic abnormality. (Marsh and Grimstad 2014) In addition, all causes of secondary amenorrhea, such as polycystic ovarian syndrome (PCOS), may present initially as primary amenorrhea. (Welt and Barbieri 2022b)

Presentation: Females present in early teens with the absence of menarche with or without initial development of secondary sex characteristics. If the development of secondary sex characteristics associated with puberty has not begun by age 13, evaluation for primary amenorrhea should be considered at this time. Some patients will present with cyclic pelvic pain.

Risk Factors: A family history of amenorrhea, genetic conditions that affect the menstrual cycle, obesity, being underweight, anorexia nervosa, over-exercising, poor diet, stress, and other chronic illness are all risk factors for primary amenorrhea.

Pathophysiology: The menstrual cycle requires functional coordination among four functionally distinct anatomical components, namely the uterus, hypothalamus, pituitary, and ovaries. Coordinated neuroendocrine events lead to the growth of follicles within the ovary and ovulation. Ovarian hormones regulate the growth and maturation of the endometrial lining in preparation for pregnancy. If an egg is not fertilized, the ovarian corpus luteum will regress, and without progesterone support, the endometrial lining sheds, and the cycle begins anew. Malfunction of any of the components prevents menstruation. (Marsh and Grimstad 2014)

Examination: Breast development can assess estrogen action, which indicates ovarian function. The presence or absence of a uterus can also be evaluated by physical examination. Imaging and laboratory studies are used to determine the cause of amenorrhea.

Laboratory: FSH levels, testosterone levels, and karyotyping help differentiate the causes of primary amenorrhea. (Current evaluation of amenorrhea 2008) hCG should be measured to rule out pregnancy. TSH and PRL levels explore central hypothyroidism and hyperprolactinemia, respectively. (Majumdar and Mangal 2013; Welt and Barbieri 2022b) Free T4 may also be measured if central hypothyroidism is suspected. Estradiol levels can assist with the interpretation of FSH results. (Welt and Barbieri 2022b)

Imaging: Ultrasound and MRI studies can determine the presence or absence of a uterus, cervix, vagina, and ovaries. Vaginal and cervical obstruction can also be identified in women with cyclic pain and amenorrhea.

Associated Symptoms/Conditions: Decreased estrogen levels in the presence of primary amenorrhea increase the risk of osteoporosis and bone fractures due to decreased bone density.

Diagnosis: Elevated serum FSH indicates ovarian failure, which occurs most commonly due to congenital gonadal malformations and can be diagnosed with a karyotype. Normal FSH without a uterus suggests congenital Mullerian agenesis causing failure of the uterus to form or androgen insensitivity. High levels of testosterone point to androgen insensitivity. Low or normal FSH with a uterus present necessitates further investigation to differentiate between an "extreme of normal" pubertal delay and causes of secondary amenorrhea, such as PCOS, that may present in this age range. The findings of normal FSH with breast development and a uterus require imaging for blood in the uterus, as these signs are commonly associated with obstruction of the outflow tract.

Treatment: Therapeutics target the underlying cause of primary amenorrhea. For primary amenorrhea with a structural origin, surgery is indicated. For those diagnosed with any form of gonadal failure, or hypergonadotropic hypogonadism, treatment with ovarian steroids (estrogens and progestins), given to mimic the natural menstrual cycle, is required for pubertal changes, and maintenance of secondary sex characteristics. (Welt and Barbieri 2022b)

Management: Management of primary amenorrhea varies according to the underlying cause. Counseling is an essential management component due to the psychological issues of fertility and gender identity. For patients with Y chromosomal material, gonadectomy following puberty is required to prevent gonadal neoplasia. The benefits and risks of hormone replacement therapy must be discussed for those with low estrogens. Prevention of osteoporosis and coronary heart disease is vital in this population. Assisted reproductive technologies are available for those who wish to conceive.

Secondary Amenorrhea:

Irregular periods or some disruption of the regularity of the menstrual cycle occur in almost every woman at some point in the reproductive lifespan. However, secondary amenorrhea is defined as a cessation of menstruation for at least three months after menarche. Although a single missed menstrual period is not cause for concern, having fewer than nine cycles per year, and intermenstrual intervals of longer than 45 days in females who are > 2 years post menarche, require investigation. (Welt and Barbieri 2022a)

Presentation: Women present with an absence of menstruation that persists for longer than three months in those with previously regular cycles or greater than six months in women with previously irregular cycles.

Risk Factors: The most prevalent cause of secondary amenorrhea is pregnancy. Other risk factors include obesity, eating disorders, a family history of amenorrhea or early menopause, excessive exercise and weight loss, and genetics, such as alterations of the *FMR1* gene. (Master-Hunter and Heiman 2006; Current evaluation of amenorrhea 2008)

Pathophysiology: Secondary amenorrhea can occur due to multiple factors originating in any part of the reproductive axis, including the hypothalamus, pituitary, ovary, uterus, and vagina. In addition, pathologies associated with the thyroid and adrenal gland may be the cause.

Examination: The first step is to rule out pregnancy. Menstrual cycle history and the appearance of menopausal symptoms are assessed. The skin should be evaluated for acne and hirsutism. Symptoms of headaches, visual field defects, fatigue, and polydipsia should be assessed to look for hypothalamic causes of amenorrhea. Galactorrhea may be a sign of prolactinoma. Hot flashes, vaginal dryness, poor sleep, and changes in libido may be signs of low estrogen levels. Pelvic examinations to evaluate vaginal atrophy are performed for any reports of vaginal dryness, dyspareunia, or sexual dysfunction. Changes in stress levels, weight, diet, and exercise habits should be considered. Additional laboratory studies are required for diagnostic purposes.

Laboratory: Pregnancy can be evaluated by measuring hCG. FSH should be measured to assess for premature ovarian failure. Prolactin levels can point to the presence of a prolactinoma, and TSH can determine a thyroid abnormality. Estradiol levels are frequently measured along with FSH to determine if the ovaries are responding to hypothalamic-pituitary signaling. Testosterone may also be measured if there is clinical evidence of hyperandrogenism.

Imaging: Ovarian ultrasound may be helpful.

Associated Symptoms/Conditions: Various associated conditions may co-exist with secondary amenorrhea. Neoplasms may disrupt menstrual cycles, including astrocytoma, craniopharyngioma, glioma, and prolactinoma. Other endocrine disorders such as thyroid disease, diabetes mellitus, Cushing syndrome, congenital adrenal hyperplasia, and growth hormone deficiency may contribute to menstrual irregularity. Secondary amenorrhea may also occur due to chronic renal disease, AIDS, trauma, asthma, and after cancer treatments.

Diagnosis: Criteria for a diagnosis of secondary amenorrhea have not been established. However, the diagnosis is given after the absence of menstrual cycles over time, as described above. Establishing the cause, when possible, helps determine appropriate treatment plans.

Treatment: Appropriate treatment must align with the underlying pathology when possible. Estrogen deficiency treatment is desirable for osteoporosis prevention in women with primary ovarian insufficiency. Depending on the woman's goals, this can be oral contraceptives or estrogen and progesterone replacement therapy. If menstrual cycle abnormalities result from other hormonal systems (thyroid or adrenal gland), treatment of those underlying conditions must be employed to regain menstrual cycle function.

Management: The first goals are to correct the underlying pathology, if possible, and to prevent downstream complications. Subsequent considerations should be made based on the family planning needs of the patient. If desired, goals should be designed to assist in achieving fertility. This plan may include hormone replacement therapy or assisted reproductive technologies when necessary. Lifestyle changes that include appropriate caloric intake and balanced exercise may be required. (Welt and Barbieri 2022a)

Polycystic Ovarian Syndrome (PCOS):

PCOS is an endocrine disorder that manifests as oligomenorrhea and hyperandrogenism. As one of the most common endocrine pathologies, it may affect up to 15 percent of women. (Norman and Teede 2018) Although the causes of PCOS remain unknown, it is clearly associated with hormonal imbalances originating within and beyond the reproductive system. (Puttabyatappa and Padmanabhan 2018) Development usually begins around the time of menarche but may develop later when associated with substantial weight gain.

Presentation: Women can present during puberty or any time after that with irregular menses or amenorrhea and symptoms of hyperandrogenism, which may include acne, hirsutism, and male-patterned hair loss. Many patients will also present with an elevated body mass index and central obesity. Oligomenorrhea or hyperandrogenism may present in the absence of other symptoms.

Risk Factors: PCOS is linked to both genetic and environmental factors. There is an 8-fold increased risk of PCOS in female children of afflicted women. Risk is enhanced in this group if the mother smoked during pregnancy. Variants in the anti-Mullerian hormone gene are associated with increased incidence of PCOS, (Gorsic et al. 2017) Type 1 diabetes, type 2 diabetes, and an elevated BMI may also increase risk.

Pathophysiology: PCOS is a self-perpetuating cycle of endocrine and metabolic dysfunction perpetuated by complex interactions among a network of neuroendocrine, metabolic, genetic, and environmental influences. The most important pathophysiological findings in PCOS are irregular menstrual cycles accompanied by increased androgens, increasingly frequent LH pulses, and insufficient levels of FSH. (Witchel et al. 2019)

Although the initial causes remain unknown, many interacting factors in PCOS have been identified. Within the ovary, PCOS is characterized by an increased number of growing follicles. Abnormal acceleration of growth of primordial follicles to the small antral follicle stage may be due to changes in AMH in an environment of elevated androgens and insulin, accompanied by insufficient FSH. Altered steroidogenesis in the ovary and adrenal gland leads to increased levels of androgens.

In PCOS, the hypothalamus has increased amplitude and frequency of pulsatile LH release, likely due to an impaired negative feedback mechanism. (Witchel et al. 2019) Women with PCOS have inherent insulin resistance independent of body mass index. They also exhibit a 3-fold higher incidence of metabolic syndrome. (Witchel et al. 2019) Insulin increases ovarian/adrenal androgen production. In addition, it decreases SHBG production by the liver, leading to elevated androgen levels in the blood.

Paradoxically, fat, liver, and skeletal muscle are insulin resistant in women with PCOS, whereas steroidogenic tissues retain insulin sensitivity so that insulin promotes steroidogenesis. (Geffner and Golde 1988; Wu et al. 2012) Increased BMI exacerbates insulin resistance in PCOS. Adipose tissue function is also altered in women with PCOS, regardless of BMI. Normal-weight women with PCOS have increased abdominal fat and a suppressed capacity of subcutaneous fat to expand to meet metabolic demands. (Dumesic et al. 2019) Increased insulin resistance in subcutaneous fat is directly related to serum androgen levels in these women.

Examination: Patients with PCOS often have central obesity from metabolic syndrome. They are likely to have hirsutism with hair growing on the chin, chest, lower abdomen, back, or thighs. The level of hirsutism is evaluated using the Ferriman-Gallway scoring system. (Hatch et al. 1981) Blood pressure should be measured.

Laboratory: Symptoms of hyperandrogenism should be evaluated further with measurements of total testosterone, SHBG, and dehydroepiandrosterone sulfate (DHEA-S). PRL levels are determined to assess the presence of a pituitary adenoma. Fasting glucose, hemoglobin A1c, and a lipid panel will determine metabolic dysfunction. 17-hydroxyprogesterone levels are assessed to rule out non-classical congenital adrenal hyperplasia from 21-hydroxylase deficiency; if levels are greater than 200 ng/dl, an ACTH stimulation test can further evaluate the presence of congenital adrenal hyperplasia. Beta hCG, TSH, and LH can be used to rule out other causes of oligomenorrhea. (Witchel et al. 2019)

Imaging: Transvaginal ultrasound is frequently used as a part of the diagnostic criteria for PCOS. Using the Rotterdam criteria, follicle number and size, rather than the presence of cysts, determines the presence of polycystic ovarian morphology (PCOM). PCOM is defined as 12 or more follicles that are 2-9 mm in diameter in an individual ovary, together with increased ovarian size. However, it is important to note that this number of follicles can occur in normal women, so the ultrasound cannot be used in isolation. Furthermore, ultrasound may not be necessary if other diagnostic criteria are met. Because the presence of multiple follicles on ultrasound is common, additional criteria are essential for diagnostic purposes. Adrenal imaging may also be implicated if congenital adrenal hyperplasia remains a consideration.

Associated Symptoms/Conditions: Several co-morbidities can be associated with PCOS. Metabolic issues, including insulin resistance, type 2 diabetes, and dyslipidemia, may be present independent of BMI. (Teede et al. 2018) Many women with PCOS are overweight or obese. Additional conditions that may be present include anxiety, depression, eating disorders, and sleep apnea. (Guidi et al. 2015)

Diagnosis: The most accepted mechanism for diagnosing PCOS follows the Rotterdam criteria. According to this method, a diagnosis of PCOS requires the presence of two of the following three criteria: 1) oligomenorrhea or anovulation, 2) clinical or biochemical signs of hyperandrogenism, and 3) the presence of polycystic ovaries on ultrasound. PCOS is only confirmed upon exclusion of other causes of hyperandrogenism and oligomenorrhea, which may include non-classical congenital adrenal hyperplasia, hyperprolactinemia, thyroid disease, and androgen-secreting tumors.

Treatment: Combined estrogen-progestin hormonal contraceptives are the primary treatment for patients with PCOS who do not desire to achieve pregnancy. Treatment of hirsutism may require the addition of an anti-androgen therapy if contraceptives alone do not achieve the desired effect. Weight loss and other lifestyle changes may assist with menstrual cycle regularity in women with elevated BMI. For women wanting to conceive, ovulation-inducing medications, including letrozole and clomiphene citrate, may stimulate ovulation.

Management: The Endocrine Society Clinical guidelines (Legro et al. 2013) and international, evidence-based guidelines (Teede et al. 2018) provide guidance for managing multiple issues associated with PCOS. Goals must address glucose tolerance, metabolic risk, anovulation, oligomenorrhea, fertility, and hyperandrogenism. Weight loss is a first-line, non-pharmacological lifestyle change that improves metabolic parameters and can restore menstrual cycles with ovulation. Overall goals are multifold. Pharmacological treatments can reduce hirsutism, acne, and male pattern hair loss. Weight loss and drugs can address metabolic risks, improve glucose intolerance, and balance healthy lipid levels to ameliorate the risk of cardiovascular disease. Chronic anovulation can lead to endometrial hyperplasia and potentially uterine carcinoma; imaging and treatments, if necessary, should be undertaken to reduce this risk.

Contraception is often warranted for those who do not desire pregnancy, as ovulation may occur intermittently. Pharmacological intervention for ovulation induction may be necessary for those who desire pregnancy.

Endometriosis:

Approximately 10% of reproductive-age women across the globe are diagnosed with endometriosis (Shafrir et al. 2018; Soliman et al. 2018). Defined as the appearance of endometrial tissue outside the uterine cavity, lesions typically appear in the abdominal compartment attached to the ovary's surface or the endometrium's exterior surface. However, endometrial explants can be associated with the intestines, diaphragm, and even the pleural cavity. This benign, estrogen-dependent inflammatory disease can range in severity and can be severely debilitating. Inflammation can lead to dysmenorrhea, infertility, dyspareunia, and chronic pain. It occurs across the reproductive lifespan in women.

Presentation: Women present during their reproductive lifespan with chronic abdominal or pelvic pain and pressure, abnormal menstrual patterns, dyspareunia, heavy menses, and fertility problems. (Brawn et al. 2014) Bowel and bladder problems, lower back pain, and chronic fatigue may also be present. (Sinaii et al. 2008; Vercellini et al. 2014; Engemise et al. 2010)

Risk Factors: Various factors may influence endometriosis risk, which include: 1) having an immediate family member diagnosed with endometriosis, 2) menarche before the age of 11, 3) long and heavy menses, 3) menstrual cycles shorter than 27 days, and 4) infertility. (Peterson et al. 2013)

Pathophysiology: Endometriosis develops when ectopic endometrial tissue grows outside the uterine cavity and elicits an inflammatory response. (Giudice 2010) Pathogenesis is multifactorial. Genetic abnormalities in cancer genes (PIK3CA, KRAS, ARID1A) have been associated with endometriosis and may drive the invasiveness of the ectopic cells. (Rahmioglu et al. 2014; Anglesio et al. 2017; Bulun et al. 2019) Cells are transported from the uterine cavity to the peritoneum, where they attach and grow. Imbalances in cell proliferation and apoptosis, altered immunity, and aberrant endocrine signaling may all contribute.

The most popular theory for the appearance of endometrial cells in the peritoneum posits that cells arrive due to retrograde flow during menses. However, up to 90% of women experience some retrograde flow. Because the percentage of endometriosis is much lower, additional factors must be involved. (Vercellini et al. 2014) Furthermore, endometriosis may present before menarche, suggesting that alternative sources of endometrial cells may exist. These may include Mullerian rests, mesothelium, bone marrow stem cells, and embryonic vestiges. (Burney and Giudice 2012; Du and Taylor 2007)

Once present, explant growth is estrogen-dependent. Inflammatory changes associated with explant growth and altered sympathetic sensory innervation within the explants lead to increased pain. (Du and Taylor 2007; Arnold et al. 2012; Arnold et al. 2013) A combination of inhibition of sympathetic nerve fibers by estrogen, nerve sensitization by inflammatory cytokines, and central nervous system changes associated with chronic pain all contribute to pain. (Liang and Yao 2016; Wheeler et al. 2014; As-Sanie et al. 2012) Infertility likely derives from anatomical changes due to pelvic adhesions and the production of biochemical mediators that inhibit ovarian function, fertilization, and implantation.

Examination: Focal tenderness in the vagina during pelvic examination may suggest endometriosis. Adnexal masses and displacement of the uterus or cervix are indicative of lesions. However, the pelvic examination may be completely unremarkable.

Laboratory: No pathognomonic laboratory studies are definitive for the diagnosis of endometriosis.

Imaging: Transvaginal ultrasound, transabdominal ultrasound, CT, and MRI may all be useful in suspected cases of endometriosis. The imaging modality most helpful depends on the site of the lesions.

Associated Symptoms/Conditions: Women with endometriosis are more likely to suffer from autoimmune disorders, including lupus, Sjogren's syndrome, rheumatoid arthritis, and hypothyroidism. Chronic fatigue syndrome, multiple sclerosis, fibromyalgia, asthma, allergies, and eczema are also more common in this population.

Diagnosis: Surgical diagnosis has long been the gold standard for endometriosis. However, a presumptive clinical diagnosis based on symptoms, physical examination, and imaging is less invasive and facilitates the initiation of treatment. (Agarwal et al. 2019) This option is preferred in patients with mild to moderate disease symptoms. This diagnosis is sufficient to begin low-risk therapies, such as hormonal treatments. Treatment response, however, is not a definitive diagnosis. Definitive diagnosis requires histologic evaluation of lesions biopsied during surgery.

Treatment: For optimal effect, NSAIDs are combined with contraceptives containing estrogen and progestin. In patients where estrogen is contraindicated, progestin-only contraceptives can be used. In severe diseases, gonadotropin-releasing hormone analogs or aromatase inhibitors (aromatase is the rate-limiting enzyme in estrogen formation) can be used.

Management: Endometriosis is a chronic disease that requires long-term management. Goals are designed to reduce the number of repeated surgical procedures using medical management where possible. Treatments are personalized to clinical presentation considerations, symptom severity, patient age, and family planning needs. Medical management is first-line therapy, starting with NSAIDs combined with hormonal contraceptives. Surgical interventions may be necessary, but medical treatment can reduce the lifetime number of surgeries needed, avoid surgical complications, and treat endometrial explants that escape visualization during surgery. Adverse reactions to medications and a high recurrence rate upon discontinuation of treatment limit medical interventions. Hormonal contraceptives prevent ovulation and cannot be used for women who desire to become pregnant.

For patients who do not respond to a combination of NSAIDs and hormonal contraceptives, medications that suppress pituitary function and ultimately produce a hypoestrogenic state may be used. Aromatase inhibitors may be used for those with severe symptoms that do not respond to other treatments. Long-term use of aromatase inhibitors is associated with bone loss. Surgery to resect endometrial implants is required when medical therapies become ineffective.

General Treatment Strategies by Drug Class

Estrogens

Estrogens are derived through cholesterol metabolism in a series of cytoplasmic and mitochondrial enzymatic reactions. Aromatization of the A ring of androstenedione or testosterone, mediated by the aromatase enzyme within the endoplasmic reticulum, produces estrogens. 17β-estradiol (E2) is the most abundant circulating estrogen, followed by estrone (E1) and estriol (E3). Common features are a phenolic A ring carrying a hydroxyl group at carbon 3 and either a hydroxyl group or ketone at carbon 17 in ring D.

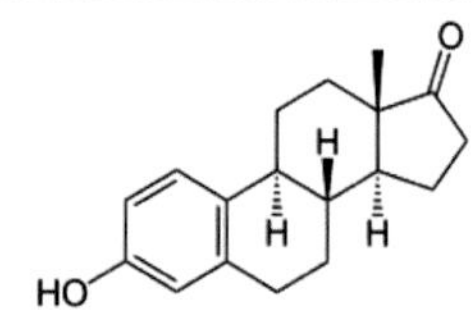

Estrone (E1)

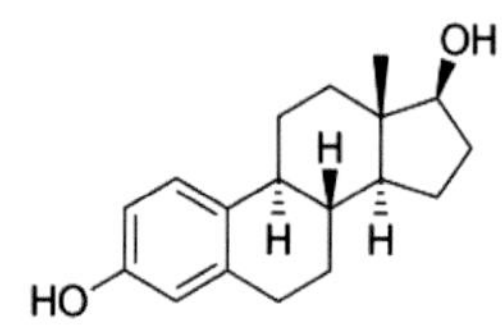

17β-estradiol (E2)

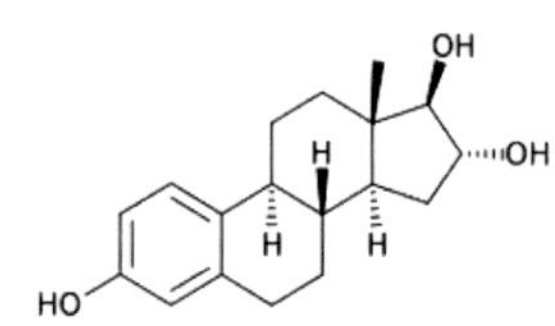

Estriol (E3)

Female secondary sex characteristics result from estrogen production induced upon activation of the hypothalamic-pituitary-gonadal axis at puberty. Estrogen acts as a growth factor to cause the pubertal long bone growth spurt followed by epiphyseal closure, promotes the development of the fallopian tubes, uterus, and vagina, and contributes to breast development. Thus, estrogenic compounds may encourage the development of secondary sex characteristics in delayed puberty. They are also used to treat various disorders associated with dysmenorrhea.

Outside the reproductive system, estrogens act in a cell-specific manner. Estrogen binds to estrogen receptor α or β (ERα or ERβ), and the ratios of the two receptors vary in bone, central nervous system, GI tract, heart, liver, immune system, and vascular endothelium. These differences result in altered function in different tissues.

Most actions of estrogen are mediated by specific, ligand-activated transcription factors of the nuclear receptor superfamily, which have widespread distribution. ERα and ERβ have distinct tissue expression patterns and diverse functions in response to ligand binding. The similarity in the DNA binding domains demonstrates recognition of common promoter elements and regulation of similar sets of target genes. However, based on the physiological context, the actions differ depending on the recruitment of co-activators and co-repressors to the promoter.

ERα is abundant throughout the reproductive tract, including the ovary, uterus, and vagina; it is also found in the breast, hypothalamus, vascular endothelium, and smooth muscle. In the reproductive tract, ERβ is mainly restricted to the ovaries but is also expressed in bone, brain, lung, and vasculature. Individual cells may express only one form of ER or both ERα and ERβ.

Unbound ER exists as monomers bound to heat shock proteins (HSP) in the cell nucleus. Lipophilic estrogens diffuse across cell membranes and bind ER, initiating a conformational change that displaces HSP90, leads to receptor dimerization (homodimers or heterodimers) and promotes binding to estrogen response elements (ERE) in the proximal promoters of target genes. Protein-protein interactions between ERs and other transcription factors, such as SP1 and AP-1, mediate alternative actions through interactions with non-ERE sites on target gene promoters.

ERα and ERβ also exist within caveolae on the plasma membrane. Activation of these receptors leads to alternative cell signaling and cross-talk with MAPK and cAMP pathways. Finally, MAPK and Akt may activate ERs independent of estrogen, further complicating the cross-talk among cellular signaling cascades.

ERα is abundant within the female reproductive tract, including the hypothalamus, ovaries, uterus, and vagina, and can also be found in vascular endothelium and smooth muscle. Although also expressed in the ovaries, ERβ is found in bone, brain, liver, and vasculature. Breast cancers express both forms of ER, although Erα predominantly mediates tumor growth. Thus, estrogens have numerous effects on multiple physiological systems.

Within the reproductive tract, estrogen acts predominantly as a growth-promoting agent, particularly in the endometrium, where it promotes thickening throughout the follicular phase of the menstrual cycle.

Estrogens have metabolic effects outside the reproductive system. In bone, estrogen promotes increased mass by regulating cytokine production and osteoblasts as well as inhibiting osteoclast activity. Estrogens also stimulate epiphyseal plate closure.

Estrogens can affect lipid and cholesterol profiles. A desirable increase in the HDL: LDL ratio occurs due to both increased HDL and decreased LDL in response to estrogen. Serum triglycerides may be slightly elevated, whereas estrogens suppress cholesterol levels. In the liver, estrogens positively affect lipoprotein metabolism, increase cholesterol secretion, and reduce bile acid secretion.

Importantly, estrogens alter clotting by affecting the production of plasma proteins, stimulating coagulation factors, suppressing anticoagulation factors, and increasing fibrinolysis. These effects contribute significantly to some of the most serious adverse events associated with estrogen therapies.

Estrogen therapies:

Estrogen therapies are administered through a variety of preparations, including pills, injectables, patches, and creams. The lipophilic nature of estrogen compounds assures easy absorption. Many of the available estrogens are modifications of the endogenous hormone through conjugation or esterification. Micronized forms of estradiol are also used. These preparations increase bioavailability by reducing first-pass metabolism.

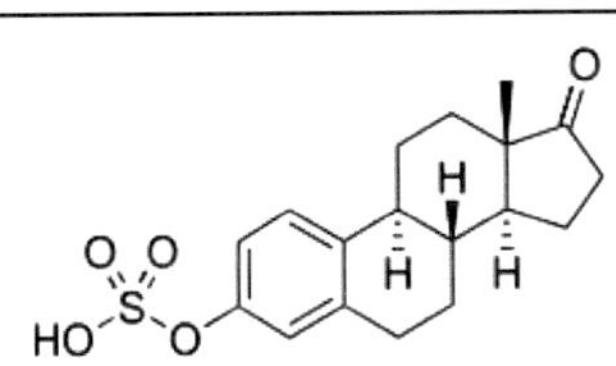

Estrone sulfate

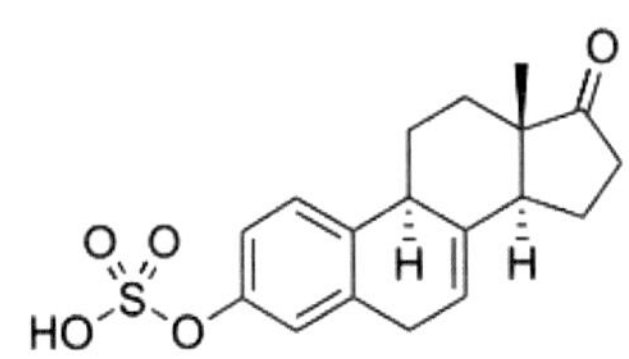

Equilin sulfate

Conjugated and esterified Estrogens: Conjugated equine estrogens (purified from the urine of pregnant horses) contain a combination of estrone sulfate, equilin sulfate, 17 α-dihydroequilin, 17 α-estradiol, and 17 β-dihydroequilin. This drug is approved for short-term use for idiopathic abnormal uterine bleeding to temporarily elevate estrogen levels, restore physiologic hormone balance, and reset the menstrual cycle.

Conjugated equine estrogens are also used to elevate estrogens in cases of hypogonadism and primary ovarian insufficiency. In menopausal women, conjugated equine estrogens are indicated for the prevention of osteoporosis, genitourinary syndrome of menopause, (Portman and Gass 2014), and alleviation of menopausal vasomotor symptoms. A vaginal preparation is available for the treatment of genitourinary syndrome of menopause.

Estradiol and Estrone: Estradiol is the main form of estrogen secreted in premenopausal women. After menopause, the primary estrogen in women is estrone. Estradiol is available in long-acting depot formulation (estradiol cypionate), oral, transdermal, and vaginal forms for treating hypogonadism due to primary ovarian insufficiency. In menopause, it alleviates genitourinary symptoms such as vaginal dryness/irritation, frequent urinary tract infections, and vasomotor symptoms. A vaginal cream of estrone treats genitourinary syndrome of menopause.

Adverse Reactions and Concerns:

Estrogen therapy does carry significant breast cancer risk in postmenopausal patients. Conjugated equine estrogens, combined with medroxyprogesterone acetate, also increase the risk of invasive breast cancer. However, there was no increased risk of invasive breast cancer in patients after surgical menopause (oophorectomy) treated with conjugated estrogens alone. Breast cancer risk in postmenopausal patients on hormone therapy likely depends upon multiple factors, including estrogen and progestin compound, dose, initiation and duration of therapy, and route of administration. Treatment for menopausal symptoms is highly dependent upon individual characteristics and must be carefully considered on a case-by-case basis. Breast density may be increased with conjugated estrogen therapy.

Unopposed estrogens are associated with exacerbation of endometriosis, malignant transformation of endometrial explants, and increased risk of endometrial cancer. Thus if the woman still has her uterus, they should be combined with progestin.

Using conjugated estrogens in conjunction with medroxyprogesterone acetate is associated with an increased risk of dementia in women over 65. Estrogen compounds increase high-density lipoproteins, decrease low-density lipoproteins and, to a lesser extent, increase triglycerides. Estrogens may cause retinal vascular thrombosis.

Estrogens with or without progestin increase the risk of deep vein thrombosis (DVT), stroke, pulmonary emboli, myocardial infarction, and breast cancer. Other conditions that can be exacerbated with estrogen use include diabetes, asthma, epilepsy, hepatic dysfunction, hereditary angioedema, migraine, porphyria, and systemic lupus erythematosus.

Common Adverse Reactions to Estrogen Treatment:

a) Headache
b) Abdominal pain
c) Vaginal hemorrhage
d) Back pain
e) Arthralgia
f) Pharyngitis
g) Sinusitis
h) Depression
i) Dizziness
j) Pruritus
k) Diarrhea or flatulence
l) Vaginitis
m) Leukorrhea
n) Vulvovaginal candidiasis
o) Leg weakness or cramps

Progestins:

Natural and synthetic compounds with activities like the native hormone, progesterone, are classified as progestins. The natural group is produced early in the steroidogenic pathway by cleavage of the side chain from the D ring of the cholesterol molecule by the P450 side chain cleavage enzyme to form pregnenolone. Subsequently, 3β-hydroxysteroid dehydrogenase converts pregnenolone to progesterone, the primary circulating progestin in women.

Stimulated by the pituitary gonadotropin luteinizing hormone, progesterone is produced mainly by the ovarian corpus luteum throughout the secretory phase of the menstrual cycle. The corpus luteum continues producing progesterone during the first trimester of pregnancy, after which the placenta takes over progesterone production. The zona fasciculate of the adrenal gland also makes progesterone.

Progesterone has many functions related to the female reproductive system. In the normal menstrual cycle, it induces secretory changes in the endometrium secondary to the proliferative effects of estrogen. It is required to maintain pregnancy, during which it inhibits ovarian follicle maturation and ovulation which prevents menstruation, promotes mammary gland development, and relaxes uterine smooth muscle. Progesterone suppresses GnRH pulsatility, which blocks the LH surge and prevents ovulation. The prevention of the LH surge is the mechanism of action of progestins in contraceptives.

Like estrogens, progestins also have metabolic effects. Progesterone may increase insulin secretion after the consumption of carbohydrates, increase lipoprotein lipase activity to promote fat deposition, and increase low-density lipoprotein levels.

Synthetic progestins are classified as pregnanes (17α-acetoxyprogesterone derivatives), estranes (19-nortestosterone derivatives), and gonanes (18-homologated 19-nortestosterone derivatives). Another class of progestins is derived from spironolactone. This class has anti-mineralocorticoid and antiandrogen activities characteristic of all progestins.

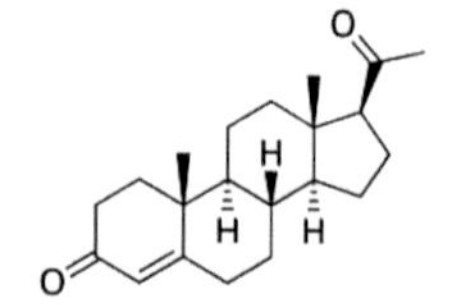

Progesterone

Two nuclear receptor superfamily members mediate most of the progesterone's actions: Progesterone receptors A and B (PR-A and PR-B). They are products of the same gene and have identical ligand binding domains; PR-A exists as a shortened form of PR-B that is missing 165 amino acids from the N-terminal. Isoform expression depends on tissue type, developmental stage, and hormone status and is driven by estrogen-dependent promoter elements in the PR gene. Unbound PR monomers translocate to the nucleus bound to HSP90, HSP70, and p59. Progesterone binding induces the release of the chaperones, phosphorylation, homo- or hetero-dimerization, and binding to progesterone-responsive elements in the promoters of target genes. Recruitment of co-activators or co-repressors is isoform and context-specific, leading to changes in gene expression. PR-B mediates most of the stimulatory activities of progesterone; PR-A antagonizes the effects of PR-B, as well as inhibits other steroid receptors.

Progestin Therapies:

Like estrogens, progestin therapies are available in a variety of preparations, including pills, injectables, patches, and creams. These steroidal compounds are readily absorbed due to their lipophilic nature. Although the native form of the hormone is used for some indications, other hormonal preparations that target the PR are derivatives of progesterone, testosterone, and glucocorticoids to reduce first-pass metabolism. Synthetic derivatives (pregnanes, estranges, and gonanes) also increase bioavailability by reducing first-pass metabolism.

Progesterone: Progesterone is the primary circulating progestin in women. Progesterone is available in multiple forms, including capsules, gels, vaginal suppositories, and injectables. It is used to treat amenorrhea or abnormal uterine bleeding without organic pathology (fibroids or uterine cancer), as a supplement in assisted reproductive technologies, and to prevent endometrial hyperplasia in postmenopausal women with an intact uterus receiving oral conjugated estrogens.

Medroxyprogesterone Acetate: With the addition of an acetate group to carbon 17 in the D ring of the steroid, medroxyprogesterone acetate is a modification of the native hormone that is available for use in injectable and oral formulations. In addition to its use as a hormonal contraceptive (see below), it is also approved for use in the treatment of secondary amenorrhea and abnormal uterine bleeding in the absence of organic pathologies (fibroids or uterine cancer), prevention of endometrial hyperplasia in postmenopausal women receiving oral conjugated estrogens, and in the management of pain associated with endometriosis.

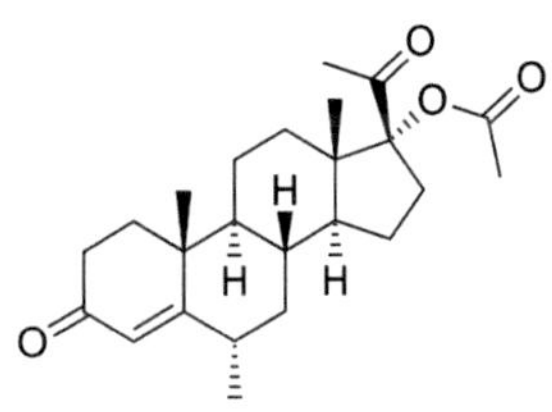

Medroxyprogesterone Acetate

Norethindrone Acetate: Norethindrone acetate is a pro-drug, which is converted upon ingestion into norethindrone for use in the treatment of abnormal uterine bleeding, amenorrhea, and endometriosis. It is also used in contraception (see below).

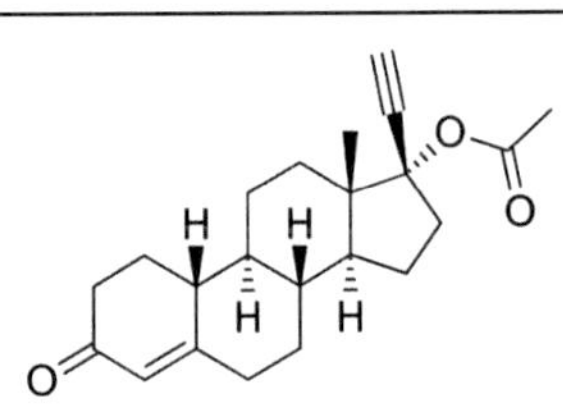

Norethindrone Acetate

Hydroxyprogesterone caproate: With the addition of a hexane-derived carboxylic acid to C17 of the D ring of the native hormone, this drug is available for use as a depot injectable for the treatment of primary and secondary amenorrhea, as well as abnormal uterine bleeding without organic pathologies (fibroids or uterine cancer). It is also used to prevent pre-term birth in pregnant women with a history of this issue.

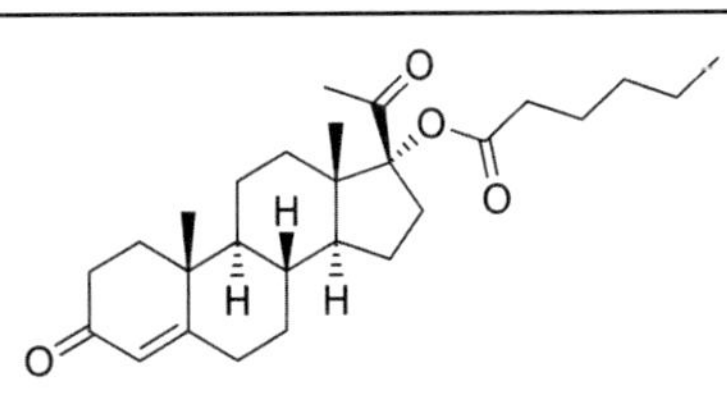

Hydroxyprogesterone caproate

Levonorgestrel: Levonorgestrel is commonly used in combination with estrogen/progestin oral contraceptives. It also comes as an IUD (intrauterine device) formulation, which releases Levonorgestrel daily for up to 8 years. Another preparation of Levonorgestrel, available over the counter as Plan B, is used as an emergency contraceptive. Levonorgestrel is more androgenic than newer progestins, but its risk of deep venous thromboembolism is less.

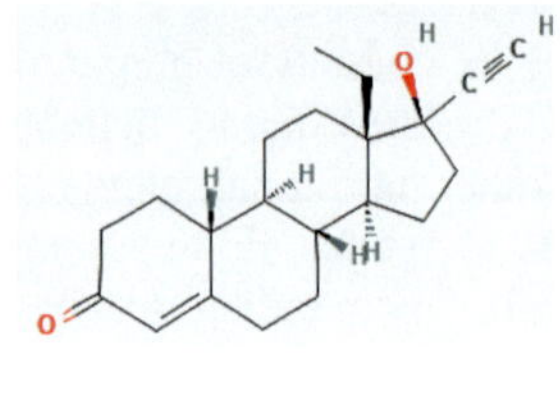

Levonorgestrel

Common Adverse Reactions to Progestin Treatment:

a) Acne
b) skin rash
c) change in menstrual flow, breakthrough bleeding
d) galactorrhea
e) weight changes
f) nausea
g) breast tenderness
h) abdominal pain
i) mood changes/depression

Contraception

Prevention of pregnancy is a primary therapeutic use for estrogens and progestins. Hormonal contraceptives are among the most widely prescribed drugs in the world. Contraceptives containing either progestin alone or a combination of estrogen and progestin are widely available. The effectiveness of hormonal contraceptives varies with the type of contraceptive employed and the user's vigilance in adhering to use guidelines. Hormone-containing IUDs and implants, whose success is largely independent of the users' actions, are 99.9% effective. Similarly, patches, injections, vaginal rings, and oral contraceptives are above 99% effective with perfect use. However, effective use declines as dependence on user compliance increases, such that the typical failure rates are 6% for injectables and 9% for patches, vaginal rings, and oral forms of birth control. Women should be given this information as they decide which contraceptive is most appropriate for them.

Combination Oral Contraceptives (COC)

Oral contraceptives that combine estrogen and progestin remain the most prescribed form of birth control in the U.S. A variety of formulations are available; most contain ethinyl estradiol combined with one of a dozen progestins. Progestins can be classified by generation (based on approval timing) or structural properties. First and second-generation progestins have less receptor specificity, with crossover binding to the ER, androgen receptor, and glucocorticoid receptor. Newer, fourth-generation progestins (Drospirenone, Norethindrone Acetate) have anti-androgen properties that can be useful for patients who experience hirsutism. In general, first and second-generation progestins have increased safety as they counteract the clotting effects of estrogens.

Structurally, progestins in COCs are classified as estranes, gonanes, or pregnanes, which are synthetic derivatives of testosterone (estranes and gonanes), or progesterone (pregnanes), with the 17α-alkyl-19-nortestosterone derivatives most common. Typically, COCs are provided in a daily dosage 28-day pack that mimics the average length of the menstrual cycle, with the last seven pills devoid of hormones to allow for menstruation. Monophasic preparations contain pills with a fixed amount of estrogen and progestin. Multiphasic packs contain 2 or 3 different types of drugs with amounts of the hormone that vary across the 21 days of hormone exposure. These preparations reduce overall hormone exposure and more accurately reflect estrogen/progesterone ratios across the menstrual cycle. More recently, continuous dosing of COCs is used that allows progestin withdrawal, and thus induction of menstruation, only every three months.

Contraceptives containing estrogen and progestin are also available as vaginal rings and transdermal patches. The hormones work synergistically to suppress reproductive cycles. While the primary effect is to stop the pulsatility of GnRH, estrogens, and progestins also directly suppress gonadotropin production by the pituitary. Estrogens reduce FSH and inhibit ovarian follicular growth, whereas progestins suppress the LH surge required for ovulation. In addition, progestins cause uterine endometrium atrophy, prevent implantation, increase cervical mucous viscosity to prevent sperm penetration and impair tubal motility.

Adverse Reactions to COCs

a) nausea
b) breast tenderness
c) headaches
d) breakthrough bleeding
e) hypertension
f) venous thromboembolism
g) increased triglycerides
h) reduced glucose tolerance

Progesterone-only Contraceptives

Specific forms of contraceptives contain only progestin. These are available in mini-pills, depot injectables, subcutaneous implants, and IUDs. The mechanism of action depends on the dose of the progestin. All forms thicken the cervical mucous to inhibit sperm transit and alter the uterine endometrium to inhibit implantation. Feedback to the hypothalamus and pituitary axis to inhibit the LH surge and prevent ovulation remains the primary mechanism of action for the injectable and subcutaneous forms. The mini-pill reduces or delays the LH surge but may not always inhibit ovulation. Local uterine effects are the primary mechanism of action for the progestin-containing IUD. Breakthrough bleeding is the most common side effect of progestin-only contraceptives. Adverse effects on lipid profiles, glucose tolerance, and headaches are also reported. Some progestin-only contraceptives also increase the risk of venous thromboembolism, especially medroxyprogesterone acetate depot form. The progestin-only mini-pills do not increase the risk of venous thromboembolism.

Common Progestins in Monophasic Combined Oral Contraceptives

Name	Structural Class	Generation	Chemical Structure
Cyproterone	Pregnane	1st	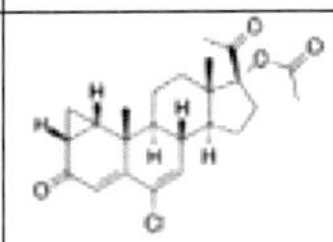
Ethynodiol Acetate	Estrane	1st	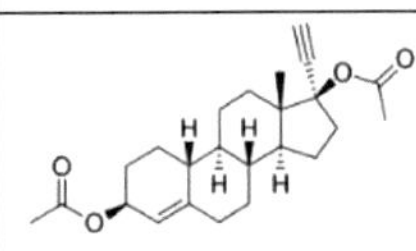
Nomegestrel Acetate	Pregnane	4th	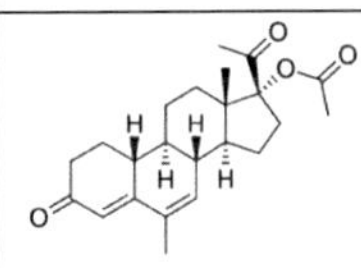
Norethindrone	Estrane	1st	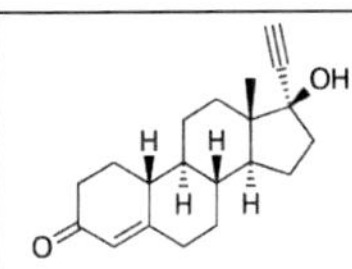
Norgestimate	Gonane	3rd	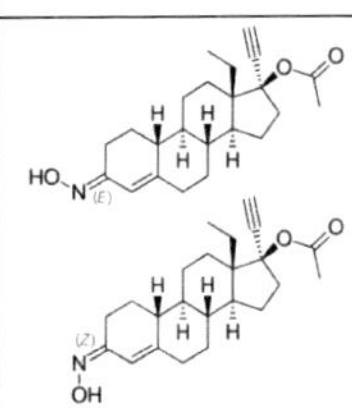
Norgestrel	Gonane	3rd	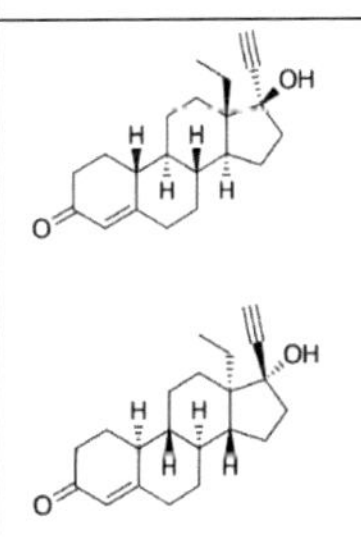

Drospirenone	Spironolactone	4th	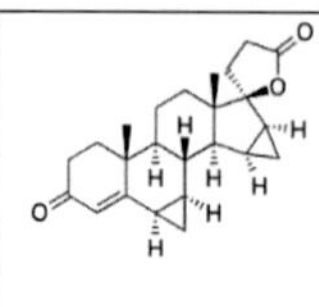
Common Progestins in Multiphasic Combined Oral Contraceptives			
Name	Structural Class	Generation	Chemical Structure
Desogestrel	Gonane	2nd	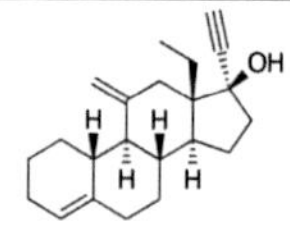
Dienogest	Estrane	4th	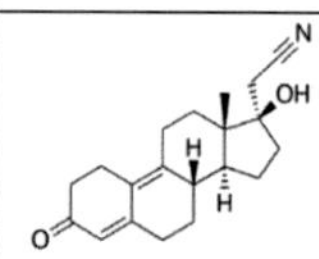
Levonorgestrel	Gonane	2nd	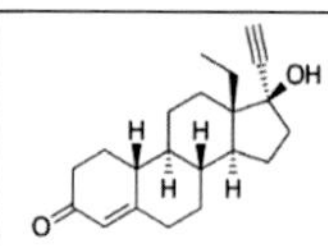
Norethindrone Acetate	Estrane	4th	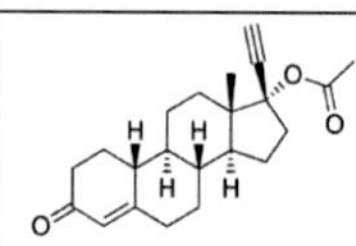
Norgestimate	Gonane	3rd	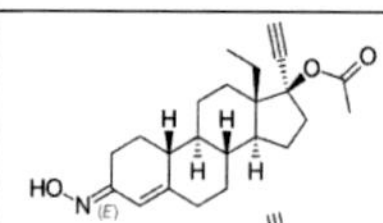 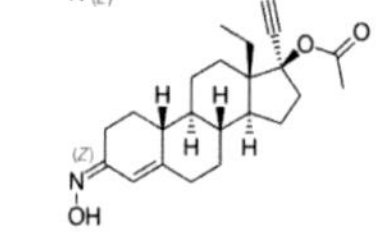
Progestins in Combination Patches			
Norgelstromin	Gonane	3rd	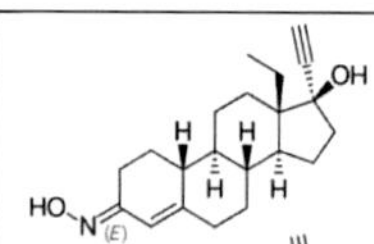 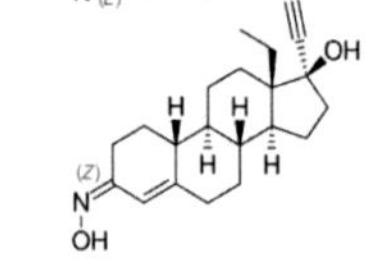
Progestins in Combination Vaginal Rings			
Etonogestrel	Gonane	3rd	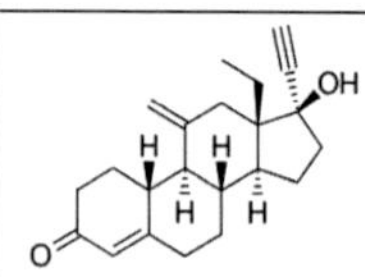
Segesterone Acetate	Pregnane	4th	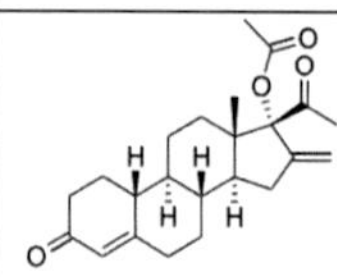

Progestin-only Contraceptives				
Name	Method	Structural Class	Generation	Chemical Structure
Desogestrel	Pill	Gonane	2nd	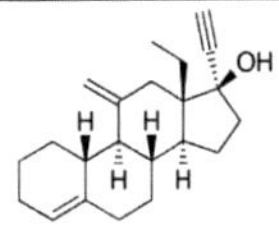
Drospirenone	Pill	Spironolactone	4th	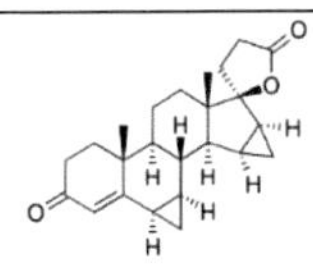
Etonogestrel	Implant	Gonane	3rd	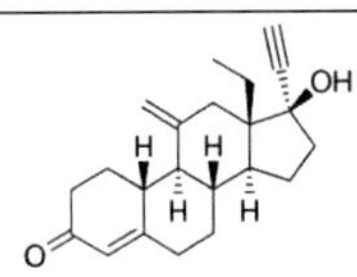
Levonorgestrel	Implant/IUD	Gonane	2nd	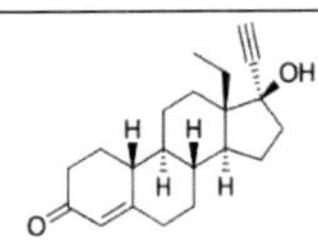
Medroxyprogesterone acetate	Injectable	Pregnane	1st	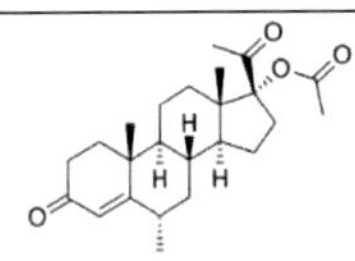
Norethindrone enanthate	Injectable/pill	Estrane	1st	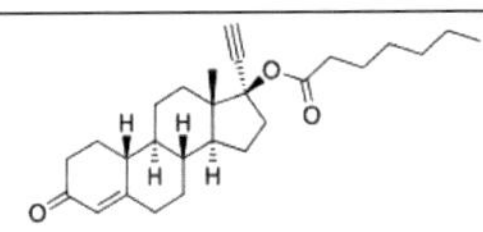

Selective Estrogen Receptor Modulators (SERMs) and Selective Estrogen Receptor Down Regulators (SERDs)

Compounds that bind intracellular ERs modify their activity by altering how ERs engage dimerization partners, bind DNA promoter elements, and recruit co-activators and co-repressors to regulate target gene expression in a cell-specific manner. SERMs/SERDs competitively inhibit estrogen binding to the ERs, but in contrast to pure ER agonists and antagonists, they have mixed agonist and antagonist activity, which is tissue-specific depending on the type of ER present. Molecules that interact with ERs can be anti-estrogenic in all tissues, estrogenic in all tissues, or antiestrogenic in some tissues, with mixed effects in others. SERMs are available orally, whereas the only approved SERD, fulvestrant, must be delivered by intramuscular injection.

SERM and SERD Therapies:

Tamoxifen: This non-steroidal, triphenylethylene SERM is indicated to treat ER-positive breast cancer and to reduce breast cancer risk in women at high risk for developing breast cancer. Tamoxifen competes with estrogens for binding to ER, inhibits estrogen effects, and contributes to cell cycle arrest in G_0 and G_1. These effects are mediated by recruiting a co-repressor to the ER-DNA complex. Tamoxifen has anti-resorptive properties in bone and reduces total cholesterol, LDL, and LPA in postmenopausal women. When using tamoxifen, venous thromboembolism, and endometrial cancer risk increases 2-3 fold. Endometrial cancer risk is caused by the agonist activity of tamoxifen on ERα in the endometrium. Other adverse effects include hot flashes, cataracts, and nausea.

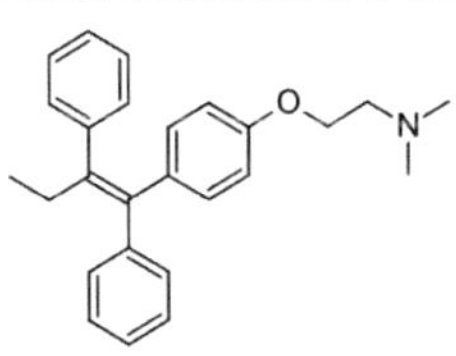

Tamoxifen

Toremifene: This non-steroidal, chlorinated derivative of tamoxifen is indicated for use in the treatment of postmenopausal women with ER-positive metastatic breast cancer. Adverse effects are similar to tamoxifen.

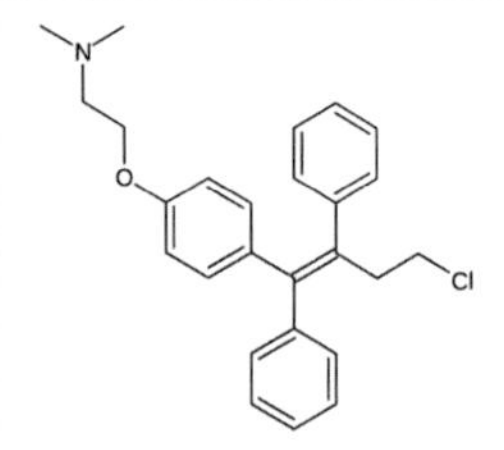

Toremifene

Ospemifene: This metabolite of toremifene is indicated for treating dyspareunia in postmenopausal women. Adverse effects are similar to tamoxifen.

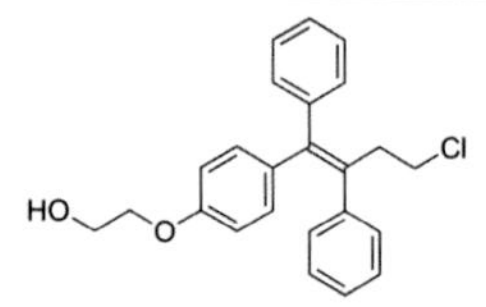

Ospemifene

Bazedoxifene: This third-generation SERM is used with conjugated equine estrogens to prevent osteoporosis in postmenopausal women with a significant risk for bone loss. It is an estrogen receptor agonist in bone. Adding the SERM to the conjugated estrogen can also reduce the risk of endometrial hyperplasia caused by unopposed estrogens.

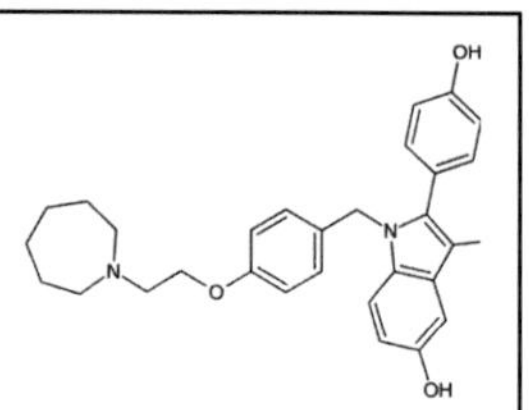

Bazedoxifene

Raloxifene: This non-steroidal, polyhydroxylated compound with a benzothiophene core binds with high affinity to both types of ER and prevents estrogen binding. Recruitment of co-activators and co-repressors to the ER-DNA complex differs from those observed with tamoxifen. As an estrogen agonist in the bone, it is indicated for treating and preventing osteoporosis in postmenopausal women. Raloxifene is an ER antagonist in the breast and is indicated for risk reduction and invasive breast cancer treatment. Raloxifene blocks estrogen action in the uterus and thus does not increase endometrial proliferation. Adverse reactions include an increased risk of venous thromboembolism and stroke. It should be avoided in patients with an increased risk of stroke.

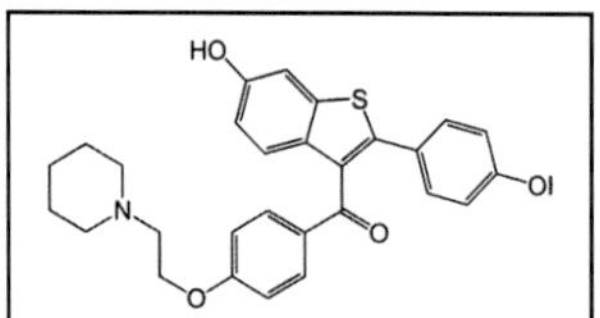

Raloxifene

Fulvestrant: This 7α-alkylamide derivative of estradiol has an affinity to ER comparable to the native hormone. As opposed to SERMs, fulvestrant is a pure ER antagonist. Fulvestrant binding alters the conformation of ER, which impairs dimerization, impedes nuclear localization, inhibits transcriptional activity, and increases hydrophobicity, which enhances degradation. This drug treats hormone receptor-positive breast cancer, including advanced cancers that are HER2-negative in postmenopausal women. It may also be combined with kinase inhibitors to treat advanced breast cancers. Adverse effects include an increased risk of venous thromboembolism, hot flashes, and increased liver transaminases.

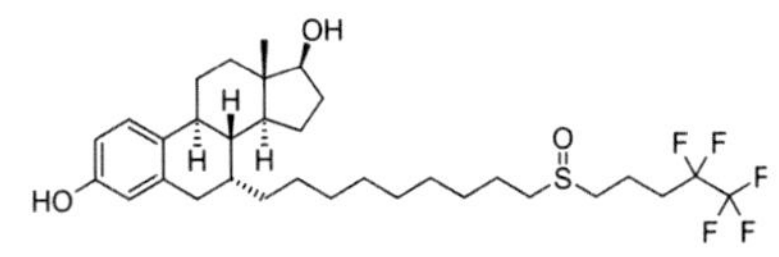

Fulvestrant

Selective PR Modulators (SPRMs) and Anti-progestins

Progesterone Receptor (PR) modulators and anti-progestins may act as partial agonists/antagonists at the intracellular PR to alter transcriptional activity. Whether a compound is a pure antagonist or has mixed agonist/antagonist activities depends mainly on cell context. The availability of co-activators and co-repressors within specific cell types may influence any PR-binding compound's agonist/antagonist activity. Pure antagonists inhibit PR from recruiting co-activators to the PR-DNA interface, thereby allowing increased interactions with co-repressors and blocking the initiation of target gene transcription. A mixed agonist/antagonist recruits both co-activators and co-repressors. SPRMs and anti-progestins antagonize all the physiological effects of progesterone, which include: initiation and maintenance of pregnancy, transformation to secretory uterine endometrium, inhibition of uterine muscle contraction, and facilitation of the LH surge.

Mifepristone: This derivative of the 19-norprogestin norethindrone is a competitive antagonist of the PR and glucocorticoid receptor, where it acts by recruiting co-repressors to the receptor-DNA complex. It is prescribed (together with Misoprostol) for early pregnancy termination. In this context, mifepristone blocks uterine PRs to induce decidual breakdown and induction of myometrial uterine contractions. In addition, mifepristone delays or blocks ovulation through actions at the hypothalamus and pituitary gland. The combination of Mifepristone and Misoprostol is available in the US only by prescription and under a REMS (risk evaluation and management strategy) program, which requires providers to undergo special education.

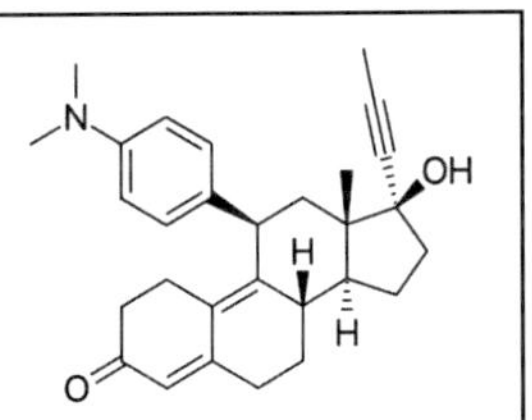

Mifepristone

During the second (luteal) half of the menstrual cycle, PR antagonism with mifepristone induces menstruation by initiating the events associated with progesterone withdrawal during the secretory phase of the cycle. It can also treat uterine fibroids.

High doses of mifepristone can also control hyperglycemia in people with type 2 diabetes with hypercortisolism (Cushing's syndrome) by acting as an antagonist at the glucocorticoid receptor.

Adverse events of Mifepristone include abdominal and uterine cramps, vaginal hemorrhage, and back pain when used for termination of pregnancy. Use in the treatment of Cushing's syndrome is associated with abdominal cramping, fatigue, headache, and endometrial hypertrophy.

Ulipristal acetate: This derivative of 19-norprogesterone is classified as a selective PR modulator with partial agonist activity at the PR and weak antagonist activity at the glucocorticoid receptor. It competes with progesterone for binding to the receptor. It may inhibit ovulation and alter the uterine endometrium to inhibit implantation. It is approved as a prescription emergency contraceptive following unprotected intercourse or in cases of suspected contraceptive failure. Common adverse effects include delayed menstruation, abnormal uterine bleeding, abdominal pain, and headache.

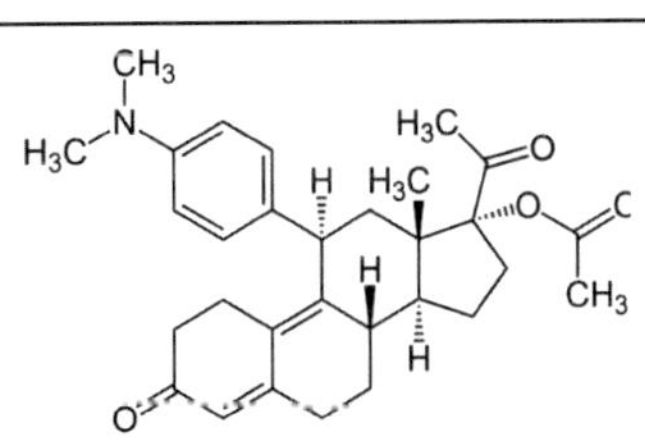

Ulipristil acetate

References

Agarwal, S. K., C. Chapron, L. C. Giudice, M. R. Laufer, N. Leyland, S. A. Missmer, S. S. Singh, and H. S. Taylor. 2019. Clinical diagnosis of endometriosis: a call to action. *Am J Obstet Gynecol* 220 (4):354.e351-354.e312.

Anglesio, M. S., N. Papadopoulos, A. Ayhan, T. M. Nazeran, M. Noë, H. M. Horlings, A. Lum, S. Jones, J. Senz, T. Seckin, J. Ho, R. C. Wu, V. Lac, H. Ogawa, B. Tessier-Cloutier, R. Alhassan, A. Wang, Y. Wang, J. D. Cohen, F. Wong, A. Hasanovic, N. Orr, M. Zhang, M. Popoli, W. McMahon, L. D. Wood, A. Mattox, C. Allaire, J. Segars, C. Williams, C. Tomasetti, N. Boyd, K. W. Kinzler, C. B. Gilks, L. Diaz, T. L. Wang, B. Vogelstein, P. J. Yong, D. G. Huntsman, and I. M. Shih. 2017. Cancer-Associated Mutations in Endometriosis without Cancer. *N Engl J Med* 376 (19):1835-1848.

Arnold, J., M. L. Barcena de Arellano, C. Rüster, G. F. Vercellino, V. Chiantera, A. Schneider, and S. Mechsner. 2012. Imbalance between sympathetic and sensory innervation in peritoneal endometriosis. *Brain Behav Immun* 26 (1):132-141.

Arnold, J., G. F. Vercellino, V. Chiantera, A. Schneider, S. Mechsner, and M. L. Barcena de Arellano. 2013. Neuroimmunomodulatory alterations in non-lesional peritoneum close to peritoneal endometriosis. *Neuroimmunomodulation* 20 (1):9-18.

As-Sanie, S., R. E. Harris, V. Napadow, J. Kim, G. Neshewat, A. Kairys, D. Williams, D. J. Clauw, and T. Schmidt-Wilcke. 2012. Changes in regional gray matter volume in women with chronic pelvic pain: a voxel-based morphometry study. *Pain* 153 (5):1006-1014.

Baber, R. J., N. Panay, A. Fenton, and I. M. S. Writing Group. 2016. 2016 IMS Recommendations on women's midlife health and menopause hormone therapy. *Climacteric* 19 (2):109-150.

Bakalov, V. K., J. N. Anasti, K. A. Calis, V. H. Vanderhoof, A. Premkumar, S. Chen, J. Furmaniak, B. R. Smith, M. J. Merino, and L. M. Nelson. 2005. Autoimmune oophoritis as a mechanism of follicular dysfunction in women with 46,XX spontaneous premature ovarian failure. *Fertil Steril* 84 (4):958-965.

Bakalov, V. K., L. Gutin, C. M. Cheng, J. Zhou, P. Sheth, K. Shah, S. Arepalli, V. Vanderhoof, L. M. Nelson, and C. A. Bondy. 2012. Autoimmune disorders in women with turner syndrome and women with karyotypically normal primary ovarian insufficiency. *Journal of Autoimmunity* 38 (4):315-321.

Bakalov, V. K., V. H. Vanderhoof, C. A. Bondy, and L. M. Nelson. 2002. Adrenal antibodies detect asymptomatic auto-immune adrenal insufficiency in young women with spontaneous premature ovarian failure. *Hum Reprod* 17 (8):2096-2100.

Brawn, J., M. Morotti, K. T. Zondervan, C. M. Becker, and K. Vincent. 2014. Central changes associated with chronic pelvic pain and endometriosis. *Hum Reprod Update* 20 (5):737-747.

Bulun, S. E., Y. Wan, and D. Matei. 2019. Epithelial Mutations in Endometriosis: Link to Ovarian Cancer. *Endocrinology* 160 (3):626-638.

Burney, R. O., and L. C. Giudice. 2012. Pathogenesis and pathophysiology of endometriosis. *Fertil Steril* 98 (3):511-519.

Casper, R.F. 2022. *Clinical manifestations and diagnosis of menopause*. UpToDate 2022 [cited February 2, 2023 2022]. Available from https://www.uptodate.com/contents/clinical-manifestations-and-diagnosis-of-menopause.

Current evaluation of amenorrhea. 2008. *Fertil Steril* 90 (5 Suppl):S219-225.

De Vos, M., P. Devroey, and B. C. Fauser. 2010. Primary ovarian insufficiency. *Lancet* 376 (9744):911-921.

Du, H., and H. S. Taylor. 2007. Contribution of bone marrow-derived stem cells to endometrium and endometriosis. *Stem Cells* 25 (8):2082-2086.

Dumesic, D. A., J. D. Phan, K. L. Leung, T. R. Grogan, X. Ding, X. Li, L. R. Hoyos, D. H. Abbott, and G. D. Chazenbalk. 2019. Adipose Insulin Resistance in Normal-Weight Women With Polycystic Ovary Syndrome. *J Clin Endocrinol Metab* 104 (6):2171-2183.

Elizur, S. E., M. Friedman Gohas, O. Dratviman-Storobinsky, and Y. Cohen. 2019. Pathophysiology Mechanisms in Fragile-X Primary Ovarian Insufficiency. *Methods Mol Biol* 1942:165-171.

Engemise, S., C. Gordon, and J. C. Konje. 2010. Endometriosis. *Bmj* 340:c2168.

Geffner, M. E., and D. W. Golde. 1988. Selective insulin action on skin, ovary, and heart in insulin-resistant states. *Diabetes Care* 11 (6):500-505.

Giudice, L. C. 2010. Clinical practice. Endometriosis. *N Engl J Med* 362 (25):2389-2398.

Gorsic, L. K., G. Kosova, B. Werstein, R. Sisk, R. S. Legro, M. G. Hayes, J. M. Teixeira, A. Dunaif, and M. Urbanek. 2017. Pathogenic Anti-Müllerian Hormone Variants in Polycystic Ovary Syndrome. *J Clin Endocrinol Metab* 102 (8):2862-2872.

Guidi, J., A. Gambineri, L. Zanotti, F. Fanelli, G. A. Fava, and R. Pasquali. 2015. Psychological aspects of hyperandrogenic states in late adolescent and young women. *Clin Endocrinol (Oxf)* 83 (6):872-878.

Harlow, S. D., M. Gass, J. E. Hall, R. Lobo, P. Maki, R. W. Rebar, S. Sherman, P. M. Sluss, T. J. de Villiers, and Straw Collaborative Group. 2012. Executive summary of the Stages of Reproductive Aging Workshop + 10: addressing the unfinished agenda of staging reproductive aging. *Journal of Clinical Endocrinology and Metabolism* 97 (4):1159-1168.

Hatch, R., R. L. Rosenfield, M. H. Kim, and D. Tredway. 1981. Hirsutism: implications, etiology, and management. *Am J Obstet Gynecol* 140 (7):815-830.

Johnston-MacAnanny, E. B.;, B. G.; Patel, and R. N. Taylor. 2022. Chapter 22: Disorders of the Female Reproductive Tract. In *Pathophysiology of Disease: An Introduction to Clinical Medicine*, edited by G. D. Hammer and S. J. McPhee. New York: McGraw-Hill.

Legro, R. S., S. A. Arslanian, D. A. Ehrmann, K. M. Hoeger, M. H. Murad, R. Pasquali, and C. K. Welt. 2013. Diagnosis and treatment of polycystic ovary syndrome: an Endocrine Society clinical practice guideline. *J Clin Endocrinol Metab* 98 (12):4565-4592.

Liang, Y., and S. Yao. 2016. Potential role of estrogen in maintaining the imbalanced sympathetic and sensory innervation in endometriosis. *Mol Cell Endocrinol* 424:42-49.

Majumdar, A., and N. S. Mangal. 2013. Hyperprolactinemia. *J Hum Reprod Sci* 6 (3):168-175.

Marsh, C. A., and F. W. Grimstad. 2014. Primary amenorrhea: diagnosis and management. *Obstet Gynecol Surv* 69 (10):603-612.

Martin, K. A., and J. E. Manson. 2008. Approach to the patient with menopausal symptoms. *Journal of Clinical Endocrinology and Metabolism* 93 (12):4567-4575.

Martin, K.A. MD, and R.L. MD Barbieri. 2022. *Treatment of menopausal symptoms with hormone therapy*. UpToDate 2022 [cited February 2, 2023 2022]. Available from https://www.uptodate.com/contents/treatment-of-menopausal-symptoms-with-hormone-therapy/print.

Master-Hunter, T., and D. L. Heiman. 2006. Amenorrhea: evaluation and treatment. *Am Fam Physician* 73 (8):1374-1382.

Nelson, L. M. 2009. Clinical practice. Primary ovarian insufficiency. *N Engl J Med* 360 (6):606-614.

Norman, R. J., and H. J. Teede. 2018. A new evidence-based guideline for assessment and management of polycystic ovary syndrome. *Med J Aust* 209 (7):299-300.

Peterson, C. M., E. B. Johnstone, A. O. Hammoud, J. B. Stanford, M. W. Varner, A. Kennedy, Z. Chen, L. Sun, V. Y. Fujimoto, M. L. Hediger, and G. M. Buck Louis. 2013. Risk factors associated with endometriosis: importance of study population for characterizing disease in the ENDO Study. *Am J Obstet Gynecol* 208 (6):451.e451-411.

Puttabyatappa, M., and V. Padmanabhan. 2018. Ovarian and Extra-Ovarian Mediators in the Development of Polycystic Ovary Syndrome. *J Mol Endocrinol* 61 (4):R161-r184.

Portman, DJ., and ML Gass. 2014. Vulvovaginal Atrophy Terminology Consensus Conference Panel. Genitourinary syndrome of menopause: new terminology for vulvovaginal atrophy from the International Society for the Study of Women's Sexual Health and the North American Menopause Society. *Menopause* 21(10):1063-8.

Rahmioglu, N., D. R. Nyholt, A. P. Morris, S. A. Missmer, G. W. Montgomery, and K. T. Zondervan. 2014. Genetic variants underlying risk of endometriosis: insights from meta-analysis of eight genome-wide association and replication datasets. *Hum Reprod Update* 20 (5):702-716.

Santen RJ, Loprinzi CL, and Casper RF. 2022. *Menopausal hot flashes*. UpToDate 2022 [cited February 2, 2023 2022]. Available from https://www.uptodate.com/contents/menopausal-hot-flashes.

Santoro, N., C. N. Epperson, and S. B. Mathews. 2015. Menopausal Symptoms and Their Management. *Endocrinol Metab Clin North Am* 44 (3):497-515.

Shafrir, A. L., L. V. Farland, D. K. Shah, H. R. Harris, M. Kvaskoff, K. Zondervan, and S. A. Missmer. 2018. Risk for and consequences of endometriosis: A critical epidemiologic review. *Best Pract Res Clin Obstet Gynaecol* 51:1-15.

Sinaii, N., K. Plumb, L. Cotton, A. Lambert, S. Kennedy, K. Zondervan, and P. Stratton. 2008. Differences in characteristics among 1,000 women with endometriosis based on extent of disease. *Fertil Steril* 89 (3):538-545.

Soliman, A. M., E. Surrey, M. Bonafede, J. K. Nelson, and J. Castelli-Haley. 2018. Real-World Evaluation of Direct and Indirect Economic Burden Among Endometriosis Patients in the United States. *Adv Ther* 35 (3):408-423.

Talaulikar, V. 2022. Menopause transition: Physiology and symptoms. *Best Pract Res Clin Obstet Gynaecol* 81:3-7.

Teede, H. J., M. L. Misso, M. F. Costello, A. Dokras, J. Laven, L. Moran, T. Piltonen, and R. J. Norman. 2018. Recommendations from the international evidence-based guideline for the assessment and management of polycystic ovary syndrome. *Clin Endocrinol (Oxf)* 89 (3):251-268.

Vercellini, P., P. Viganò, E. Somigliana, and L. Fedele. 2014. Endometriosis: pathogenesis and treatment. *Nat Rev Endocrinol* 10 (5):261-275.

Welt, C. K. 2022. Management of spontaneous primary ovarian insufficiency (premature ovarian failure). In *UpToDate*, edited by K. A. Martin.

Welt, C. K., and R.L. Barbieri. 2022a. Evaluation and management of secondary amenorrhea. In *UpToDate*, edited by K. A. Martin.

Welt, C.K., and R.L. Barbieri. 2022b. Evaluation and management of primary amenorrhea. In *UpToDate*, edited by K. A. Martin.

Wheeler, M. A., D. L. Heffner, S. Kim, S. M. Espy, A. J. Spano, C. L. Cleland, and C. D. Deppmann. 2014. TNF-α/TNFR1 signaling is required for the development and function of primary nociceptors. *Neuron* 82 (3):587-602.

Witchel, S. F., S. E. Oberfield, and A. S. Peña. 2019. Polycystic Ovary Syndrome: Pathophysiology, Presentation, and Treatment With Emphasis on Adolescent Girls. *J Endocr Soc* 3 (8):1545-1573.

Wu, S., S. Divall, F. Wondisford, and A. Wolfe. 2012. Reproductive tissues maintain insulin sensitivity in diet-induced obesity. *Diabetes* 61 (1):114-123.

Case Study Question

Case Study

A 25-year-old woman in a monogamous relationship with her husband of 4 years presents to her primary care physician complaining of an inability to get pregnant. She discontinued her hormonal contraceptives six months ago and then waited three months before trying to conceive. However, she has had no menstrual periods since stopping birth control. She says that before starting birth control at age 16, her periods occurred on a regular schedule at approximately 30 days intervals, but sometimes with heavy bleeding and pain during menses. She does report a weight gain of 20 lbs over the past two years. Her current BMI is 32. Physical examination shows a well-developed female with appropriate secondary sex characteristics. There is a darkening and thickening of the hair over her lower abdomen. She reports that she regularly bleaches the hair above her upper lip. A pelvic examination is unremarkable. What should the physician do?

Quiz Questions

1. Analysis of a uterine biopsy of a patient with fertility issues reveals a very thin endometrial layer. Which treatment may promote the development of a thickened endometrium to increase the chances of a successful pregnancy?

A Drospirenone
B Ethinyl estradiol
C Fulvestrant
D Levonorgestrel
E Mifepristone

2. What is the *primary* source of progesterone?

A Corpus luteum of the ovary
B Granulosa cells of the ovary
C Theca cells of the ovary
D Zona fasciculata of the adrenal gland
E Zona glomerulosa of the adrenal gland

3. Which hormone can have a positive feedback effect on gonadotropin-releasing hormone (GnRH) pulsatility leading to the luteinizing hormone surge and ovulation?

A Androstenedione
B Estradiol
C Follicle stimulating hormone (FSH)
D Luteinizing hormone (LH)
E Progesterone

4. Maturation of blood vessels and stimulation of epithelial secretions during the luteal phase of the menstrual cycle is primarily controlled by which hormone?

A Androstenedione
B Estradiol
C Follicle stimulating hormone
D Luteinizing hormone
E Progesterone

5. A 50-year-old woman presents for her annual primary care check-up with increasingly irregular periods. Her last menstrual period was three months ago, and it was very light. She also complains of waking up in the middle of the night with the back of her pajama top soaking wet. What is the best initial treatment for this patient's condition?

A Ethinyl estradiol injections
B Estrogen/progestin-containing contraceptives
C Medroxyprogesterone acetate injections
D Oral estrogen receptor antagonist
E Progestin-only mini-pill

6. Which hormone is frequently elevated in postmenopausal women?

A 17β-Estradiol
B Estrone
C Follicle stimulating hormone (FSH)
D Progesterone
E Testosterone

7. A 52-year-old woman presents to her primary care physician for her annual evaluation. She complains of poor sleep, feeling tired and irritable, and has been experiencing hot flashes with increased frequency. Approximately four years ago, she had a hysterectomy, but her ovaries were not removed at that time. She is interested in trying hormone replacement therapy to assist with her symptoms. Her primary care doctor sends her home with a prescription for which medication?

A Conjugated equine estrogens
B Estrogen/progestin-containing contraceptives
C Medroxyprogesterone acetate injections
D Oral estrogen receptor antagonist
E Progestin-only mini-pill

8. A 53-year-old woman has been on hormone replacement therapy to alleviate the vasomotor and genitourinary symptoms of menopause for three years. She is concerned about the risks of hormone replacement on metabolic health. At this visit, her hemoglobin A1c, blood pressure, and triglycerides are within normal limits. Her doctor advises that it is safe to continue hormone replacement therapy until:

A Age 55
B Age 65
C Blood pressure and triglycerides rise above normal levels
D Indefinitely
E She completes five years of treatment

9. A 37-year-old woman presents to her primary care doctor complaining of irregular menses since discontinuing hormonal contraceptive use nine months ago in an attempt to get pregnant. The first laboratory study that her doctor performs is to measure which hormone?

A β-hCG
B Estradiol
C FSH
D Prolactin
E Testosterone

10. A 38-year-old woman presents with complaints of amenorrhea for four months. Prior to this time, she has had light and irregular periods for the last year. She also has dry skin, irritability, trouble sleeping, and discomfort during intercourse due to vaginal dryness. Serum hCG, prolactin, and thyroid stimulating hormone are all within normal limits. Further laboratory studies indicate elevated levels of FSH and low levels of 17-β estradiol, leading to a definitive diagnosis. Because the woman is interested in getting pregnant, a determination of ovarian reserve is performed to predict responsiveness to fertility treatment. Which hormonal level predicts a higher likelihood of success for ovulation using superovulation treatments?

A High levels of androstenedione
B High levels of anti-Mullerian hormone
C High levels of 17-OH progesterone
D Low levels of anti-mullerian hormone
E Low levels of steroid hormone binding globulin

11. A 37-year-old woman presents to her primary care physician with amenorrhea, hot flashes, and vaginal dryness. She has a BMI of 22; her blood pressure is 110/70. HDL, LDL, and triglycerides are all within normal limits. Laboratory studies indicate that FSH is elevated and 17-β estradiol is low. Imaging studies reveal that the ovarian reserve is depleted. The physician prescribes hormonal contraceptives. Which observation is NOT a benefit of this treatment in this woman?

A Decreased hot flashes
B Decreased risk of lipid abnormalities (low HDL/LDL)
C Improvement in vaginal dryness
D Maintenance of bone density
E Preservation of fertility

12. A 16-year-old female presents to her pediatrician for an annual examination. Although she has developed secondary sex characteristics appropriate for her age, her mother is concerned because she has not started menstruating. She also has central obesity and fine, dark hair on her lower abdomen. hCG testing is negative. Upon further testing, which lab finding is likely to be elevated in this patient?

A Androstenedione
B 17-hydroxyprogesterone
C Progesterone
D Prolactin
E Steroid hormone binding globulin

13. A 27-year-old female presents to her gynecologist with irregular periods, but with pain and heavy flow when menses do occur. Her periods are often 25 days apart and last for seven days, although there will be months when she skips her period entirely. Her last menstrual period was 40 days prior to this visit. hCG testing is negative for pregnancy. She has also experienced fatigue and weight gain over the past year. Her current BMI is 35, which is increased from her last visit one year ago when it was 27. Her past medical history is positive for a deep vein thrombosis suffered after taking a long transatlantic flight 2 years ago. She just started a new relationship and is seeking advice on the best way to avoid pregnancy. After further testing, all laboratory values fall within normal limits. The physician recommends which treatment plan?

A Laparoscopic surgery
B NSAIDs and ethinyl estradiol
C NSAIDs and an estrogen-progestin-containing contraceptive
D NSAIDs and medroxyprogesterone acetate injectable contraceptive
E NSAIDs and the progestin-containing mini pill

14. Which enzyme directly results in the formation of estrogens from androgens?

A 5α Reductase
B 11β Hydroxylase
C 17α Hydroxylase
D Aromatase
E Steroidogenic acute regulatory protein

15. A 55-year-old woman had her last menstrual period 18 months ago. Her primary care physician has prescribed a hormonal replacement therapy containing estrogen and progestin. The progestin in the regimen treats which issue?

A Endometrial hyperplasia
B Genitourinary syndrome
C Hot flashes
D Joint pain
E Osteoporosis

16. A 20-year-old college student inquires about birth control methods. She is healthy, has a BMI of 24, and does not smoke. She has no family history of stroke, pulmonary embolism, or deep vein thrombosis. She has regular periods every 30 days, with little menstrual discomfort and light flow lasting four days. She does have some fine dark hair above her upper lip that concerns her. Her doctor prescribes a method of birth control that could have the added benefit of reducing her facial hair. The prescription is most likely for which medicine?

A Injectable medroxyprogesterone acetate
B Oral ethinyl estradiol combined with drospirenone
C Oral estrone sulfate combined with levonorgestrel
D Oral ethinyl estradiol combined with norgestimate
E Transdermal ethinyl estradiol combined with norelgestromin

17. A 51-year-old postmenopausal woman has been treated with conjugated estrogens to relieve vasomotor symptoms for one year. Her past medical history is significant for a surgical hysterectomy at age 45. She is small and has a BMI of 19. A bone scan performed this year shows a substantial decrease in bone mineral density over the past year. Which pharmaceutical can be added to her current treatment to assist with protection against further bone loss?

A Bazedoxifene
B Fulvestrant
C Levonorgestrel
D Mifepristone
E Tamoxifen

18. The safety of combined estrogen: progestin hormonal contraceptives is decreased when the formulation includes a third or fourth-generation progestin. The reduced safety is due to which observation?

A Increased androgenization
B Increased LDL
C Increased risk of pregnancy
D Increased risk of thromboembolic events
E Increased triglycerides

19. A 32-year-old woman is interested in using hormonal birth control. She is obese and does not smoke. Approximately 20 years ago, her mother suffered a deep vein thrombosis after taking a flight to Europe from the US. Her physician prescribes which contraceptive?

A Vaginal ring with ethinyl estradiol and etonogestrel
B Mini pills with norethindrone
C Injectable medroxyprogesterone acetate
D Combined hormonal pills with ethinyl estradiol and levonorgestrel
E Transdermal patch with ethinyl estradiol and norethindrone

20. Termination of early pregnancy can be achieved by administering a combination of two drugs. One drug acts to increase myometrial contractions. In this context, the second drug acts as which effector?

A Estrogen receptor reverse agonist
B Glucocorticoid receptor antagonist
C Glucocorticoid receptor partial agonist
D Progesterone receptor agonist
E Progesterone receptor antagonist

Case Study Answer

The first step in evaluating secondary amenorrhea is to rule out pregnancy. Once the hCG test is negative, the next steps involve determining the source of the pathology within the hypothalamic-pituitary axis. A thorough history should investigate changes in diet, exercise, weight, and other illnesses that may contribute to menstrual dysfunction. This woman just discontinued contraceptives; sometimes, returning to fertility can take several months. Although she has a history of regular menses, changes in body hair indicate hyperandrogenism and require further evaluation. History questions should also investigate potential hypothalamic-pituitary sources of pathology, such as visual changes, headaches, fatigue, polyuria, and polydipsia. Symptoms of estrogen deficiency, including hot flashes, vaginal dryness, sleep changes, and decreased libido, must also be discussed. This patient has an elevated BMI and evidence of hirsutism. Endocrine laboratory studies are needed for further evaluation. TSH and PRL should be obtained to rule out thyroid dysfunction and hyperprolactinemia, respectively. Serum FSH levels can test for hypoestrogenism associated with premature ovarian failure. Estrogen levels can also be helpful. The evidence of hirsutism necessitates total testosterone, SHBG, and DHEA-S measurements. 17-hydroxyprogesterone can be measured to rule out non-classical congenital hyperplasia.

The most common diagnosis with this presentation is PCOS. In this case, relevant endocrine lab values might include elevated androgens with suppressed SHBG, FSH levels that are normal or low, and normal levels of estrogen. Follow-up laboratory studies are necessary. These might consist of an LH level, which may be elevated. An elevated LH: FSH ratio is frequently observed in these patients. The patient should be evaluated for metabolic dysfunction by examining fasting blood glucose, HgA1C, and triglycerides. Transvaginal ultrasound may show the presence of multiple developing follicles, with or without cysts, in the ovary. The first line of treatment for this patient, who desires to get pregnant, should be a recommendation for lifestyle modifications that target weight loss. Even a 5% reduction in BMI may be sufficient to initiate ovulatory menstrual cycles. If amenorrhea persists, treatment with ovulation-inducing agents may be required.

Quiz Answers

1. B. Ethinyl estradiol is a form of estrogen that works during the cycle's first (follicular) phase to increase uterine thickness. Drospirenone is a fourth-generation synthetic progestin derived from spironolactone, which blocks the LH surge, ovulation, and menstruation. The SERD (selective estrogen receptor down regulator) Fulvestrant is a pure ER antagonist used in hormone-positive breast cancer. Levonorgestrel is a second-generation synthetic progestin that alters uterine endometrium to inhibit implantation, preventing conception. Mifepristone is a progestin that blocks uterine progesterone receptors and induces uterine contractions.

2. A. During normal menstrual cycles and the first trimester of pregnancy, progesterone is produced in the ovary's corpus luteum. Later in pregnancy, it is made by the placenta. The granulosa and thecal cells of the ovary do produce progesterone (as well as estrogen and other steroids) but in much smaller amounts than the corpus luteum. In normal conditions, the zona fasciculata of the adrenal gland makes only a small amount of progesterone. The zona glomerulosa of the adrenal gland makes mineralocorticoids.

3. B. Early in the menstrual cycle, small amounts of estradiol inhibit the GnRH pulsatility. However, as the dominant follicle progresses to making large amounts of estradiol just before ovulation, there is a switch from negative feedback to positive feedback. On the day of the LH surge, estradiol stimulates GnRH pulsatility. Progesterone blocks this pulsatile GnRH release. Androstenedione is a precursor of estrogen and does not have significant estrogenic activity. FSH and LH are both released from the anterior pituitary following pulsatile GnRH stimulation.

4. E. Progesterone slows the endometrial growth caused by estrogen and stimulates blood vessel development in the endometrium. Endometrial secretions which facilitate embryo implantation are stimulated by progesterone. Androstenedione is a precursor of estradiol. Neither estradiol nor androstenedione helps the endometrium mature in preparation for an embryo. FSH and LH lead to ovulation; thus, their main target is the ovary.

5. B. Since the patient is having problems with sleep because of night sweats, hormonal therapy would be appropriate. Usually, this would be continued for five years or less or be stopped at age 60 if this comes first. The reasons for stopping therapy are to prevent the increased risk of venous thrombosis, stroke, heart attack, and breast cancer. As she still has her uterus (her last period was three months ago), she requires the addition of progestin to protect against uterine cancer. Ethinyl estradiol injections do not provide any progestin. Medroxyprogesterone is a progestin and will not treat the perimenopausal symptoms the woman is having. Fulvestrant is a SERD (selective estrogen receptor down-regulator) and antagonizes estrogen. Thus it would not help perimenopausal symptoms and might make them worse. The progestin-only mini-pill lacks estrogen activity and would not alleviate perimenopausal symptoms.

6. C. In menopause, a woman's ovaries have decreased responsiveness to FSH, and in an attempt to compensate, the pituitary produces more FSH. Thus, an elevated FSH level can be taken as evidence that menopause may be approaching. Estrogen, estrone, and progesterone levels decrease because the ovaries and corpus luteum are not producing them. Testosterone levels gradually decline in menopause.

7. A. The patient is experiencing symptoms of menopause that will be relieved by estrogen therapy. As she does not have a uterus, she does not need progestins, and estrogen/progestin-containing contraceptives would be inappropriate. The progestin-only choices of medroxyprogesterone acetate injections or progestin-only mini-pill would not treat her symptoms as they lack estrogen. An estrogen receptor antagonist would block estrogen's effects and likely worsen her symptoms.

8. E. Since long-term treatment with estrogen increases the risks of pulmonary embolism, stroke, heart attack, and breast cancer, it is currently advised that treatment be limited to 5 years and not be continued after age 60. Exceptions can be made depending on the individual circumstances of the patient.

9. A. The first test should rule out pregnancy as if it is present, no other testing is needed, but prenatal care is necessary. FSH and estradiol can then be measured to test for ovarian function, which would cause elevated FSH and low estradiol. Prolactin can be measured to assess whether an active prolactinoma in the pituitary is blocking the LH surge and ovulation. If there are signs of excess androgens, testosterone can be measured. TSH testing would also be helpful.

10. B. Anti-Mullerian hormone is secreted by undeveloped, small follicles. If these are present in sufficient numbers, anti-mullerian hormone will be high. Low levels of this hormone would indicate decreased fertility from insufficient follicles. Androstenedione is a precursor of testosterone and does not evaluate follicular reserve. It likely indicates adrenal problems. 17-OH progesterone is a precursor of cortisol and would most likely indicate adrenal malfunction. It says nothing about the follicular reserve. Low levels of steroid hormone-binding globulin are seen in PCOS but do not directly reflect ovarian follicular reserve.

11. E. This woman has secondary amenorrhea with menopause symptoms. Treatment with hormonal contraceptives can do nothing for her infertility, as her ovarian reserve is depleted. Estrogen will help with her hot flashes. It will

improve her lipid profile by increasing HDL (the "good cholesterol") and decreasing LDL (the "bad" cholesterol). It will help with vaginal lubrication and will also help maintain bone density by stimulating osteoclasts and inhibiting osteoblasts.

12. A. This girl has primary amenorrhea, likely due to polycystic ovary syndrome (PCOS). In PCOS, the adrenal glands secrete excess androgens, including androstenedione, which can be transformed into testosterone. 17-Hydroxyprogesterone would be elevated only if there were a congenital 21-hydroxylase deficiency causing non-classical congenital adrenal hyperplasia, which is rare but essential to rule out. Progesterone levels are low because in PCOS there is a failure of ovulation, resulting in a lack of corpus luteum, where the bulk of progesterone is made. Elevated prolactin levels would indicate a pituitary problem, which is not usually seen in PCOS. Steroid hormone binding globulin is low in PCOS, contributing to elevated androgen levels.

13. E. This woman likely has endometriosis. To definitively make this diagnosis would require laparoscopic surgery and visualization of endometrial implants outside the uterus. That isn't necessary for this woman who does not have severe symptoms. A trial of NSAIDs during menstruation may provide significant relief. In addition, she wants contraception, and it is advisable to see if this will help her pain and heavy bleeding. She is obese and has a history of deep vein thrombosis, making estrogen risky as she could have further clot formation. Ethinyl estradiol or estrogen-progestin pills would not be appropriate. Most progestin-only methods of contraception do not have an increased risk of deep vein thrombosis, but Medroxyprogesterone acetate injectable contraception is an exception and does have an increased clotting risk. Thus NSAIDS to treat her pain and a progestin-only contraceptive is the best treatment for this woman.

14. D. The enzyme Aromatase completes the final step in estrogen synthesis. 5α Reductase is an enzyme involved in the breakdown of testosterone which converts testosterone into dihydrotestosterone. 11β Hydroxylase and 17α Hydroxylase are adrenal enzymes involved in the formation of DHEA. Steroidogenic acute regulatory protein facilitates cholesterol transfer within adrenal cells to form steroids.

15. A. Estrogen stimulates endometrial proliferation; progesterone blocks this proliferation. Without progestin, a woman treated with estrogen is at risk of developing uterine cancer (unless she has already had a hysterectomy). Genitourinary syndrome, hot flashes, joint pain, and osteoporosis are all symptoms caused by a lack of estrogen.

16. B. Fine dark hair above the upper lip of a 20-year-old woman is an example of hirsutism. Fourth-generation progestins have anti-androgen effects, which can treat hirsutism. Medroxyprogesterone acetate and levonorgestrel are 2nd generation progestins. Norgestimate and norgelstromin are third-generation progestins.

17. A. Bazedoxifene is a SERM (selective estrogen receptor modulator). It is a tissue-specific estrogen receptor agonist in bone and hence treats osteoporosis. In the US, it is only available combined with conjugated equine estrogen. Fulvestrant is the only commercially available SERD (selective estrogen receptor down regulator) in the US. It is a pure estrogen receptor antagonist, which would help neither her vasomotor nor decreasing bone density issues. Levonorgestrel is a second-generation progestin that would not treat menopausal symptoms nor increase bone density. Mifepristone is a progesterone receptor antagonist used to terminate early pregnancy. Tamoxifen is a SERM which is an estrogen receptor antagonist used to treat breast cancer. It would lower bone density and increase vasomotor symptoms, which is inappropriate for this patient.

18. D. The 3rd and 4th generation progestins were created to decrease androgenic effects and to help with premenstrual symptoms. They do not stop the prothrombotic effects of estrogen and have the highest rate of extremely rare but life-threatening venous thromboembolism. Hence 1st and 2nd generation progestins are considered to be the safest. Decreased androgenization is a hallmark of 3rd and 4th generation progestins. All oral contraceptives are about 99% effective in perfect use and 91% effective in general use. The type of progestin used does not change this. In general oral contraceptives currently in use do not affect LDL or TG very much. If anything, 3rd and 4th generation progestins may cause a beneficial mild elevation of HDL.

19. B. This woman is obese with a family history of deep vein thrombosis. She is also 32, which raises her risk of deep vein thrombosis. She needs a contraceptive that will not further increase the risk of clotting. Estrogen is the primary cause of the increased risk of deep vein thrombosis in women taking contraceptives; thus, all the options with ethinyl estradiol would be poor choices for this patient. Although both the mini pills with norethindrone and injectable medroxyprogesterone acetate contain only progestins, the 1st generation mini pill with norethindrone is the safest choice. Some studies have suggested a slight risk with the injectable medroxyprogesterone acetate.

20. E. Progesterone is what induces ovulation and helps maintain pregnancy. A progesterone receptor antagonist will prevent ovulation and maintenance of pregnancy. Neither estrogen nor glucocorticoid receptors are involved in the termination of early pregnancy.

MISCELLANEOUS – BENZODIAZEPINES – OPIOIDS

CHAPTER 23

BENZODIAZEPINES

LEAH W. HAMMER, PHD

West Virginia University, Morgantown, West Virginia, USA

Benzodiazepines have enjoyed a remarkably successful history in medicine. Since the first member of this group, **chlordiazepoxide** was introduced in 1960, benzodiazepines have become one of the most frequently prescribed groups of drugs in the US, with **diazepam** being the top-selling prescription medicine in the 1970s. Although their use as **sedatives** (calming or sedating agents), **hypnotics** (sleeping agents), and **anxiolytics** (anxiety-reducing agents) is declining, several benzodiazepines continue to be prescribed in the US for their anxiolytic and sedative-hypnotic actions, and some are used for their anticonvulsant and muscle relaxant properties. Thus, the clinical indications for specific benzodiazepines are not absolute, and their uses overlap considerably. The basic chemical structure of the benzodiazepines consists of a benzene ring coupled to a seven-member heterocyclic structure containing two nitrogens (diazepine) at positions 1 and 4 (Fig. 23.1). Of the more than 2,000 benzodiazepines that have been synthesized, 13 clinically useful compounds are currently on the market in the United States (Table 23.1). Currently, **alprazolam** is the most frequently prescribed benzodiazepine in the outpatient setting in the US. Clobazam is also available in the US to treat seizures associated with Lennox-Gastaut syndrome. It is chemically distinct from the 13 other benzodiazepines available.

Figure 23.1. General structure of 1,4 benzodiazepines.

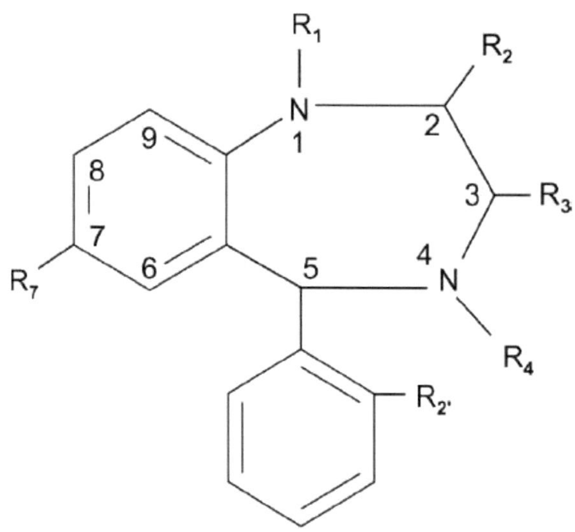

Table 23.1. Clinical uses of benzodiazepines

Drug Name	FDA Indications	Non-FDA Indications
Alprazolam	**Anxiety**, panic disorder	Insomnia, PMS, PMDD
Chlordiazepoxide	**Anxiety**, ethanol withdrawal	
Diazepam	Amnesia induction, **anxiety**, drug-induced seizures, ethanol withdrawal, muscle spasm, partial seizures, sedation induction, status epilepticus, tetanus, tonic-clonic seizures	Agitation, benzodiazepine withdrawal, chloroquine overdose, insomnia, seizure prophylaxis
Clorazepate	**Anxiety**, ethanol withdrawal, partial seizures	Insomnia
Flurazepam	**Insomnia**	Anxiety
Lorazepam	Amnesia induction, **anxiety**, sedation induction	Agitation, ethanol withdrawal, insomnia, sedation maintenance, seizure prophylaxis, status epilepticus
Midazolam	Amnesia induction, **anxiety**, general anesthesia induction and maintenance, sedation induction, and maintenance	Agitation, status epilepticus
Clonazepam	Absence seizures, Lennox-Gastaut syndrome, myoclonic seizures, panic disorder	Anxiety, insomnia, nystagmus, restless leg syndrome
Oxazepam	**Anxiety**, ethanol withdrawal	Insomnia
Temazepam	**Insomnia**	
Triazolam	**Insomnia**	
Quazepam (*Doral*)	**Insomnia**	Anxiety
Estazolam	**Insomnia**	Anxiety

Clinical Uses and Therapeutic Effects

Benzodiazepines are used interchangeably across several clinical disorders regardless of their FDA-approved use. However, individual drugs do exhibit clinically distinguishable features such as their pharmacokinetic profiles, which may support their first-line use for a particular disorder. Unfortunately, a pharmacokinetic feature that makes an individual benzodiazepine useful for a clinical disorder may also predispose the patient to adverse effects that limit its use. For example, the ideal hypnotic agent to produce sleep would be a fast-acting compound. However, such drugs usually have a short half-life and may allow early awakening. They are also associated with a greater abuse liability and higher risk of rebound insomnia upon abrupt discontinuation of their use. On the other hand, the therapeutic action of a benzodiazepine with a longer half-life may be better maintained, but longer half-lives increase the risk of drug accumulation and therefore excessive daytime sedation. This can result in confusion, dizziness, and falls, especially in the elderly. The main clinical uses of benzodiazepines are discussed below.

Anxiety

Anxiety disorders are comprised of several acute and chronic conditions including generalized anxiety disorder, panic disorder, obsessive-compulsive disorder (OCD), posttraumatic stress disorder (PTSD), agoraphobia, and specific phobias. Due to their depressant action on the central nervous system (CNS), benzodiazepines are effective for most anxiety states, although they may be less useful as monotherapies for OCD and are not recommended for PTSD. Although still popular, the use of benzodiazepines for anxiety disorders has declined since the introduction of selective serotonin reuptake inhibitors in the 1980s (Chapter 17).

The pharmacokinetic properties of individual benzodiazepines may be considered when choosing treatment for a particular disorder (see Table 23.2). For example, a patient suffering from intense, chronic anxiety may benefit from a benzodiazepine with a long half-life, whereas a patient experiencing situational anxiety with a definable stimulus may benefit from a benzodiazepine with a short half-life. Regardless of which benzodiazepine is chosen to treat anxiety, it should be used in the lowest effective dose for the shortest duration of therapy to provide maximum benefit to the patient while minimizing the potential for adverse reactions. The benzodiazepines that are FDA-approved for the treatment of anxiety are listed in Table 23.1. Clobazam is used to treat anxiety in various countries outside of the US.

Insomnia

Due to their greater margin of safety and more favorable effect on the sleep cycle, benzodiazepines replaced barbiturates as the mainstay of treatment for insomnia in the 1970s. They remained the most commonly prescribed drugs for insomnia until the 1990s, at which time more selective non-benzodiazepine hypnotics, commonly referred to as **benzodiazepine receptor agonists** or "**Z-drugs**," were developed.

The ideal hypnotic drug would have a fast onset of action and a duration of action that is sufficient to maintain sleep throughout the night without causing sedation, or a "hangover," the next day. While the effects of sedative-hypnotic agents on the phases of the sleep cycle are complex, the ideal hypnotic agent should not suppress REM sleep. One of the many reasons that barbiturates are no longer used for chronic treatment of insomnia is their ability to suppress REM sleep. Benzodiazepines are much less likely to cause an overall decrease in the time associated with REM sleep, and the newer benzodiazepine receptor agonists produce even less suppression.

The benzodiazepines approved in the US for insomnia are listed in Table 23.1. As with the treatment of anxiety, the choice of a particular benzodiazepine to treat a sleep disturbance is generally based on pharmacokinetic criteria. Longer-acting compounds such as **flurazepam** ensure that a patient will sleep through the night, but they also may cause cumulative effects resulting in daytime sluggishness or drug hangover. Shorter-acting compounds like **triazolam** avoid the hangover problem, but their use may be associated with early awakening, an increase in daytime anxiety, and rebound insomnia.

Epilepsy and Seizures (see also Chapter 18)

Nearly all CNS depressants have some capacity to suppress seizures because of their depressant activity on the brain and spinal cord. Among the benzodiazepines approved for the treatment of seizures are diazepam, **clonazepam**, and **clorazepate,** while off-label use of **lorazepam** is becoming increasingly popular (Table 23.1). Lorazepam and diazepam are available in parental formulations, making them ideal drugs for the life-threatening condition of status epilepticus. Lorazepam is the drug of choice for status epilepticus because it persists longer in the CSF than diazepam. A more recently approved drug in the US, clobazam, may be used to treat seizures associated with Lennox-Gastaut syndrome. Clobazam is also commonly used in the treatment of Dravet syndrome, although this is not an approved use.

Sedation, Amnesia, and Anesthesia

Benzodiazepines can produce a calming effect and in higher doses will produce hypnosis and/or anesthesia. **Anterograde amnesia** may occur with high doses and is nearly unavoidable when the drugs are used for anesthesia. Patients cannot recall events that took place for some time after such doses of the drugs are administered.

Benzodiazepine-induced sedation and amnesia are useful in the preparation of patients for anesthesia or surgery and for the relief of anxiety associated with other unpleasant medical and dental procedures. **Midazolam** is the benzodiazepine most frequently used for anesthesia and is commonly used for moderate sedation (formerly termed conscious sedation) and deep sedation. This is because its high degree of water solubility allows it to be formulated as an aqueous solution that is easily injected intravenously. The non-water-soluble benzodiazepines require formulation in viscous solutions that are more difficult to inject and which also cause painful irritation of the blood vessels.

Muscle Relaxation

In patients with cerebral palsy, benzodiazepines decrease spasticity and provide relief; however, it is uncertain whether they can relax voluntary muscles in doses that do not cause considerable CNS depression. Nevertheless, benzodiazepines, such as diazepam, are often prescribed for patients who have muscle spasms and pain as a result of injury. In these circumstances, the sedative and anxiolytic properties of the drug also may promote relaxation and relieve tension associated with the condition.

Alcohol and Sedative-Hypnotic Withdrawal

Withdrawal from long-term, high-dose use of alcohol or sedative-hypnotic drugs can be life-threatening if physical dependence is present. Benzodiazepines with longer half-lives, such as chlordiazepoxide and diazepam, are among the most commonly employed benzodiazepines to lessen the intensity of these withdrawal symptoms. However, lorazepam is preferred by some clinicians when treating patients with hepatic impairment. Unlike diazepam, the therapeutic action of lorazepam does not rely on the formation of active metabolites. Benzodiazepines are also employed to help relieve anxiety and other behavioral symptoms that may occur during rehabilitation.

Pharmacokinetics

Benzodiazepines are usually given orally and are well absorbed by this route. Since benzodiazepines are weak bases, they are less ionized in the relatively alkaline environment of the small intestine, and therefore, most of their absorption takes place at this site. Benzodiazepines also can be given parenterally for emergency treatment of seizures and use in anesthesia. Diazepam, midazolam, and lorazepam are available for intravenous administration, but midazolam may be preferred because it is water-soluble and thus more easily administered. The pharmacokinetic properties of the benzodiazepines available in the US are summarized in Table 23.2.

Table 23.2. Pharmacokinetic properties of benzodiazepines

Drug Name	Route(s) of Administration	Onset of Action (min)	Tmax (hr)	$T_{1/2}$ (hr) (active metabolites)	Active Metabolites	Comments
Alprazolam	Oral	15-30	1-2	12-15	Yes	Rapid oral absorption, extended-release formulation available.
Chlordiazepoxide	Oral	30-45	0.5-2	5-30 (14-100)	Yes	No longer commonly used.
Diazepam	Oral, Rectal Gel, IM, IV	 1-5	0.5-1.5	30-60	Yes	IM erratic bioavailability; most rapid absorption following oral dose; IV form can be used for status epilepticus.
Clorazepate	Oral	N/A	1-2	20-30 (50-100)	Yes	Prodrug - hydrolyzed to the active form (desmethyldiazepam) in stomach acid.
Flurazepam	Oral	<20 variable	0.5-1	0.5-3 (2-120)	Yes	Duration of effect ~ 7-10 hrs.
Lorazepam	Oral IM IV	 5 - 20	1-6	10-20	No	IV form is the benzodiazepine of choice for status epilepticus. Non-CYP hepatic elimination.
Midazolam	Oral (liquid only) IM IV	10-30 5-15 1.5-5	0.5	1-5	Yes	Oral form undergoes significant pre-systemic clearance.
Clonazepam	Oral	20-60	1.5	19-50	No	
Oxazepam	Oral	60-120	2-4	5-15	No	Intermediate-acting. Non-CYP hepatic elimination.
Temazepam	Oral	30-60	2-3	8-20	No	Slow absorption.
Triazolam	Oral	15-30	1.5-2	1.5-5.5	No	Rapid onset and short duration.
Quazepam	Oral	N/A	1.5	20 - 40 (20-120)	Yes	Rapid onset, long-acting.
Estazolam	Oral	1	2	10-24	Negligible	Intermediate-acting. No clinically important metabolites.

The distribution of benzodiazepines from blood to tissues and back again is a dynamic process with considerable influence on the onset and duration of the therapeutic effects produced by these compounds. Those having greater lipid solubility tend to enter the CNS more rapidly and thus produce their effects more quickly. Several benzodiazepines have therapeutic effects that are much shorter in duration than would be predicted based on their rates of metabolism and excretion; redistribution away from the CNS is of primary importance in terminating their therapeutic effects.

Although tissue redistribution of benzodiazepines may be an important means of terminating the actions of selected members of this class of drugs, many benzodiazepines undergo extensive biotransformation. Metabolism takes place both by dealkylation and conjugation reactions. In many instances, dealkylation can result in the formation of pharmacologically active compounds. Indeed, most clinically available benzodiazepines are converted in the liver to one or more active metabolites (Table 23.2). In several cases, the active metabolites have a much longer half-life than the parent compound. Clorazepate is the only benzodiazepine that is an inactive prodrug. Acid hydrolysis in the stomach is required to convert clorazepate to the active drug, desmethyldiazepam (nordiazepam). The water-soluble metabolites of benzodiazepines are excreted primarily in the urine.

Since most benzodiazepines undergo biotransformation, changes in liver function may alter the duration of the therapeutic effect produced by these drugs. Although few clinical studies have demonstrated serious toxicities associated with benzodiazepine administration in individuals with compromised liver function, prudence in the use of these compounds in the elderly and individuals with liver disease is advisable. Drugs such as lorazepam, **temazepam**, and **oxazepam**, which are not metabolized by cytochrome P450 (CYP450) enzymes and do not have active metabolites, may be advantageous in individuals with compromised liver function and patients taking other drugs metabolized by the CYP450 enzymes.

One of the great disadvantages associated with many of the sedative and hypnotic drugs that have now largely been replaced by benzodiazepines (e.g., barbiturates) is that those drugs are very effective inducers of hepatic drug-metabolizing enzymes. Since benzodiazepines are only weak inducers of hepatic microsomal enzymes, they cause relatively few clinically significant drug interactions related to the metabolism of other drugs.

Mechanism of Action

The benzodiazepines bind to a receptor site located on the $GABA_A$ receptor complex, a ligand-gated chloride (Cl^-) channel that consists of five protein subunits (Chapters 16-17). The binding of a benzodiazepine to its receptor enhances the increase in Cl^- conductance that is initiated by GABA binding to its own, separate receptor site. *Thus, a benzodiazepine, acting through its distinct binding site, facilitates this action of GABA to intensify the inhibition of neuronal function by allowing a greater hyperpolarization of the cells.*

Each of the five subunits of the $GABA_A$ receptor complex may be one of eight different proteins, designated α, β, γ, δ, ε, θ, π, and ρ, which may exist in different isoforms (e.g., α_1). The receptor for benzodiazepines is located at the interface between an α subunit and a γ subunit. In the CNS, the most common form of the $GABA_A$ receptor complex consists of two α_1 subunits, two β subunits, and one γ_2 subunit. The subunit composition of the $GABA_A$ receptor complex determines the effect of drugs on its function. For example, for benzodiazepines to bind to the $GABA_A$ receptor complex, an α_1, α_2, α_3, or α_5 protein must be adjacent to a γ_2 subunit. The α_1 subunit appears to confer the ability of benzodiazepines to produce sedation and hypnosis, anterograde amnesia, and anticonvulsant effects. The presence of α_2 is reported to be responsible for benzodiazepines' anxiolytic and muscle relaxant effects, whereas the α_3 subunit is believed to mediate benzodiazepines' anxiolytic, muscle relaxant, and anticonvulsant effects.

Adverse Effects and Contraindications

Most adverse effects of benzodiazepines are related to their ability to produce CNS depression. These include drowsiness, excessive sedation, impaired motor coordination, confusion, and memory loss. The effects subside after the first two weeks of continuous use, thus producing less difficulty for patients as they become tolerant. Although for most individuals these symptoms are mild, patients should be cautioned against engaging in potentially dangerous tasks that require vigilance, such as operating machinery or driving a car.

Less common adverse effects include blurred vision, hallucinations, and paradoxical reactions consisting of excitement, stimulation, and hyperactivity. Also, a variety of gastrointestinal complaints can occur, and blood dyscrasias have been reported, but these are rare. Most benzodiazepines were classified in FDA pregnancy risk category D, before the abolishment of these categories; an increased risk of congenital malformations is associated with the use of these drugs during the first trimester. Benzodiazepine administration during labor, delivery, or lactation has the potential to produce adverse effects in the infant (e.g., sedation, respiratory depression) and should be avoided.

One of the major reasons for the popularity of benzodiazepines is their relative safety in overdose. Overdoses with benzodiazepines occur commonly, but fatal toxic occurrences are rare. After an overdose, the patient begins a deep sleep that may last for 24 to 48 hours, depending on the dose. Unlike many other drugs in the sedative-hypnotics class, *fatal respiratory depression rarely occurs with benzodiazepine use in the absence of other CNS depressing drugs.* Fatal intoxications are more likely in children or individuals with pre-existing respiratory insufficiency.

Tolerance and dependence occur with chronic use of benzodiazepines. A greater risk of drug dependence has been associated with longer durations of treatment with drugs of this class. Discontinuation of drug administration, particularly abrupt withdrawal, can be associated with a variety of symptoms, including rebound insomnia and rebound anxiety. The level of insomnia or anxiety may even exceed that which preceded the treatment. To minimize withdrawal reactions, it is common to gradually taper the drug as it is discontinued. Nonetheless, in some individuals, even this method of drug removal can result in anxiety, apprehension, tension, insomnia, and loss of appetite. More severe symptoms may occur when an individual withdraws from a high dose, particularly if the drug has been taken for months or years. These symptoms can include, in addition to those already mentioned, muscle weakness, tremor, seizures, hyperalgesia, nausea, vomiting, and weight loss.

Drug Interactions

The actions of benzodiazepines are additive with those of other drugs that produce CNS depression, such as other sedative-hypnotics, opioids, alcohol, and sedating antihistamines. Such combinations may produce respiratory depression, which may be so severe as to lead to death. Because of this, it is recommended that doses of opioids be carefully adjusted (or avoided) when used in combination with benzodiazepines. Also, patients should be warned that ethanol-containing beverages may produce a more profound CNS depression when taken simultaneously with a benzodiazepine.

Oxidative metabolism by CYP3A4 is common to many benzodiazepines. Therefore, drugs that inhibit or induce this metabolic enzyme may potentially alter the metabolism of many benzodiazepines. CYP3A4 is inhibited by grapefruit juice and by drugs such as ketoconazole, itraconazole, nefazodone, erythromycin, and ritonavir. Coadministration of these substances along with a benzodiazepine may result in intensification and prolongation of the benzodiazepine effect. Conversely, rifampin, carbamazepine, and phenytoin can induce the CYP3A4 enzyme, and therefore their coadministration can reduce the therapeutic effect of the benzodiazepines.

Flunitrazepam

Although many countries around the world allow the use of **flunitrazepam** therapeutically for the treatment of insomnia, its use in the US is illegal. Flunitrazepam has earned its nickname as a "date rape drug" because it makes victims of abuse unable to protect themselves due to an altered state of consciousness caused by this benzodiazepine. Furthermore, the victim may be unable to recall the abuse as a result of the drug's potent amnestic properties. In the US, those who are found in possession of the drug are subject to prison terms per the provisions of the *Drug-Induced Rape Prevention and Punishment Act of 1996*. The street name for flunitrazepam is "roofie," derived from the original trade name, Rohypnol, and someone is said to be "roofied" when they unwittingly ingest a spiked drink. Although flunitrazepam is a schedule IV drug in the US, the DEA has considered reclassifying the drug to schedule I, and many states already consider it regulated at that level.

Benzodiazepine Antagonists

Flumazenil is an antagonist of benzodiazepine receptors that is available for parenteral administration. It can be used for the treatment of benzodiazepine overdose or the reversal of benzodiazepine-induced sedation. Flumazenil does not reverse the effects of other CNS depressants, such as opioid agonists or barbiturates. While its efficacy for reversing benzodiazepine-induced sedation is well established, its ability to reverse respiratory depression is variable. *Ventilatory support is the standard treatment for hypoventilation associated with benzodiazepine overdose.*

Flumazenil is administered intravenously and is highly irritating, so care must be taken to avoid extravasation into the tissue surrounding the injection site. It has a terminal half-life of approximately 1 hr, which is shorter than the majority of benzodiazepines. Thus, re-sedation is a serious risk, and multiple doses may need to be administered while the benzodiazepine is being eliminated from the body. Flumazenil is metabolized in the liver, and clearance can be dramatically altered by decreased hepatic blood flow or severe hepatic dysfunction. The excretion of metabolites is mostly by the kidneys.

Seizures are one of the most serious adverse effects associated with the use of flumazenil. Seizures are more common in patients who are already taking benzodiazepines to treat a seizure disorder, and in individuals who chronically use or misuse benzodiazepines, have increased intracranial pressure, or are taking other drugs which may precipitate a seizure. For this reason, *flumazenil is only recommended for overdose if the patient is known to have overdosed on a benzodiazepine and is taking no other drugs that may precipitate seizures*. Blockade of benzodiazepine receptors reduces treatment options in a patient experiencing emergent seizures. Flumazenil should be avoided in status epilepticus and other seizure disorders, and patients with increased intracranial pressure. In addition to precipitating seizures, flumazenil should also be avoided in cases of known tricyclic antidepressant overdose (Chapter 17) due to the possibility of cardiac dysrhythmias. As flumazenil is a benzodiazepine receptor antagonist, it will antagonize the effects of other drugs that exert their effects by interacting with benzodiazepine receptors, such as zolpidem and zaleplon. Less serious adverse effects of flumazenil include dizziness, vertigo, ataxia, pain at the injection site, diaphoresis, headache, visual disturbances, and nausea.

Case study

An unidentified man who appeared to be in his 60s was transferred to the emergency department after a good Samaritan found him in a confused, sedated state and called the police. Upon examination, he was found to have a dramatically decreased respiratory rate, hypotension, and decreased oxygen saturation levels. He was ataxic, his speech slurred and his pupils constricted. He was identified and his daughter was contacted. She informed the ED doctor that her father was a recovering heroin addict who had been on an opioid replacement program. A consultation with the man's psychiatrist confirmed that the patient has been taking buprenorphine for the past 3 months and was urine-screened for other drugs regularly. Urine and blood tests done in the ED confirmed buprenorphine in his system along with a benzodiazepine. The daughter also indicated that her father had suffered from long-term alcohol abuse and had experienced occasional seizures but that he had not had any alcohol or had a seizure for at least 2 years. What is the likely cause of this man's symptoms and what treatment options are available for him?

Discussion

Buprenorphine is a partial agonist at the μ-opioid receptor; this limits its respiratory depressing effects. When taken alone, as prescribed, buprenorphine is not as likely as a full or pure μ opioid agonist (morphine-like drug) to cause symptoms of overdose. Further, buprenorphine reduces the likelihood of overdose by full μ opioid agonists. However, because their effects on respiration are via different yet synergistic mechanisms, if enough buprenorphine is taken with a benzodiazepine, an overdose can occur and his symptoms are consistent with opioid overdose. If this man has cirrhosis of the liver due to his prior years of alcohol use, the metabolism of both the opioid and the benzodiazepine may be impaired, resulting in higher-than-expected blood levels of both drugs. This would further contribute to the synergistic CNS effects.

Opioid overdose, even with buprenorphine, is treated with naloxone. However, because of buprenorphine's slow rate of dissociation from opioid receptors, the patient may not respond well or quickly to the antagonist and high doses of naloxone will be necessary. If effective, naloxone will likely precipitate symptoms of opioid withdrawal. Flumazenil, the benzodiazepine receptor antagonist, presents a risk of benzodiazepine overdose because of its unpredictable effect on reversing respiratory depression and its risk of inducing seizures. It is also contraindicated for this man because he has a history of seizures. Pharmacotherapeutic interventions may also be limited by the degree of liver damage that is likely to have occurred due to a history of alcohol abuse.

Since this man is not unconscious, nor is he vomiting, the most appropriate action would be to keep him under observation and provide respiratory support if necessary. The duration of time that the patient should be observed would depend partially on which benzodiazepine he ingested.

The man is already under the care of a psychiatrist. If he wasn't, psychotherapy would be indicated and he should be screened to rule out a suicide attempt. Many buprenorphine prescribers will withhold further prescriptions of the opioid from patients who obtain drugs such as benzodiazepines without their knowledge.

Acknowledgments: The author would like to acknowledge the contribution of David J. Smith, Ph.D.to an early version of this chapter. Dr. Smith provided an earlier version of a case study used in this chapter and reviewed the materials written by the author.

References and Additional Literature

Olsen R, Sieghart W. International Union of Pharmacology LXX. Subtypes of γ-aminobutyric acid A receptors: classification on the basis of subunit composition, pharmacology, and function update. Pharmacol. Rev. 2008;60(3):243.

Passarella S, Duong M-T. Diagnosis and treatment of insomnia. Am J Health-Syst Pharm., 2008;65:927.

Ramakrishnan K, Scheid DC. Treatment options for insomnia. Am Fam Phys. 2007;76(4):517.

The Medical Letter. Drugs for Psychiatric Disorders. Treatment Guidelines from The Medical Letter. 2006;4(46):35.

US Department of Justice. Drug-Induced Rape Prevention and Punishment Act of 1996. http://www.usdoj.gov/dea/concern/flunitrazepam.htm.

Yuan R, Flockart, DA, Balian JD. Pharmacokinetic consequences of metabolism-based drug interactions with alprazolam, midazolam and triazolam. J Clin Pharmacol. 1999;39:1109.

Quiz Questions

1. A 35-year-old woman who suffers from insomnia is taking “sleeping pills” that are left over from an old prescription that her mother took in the 1960s. She comes complaining that even though she sleeps she wakes feeling tired and sluggish. Based on the label on the pills, it is determined that she is using pills that suppress REM sleep. She is given a new prescription for a drug that has a more favorable effect on REM sleep. Which drug is likely to be the newly prescribed drug?

A Midazolam
B Flurazepam
C Flumazenil
D Secobarbital
E Propofol

2. A 55-year-old man who is having coronary angiography is given midazolam to produce a state of moderate sedation. What is most likely to occur as a result of this drug?

A Anterograde amnesia
B Adjustment of doses of his other medications
C A need for assisted ventilation
D Hyperactivity
E Hallucinations

3. A 25-year-old woman who has a substance use disorder takes diazepam nearly every night “to take the edge off.” Today, she is brought to the Emergency Department in a coma and is suffering from an apparent overdose of an unknown substance. What is the major risk associated with the administration of flumazenil to treat this woman?

A Pain at the injection site
B Headache
C Visual disturbances
D Seizures
E Respiratory depression

4. A 31-year-old man with a suspected labral tear of the hip joint is to undergo an MRI for diagnostic purposes. This procedure will involve the intraarticular injection of a fluorescent dye followed by an MRI. He is prescribed oral diazepam, which is to be taken 15 minutes before the injection. He is not taking any other medicines and is otherwise healthy. Which statement applies to this situation?

A An anesthesiologist must be present
B The man should not drive home
C Diazepam should not be taken before the dye injection
D Naloxone should be readily available
E Emergency anti-seizure medicine should be readily available
F Cardiac and respiratory function should be constantly monitored

Quiz Answers

1. B is correct. Based on the date of her mother's prescription she was very likely to have been taking a barbiturate similar to secobarbital. Benzodiazepines and more recently, benzodiazepine receptor agonists are the preferred, and safer, drugs for insomnia. Flumazenil is a benzodiazepine antagonist and would not be useful as a sleep aid. Midazolam is a water-soluble benzodiazepine that is used for moderate sedation (previously termed conscious sedation) and is not indicated for insomnia. Flurazepam is the best choice of the available options. An even better choice would be zolpidem, which has the most favorable effect on the sleep cycle and REM sleep. Propofol is a general anesthetic delivered by intravenous injections and should not and cannot be used as a "sleeping pill".

2. A is correct. Anterograde amnesia of events surrounding the peri-operative procedure is common with the higher doses of benzodiazepines adequate to produce moderate sedation. Less common side effects that may occur include hallucinations and hyperactivity. An advantage of benzodiazepines in doses needed for moderate sedation is low liability for respiratory depression requiring assisted ventilation. Benzodiazepines do not induce liver enzymes, so drug dose adjustment of other medications is not likely to be a problem. On the other hand, since benzodiazepines are metabolized by CYP enzymes, alterations of the benzodiazepine dose may be required when a patient is taking a CYP inducer or inhibitor.

3. D is correct. All but respiratory depression are side effects of administering the benzodiazepine antagonist, flumazenil, and these effects may occur in patients who abuse benzodiazepines or take them therapeutically. However, the induction of seizures is a major precaution and should be carefully considered. Respiratory depression should not occur after the administration of flumazenil, nor does the drug reliably reverse benzodiazepine-induced respiratory depression.

4. B is correct. In this situation, the patient is taking diazepam as an anxiolytic before a medical procedure. Since the patient may be sedated after the procedure, he should not drive himself home. This is not moderate sedation, so an anesthesiologist is not necessary nor is continuous monitoring of respiratory and cardiac function. Naloxone is an opioid antagonist and is not useful should hypersensitivity to diazepam be experienced by the patient. Diazepam is used to treat seizures so emergency anti-seizure medicine will not be necessary.

CHAPTER 24

OPIOID ANALGESICS AND ANTAGONISTS

KENDRA E. UNGER, MD AND LEAH W. HAMMER, PHD

West Virginia University, Morgantown, West Virginia, USA

One of the most common complaints for which patients seek medical care is the experience of pain. Whether it is acute or chronic, pain has plagued humans throughout history. Primary care clinics experience many visits per day by patients seeking pain relief and medical specialties that focus solely on pain management have developed both in the ancient world and in modern times. There have been many treatment modalities, including pharmacological agents, created to alleviate pain. The analgesic properties of opiates have been known for many centuries and these drugs continue to bring pain relief today. They are potent pain relievers and, used in the appropriate context, can significantly improve quality of life.

Morphine was first isolated from the opium poppy, *Papaver somniferum*, in the early 1800s. However, cultivation of the opium poppy dates back to at least 3000 B.C. Remarkably, morphine is still considered the analgesic "gold standard" against which the efficacy of all other analgesic agents is measured. Another commercially available opioid analgesic, **codeine**, is an alkaloid that also occurs naturally in the opium poppy. In addition to the naturally-occurring opiates, there are many semisynthetic (e.g. **hydrocodone**) and synthetic (e.g. **fentanyl**) opioid analgesics available in the US and other countries. Despite their well-known analgesic efficacy, this group of drugs is also well-known for its abuse potential and as governments tighten prescribing regulations, they are no longer prescribed as widely as they once were.

The commercially available opioid drugs (and illicit opioids such as **heroin**) belong to one of 4 chemical classes. The phenanthrenes (e.g.morphine, codeine), benzomorphans (**pentazocine**), phenylpiperidines (**meperidine,** – known as **pethidine** outside of the US, and fentanyl), and diphenylheptanes (**methadone**). Most opioids (agonists and antagonists) are phenanthrene derivatives, stemming from the fact that many of the drugs used today were designed based on the structures of morphine and codeine. Structures of some of the more commonly used phenanthrene derivatives are shown in Figure 24.1. Opioid analgesics can also be classified based on the subtype of opioid receptors via which they exert their pharmacological effects. "Morphine-like" drugs refer to those that are agonists of the mu (μ) opioid receptor (MOP or MOR) while other drugs such as pentazocine, can bind to and produce at least some agonist activity at both MOR and kappa (κ) opioid receptors (KOP or KOR; see below). Others may have agonist or partial agonist activity at one type of opioid receptor and antagonist action at other subtypes. The effects mediated by these different subtypes of opioid receptors may determine the clinical use of each drug in limited clinical scenarios (e.g., KOR agonists may be safer to use during childbirth than a pure MOR agonist), however, of more use to the clinician who is treating pain, is the classification based on the duration of action or potency of the drug (see Clinical Use). A third subtype of the opioid receptor is the delta (δ) opioid receptor (DOP or DOR). Although some commercially available opioid analgesics have affinity for the delta opioid receptor, they are not currently a target for pharmacotherapy.

Antagonists of opioid receptors have also been developed. **Naloxone** and **naltrexone** are antagonists of all subtypes of opioid receptors. Naloxone is used primarily for opioid analgesic overdose. The antagonists are also combined with some agonists to deter tampering (e.g., dissolving an oral tablet for injection) and this is an intense field of drug development at present. This topic is discussed in more detail in Anti-Diversion Forms of Opioids at the end of the chapter.

Endogenous Opioid Peptides

The endogenous ligands for opioid receptors are peptides that are often referred to as "*endorphins,*" although endorphins are only one of several families of endogenous opioids. Each family is derived from a large precursor molecule; opiomelanocortin (POMC), preproenkephalin, and preprodynorphin. POMC gives rise to β-lipotropin which is further cleaved to give rise to β-endorphin. Non-peptide sequences contained within POMC include adrenocorticotropic hormone (ACTH) and melanocyte-stimulating hormone. Preproenkaphalin (proenkaphalin A) gives rise to two endogenous opioid peptides, methionine-enkephalin (met-enkephalin) and leucine-enkephalin (leu-enkephalin). Preprodynorphin (also known as proenkephalin B) undergoes cleavage to yield dynorphin A, dynorphin B, and neoendorphins. All three families have affinity for all three opioid receptor subtypes, although endorphins, dynorphins, and enkephalins have the greatest affinity for MOR, KOR, and DOR, respectively. Distribution and function of endogenous opioids vary throughout the central nervous system (CNS) and while the analgesic activities of endorphins (via MOR) and enkephalins (via DOR) are well established, the physiologic function of dynorphins has not been fully elucidated. Opioid receptors are also present in peripheral tissues. Their physiological role has not been established, however, peripheral receptors mediate some of the adverse effects associated with exogenous opioid agonists (see Adverse Effects). Endogenous opioids are also secreted by various endocrine organs, e.g. pituitary, and can be detected circulating in blood under certain conditions.

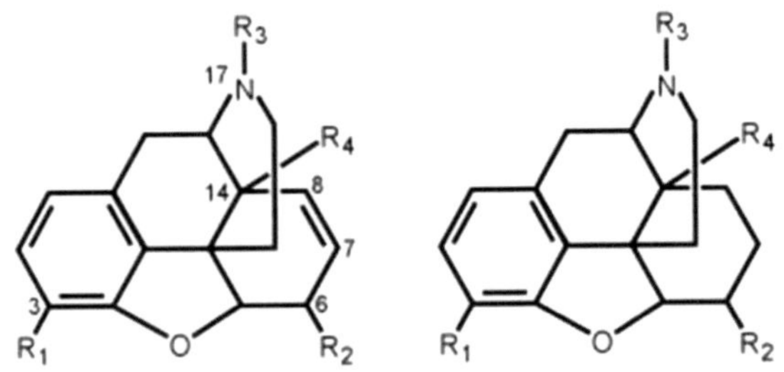

"A" template "B" template

Drug	Template	R1	R2	R3	R4
Mu Agonists					
Morpine	A	—OH	—OH	—CH_3	—H
Codeine	A	—CH_3	—OH	—CH_3	—H
Heroin	A	—$OCOCH_3$	—$OCOCH_3$	—CH_3	—H
Hydrocodone	A	—OCH_3	=O	—CH_3	—H
Oxycodone	B	—OCH_3	=O	—CH_3	—OH
Hydromorphine	B	—OH	=O	—CH_3	—H
Oxymorphine	B	—OH	=O	—CH_3	—OH
Mixed Agonists / Antagonists					
Nalbuphine	B	—OH	—OH	—CH_2—◁	—OH
Buprenorphine	B	—OH	—OCH_3	—CH_2—◁	—OH
Antagonists					
Naloxone	B	—OH	=O	—CH_3CH_2=CH_3	—OH
Naltrexone	B	—OH	=O	—CH_2—◇	—OH

Figure 24.1. Chemical structures of commonly used phenanthrene opioids

Pathophysiology of Pain (see also Chapters 9 and 14)

A thorough description of the pathophysiology of pain is beyond the scope of this textbook. However, since this pathophysiology is integral to understanding the mechanism of action of opioid analgesics, we present a simplistic summary here and in Figure 24.2. Pain is detected by specialized nerves called primary afferent sensory nerves, or nociceptors. Action potentials initiated by painful stimuli are relayed by the primary afferent nerves to the brain via secondary afferent nerves whose cell bodies are located in the spinal cord or trigeminal nucleus (stimuli originating in the facial region). These secondary afferent nerves send the signal to integration centers (e.g. thalamus) higher in the brain. These signals are then processed and appropriate responses are elicited. Opioid receptors are located at all levels of these pain pathways.

The primary afferent nerves enter the spinal cord at the level of the dorsal horn and are part of the dorsal root. Transmission of the signal between primary and secondary afferent nerves is of great significance to the experience of pain. This synapse between the primary and secondary nerves receives input from other nerves including local intraspinal nerves (interneurons) and those that comprise the inhibitory descending pathways (see below). Substances released from these other nerves can be excitatory or inhibitory and help determine the strength of the signal transmitted to the brain. Large populations of opioid receptors are found in the dorsal horn, both presynaptically and postsynaptically, and are a major target for opioid analgesics. The presence of these receptors in the spinal cord allows for the intraspinal administration of opioid drugs for certain surgical procedures.

Descending inhibition

Modulatory nerve pathways descend from the cortex to the periaqueductal gray (PAG) where neurons containing GABA project to the medulla. GABA is released onto nerves that project from the medulla to the dorsal horn of the spinal cord. These latter nerves are usually quiescent due to the tonic activity of the GABA-ergic nerves arising from the PAG. When the opioids (endogenous or exogenous) bind to MORs on the terminals of the GABA-ergic nerves, GABA release is inhibited and the nerves projecting from the medulla to the dorsal horn are activated. The neurotransmitters released at the level of the dorsal horn are serotonin and norepinephrine (a.k.a. noradrenaline). Here, these two neurotransmitters inhibit pain signals traveling from primary afferent nerves (Figure 24.2).

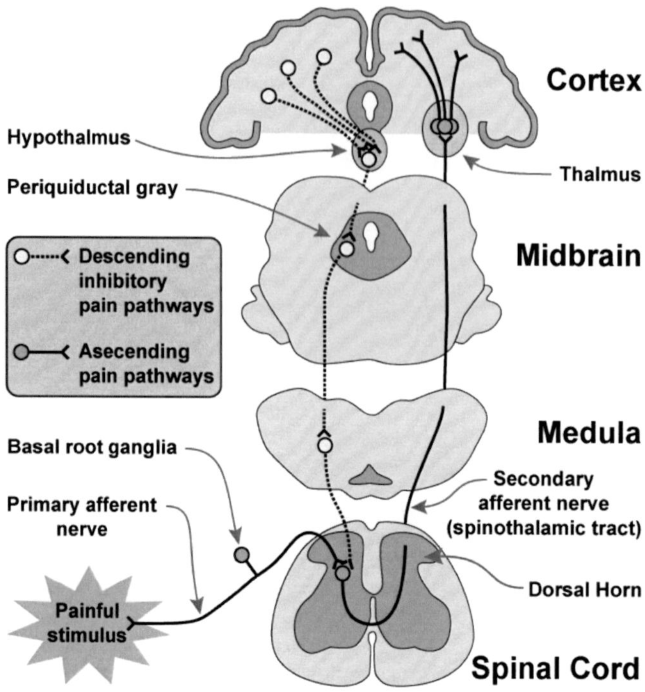

Figure 24.2. Simplistic representation of neuronal pain pathways. Pain signals travel from the periphery via the primary afferent nerve and then ascend to the brain via the ascending pathways (solid lines). In response to pain, descending inhibitory pathways (dashed lines) reduce signaling in the ascending pathways.

Clinical Use and Therapeutic Applications

A. Analgesia

In the clinical setting, a detailed evaluation of pain is very important for the development of an appropriate treatment plan. Evaluation of pain can be frustrating for a practitioner because most pain is subjective and is reported by the patient. A detailed history including the location, chronicity, quality, and severity of the pain is very important. Physical examination findings, such as elevated blood pressure or facial grimace with palpation of the affected area, can help objectify pain. Once the history and physical examination results have been obtained, the pain can be classified on a pain scale (see Table 24.1 for the commonly used Numeric Rating Scale 11). This will help the practitioner plan treatment that is most appropriate for the character and severity of the pain. If the patient is a child or has difficulty rating his or her pain, a visual scale, such as the Wong-Baker Faces Rating Scale (see wongbakerfaces.org), can be used to categorize the pain.

The World Health Organization has developed a pain relief ladder, based on the pain scale, to act as a guideline for treating pain (see (Anekar et al. 2023) for more details; last viewed on 7-27-2023). The first rung of the ladder is for mild pain and involves the use of non-opioid and adjunctive analgesics such as acetaminophen (a.k.a. paracetamol), non-steroidal anti-inflammatory drugs (NSAIDs) or aspirin (see Chapters 9 and 14). Subsequent rungs see the addition of opioids ranging from weak opioids to the strongest opioids, along with non-opioids and adjuvant drugs as the level of pain increases. Although this approach is effective for the treatment of simple pain conditions, it isn't appropriate for all painful conditions. Non-pharmacologic approaches to pain (e.g., physical therapy), and non-opioid analgesics are now considered more appropriate approaches for early interventions, with opioids reserved for the most painful of cases. In addition, neuropathic pain requires a different approach, usually with the use of non-analgesic medicines. Minimally invasive interventions can also be used in many instances instead of, or before moving on to, systemic opioids. Lastly, mental health professionals can play an important role in the treatment of chronic pain. Depression and anxiety commonly accompany chronic pain. Treating these conditions can often help reduce the perception of pain and thus reduce the overall need for analgesic medicines.

Table 24.1: Numeric Rating Scale 11 is commonly used in medical practice to determine the degree to which a patient is experiencing pain.

Rating	Pain level
0	No pain
1-3	Mild pain (annoying pain, can be ignored)
4-6	Moderate pain (difficult to ignore, interferes with ADLs)
7-10	Severe pain (disabling)

ADL= activities of daily living

a. Opioids for Acute Pain (see also Chapter 14)

Acute pain is typically defined as pain lasting for less than 3 months, or pain that does not extend beyond the expected time of healing for a particular illness or injury. The onset of acute pain is often swift and can be severe. Some examples of acute pain include pain associated with trauma, or medical illness such as appendicitis or pancreatitis, dental pain, and post-surgical pain. Healthcare providers should keep in mind that patients with chronic pain can also develop acute pain which may require treatment in addition to chronic pain treatment.

Treatment of acute pain is based on clinical evaluation of the patient. Mild pain can be treated conservatively with non-opioid and adjunct medications. Pain that is associated with inflammation is best treated with anti-inflammatory drugs alone (see Chapters 9 and 14), or in combination with an opioid, since opioid analgesics are devoid of anti-inflammatory action (see also Chapter 14). For moderate to severe pain, opioids play a major role. Because acute pain is usually short-lived, fast-acting opioids with a half-life of 1-4 hours are the drugs of choice. For mild to moderate, or episodic pain, lower-potency opioids such as codeine, hydrocodone, and **oxycodone**, can be used. Another option is **tramadol**, a weak MOR agonist that additionally inhibits the reuptake of serotonin and norepinephrine. These drugs can be dosed as needed rather than continuously. For severe acute pain, higher-potency opioids such as hydromorphone, **oxymorphone**, or fentanyl, can be used. These can be used as needed or can be taken on a regular 24-hr schedule if the patient is experiencing constant pain. Most opioids used for acute pain are available as oral formulations. Parenteral dosage forms are available for those who are unable to take medicine orally or for those patients experiencing intense severe pain requiring rapid treatment.

b. Opioids for Chronic Pain (see also Chapter 14)

Chronic pain is defined as pain lasting more than 3 months or pain that extends beyond the expected time of healing. The onset of chronic pain is gradual and can be a result of acute pain that has become chronic or can stem from an illness. Chronic pain is often described as dull and aching, but can occasionally be burning or shooting in nature. Conditions associated with chronic pain include chronic low back pain, pain due to malignancy, and arthritic joint pain. Most chronic pain is mild to moderate but it can be severe in some instances. Patients who experience chronic pain may also experience flare-ups of their underlying condition, which can exacerbate pain.

Treatment of chronic pain can be difficult at times and **non-opioid treatment should always be considered the first choice**. One must take into account the quality and severity of pain, as well as the effect that chronic pain has on the patient, to devise an appropriate treatment plan. Mild chronic pain can often be treated conservatively with physical therapy, non-opioid analgesics, and adjunct medications. Moderate chronic pain may require the addition of an opioid to control the pain and to improve the patient's quality of life. Short-acting pain medications used for acute pain (see above) can be used for episodic pain. These medications are usually given at 4, 6, or 8-hour intervals, depending on the severity and duration of pain. In general, if a patient is taking a fast-acting opioid every 4 to 6 hours regularly (120-180 tabs per month), is reporting pain that is still moderate to severe, and is experiencing functional deficits, this patient could be considered for a long-acting opioid such as extended-release morphine or oxycodone. For severe chronic pain, short-acting opioids can be used for breakthrough pain. However long-acting opioids (or extended-release formulations) are often needed to provide relief and increase the quality of life. These include the previously mentioned preparations, as well as extended-release hydromorphone and methadone. Most are given orally, however, a fentanyl patch replaced every 72 hours can also be very effective. All chronic pain patients require close monitoring to assess for pain and the safety of opioid use. The use of a pain contract between a patient and prescribing physician is common in chronic pain management. Suggestions for the safe administration of opioids to patients with chronic pain can be found at the end of the chapter.

End-of-life care is a special area that may necessitate the use of opioids. Patients who are in the active dying process deserve evaluation and adequate pain control. **Addiction should not be a concern when treating a dying patient.** Providers should not hesitate to treat this population with opioids.

B. Opioid Use Disorder

Opioid analgesics play an important role in the treatment of opioid use disorder. Patients who misuse opioid analgesics are seeking euphoria, an effect associated with the use of these drugs. Pure MOR agonists that have a rapid onset of action and a relatively short duration of action are most often associated with this well-known effect. Such use of opioid agonists can lead to deterioration of lifestyle and an increased risk of overdose. Opioid drugs with a slow onset and long duration of action, such as methadone and **buprenorphine**, are used to manage patients diagnosed with opioid use disorder.

C. Inappropriate Use Deterrence and Overdose

To reduce the risk of opioid misuse, many opioid agonists are now formulated with an opioid receptor antagonist. Such formulations are described in more detail at the end of this chapter.

Naloxone is the drug of choice to reverse respiratory depression due to opioid agonist overdose. It is administered intravenously and causes a rapid reversal of the opioid agonist resulting in improved respiration. Naloxone is described in more detail below.

D. Cough

Codeine is commonly used as an antitussive in the United States and other countries. Structural analogs of opioid analgesics have been developed as antitussives with lower abuse liability. **Dextromethorphan** is available in over-the-counter cough medicines in many parts of the world and is chemically related to opiates. Its mechanism of antitussive action is not clear (see Chapter 6). Interestingly, dextromethorphan is currently being investigated for use in pain management, and this effect is thought to be mediated via antagonism of the N-methyl-D-aspartate (NMDA) glutamate receptor. **Dihydrocodeine** is another opioid analgesic that is formulated in cough medicines. Its use is not common in the US but, like codeine, it is available without a prescription in numerous countries around the world.

E. Diarrhea

Constipation is a well-known and common adverse effect associated with opioid analgesics (see Chapters 21). Opioid receptors in the gastrointestinal tract mediate this unwanted effect. **Loperamide** is an over-the-counter opioid agonist that does not readily cross the blood brain barrier. It is used to treat diarrhea. Diphenoxylate is another opioid agonist used to treat diarrhea (see Chapters 21). It can get into the brain and is formulated with atropine to prevent misuse. It is only available via prescription.

Mu Opioid Receptor Agonists

Mu opioid receptor (MOR) agonists, also known as pure opioid agonists or morphine-like drugs, are a mainstay of pain management. All drugs in this class have the same mechanism of action and can result in the same adverse effects. Differences in pharmacokinetics and drug formulation often determine the drug choice.

Pharmacokinetics

Most MOR agonists are readily absorbed from the gastrointestinal tract, but several undergo clinically significant first-pass metabolism. Drugs such as morphine and meperidine can be administered orally, but doses are typically higher than those required by parenteral routes. Fentanyl is a substrate for intestinal CYP3A4 and P-glycoprotein, thus, oral administration does not typically yield high enough plasma concentrations to be beneficial. It is administered via parenteral routes (e.g IV, transdermal) and is also available in a variety of formulations for buccal administration (e.g. lozenge), a nasal spray, and a sublingual tablet and spray. Fentanyl distributes rapidly into tissues (especially fat) and thus remains longer in the body than its duration of action would indicate. However, it is rapidly metabolized in the liver to inactive metabolites. Accumulation is only likely to occur with hepatic dysfunction. Unlike fentanyl and its other derivatives which undergo metabolism by CYP3A4, **remifentanil** is metabolized by non-specific esterases in the blood and is thus even more rapidly eliminated.

MOR agonists with free hydroxyl groups can be directly conjugated. Morphine has a free hydroxyl group at two positions (3 and 6 - see Figure 24.1) and is conjugated, mostly with glucuronic acid, to form the metabolite morphine-3-glucuronide (M3G), and to a lesser extent, the metabolite morphine-6-glucuronide (M6G). M3G does not penetrate the CNS and has no analgesic activity whereas M6G can slowly penetrate the CNS and does have analgesic efficacy. If allowed to accumulate, M3G may cause seizures and M6G may contribute to respiratory depression.

Codeine is a prodrug that is readily absorbed when administered orally but has a low affinity for the opioid receptor in its parent form. Its action is increased by methylation at the 3-position by hepatic CYP2D6 to form morphine. Patients who exhibit the poor metabolizer phenotype for CYP2D6 will be unlikely to experience pain relief from codeine. Oxycodone and hydrocodone are also substrates for CYP2D6, although this enzyme most likely inactivates these compounds. Poor metabolizers would be expected to experience greater levels of analgesia and have an increased risk of adverse reactions when taking these drugs.

Meperidine is metabolized to the active metabolite normeperidine (a.k.a. norpethidine). This metabolite is also neurotoxic and this has resulted in a decline in meperidine use. Accumulation of the metabolite may result in seizures.

Table 24.2 Pharmacokinetic data for select opioids

Drug	Receptor Subtype			^Equianalgesic Equivalencies Parenteral/Oral (mg)	Duration of Therapeutic Effect (hr)	Metabolism[#]	Comment
	MOR	KOR	DOR				
MOR Agonists							
Morphine	+++			10/30	4 - 6	Hepatic; conjugation	Active metabolite; Pgp Substrate; ER available
Codeine	+			130*/200	2.5 - 3	Hepatic conjugation; CYP3A4	Prodrug – CYP2D6 conversion to active metabolite (morphine)
Fentanyl	+++			0.1/NA	0.5	Hepatic; CYP3A4	Pgp substrate; formulations incl. SL, TD, buccal, parenteral
Hydrocodone	+++			NA/30-45	4-6	Hepatic; CYP3A4 & 2D6	ER available
Hydromorphone	+++			1.5-3/7.5	4-5	Hepatic; conjugation	
Meperidine (pethidine)	++	+	+	75-100/300	3-5	Hepatic; hydrolysis, conjugation, CYP450	Active, neurotoxic metabolite; anticholinergic effects
Methadone	+++	+	+	Variable	4-6	Hepatic; CYP3A4	Long half-life; may inhibit reuptake of serotonin
Oxymorphone	+++			1/10	3-4	Hepatic; conjugation, reduction	ER available;
Oxycodone	+++			8-11*/15-20	3-4	Hepatic; CYP3A4, CYP2D6	ER available; rectal and parenteral formulations available outside the US
Mixed Agonists/Antagonists							
Buprenorphine	P	-	+	0.4/NA	4-8	Hepatic; CYP3A4	Active metabolite; SL, TD, buccal, parenteral formulations available; used for treatment of opioid dependence
Butorphanol	P/-	++		2/NA	3-4	Hepatic	Available as nasal spray
Nalbuphine	-	+++		10/NA	3-6	Hepatic	
Pentazocine	P/-	++		10/150	3+	Hepatic	Oral formulation is only available with naloxone in the US, dysphoria limits use

ER=extended release formulation; SL=sublingual; TD=transdermal; *Not available in the US; #Major pathway; Pgp=p-glycoprotein; NA=not available; + indicates the degree of agonism at receptor subtype; P=partial agonist at receptor subtype; P/- = weak antagonist or partial agonist; - = antagonist at receptor subtype; ^Information not intended for switching from one opioid to another. Cross-tolerance between opioids is variable and often incomplete, and the hepatic and renal status of patients may vary considerably. Opioid switching should be done by experienced clinicians using current clinical guidelines. Reduction of an equianalgesic dose is often necessary when switching from one opioid to another.

Mechanism of Action

All pure opioid agonists bind to MORs to produce analgesia. They reduce pain signaling from the periphery to the brain and they enhance the activity of the descending inhibitory pathways described above. The binding of a MOR agonist to presynaptic receptors on primary afferent neurons results in the closure of voltage-gated Ca^{2+} channels. This subsequently results in the inhibition of neurotransmitter release (glutamate and neuropeptides such as substance P) in the dorsal horn of the spinal cord. The binding of agonists to postsynaptic MORs mediates hyperpolarization of nerve cells. Both of these mechanisms serve to reduce ascending pain signals to the brain (see Figure 24.2).

The descending inhibitory pathways are usually rendered quiescent by GABA-ergic nerves within the brainstem. When a MOR agonist binds to its presynaptic receptor on these GABA-ergic nerves, it inhibits the release of GABA. Thus, activation of the presynaptic MORs removes the inhibitory influence on the descending inhibitory nerves, leading to the release of serotonin and norepinephrine in the dorsal horn of the spinal cord. These neurotransmitters have an inhibitory effect at this level of the CNS and reduce transmission of the pain signal from the periphery to the CNS. *Opioid analgesics thus indirectly activate descending inhibitory pain pathways.*

During inflammation, peripheral opioid receptors on the sensory nerve endings of the primary afferent nerves are thought to be upregulated. Thus, opioid analgesics may also produce a local effect in the periphery. Although this action of opioid analgesics is not as well understood as their central actions, evidence continues to accumulate in support of the involvement of endogenous opioids in inflammation. In addition to sensory nerve endings, opioid receptors have been identified on various immune cells including lymphocytes, monocytes, macrophages, and granulocytes, and in tissues of the skin.

Adverse Effects and Contraindications

The adverse effects caused by MOR agonists are typically extensions of their well-characterized pharmacological effects. As with their analgesic effects, tolerance develops to most of these unwanted effects, except for miosis and constipation.

Respiratory depression can occur with all opioid analgesics and is usually the cause of death in opioid overdose. This effect is amplified in patients who concurrently take other CNS depressing drugs, especially sedative-hypnotics, and is thought to be due to a depressed response of the medullary respiratory center to CO_2.

Constipation is a well-known adverse effect of opioids and is often responsible for non-adherence to opioid drug regimens. A high density of opioid receptors is present in the gastrointestinal tract and is largely responsible for this effect. Opioids can decrease gastric motility while increasing tone. Peripherally-acting opioid antagonists are being used to treat this adverse effect in those taking opioids chronically (see below).

Opioid-induced hyperalgesia (OIH): Opioid use has been associated with a paradoxical increase in pain sensation in some patients, especially in those who take them chronically; although the condition has also been observed in the acute setting. While OIH was first documented in 1870, the mechanism underlying this adverse effect is not well understood. Currently, no treatment guidelines have been established for this condition and management may include cessation of opioid therapy, rotation to a different class of opioid, or use of NMDA antagonists. The latter treatment suggests a role for glutamate in the etiology of OIH and there is some support for this in the literature.

Euphoria is a feeling of pleasure that is sought by people who take opioid analgesics and heroin outside of the medical setting. This effect is mediated by MORs. In some cases, opioid analgesics produce an unpleasant experience, termed *dysphoria*. Dysphoria is thought to be mediated by KORs.

Sedation is produced to some degree by all opioid analgesics. Patients who are particularly susceptible to this effect should be cautioned not to drive or operate heavy machinery. High oral doses or parenteral administration may result in deep sedation such that the patient may lose the ability to protect the airways.

Miosis or *pinpoint pupils* is a classic symptom of opioid use as tolerance rarely develops to this effect. Opioid-induced miosis can be blocked by opioid receptor antagonists, and by the muscarinic receptor antagonist atropine.

Rigidity of muscles, especially those of the chest wall, can occur with any opioid analgesic but is most likely to occur with intravenous use of fentanyl and its congeners. Rigidity is sensitive to naloxone, however, if preservation of analgesia is desirable, neuromuscular blocking agents may be used to treat the rigidity and care must be taken to maintain the airway.

Nausea and vomiting (see Chapter 8), common to all opioid agonists, are thought to be due to direct stimulation of the chemoreceptor trigger zone. Although older antiemetic drugs can be used to counter this effect, the newer $5HT_3$ receptor antagonists are the drugs of choice today. Nausea and vomiting are significantly more prevalent in ambulatory patients, suggesting a strong vestibular component.

Itching: Some opioids can cause peripheral vasodilation of vessels in the skin which may be accompanied by itching, urticaria, and sweating. Histamine plays a role in this effect and some opioids have a greater propensity to release histamine than others. Antihistamines may help reduce this type of itching, although their effect is somewhat variable. Intense itching can limit the use of these drugs when administered via parenteral routes. The mechanism for this intense itching may involve pruritoceptive neural circuits and for some patients, is unbearable. Histamine is thought not to be involved in centrally-mediated pruritus. Interestingly, there is sound evidence in the medical literature supporting the use of the KOR agonist/MOR antagonist, nalbuphine, for treating opioid-induced itching. A review of the literature published in 2016 concluded that low-dose nalbuphine is superior to other drugs for treating this unwanted effect.

Cardiovascular Effects: Even at the high doses used in anesthesia, the cardiovascular effects of opioid analgesics are limited. Nearly all can cause bradycardia (except meperidine, presumably due to its anticholinergic properties) and may worsen hypotension in conditions where the circulatory system is already stressed (e.g. volume depletion). Pentazocine is an exception and increases blood pressure and heart rate.

Drug Interactions

Any drug that depresses the central nervous system can interact physiologically with opioid analgesics to depress respiration.

CYP interactions may occur when opioids are administered in the presence of inducers or inhibitors of these enzymes. Codeine is metabolized to its active form by CYP2D6 and inhibitors of this isoenzyme, such as paroxetine, would be expected to result in the reduction or absence of analgesia to this opiate. Several opioids (e.g. fentanyl and methadone) are metabolized to inactive metabolites by CYP3A4 and inhibitors of this isoform may result in higher-than-expected plasma levels of these opioids.

Some opioid drugs are thought to inhibit serotonin reuptake and may increase the risk of serotonin syndrome when administered with other serotonergic drugs. MOR opioid agonists associated with this risk include fentanyl, methadone, and meperidine.

Opioid Drugs with Mixed Agonist/Antagonist Activity

Efforts to develop drugs with strong analgesic properties but reduced abuse liability and fewer adverse effects (especially respiratory depression) resulted in the development of a mixed group of drugs with varying degrees of MOR and KOR agonist and antagonist activities. Despite these efforts, these drugs have all been associated with respiratory depression and abuse potential so, while finding some niches in medicine (see below), have not replaced MOR agonists in the management of pain.

Clinical Uses and Therapeutic Effects

Buprenorphine is a phenanthrene derivative that is a potent analgesic. It has a long duration of action due to its slow dissociation from the MOR. It is a partial MOR agonist and a KOR antagonist. It is mostly used in the management of opioid dependence and, in theory, is easier for patients in remote areas to access than methadone because it can be dispensed from pharmacies. In the US, up until recently, prescribers were required to obtain a special license to prescribe buprenorphine for addiction. Recently, this requirement was removed in order for patients with opioid use disorder to have increased access to this medicine. It is also indicated for pain management but is used less frequently for this purpose. Buprenorphine is a Schedule III substance in the US.

Nalbuphine is also a phenanthrene derivative but is a strong KOR agonist and a MOR antagonist. In the US, its major use is for pain during labor and delivery. Because of its antagonist activity at MOR opioid receptors, nalbuphine is thought to have less of an effect on respiration and is thus a safer option for mother and baby. Its use is not limited to labor pain, however, and it is indicated to treat pain from other sources. In addition, it is used to antagonize severe itching produced by parenterally administered MOR agonists in the hospital setting. Nalbuphine is the only opioid analgesic that is not a controlled substance in the US.

Pentazocine and butorphanol are used less frequently. Both are KOR agonists and have partial agonist or antagonist effects at the MOR opioid receptor. Pentazocine is available for oral administration only in combination with acetaminophen, aspirin, or naloxone. Its most common use is as part of a general anesthetic regimen, where it is administered intravenously. Similarly, butorphanol is also used in general anesthesia for induction, maintenance, and preoperatively for sedation and analgesia. It has an additional indication for migraine and is available as a nasal spray for these patients. Clinical use of KOR agonists is limited by their propensity to cause dysphoria and psychomimetic effects.

Pharmacokinetics

Buprenorphine is administered via several routes that avoid first-pass metabolism (e.g sublingual, transdermal, buccal, parenteral). Buprenorphine is metabolized, mostly by CYP3A4, to the active metabolite norbuprenorphine. Norbuprenorphine does not readily penetrate the blood-brain barrier and thus exerts its effects in the periphery. Conversion to norbuprenorphine is not necessary for the drug's analgesic effect and in fact, decreases the bioavailability of the centrally-acting parent compound. Buprenorphine and norbuprenorphine undergo glucuronidation to less active metabolites. Fecal excretion appears to be the major route of elimination of the conjugated metabolites of buprenorphine and norbuprenorphine, although these metabolites are found in the urine in smaller quantities Hepatic metabolism is impaired to a clinically significant degree in patients with severe hepatic disease.

Nalbuphine also undergoes significant first-pass metabolism in both the liver and the gut. It is administered IV, IM, or SC. Metabolites are excreted in the urine, bile, and feces. The half-life of nalbuphine is around 3-6 hrs in healthy subjects but is reduced in women in active labor (approximately 2-4 hrs).

Pentazocine and butorphanol are both metabolized in the liver and metabolites are mostly excreted in the urine. The duration of analgesia is slightly longer for butorphanol and is dependent upon the route of administration. Analgesia may last up to 5 hours following intranasal administration of butorphanol.

Mechanism of Action

Buprenorphine is a partial agonist of MORs and an antagonist of KORs. Analgesia is mediated by its action at MORs.

Nalbuphine, pentazocine, and butorphanol are all agonists at KORs and this activity is thought to mediate their analgesic actions. Nalbuphine is an antagonist at MORs while pentazocine and butorphanol exhibit weak antagonism and are likely partial agonists of the MOR. The analgesic response mediated by KORs is thought to be via mechanisms similar to those described for pure MOR agonists.

Adverse Effects and Contraindications

All drugs in this mixed activity class of opioid analgesics can cause adverse effects similar to those listed for the pure MOR agonists. Respiratory depression occurs with nalbuphine, but unlike the pure MOR agonists, it appears to have a ceiling effect. Buprenorphine is a partial MOR agonist and also has a lower potential to cause respiratory depression.

Additional adverse effects associated with buprenorphine include neurologic and psychiatric effects. The incidence of these effects appears to be relatively small and affected by dosage form. Nalbuphine, pentazocine, and butorphanol are also associated with psychomimetic effects such as delusions, hallucinations, and depersonalization, although these effects may be less likely with nalbuphine. They are thought to be mediated by KOR as they are significantly less frequent for pure MOR agonists. Sedation produced by KOR agonists has also been reported to be qualitatively different from that reported for MOR agonists, being more severe for KOR agonists.

Unlike other opioid analgesics, pentazocine can increase blood pressure and heart rate.

Misuse of mixed agonists/antagonists occurs. Buprenorphine and pentazocine are both available in formulations that include the opioid antagonist, naloxone which aims to deter people from injecting oral or sublingual formulations. Buprenorphine is absorbed sublingually but the naloxone in these formulations is not. When administered orally, naloxone is not biologically active. However, when administered parenterally, it blocks opioid receptors and antagonizes the euphoric (and other) effects of the drug.

Drug Interactions

Drugs with partial MOR agonist or MOR antagonist activity should not be administered to patients who are currently using pure MOR agonists (either for medical reasons or illicitly) due to the risk of precipitating acute withdrawal.

Use with other CNS depressing drugs including sedative-hypnotics, may result in additive CNS depressive effects, including respiratory depression. Dose reduction may be necessary for such patients. When bound to MORs, buprenorphine prevents other opioid agonists from binding, thus protecting against fatal respiratory depression. However, it is important for clinicians to remember that *non-opioid drugs (especially benzodiazepines) that depress the CNS may still have a physiological synergistic effect on respiration in the presence of buprenorphine.* Patients with opioid use disorder who are co-prescribed buprenorphine and a benzodiazepine should be closely monitored. Interestingly, the respiratory depressant effects of buprenorphine are thought to be due to its metabolite, norbuprenorphine which doesn't readily enter the CNS. Animal studies have shown that norbuprenorphine is a substrate for the p-glycoprotein efflux transporter on cells of the blood-brain barrier and that blockade of the transporter enhances the respiratory depressant effect of buprenorphine. This interaction has not been reported in humans.

Attempts to administer naloxone (an opioid antagonist, see below) to rescue a patient from an overdose of buprenorphine may be limited due to the slow dissociation of buprenorphine from the MOR receptor.

Pentazocine, like some of the pure MOR agonists, and tramadol (see below) may increase serotonin levels. Use with other serotonergic drugs may, therefore, precipitate serotonin syndrome.

Tramadol and Tapentadol

Tramadol and **tapentadol** are opioid analgesics that have additional mechanisms of action. Tramadol is a synthetic analog of codeine but has a weaker affinity for the MOR receptor. It has been widely available in Europe since the 1970s but was only approved for use in the US in 1995. When first approved in the US, it was a non-controlled substance. However, as discussed below, tramadol has higher abuse potential and a greater risk of respiratory depression than originally predicted. As a result, the FDA moved it into schedule IV of the Controlled Substances Act in July 2014. The UK made a similar move that same year, with the drug moving to Schedule 3. Although it requires a prescription in most countries, regulation varies widely.

Tapentadol has a similar mechanism of action to tramadol but, due to greater affinity for opioid receptors and thus higher abuse liability, scheduling is more uniform throughout the world. In the US, it is on Schedule II.

Clinical Uses and Therapeutic Effects

Both tramadol and tapentadol are approved for use in moderate to severe pain. Tapentadol has an additional indication for neuropathic pain in the US. Tramadol has a variety of off-label uses including post-anesthesia shivering, diabetic neuropathy, and restless leg syndrome.

Pharmacokinetics

Pharmacokinetic properties of tramadol and tapentadol are summarized in Table 24.2. In the US, tramadol is only available for oral administration. However, rectal and parenteral formulations are available elsewhere in the world. Tramadol is subject to significant first-pass metabolism in the liver where it is metabolized by either CYP3A4, CYP2D6, or CYP2B6. Several metabolites result, but only one, M1, is significantly active and contributes to its analgesic activity. M1 is formed by CYP2D6-mediated O-demethylation of the (-) enantiomer. M1 activity may, therefore, be affected by CYP2D6 polymorphism and by inhibitors or inducers of this isoenzyme. The excretion of tramadol and its metabolites is mostly renal and both liver and kidney dysfunction may require dosage adjustments.

Tapentadol is eliminated mostly via phase II metabolism. Approximately 70% of the parent compound is conjugated with glucuronic acid. Minor metabolic pathways include CYP2C9, CYP2C19, and CYP2D6. The excretion of metabolites is via the kidney.

Mechanism of Action

Tramadol is a weak MOR opioid agonist with norepinephrine and serotonin reuptake-blocking activity. The analgesic effect is thought to be mediated mostly by the inhibition of serotonin reuptake. Tapentadol has greater efficacy for the MOR opioid receptor and inhibits norepinephrine reuptake.

Adverse Effects and Contraindications

Tramadol and tapentadol have been associated with respiratory depression. The risk seems to be lower for tramadol, likely due to its lower efficacy for MORs. Both drugs may lower seizure threshold and should be used with caution, if at all, in patients with seizure disorders. Serotonin syndrome can also be precipitated, especially with tramadol. Coadministration of tramadol with drugs that enhance serotonin levels is therefore cautioned.

Drug Interactions

Concurrent administration of tramadol and tapentadol with monoamine oxidase (MAO) inhibitors, including MAO-B inhibitors such as rasagiline and selegiline, should be avoided. Interactions can result in increased levels of serotonin and norepinephrine leading to an increased risk of serotonin syndrome and cardiovascular complications such as hypertension. A 14-day washout period is recommended for MAO-A inhibitors, such as the antidepressant phenelzine, before administering either drug.

Inhibition of the metabolism of tramadol by CYP3A4 inhibitors is expected to increase plasma concentrations of the parent compound. Inhibition of CYP2D6 inhibits metabolism to the active metabolite MI, thus decreasing levels of this metabolite while increasing the plasma levels of the parent compound. These effects are likely to enhance adverse effects associated with the parent compound, including serotonin syndrome.

As with all opioid agonists, concurrent use with other drugs that depress the CNS, including alcohol, is discouraged. Coadministration of these opioids with other CNS depressants increases the risk of respiratory depression.

Opioid Receptor Antagonists

There are several commercially available opioid receptor antagonists in the US, with naloxone and naltrexone being the most commonly used. Naloxone is administered parenterally and can rapidly reverse the respiratory depression caused by opioid overdose. Naltrexone is available in oral preparations and has a longer duration of action than naloxone.

Naloxone

Naloxone is a rapidly-acting antagonist of opioid receptors. Naloxone antagonizes all three subtypes of opioid receptors but has the greatest affinity for the MOR receptor. It exhibits no agonist activity and therefore has little pharmacological activity in the absence of opioid receptor ligands or drugs. Naloxone very rapidly and very specifically reverses opioid-induced respiratory depression and is used in emergency overdose situations. *Naloxone will not reverse respiratory depression caused by agents other than opioid agonists*. Because it has a relatively short duration of action, *patients who have overdosed on an agonist that has a longer duration of action than naloxone will require re-dosing with the antagonist to avoid recurrent intoxication.* Naloxone undergoes rapid glucuronidation in the liver and its half-life is approximately 1 hr.

In the US, naloxone is available to the consumer for emergency use and a nasal spray formulation was recently approved for use without a prescription. It is also available in an auto-injector. In addition, naloxone is formulated with several opioid agonists to avoid misuse of oral and sublingual preparations (see below).

Low doses of naloxone have been used off-label in an attempt to reduce some of the unwanted effects of opioid analgesia, especially with intravenous and epidural administration. Itching, nausea, and vomiting may be reduced when naloxone is used in this manner.

Naloxone is generally well-tolerated. It may precipitate acute withdrawal symptoms in patients who are chronic users of opioid analgesics for legitimate or recreational use.

Naltrexone

Like naloxone, naltrexone is an opioid receptor antagonist. However, it is administered orally and has a longer duration of action than naloxone. The half-life of naltrexone is around 4 hrs but it has an active metabolite that has a half-life of around 14 hrs. Thus, a single oral dose of naltrexone can cause a prolonged block of opioid receptors and deter further misuse of agonists. In addition to its use in the treatment of opioid dependence, it is approved in the US for the treatment of alcohol use disorder. Endogenous opioids are thought to be involved in alcohol abuse and treatment with naltrexone has met with success in some patients. Like naloxone, naltrexone is available in combination formulations with some oral opioid analgesics to prevent misuse of these preparations.

As with naloxone, naltrexone can precipitate acute withdrawal in chronic opioid users. In addition, excessive doses are associated with hepatoxicity.

Nalmefene is an analog of naltrexone that is approved for opioid overdose and alcohol use disorder. It is available for injection and a nasal spray was recently approved for prescription use in the US. Its half-life is comparable to naltrexone's and thus results in a longer reversal of overdose than naloxone.

A peripherally-acting derivative of naltrexone, **methylnaltrexone**, is available in the US to treat opioid-induced constipation. This drug is administered subcutaneously and blocks opioid receptors in the gastrointestinal tract. It does not readily cross the blood-brain barrier and is therefore not useful to reverse opioid-induced respiratory depression. It is excreted mostly unchanged in urine and feces. It is available in an oral tablet and injectable solution . **Alvimopan** is another peripherally-acting opioid antagonist. Its main use is for postoperative ileus prophylaxis but it can be used for opioid-induced constipation (off-label use). It is only used short-term in hospitals with healthcare professionals who are authorized to prescribe it.

Clinical Suggestions for Safe Administration of Opioid Agonists for Chronic Pain

Patient Evaluation and Pain Contracts

The chronic use of opioids is needed to adequately treat some patients, however, this requires close monitoring and assessment due to the potential for the patient to develop opioid tolerance, dependence, and addiction. Opioid dependence and tolerance are natural phenomena that require an assessment to assure that the patient is receiving adequate pain control. Addiction is a very serious development that must be identified and treated. The following is a suggested clinical protocol that will allow for monitoring for dependence and tolerance and for identifying addiction or other illegal use of opioids.

When considering a patient for long-term opioid use it is very important, for both clinical and legal purposes, to document the medical and social history extensively and thoroughly. Documentation should include the location, quality, and chronicity of the pain, the severity of the pain as perceived by the patient using a pain scale, and any objective evidence of pain found on physical examination. The provider should also investigate any other drugs or treatments that have been used thus far to treat the pain. The etiology of the chronic pain should also be supported by any imaging or lab values, if available, that may support the diagnosis. A firm diagnosis should be established and documented.

Once a solid diagnosis is made and the consideration for chronic pain medication is determined, the patient can then be assessed for the appropriateness of chronic opioid use. Any comorbid or exacerbating factors such as depression must be identified and treated before initiation of therapy, and the patient's risk for misuse must also be assessed. This is often done by an independent evaluator and is used to assess the patient's goals for pain control and the patient's history of risk factors for substance use disorder. It includes a Board of Pharmacy search to investigate current controlled substance use and the possible use of multiple providers. A urine drug screen (UDS) should also be done at this time.

An **opioid pain contract** is a written and signed agreement between the patient and the provider and/or the provider's practice. It establishes the need for chronic opioid use based on a diagnosis. The patient is usually asked to agree to obtain his or her medication from one pharmacy which is documented in the contract. By signing the contract the patient agrees to random UDS, pill counts on provider request, and frequent face-to-face evaluation. The patient also acknowledges that the provider may discontinue prescribing the medication if the patient receives opioids from another provider (unless the patient is hospitalized or requires surgery), no opioids are found on UDS (this suggests diversion), other controlled or illegal substances are found on UDS, the patient fails to attend regular face to face monitoring, the patient requests early prescriptions, reports multiple lost prescriptions, the medication is no longer effective, or the provider feels that the medication is harmful to the patient in any way. These suggested requirements can be added or subtracted from the pain contract as deemed appropriate by providers or practices.

Opioid addiction and diversion are at the forefront of providers' minds when prescribing opioids. While these are real issues, a patient who is in pain requires proper evaluation and treatment. If addiction is identified, this too deserves appropriate evaluation and treatment by the physician. Addicted patients should be referred to appropriate services for treatment.

Anti-diversion Formulations of Opioids

The development of abuse-deterrent drug formulations is currently a very active area of drug development. The increased legitimate use of controlled substances by the general public has resulted in a concomitant increase in the abuse and misuse of these drugs. This has resulted in the reluctance of some healthcare providers to prescribe opioids for patients who need them, and some pharmacists to dispense them. Formulations that are designed to make abuse and misuse more difficult may one day become required by law and while several products are already commercially available, several more products are currently in development.

Extended-release opioid analgesics are attractive to those who seek to misuse opioids because they contain higher doses of the active ingredient than immediate-release formulations. An extended-release oral formulation of oxycodone is now available in a pill that is difficult to crush or break. In addition, attempts to dissolve the pill result in a viscous gel that is difficult to inject through a needle. Hydrocodone also comes in an extended-release tablet that forms a gel when dissolved.

Several opioid analgesics contain the antagonist, naloxone. Naloxone is not well absorbed, thus, when administered via a route that requires absorption, such as orally or sublingually, it does not impair the therapeutic effect of the opioid. However, intravenous administration of naloxone will result in antagonism of opioid receptors rendering the opioid ineffective with no resultant euphoria. Thus, attempts to crush, dissolve and inject drugs not intended for the intravenous route, are likely to be deterred. Drugs formulated with naloxone include oxycodone, pentazocine, and buprenorphine.

Extended-release morphine is available in capsules that contain a core of the opioid antagonist, naltrexone. Naltrexone is orally bioavailable, however, in these specially designed capsules, the naltrexone core is protected from breakdown in the gastrointestinal tract. Thus, when taken as prescribed, morphine is slowly released, but naltrexone is not. Attempts to crush or dissolve the capsule result in the release of naltrexone and subsequent antagonism of opioid receptors.

Acknowledgements: The authors wish to acknowledge Chris Van Dyke, Dept. Physiology, Pharmacology, and Toxicolgy, WVU, for creating the figures in this chapter.

References and Suggested Readings

Anekar, A. A., J. M. Hendrix, and M. Cascella. 2023. WHO Analgesic Ladder. In *StatPearls*. Treasure Island (FL) ineligible companies. Disclosure: Joseph Maxwell Hendrix declares no relevant financial relationships with ineligible companies. Disclosure: Marco Cascella declares no relevant financial relationships with ineligible companies.

Brown, S.M., Holtzman, M., Kim, T., and Kharasch, E.D. (2011) Buprenorphine metabolites, buprenorphine-3-glucuronide and norbuprenorphine-3-glucuronide, are biologically active. *Anesthesiology* 115(6): 1251-1260

Jannuzzi, R.G. (2016) Nalbuphine for treatment of opioid-induced pruritus: A systematic review of the literature. *Clin J Pain* (32): 87-93

Lötsch, J. (2005) Opioid metabolites. *J Pain Sym Man* 29(5S): S10-24

Nguyen, V., Raffa, R.B., Taylor, R., and Pergolizzi, J.V. (2015) The role of abuse-deterrent formulations in countering opioid misuse and abuse. *J Clin Pharm Ther*. 40:629-634

Pasternak, G. (2014) Opiate pharmacology and pain relief. *J Clin Oncol*. 32:1655-1661

Pasternak, G.W. and Ying-Xian, P. (2013) Mu opioids and their receptors: evolution of a concept. *Pharm Rev* 65:1257-1317

Case Study Question

Case Study

A 25-year-old woman administered spinal anesthesia consisting of 2% lidocaine with epinephrine (1:200,000) with fentanyl and delivers a healthy baby boy via standard cesarean. Anesthesia is halted and the mother is administered morphine every 12 hours via the epidural catheter. Several hours after stopping anesthesia, the woman develops pruritus which becomes increasingly severe. What is the cause of the pruritus and what are the options for treating this woman at this time?

Quiz Questions

1. A 22-year-old woman who is a former heavy user of heroin has voluntarily submitted to therapy in an attempt to improve her quality of life. She lives in a remote rural area of the United States, far from any health care services with the exception of a pharmacy at her local grocery store. Following inpatient treatment at a hospital that is a 9 hour drive from her home, her team of specialists decide that opioid maintenance therapy is the best option for treating opioid use disorder. Which of the following would be most appropriate drug for her treatment at this time?

A Methadone
B Buprenorphine with naloxone
C Naloxone alone
D Extended-release hydrocodone
E Codeine with acetaminophen

2. A 25-year-old man is prescribed oxycodone and acetaminophen after surgery to repair a broken arm sustained during a dirt bike race. This is the man's third broken bone due to his hobby and he knows that he will suffer a common adverse effect of this drug combination. He asks his wife to pick up an over-the-counter drug which he will begin taking as soon as he begins taking oxycodone and acetaminophen at home. What is this over-the-counter drug?

A Loperamide
B Naltrexone
C Dextromethorphan
D Docusate sodium

3. A 25-year-old woman who is in active labor is given an opioid analgesic to relieve pain during what is hoped will be a normal vaginal delivery. The opioid she is administered is considered relatively safer for her baby than most other opioid analgesics, although it can cause considerable sedation and dysphoria for the mother. What is the mechanism of action of this opioid that the mother was administered?

A Pure MOR agonist
B Partial MOR agonist, KOR antagonist
C MOR antagonist, KOR agonist
D Pure KOR agonist

4. In an animal experiment designed to examine the effect of a potential new MOR analgesic on descending inhibitory neural pain pathways, neurotransmitter levels are measured in samples of CSF collected from the PAG in the brain and the spinal cord dorsal horn following the intramuscular injection of the new drug. Which answer represents the alterations that are most likely to occur when the new drug is injected?

A No change in GABA (PAG); Enkephalin increases (Spinal Cord)
B No change in GABA (PAG); Dynorphin increases (Spinal Cord)
C GABA increases (PAG); Substance P increases (Spinal Cord)
D GABA increases (PAG); Norepinephrine increases (Spinal Cord)
E GABA decreases (PAG); Glutamate increases (Spinal Cord)
F GABA decreases (PAG); Serotonin increases (Spinal Cord)

5. A 31-year-old man who is being treated with escitalopram for depression is prescribed an analgesic following the extraction of 3 teeth. The analgesic is a weak MOR agonist that also inhibits reuptake of norepinephrine and serotonin. The man is cautioned to only take the drug as directed due to an interaction that can occur between this drug and his antidepressant. What is the drug, and what is the consequence of the drug interaction?

A Codeine; seizures
B Tramadol; seizures
C Tapentadol; seizures
D Codeine; serotonin syndrome
E Tramadol; serotonin syndrome
F Tapentadol; serotonin syndrome

Case Study Answer

Opioids administered via the spinal or epidural route are used for regional anesthesia and postoperative pain. However, pruritus is an undesirable adverse effect of neuraxial administration of opioids that occurs in up to 85% of patients. Maintaining analgesia is important, but for some patients, the opioid-induced itching is unbearable. Several drugs have been used to treat or prevent opioid-induced itching including opioid antagonists (MOR antagonists such as naloxone and mixed agonists/antagonists such as nalbuphine), antihistamines, antiemetics (5-HT_3 antagonists), NSAIDs, propofol, gabapentin, and others. Evidence supports the use of drugs that antagonize MORs, however, the dose that relieves itching is not much lower than the dose that antagonizes analgesia. Thus, when using neuraxial opioid administration for pain control, drugs such as naloxone may not have much utility. In contrast, drugs that have partial MOR agonist activity or MOR antagonist activity combined with KOR activity (e.g. nalbuphine), have been shown to reduce itching and maintain analgesia. Diphenhydramine may have some utility in reducing itching caused by opioid-induced histamine release, however, this appears not to be the mechanism of itching resulting from neuraxial opioid administration. Ondansetron and other 5-HT_3 antagonists are anti-emetics that have been examined with mixed results for relieving neuraxial opioid-induced itching. Similarly, evidence supporting the use of other non-opioid drugs, such as NSAIDs, is not convincing.

Quiz Answers

1. A. Buprenorphine with naloxone is indicated for opioid maintenance therapy and can be dispensed from pharmacies to patients who do not have access to methadone clinics. Methadone is also indicated for opioid maintenance therapy but it cannot be dispensed from community pharmacies to patients in the United States. Hydrocodone and codeine with acetaminophen are not indicated for opioid maintenance therapy.

2. D. Docusate sodium is a stool softener which is readily available without a prescription. It is available alone or in combination with a stimulant laxative. Constipation is a common adverse effect of opioid analgesics. A stimulant laxative is often a better choice than a stool softener. Naltrexone is an opioid receptor antagonist, is not available over-the-counter (OTC), and it would antagonize the analgesic effect of oxycodone. While some prescribers will prescribe naloxone for patients who take opioid analgesics (in case of overdose), naltrexone is not used in this setting. Dextromethorphan is a cough suppressant that is chemically related to some opioid analgesics. Its role in preventing opioid-induced constipation has not been established. Loperamide is a peripherally acting opioid agonist that is used to treat diarrhea. It would worsen opioid-induced constipation.

3. C. Nalbuphine is commonly used as an analgesic in obstetrics. Nalbuphine is an antagonist of MORs and agonist of KORs. Respiratory depression resulting from opioid analgesics is thought to be mediated mostly via the MOR. Thus, the risk to the baby is lower than it is with a pure MOR agonist. KOR agonists are associated with more sedation and dysphoria than MOR agonists.

4. F. MOR agonists exert their effects at numerous locations within the CNS and periphery. At the level of the periaqueductal gray, these drugs bind to presynaptic receptors that inhibit Ca^{2+}-dependent GABA release. In the absence of pain or an opioid analgesic, these GABA-ergic neurons normally release inhibitory GABA onto serotonergic and noradrenergic neurons that descend from the PAG to the spinal cord. An opioid-induced reduction of GABA in the PAG will result in increased release of serotonin and noradrenaline at the level of the spinal cord. Glutamate release from primary afferent nerves will decrease in response to activation of descending pain pathways.

5. E. Of the drugs listed, tramadol is the only one that is a weak agonist of MORs and inhibits both norepinephrine and serotonin reuptake. Codeine is a weak MOR agonist but does not have the second mechanism. Tapentadol is a stronger agonist at MORs and it appears to inhibits norepinephrine reuptake only. Since the man is already taking a selective serotonin reuptake inhibitor, the combination of escitalopram and tramadol can result in serotonin syndrome. Tapentadol is not expected to increase this risk due to its apparent lack of activity on serotonin reuptake. However, the risk of serotonin syndrome due to opioids is still not clearly defined. Tramadol does increase seizure risk, and seizures may be associated with serotonin syndrome, however, escitalopram is not likely to increase the seizure risk of tramadol in the absence of serotonin syndrome. Thus, serotonin syndrome is the best answer.